AF251958

The PHYSIOLOGIC NATURE OF SLEEP

The PHYSIOLOGIC NATURE OF SLEEP

Pier Luigi Parmeggiani
University of Bologna, Italy

Ricardo A. Velluti
Universidad de la República, Uruguay

Imperial College Press

Published by

Imperial College Press
57 Shelton Street
Covent Garden
London WC2H 9HE

Distributed by

World Scientific Publishing Co. Pte. Ltd.
5 Toh Tuck Link, Singapore 596224
USA office: 27 Warren Street, Suite 401-402, Hackensack, NJ 07601
UK office: 57 Shelton Street, Covent Garden, London WC2H 9HE

British Library Cataloguing-in-Publication Data
A catalogue record for this book is available from the British Library.

ISBN 1-86094-557-0

Typeset by Stallion Press
Email: enquiries@stallionpress.com

Printed by FuIsland Offset Printing (S) Pte Ltd, Singapore

This book is dedicated to our wives:
Luisa and Marisa

CONTENTS

II.   PHYSIOLOGICAL FUNCTIONS IN SLEEP

CONTRIBUTORS

Jorge M. Affanni
Instituto de Neurociencias, Facultad de Medicina, Universidad de Morón
Buenos Aires, Argentina

Noor Alam
V.A.G.L.A.H.S., Sepulveda, and Departments of Psychology and Medicine
UCLA, Los Angeles, CA, USA

Geneviève Albouy
Cyclotron Research Centre, University of Liège
Belgium

Mourad Akaârir
Departamento de Biología, F.I.C.S. Universitat de les Illes Balears
Palma de Mallorca, Spain

Roberto Amici
Dipartimento di Fisiologia Umana e Generale, Università di Bologna
Bologna, Italy

Véronique Bach
Physiological and Behavioural Adaptation Research Unit
Faculty of Medicine, University of Picardy Jules Verne
Amiens, France

Hélène Bastuji
Sleep Disorders Unit, Functional Neurology Department
Hôpital Neurologique
INSERM 0342 and University Claude Bernard
Lyon, France

Gabrielle Brandenberger
Laboratoire des Régulations Physiologiques et des Rythmes
Biologiques chez l'Homme
Strasbourg, France

Tijana Bojic
Dipartimento di Fisiologia Umana e Generale, Università di Bologna
Bologna, Italy

Mélanie Boly
Cyclotron Research Centre, University of Liège
Belgium

Ritchie E. Brown
In Vitro Neurophysiology Group, Laboratory of Neuroscience
Department of Psychiatry, VA Medical Center and
Harvard Medical School
Brockton, MA, USA

Daniel P. Cardinali
Department of Physiology, Faculty of Medicine
University of Buenos Aires
Buenos Aires, Argentina

Claudio O. Cervino
Instituto de Neurociencias, Facultad de Medicina, Universidad de Morón
Buenos Aires, Argentina

Raymond Cespuglio
Claude Bernard University, Av. Rockefeller
Lyon, France

Chiara Cirelli
Department of Psychiatry, University of Wisconsin, Madison
Madison, WI, USA

Carlo Cipolli
Dipartimento di Psicologia, Università di Bologna
Bologna, Italy

Damien Colas
Claude Bernard University, Av. Rockefeller
Lyon, France

Thahn Dang-Vu
Cyclotron Research Centre, University of Liège
Belgium

Martin Desseilles
Cyclotron Research Centre, University of Liège
Belgium

Susana Esteban
Departamento de Biología, F.I.C.S. Universitat de les Illes Balears
Palma de Mallorca, Spain

Carlo Franzini
Dipartimento di Fisiologia Umana e Generale, Università di Bologna
Bologna, Italy

Antoni Gamundi
Departamento de Biología, F.I.C.S. Universitat de les Illes Balears
Palma de Mallorca, Spain

Sabine Gautier-Sauvigné
Claude Bernard University. Av. Rockefeller
Lyon, France

Luis García-Larrea
INSERM 0342 and University Claude Bernard
Lyon, France

Hui Gong
V.A.G.L.A.H.S., Sepulveda, and Departments of Psychology and Medicine
UCLA, Los Angeles, CA, USA

Ruben Guzman-Marin
V.A.G.L.A.H.S., Sepulveda, and Departments of Psychology and Medicine
UCLA, Los Angeles, CA, USA

Ronald M. Harper
University of California at Los Angeles
Los Angeles, CA, USA

Luke A. Henderson
University of California at Los Angeles
Los Angeles, CA, USA

Christine A. Jones
Dipartimento di Fisiologia Umana e Generale, Università di Bologna
Bologna, Italy

James M. Krueger
Department of Veterinary and Comparative Anatomy, Pharmacology and
Physiology, Washington State University
Pullman, WA, USA

Rajesh Kumar
University of California at Los Angeles
Los Angeles, CA, USA

Steven Laureys
Cyclotron Research Centre, University of Liège
Belgium

Pierluigi Lenzi
Dipartimento di Fisiologia Umana e Generale, Università di Bologna
Bologna, Italy

Jean-Pierre Libert
Physiological and Behavioural Adaptation Research Unit
Faculty of Medicine, University of Picardy Jules Verne
Amiens, France

Paul M. Macey
University of California at Los Angeles
Los Angeles, CA, USA

Pierre A. A. Maquet
Cyclotron Research Centre, University of Liège
Belgium

Robert W. McCarley
Laboratory of Neuroscience, Department of Psychiatry
VA Medical Center and Harvard Medical School
Brockton, MA, USA

Dennis McGinty
V.A.G.L.A.H.S., Sepulveda, and Departments of Psychology and Medicine
UCLA, Los Angeles, CA, USA

Melvi Methippara
V.A.G.L.A.H.S., Sepulveda, and Departments of Psychology and Medicine
UCLA, Los Angeles, CA, USA

Adrian R. Morrison
Laboratory for Study of the Brain in Sleep, Department of Animal Biology
School of Veterinary Medicine, University of Pennsylvania
Philadelphia, PA, USA

María C. Nicolau
Departamento de Biología, F.I.C.S. Universitat de les Illes Balears
Palma de Mallorca, Spain

Ferenc Obal Jr.
Department of Physiology, A. Szent-Györgyi Medical Center,
University of Szeged
Szeged, Hungary

John M. Orem
Murray Professor of Physiology, Texas Tech University, School of Medicine
Lubbock, TX, USA

Pier Luigi Parmeggiani
Dipartimento di Fisiologia Umana e Generale, Università di Bologna
Bologna, Italy

Marisa Pedemonte
Neurofisiología, Facultad de Medicina, Universidad de la República
Montevideo, Uruguay

Philippe Peigneux
Cyclotron Research Centre, University of Liège
Belgium

Rosa Peraita-Adrados
Sleep and Epilepsy Unit, Department of Clinical Neurophysiology
Hospital General Universitario "Gregorio Marañón"
Madrid, Spain

Emanuele Perez
Dipartimento di Fisiologia Umana e Generale, Università di Bologna
Bologna, Italy

Chiara M. Portas
Department of Biomedicine, Section of Physiology
Faculty of Medicine, University of Bergen
Bergen, Norway

Rubén V. Rial
Departamento de Biología, F.I.C.S. Universitat de les Illes Balears
Palma de Mallorca, Spain

Christopher A. Richard
University of California at Los Angeles
Los Angeles, CA, USA

Perrine Ruby
Cyclotron Research Centre, University of Liège
Belgium

Jerome M. Siegel
Neurobiology Research, G.L.A.H.S., Sepulveda, and Department of
Psychiatry, UCLA Medical Center
North Hills, CA, USA

Alessandro Silvani
Dipartimento di Fisiologia Umana e Generale, Università di Bologna
Bologna, Italy

Virginie Sterpenich
Cyclotron Research Centre, University of Liège
Belgium

Natalia Suntsova
V.A.G.L.A.H.S., Sepulveda, and Departments of Psychology and Medicine
UCLA, Los Angeles, CA, USA

Ron Szymusiak
V.A.G.L.A.H.S., Sepulveda, and Departments of Psychology and Medicine
UCLA, Los Angeles, CA, USA

Giulio Tononi
Department of Psychiatry, University of Wisconsin, Madison
Madison, WI, USA

Ricardo A. Velluti
Neurofisiología, Facultad de Medicina, Universidad de la República
Montevideo, Uruguay

Mary A. Woo
University of California at Los Angeles
Los Angeles, CA, USA

Giovanni Zamboni
Dipartimento di Fisiologia Umana e Generale, Università di Bologna
Bologna, Italy

Giovanna Zoccoli
Dipartimento di Fisiologia Umana e Generale, Università di Bologna
Bologna, Italy

PREFACE

The editors of this book met for the first time in Szeged, Hungary, in 1986, at the meeting of the European Sleep Research Society. This was the beginning of an academic and scientific collaboration which has lasted for years and has progressively involved an increasing number of collaborators.

The book, a late outcome of this collaboration, addresses many aspects of sleep physiology, which are presented in 26 chapters by sleep researchers from different countries. The editors are deeply indebted to these colleagues who, by presenting their scientific expertise over such diverse fields, were instrumental in the originality of the book.

The first part of the book includes contributions of a general nature, which aim to introduce the phenomenal complexity of sleep behavior to both the experienced and the non-experienced researcher. Technical methods and epistemological problems of sleep research are also considered in order to place the physiological topics of the second part of the book within a specific framework. In particular, topics such as energy processes during sleep; humoral factors, neurotransmitters, and synaptic activity of sleep; recording techniques for the bioelectrical and vascular parameters of neuronal activity of the brain during sleep; hypothalamic control of sleep; sleep phylogenesis; and new viewpoints on sensory neurophysiology and epistemological issues of sleep research are covered.

The second part of the book deals with the specific aspects of the physiological changes characterizing the sleep cycle and, in many cases, also with respect to their medical implications. In particular, sleep-related changes in muscle tone, respiration, circulation, temperature regulation, endocrine secretion, auditory and olfactory functions, and memory processes are covered.

This analysis of sleep physiology and its medical implications is far from being exhaustive because of the still overwhelming complexity of the mechanisms underlying the functional events characterizing this behavior, the teleological significance of which is still not completely understood. Such issues are often discussed from both theoretical and practical viewpoints with the aim to provide new incentives to further basic research on sleep mechanisms.

It is the warm hope of the editors that the book may contribute to stimulating new generations of scientists to continue a research endeavor which has already been highlighted by important discoveries, particularly during the second half of the last century. On the other hand, the practical importance of clarifying sleep mechanisms is growing year after year in connection with the conspicuous changes in human habits and living environments and the recent development of a branch of medicine specific for sleep disorders. Characteristically, modern societies exert a negative influence on the free expression of a healthy sleep behavior. It is now well established that human beings, particularly those living in large cities, often suffer from a chronic deprivation of sleep that may become a morbidity factor and also a frequent cause of accidents.

The editors are deeply indebted to Imperial College Press (London, UK) for allowing the publication of an attractive and up-to-date volume dedicated not only to the large community of basic and clinical scientists, but also to other readers who wish to develop their subjective experience of sleep behavior into objective knowledge.

The editors are also grateful to the Istituto Italiano di Cultura (Montevideo, Uruguay), the Program for Basic Research Development (PEDECIBA, Montevideo, Uruguay), and the University of Bologna (Bologna, Italy) for their logistic support of the collaborative work of the editors.

Pier Luigi Parmeggiani
Ricardo A. Velluti

I. GENERAL ASPECTS OF SLEEP

Chapter 1

ENERGY PROCESSES UNDERLYING THE SLEEP–WAKE CYCLE

Raymond Cespuglio[1], Damien Colas, and Sabine Gautier-Sauvigné

A restorative role of sleep (Adams and Oswald, 1997; Adams, 1980) appears intuitively reasonable given the feeling of recovery usually present after sleep. There is now experimental evidence that sleep restoration is associated more with the brain than the body, since quiet wakefulness is sufficient for resting the body and particularly the motor systems, but insufficient for satisfying the need of sleep (Horne, 1985; Benington and Heller, 1995). Brain studies indicate that restorative processes are concerned with energy storage and production, in which glucose and glycogen play a dominant part (Walker and Berger, 1980; Benington and Heller, 1995).

In the present chapter, we first discuss some phylogenetic considerations and then recall the basic biochemical pathways through which energy is made available. The specificities of the energy metabolites for each sleep and wake state are then analysed. Finally, regulatory processes related to food intake and energy-production pathways are considered.

Phylogenetic Considerations

Pre-mammals (fish, amphibians, and reptiles) are ectothermic, cold-blooded species exposed to the ambient variations in temperature, whereas mammals and birds are endothermic, warm blooded, and capable of keeping their internal temperature constant in spite of environmental changes

---

[1] cespuglio@univ-Lyon1.fr

(Karmanova, 1982). This homeothermy in mammals is associated with lesser neurogenesis and several other aromorphoses (e.g., heart division into arterial and venous halves, and intensification of respiration) necessary for the maintenance and control of a more intense metabolism (Karmanova, 1982). For a constant body temperature, the resting metabolic rate of reptiles is lower than that of mammals (Guppy *et al.*, 1987), and homeothermy is concomitant with the appearance of rapid-eye-movement sleep (REM sleep), which, in addition to wakefulness and slow-wave sleep (SWS), constitutes a new functional state for the brain. The cost of independence towards the environmental conditions allowed by homeothermy is the permanent need for energy (Karmanova, 1982; Heller *et al.*, 1988; Berger and Phillips, 1993). The metabolic rate of an organism, even at rest, is profoundly affected by whether or not it does work to maintain its body temperature, i.e., whether it is ectothermic or endothermic. Homeotherms adapt to environmental changes in temperature by modifying their metabolism through homeostatic and behavioural adaptations, such as changes in the blood flow and posture, and the use of shivering, sudation, and panting. At low temperatures, shivering compensates for the heat loss by the exothermic hydrolysing of adenosine triphosphate (ATP) in muscles; whereas when the temperature increases, sudation and panting facilitate heat loss. All these adaptive aspects are under hypothalamic control and involve peripheral and central thermosensors (Parmeggiani, 1985; Simon *et al.*, 1986; Sawaya and Ingvar, 1989; Purves *et al.*, 1992). It is also noteworthy that in the brown adipose tissue of homeothermic mammals, mitochondria respiration is naturally uncoupled from the synthesis of ATP, and the energy produced is totally dissipated as heat. While the underlying mechanisms are not yet fully understood, brown adipose tissue is particularly useful in hibernation (mainly when emerging from hibernation), as well as for animals or humans to adapt to cold conditions (Himms-Hagen, 1976; Nicholls, 1976; Konings and Michels, 1980). Hibernation is not simply a response to a lowering in temperature, but an extreme case of temporal heterothermy resulting from a dramatic decrease in energy transaction.

It is also remarkable that evolution has resulted in the emergence of REM sleep (Jouvet, 1994), a state in which energy production in homeotherms is even more complex: energy is required both to maintain their homeothermic status and for the occurrence of REM sleep. It seems reasonable to assume that this challenge has occurred through phylogenetic evolution because determinant functional processes occur during REM sleep. These functions might be elucidated by phylogenic considerations of the precise conditions in which this state of sleep originates.

Brain Metabolism throughout the Sleep–Wake Cycle in Homeotherms

Pathways for energy production

The energy necessary for the functioning of cellular elements comes mainly from ATP. The basic difficulty of ATP renewal can be overcome only through the supply of energetic substrata represented, in the case of eukaryotic cells, by organic nutrients. The molecules constituting these nutrients represent a potential store of energy whose degradation allows the production of the energy necessary for the synthesis of ATP. While the cellular elements are capable of metabolising compounds such as sugars, proteins, amino acids, and lipids, glucose is the main energetic compound in ATP production (Siesjö, 1978; Magistretti *et al.*, 1994, 1999; Magistretti and Pellerin, 1997, 1999; Pellerin and Magistretti, 2004).

Glycolysis

Glucose is the primary source of energy for the brain, and hence its supply is of paramount importance. This molecule easily crosses the blood–brain barrier where it is transported into astrocytes and neurons via GLUT-1 and GLUT-3 glucose transporters, respectively (Brown, 2004). Glycolysis occurs mainly in glia cells and particularly in astrocytes where, irrespective of the conditions of oxygen supply (aerobic or anaerobic), 2 moles of pyruvate are produced per mole of glucose. Throughout this biochemical process, the glucose dehydrogenation performed in several successive steps ensures a transfer of protons and electrons to a transporter (e.g., the oxidised and reduced forms of nicotinamide adenine dinucleotide: $NAD^+/NADH$). In this step, the energetic balance sheet is 2 moles of ATP produced per mole of glucose metabolised (Figure 1).

The pyruvate produced by glycolysis may be subjected to lactic fermentation and transformed into lactate. In these conditions, pyruvate plays the role of a proton acceptor and the electrons produced through the glycolysis are transferred to a transporter. While lactate is an end product that can be eliminated through blood and urine, it can also be again converted into pyruvate through the activity of lactate dehydrogenase. Pyruvate produced in this way is normally used in oxidative phosphorylation to produce ATP. Other simple sugars such as mannose and fructose may also participate in glycolysis, although only to a minor extent. Glucose can also be oxidised to pentose phosphate in the cytoplasm by a sequence of enzymes, and the electron transporter is then NADPH (phosphorylated NADH) production

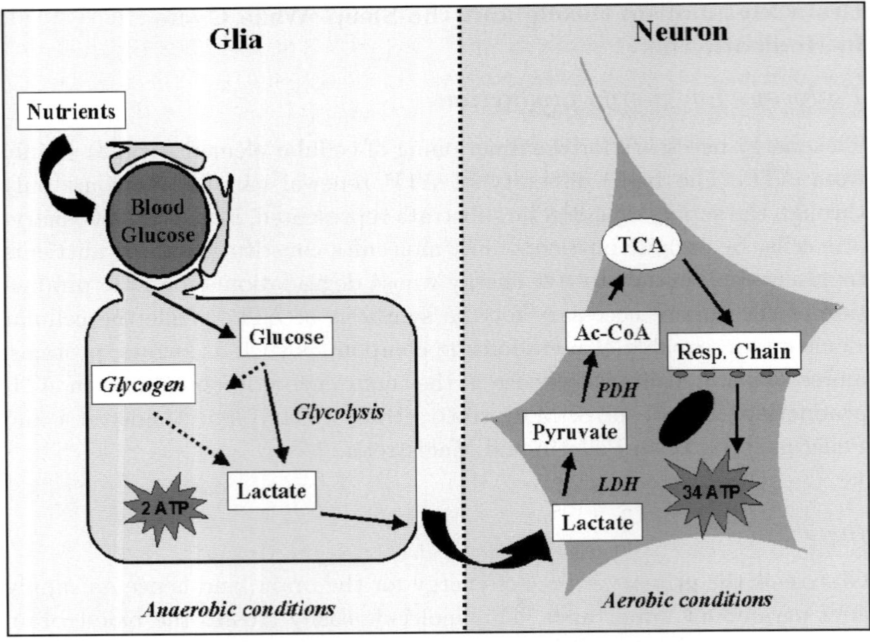

Figure 1. Glucose, derived from nutrients or polysaccharides (glycogen), is the main source for the synthesis of adenosine triphosphate (ATP) in endotherms. It is metabolised into pyruvate in anaerobic conditions and throughout glycolysis. In this step there is a positive balance of 2 moles of ATP per mole of glucose. Still in anaerobic conditions, pyruvate can be subjected to lactic fermentation and transformed into lactate. In aerobic conditions (throughout the Krebs cycle and the respiratory chain), pyruvate oxidised into CO_2 and H_2O contributes to the production of 34 additive moles of ATP. The total degradation of 1 mole of glucose therefore produces 36 moles of ATP. Lipids, proteins, and amino acids may also be involved in the production of ATP, entering in the pathway of phosphorylative oxidation in the form of acetyl-coenzyme A (acetyl CoA).

(Siesjö, 1978; Magistretti *et al.*, 1994, 1999; Magistretti and Pellerin, 1997, 1999; Pellerin and Magistretti, 2004).

Oxidative phosphorylation

This starts after glycolysis and occurs, under aerobic conditions, within the internal membrane of the mitochondria. Pyruvic acid, produced by glycolysis, is first transformed into acetyl-coenzyme A (acetyl CoA). Together with oxaloacetate, this radical contributes to the synthesis of citric acid that enters the Krebs cycle where it is subjected to successive decarboxylations and dehydrogenations. Each decarboxylation allows the release of a carbon dioxide molecule, while each dehydrogenation transfers a proton to a transporter that reduces it. Finally, through the redox processes of the proton motive respiratory chain, the reduced transporters are oxidised again, and thus regenerated; the potential energy released is converted by the ATPases into 34 additional moles of ATP per mole of glucose (Figure 1). The resulting protons and electrons, together with oxygen, produce 6 moles of water. It should be noted that lipids, proteins, and amino acids can also contribute to the formation of acetyl CoA and thus participate as nutrients in the production of ATP through oxidative phosphorylation (Siesjö, 1978; Magistretti *et al.*, 1994, 1999; Magistretti and Pellerin, 1997, 1999; Pellerin and Magistretti, 2004). Finally, in addition to its major involvement in ATP production, acetyl CoA might also cross the mitochondrial membrane to contribute together with choline to the synthesis of acetylcholine within the cytoplasm. This process, however, remains controversial (Lefresne *et al.*, 1978; Gibson and Shimada, 1980; Tucek, 1984).

In conclusion, the full degradation of 1 mole of glucose, including glycolysis, Krebs cycle, and the respiratory chain, requires 6 moles of oxygen and generates 6 moles of carbon dioxide, 6 moles of water, and 36 moles of ATP. The overall energetic yield is close to 40%, with the remaining 60% being dissipated as heat. It should be noted that the cerebral metabolic rate of oxygen consumption (CMR_{O_2}) is six times higher than the cerebral metabolic rate of glucose (CMR_{glu}), and hence the theoretical value of the CMR_{O_2}/CMR_{glu} ratio is 6.

Variations in energy metabolites related to sleep–wake states

It is difficult to identify with certainty the existence of sleep in ectotherms using the sleep criteria established in homeothermic species. While rest–activity cycles are evident in fish and amphibians, there are no reports of marked differences in their brain electrical activity between rest and activity. In reptiles, however, electroencephalographic synchronisation occurs together with a deceleration of the heart rate and a reduction in the muscle tone. Nevertheless, a correlation with the rest–activity cycle still remains controversial, and REM sleep has never been described convincingly in these species (Karmanova, 1982; Campbell and Tobler, 1984; Jouvet, 1994). Whatever the situation, it can be concluded that the rate of energy production is lower in ectotherms than in endotherms (Guppy *et al.*, 1987; Weber and Haman, 1996).

In endotherms, where the sleep–wake states are clearly defined, the energy processes are better documented due to the difficulties of evaluating the different steps of the energy metabolism in the genuine conditions of the animal being asleep or awake. Studies have used autoradiographic methods (Kennedy *et al.*, 1982; Ramm and Frost, 1983, 1986; Lydic *et al.*, 1991), positron-emission tomography (PET) (Heiss *et al.*, 1985; Maquet *et al.*, 1990), and enzymatic biosensors for glucose (Netchiporouk *et al.*, 1996) and lactate (Shram *et al.*, 1998) measurements as well as laser techniques for the detection of NADH fluorescence (Mottin *et al.*, 1997). The data that are presently available are detailed below.

Waking state

This state is associated with the search for nutrients and various other behaviours, and hence also increased brain blood flow and oxygen consumption (Reivich *et al.*, 1968; Townsend *et al.*, 1973). In humans, under conscious resting conditions, the ratio of oxygen and glucose cerebral metabolic rates (CMR_{O_2}/CMR_{glu}) is close to 5.5, near to the theoretical value of 6. This ratio decreases during activity when brain lactate and blood oxygenation are increased. These changes, indicating an increased glucose consumption without additive oxygen supply, lead to the suggestion that brain activation can be supported by anaerobic glycolysis that may involve glycogen (Magistretti and Pellerin, 1999; Magistretti *et al.*, 1999). Glucose and lactate biosensors that allow the movement of metabolites in the extracellular space to be analysed have revealed that in the frontal cortex of the freely moving rat glucose decreased concomitantly with an increase in lactate during active wakefulness versus quiet wakefulness (Figure 2). These opposing changes thus support the existence of an active consumption of glucose resulting in an increased production of lactate capable of fuelling neurons for the aerobic production of ATP (Netchiporouk *et al.*, 2001; Shram *et al.*, 2002). The ability of lactate to fuel neurons during their activation has also been recently demonstrated in the rat (Serres *et al.*, 2003).

Slow-wave sleep

Brain blood flow and oxygen consumption both decrease during SWS. Compared to wakefulness, there is a general decrease in the utilisation of glucose accompanied by hypothermia that probably results from a loss of heat (Reich *et al.*, 1972; Kennedy *et al.*, 1982; Giuditta *et al.*, 1984; Marsden and

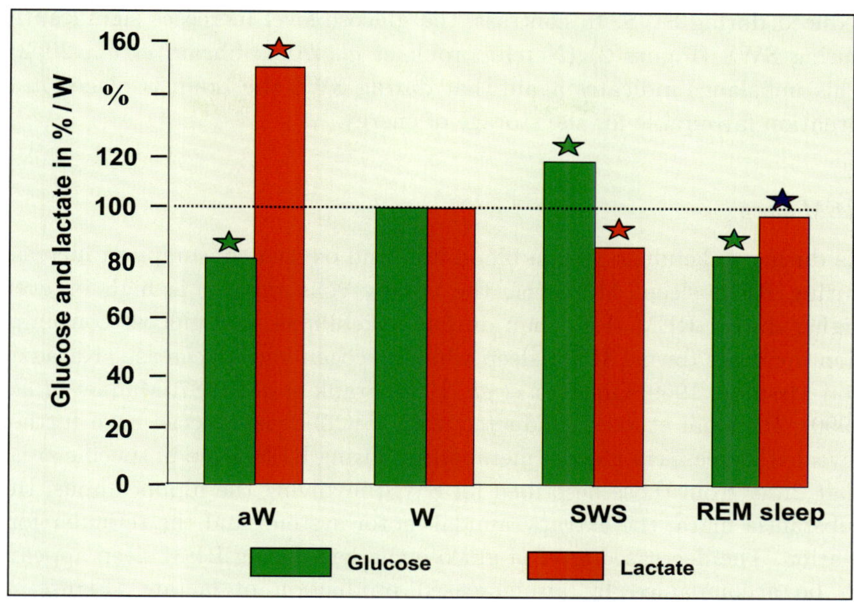

Figure 2. Changes in the extracellular glucose and lactate levels during the sleep–wake states. Voltammetric measurements were performed in freely moving animals equipped with polygraphic electrodes. The mean value obtained during the waking state (W) is normalised to 100%, while those obtained during active wakefulness (aW), slow-wave sleep (SWS), and rapid-eye-movement sleep (REM sleep) are expressed as percentages relative to W. Changes in glucose levels observed during W, SWS, and REM are significant relative to W (green*), and changes in lactate during aW and SWS are significant relative to W (red*). The increase observed during REM sleep is significant relative to SWS (blue*). Statistics: an ANOVA followed by a multiple-range test was performed ($p < 0.05$ for LSD test, states as the independent variable). For details, see Netchiporouk *et al.* (2001) and Shram *et al.* (2002).

Wildschiodtz, 1994). Studies on the regional metabolic activity during the sleep–wake cycle, performed using [^{14}C]2-deoxyglucose, also confirm that the mean cerebral metabolism during SWS reflects a condition of energy conservation (Reich *et al.*, 1972; Karnovsky *et al.*, 1983). Moreover, this general decrease in the energy metabolism is not homogeneous throughout the brain: while the metabolism is low in sensory relays, the cerebellum, the thalamus, and the cortex, it is increased in the hypothalamus and hippocampus (Ramm and Frost, 1983, 1986; Lydic *et al.*, 1991). The few studies that have investigated the changes in lactate throughout the sleep–wake cycle (Richter and Dawson, 1948; Shimizu *et al.*, 1966; Reich *et al.*, 1972), generally conducted *ex vivo*, suggest that the lactate level is reduced during SWS. In contrast, the glucose level increases significantly during SWS (Figure 2) (Netchiporouk *et al.*, 2001; Shram *et al.*, 2002). This imbalance indicates again that during SWS the brain is placed in a situation favourable for the storage of energy.

REM sleep

As during wakefulness, brain blood flow and oxygen consumption increase during REM sleep. Moreover, the energy consumption is high or even higher during REM sleep than during wakefulness, and glucose consumption increases during REM sleep while glycogen levels decrease (Karadzic and Mrsulija, 1969; Giuditta *et al.*, 1984; Frank *et al.*, 1987; Maquet *et al.*, 1990). Regional studies conducted with [^{14}C]2-deoxyglucose have further revealed increases in glucose metabolism during REM sleep in specific areas that differ from those described for SWS, involving the hippocampus, the substantia nigra, the extrapyramidal motor system, and the reticular formation. The decreased level of glucose checked during REM sleep appears to be accompanied by an increased production of lactate (Figure 2) (Netchiporouk *et al.*, 2001; Shram *et al.*, 2002), although the lactate level remains lower than that during active wakefulness. This is probably due to the brevity of REM sleep episodes. However, the lactate level remains significantly higher than that during SWS. No ATP exchange occurs between astrocytes and neurons (Magistretti *et al.*, 1999), and hence lactate might constitute an important metabolic substrate to fuel neurons, and its extracellular level might then represent the balance between astrocytic production and neuronal uptake. The rapid changes in lactate metabolism from SWS to REM sleep together with the marked enhancement of neuronal discharges during REM sleep (Sakai, 1988) might also support the existence of an astrocytic–neuronal coupling that is at least as strong as that during wakefulness. Glutamate uptake by astrocytes may stimulate glucose entry that leads to an overproduction of lactate (Tsacopoulos and Magistretti, 1996). Finally, the existence of astrocytic–neuronal coupling is also consistent with the presence of LDH-1 (lactate dehydrogenase type-1) within neuronal sets involved in REM sleep generation (Sakai, 1988; Laughton *et al.*, 2000), and with data on vasointestinal polypeptide, which is capable of stimulating glycogenolysis (Tsacopoulos and Magistretti, 1996) and lengthening REM sleep episodes (Riou *et al.*, 1982). The involvement of an oxidative metabolism is supported by the decrease in REM sleep observed during hypoxia (Huertas and McMillin, 1968; Baker and McGinty, 1979) and by the increase observed when oxygen availability is increased in "pontine cats" (Arnulf *et al.*, 1998). This view is reinforced by the administration of chloramphenicol leading to inhibition of the first site of oxidative phosphorylation and a very efficient reduction in REM sleep in cat (Petitjean *et al.*, 1979) and rat (Chastrette *et al.*, 1990), and by increased laser-induced NADH fluorescence during REM sleep within the raphe dorsal nucleus and the cortex (Mottin *et al.*, 1997).

In conclusion, the energy needs of homeotherms fluctuate with sleep–wake states. Lactate produced by astrocytic glycolysis appears to be a basic fuel for neurons to ensure the aerobic production of ATP. During wakefulness, processes for the aerobic production of energy are active. SWS appears to be a state propitious for energy saving, and REM sleep is associated with energy processes similar to those of wakefulness, and is dependent on aerobic energy.

Energy storage

Glycogen

Glycogen is a highly branched polysaccharide of D-glucose into which excess glucose can be stored or from which glucose can be rapidly released on demand. While the largest reserves are found in the liver and skeletal muscles, glycogen is also present in brain (about 0.1% of the total brain weight) (Brown, 2004) where it is localised mainly in astrocytes (Phelps, 1972; Pfeiffer *et al.*, 1990, 2003; Sorg and Magistretti, 1992; Allaman *et al.*, 2000). The greatest accumulation of astrocytic glycogen is found in areas exhibiting a high synaptic density and in grey-matter structures (Phelps, 1972; Pfeiffer *et al.*, 1990). Glycogen metabolism involves key glia regulatory enzymes such as brain glycogen synthase, glycogen phosphatase, and protein-targeting glycogen (PTG) (Pellegri *et al.*, 1996; Allaman *et al.*, 2000; Pfeiffer-Guglielmi *et al.*, 2003). Glycogen metabolism is tightly controlled by hormonal factors, e.g., insulin and vasointestinal peptide (Sorg and Magistretti, 1992), glucocorticoids (Allaman *et al.*, 2004; Gip *et al.*, 2004), neurotransmitters such as noradrenaline (Sorg and Magistretti, 1992), serotonin, and adenosine (Benington and Heller, 1995; Porkka-Heiskanen *et al.*, 1997, 2000, 2002; Allaman *et al.*, 2003). Recent studies based mainly on ^{13}C nuclear magnetic resonance (NMR) imaging and PET approaches suggest that glycogen plays either the part of an energy buffer enabling short-term energy supply (Brown *et al.*, 2003) or constitutes an energy reserve satisfying long-term energy requirements (Gruetter, 2003). Finally, it is now accepted that lactate rather than glucose is the ultimate energy substrate provided by astrocytic glycogenolysis (Dringen and Hamprecht, 1992; Dringen *et al.*, 1993).

Glycogen metabolism and sleep–wake states

Explorations of the energy metabolism throughout the sleep–wake cycle have focused mainly on glucose and oxygen consumption, but interest in glycogen is now growing. During SWS, the level of glycogen in the rat brain rises rapidly to about 70% above that during wakefulness, and it is not further increased during repetition of SWS episodes. Upon awakening, the glycogen that has accumulated rapidly dissipates (Karnovsky *et al.*, 1983). Brain glycogen decreases by about 40% in rats deprived of sleep for 12 or 24 h, and this decrease is reversed after 15 h of sleep recovery (Kong *et al.*, 2002). Replenishment of glycogen reserves appears to occur during SWS when the levels of excitatory neurotransmitters and the metabolic activity are low. Examinations of the expression levels of the three key enzymes involved in glycogen metabolism (glycogen synthase, glycogen phosphorylase, and PTG) either throughout the sleep–wake cycle or after 6 h of sleep deprivation in mice have revealed significant variations in glycogen synthase and glycogen phosphorylase mRNAs in the cerebral cortex. Sleep deprivation leads to an increase in PTG mRNA with a concomitant decrease in glycogen synthase and glycogen phosphorylase mRNAs, with the activity of the glycogen synthase increasing 2.5-fold (Petit *et al.*, 2002). These experiments appear to indicate that glycogen metabolism is affected by sleep loss. Nevertheless, the changes in brain glycogen content after sleep deprivation in mice appear to vary with genotype (Franken *et al.*, 2003), suggesting that sleep influences glycogen turnover rather than its absolute levels.

In conclusion, glycogen, which is mobilised upon waking, decreases during sleep deprivation but increases during SWS, and hence appears to represent an energy substrate during periods of tissue demand.

Integrated regulatory processes

We now consider the brain mechanisms that regulate the intake of nutrients. The main consequences of sleep deprivation are an energy loss concomitant with abnormal food-intake behaviour and body mass regulation (Rechtschaffen *et al.*, 1989). The determinant regulatory processes appear to reside in the basal forebrain, and ghrelin and leptin are key hormones in the regulation of food intake and body mass. Ghrelin originates from the gastrointestinal tract and acts at the hypothalamic level (Horvath *et al.*, 2001) to stimulate food intake and body mass gain (Tschop *et al.*, 2000; Wren *et al.*, 2001). Leptin, however, is synthesised by fatty tissues and acts also on the hypothalamus, but contributes to keeping the body mass constant despite changes in daily food intake and energy expenditure (Pelleymounter *et al.*, 1995; Meister, 2000). Ghrelin and leptin exert opposite effects on glucose-sensing neurons within the hypothalamus (Rough, 2002; Muroya *et al.*, 2004). There are also other reports on the part played by the basal forebrain (posterior–anterior parts of the hypothalamus and preoptic area) in the regulation of the sleep–wake cycle (Denoyer *et al.*, 1989; Sallanon *et al.*, 1989; McGinty and Szymusiak, 2000; Saper *et al.*, 2001). It is noteworthy that the laterodorsal hypothalamus contains a hypocretinergic system related to the waking system (Taheri *et al.*, 2002) and involved in the regulation of food intake and body mass (Sakurai *et al.*, 1998; Sakurai, 2003). Neurons of this system are inhibited by leptin and activated by ghrelin (Yamanaka *et al.*, 2003), while preprohypocretin RNA is greatly increased in the lateral hypothalamus during fasting or hypoglycaemia (Hungs and Mignot, 2001; Sakurai, 2003). Therefore, it appears likely that hypocretins are activated by fasting and inhibited by satiety through ghrelin and leptin hormonal signals. On the other hand, the hypocretinergic system can activate energy metabolism (Hungs and Mignot, 2001). Physical exercise enhances both hypocretin level and energy expenditure (Wu *et al.*, 2002), while in narcoleptic patients the deficiency in hypocretins could result in obesity due to diminished energy expenditure (Yamanaka *et al.*, 2003). It has also been observed that sleep deprivation in rats decreases circulating anabolic hormones, thus increasing their energy expenditure (Everson and Crowley, 2004). Finally, adenosine, formed from AMP and produced during wakefulness when energy reserves are low (Benington and Heller, 1995), might play an important role in the above regulatory mechanisms by favouring the transition from wakefulness to SWS, which is a state of energy conservation (Kalinchuk *et al.*, 2003).

In conclusion, functional relationships exist between sleep–wake states and the endocrine elements that regulate food intake and the production, expenditure, or storage of energy. The reality of such cross-linked processes ensuring the integration of a great variety of influences still remains to be confirmed.

Conclusion and Perspectives

It is noteworthy that evolution has allowed the emergence of REM sleep, thereby requiring homeothermic species to supply the energy required for the occurrence of this state of sleep as well as that necessary for the maintenance of their homeothermic status. This challenge suggests the importance of REM sleep. Lactate produced by astrocytic glycolysis appears capable of ensuring the aerobic neuronal production of ATP necessary for the maintenance of an active physiological wakefulness and the occurrence of REM sleep. SWS, however, is propitious for energy saving. Moreover, glycogen, a storage form of energy, appears to represent a source of energy substrate during periods of tissue demand. Finally, it appears that functional relationships exist between sleep–wake states and endocrine elements that regulate food intake.

Studying the energy metabolism of the brain relative to the sleep–wake cycle remains difficult due to the absence of specific pharmacological tools for *in vivo* approaches. One new methodology that may lead to a better understanding of the physiological and pathological processes is combining polysomnographic measurements with NMR micro-imagery and spectroscopic methods.

Summary

Evolution, by allowing the emergence of REM sleep, rendered more complex the energy-production situation of homeotherms. These species must supply the energy required for both their homeothermic status and the occurrence of REM sleep. Pathways for energy and heat production are thus crucial to the existence of homeotherms, and glucose is generally accepted as the main fuel for the synthesis of ATP. Throughout astrocytic glycolysis and in the absence of oxygen demand, glucose is first metabolised into pyruvate, which results in a positive balance of 2 moles of ATP per mole of glucose. Still in anaerobic conditions, pyruvate can be subjected to lactic fermentation and transformed into lactate. After transport into neurons, lactate contributes — through the aerobic conditions of the Krebs cycle and the respiratory chain — to the production of 34 additional moles of ATP per mole of glucose. The degradation of 1 mole of glucose thus produces 36 moles of ATP, the cerebral metabolic rate of oxygen consumption thus being six times higher than that of glucose. Glucose is actively consumed during wakefulness and particularly during active wakefulness, which contributes to the production of lactate that ensures, through an astrocytic–neuronal coupling, the aerobic production of ATP. It is likely that such processes also occur during REM sleep. During SWS, a state propitious for energy saving, glucose consumption, and lactate production are decreased and the glycogen level is increased. Glycogen, a storage form of energy, appears to represent a source of energy substrate during periods of tissue demand. Finally, it appears that hypocretins together with other hormonal signals contribute to the regulation of food intake and body mass in balance with the production, storage, and expenditure of energy. The reality of such processes remains to be confirmed.

References

Adams, K. and Oswald, I. (1997). Sleep is for tissue restoration. *J. R. Coll. Physicians Lond.*, 11: 376–388.

Adams, K. (1980). Sleep as a restorative process and a theory to explain why. *Prog. Brain Res.*, 53: 289–305.

Allaman, I., Pellerin, L., and Magistretti, P.J. (2000). Protein targeting to glycogen mRNA expression is stimulated by noradrenaline in mouse cortical astrocytes. *Glia*, 30: 382–391.

Allaman, I., Lengacher, S., Magistretti, P.J., and Pellerin, L. (2003). A_{2B} receptor activation promotes glycogen synthesis in astrocytes through modulation of gene expression. *Am. J. Physiol. Cell. Physiol.*, 284: C696–C704.

Allaman, I., Pellerin, L., and Magistretti, P.J. (2004). Glucocorticoids modulate neurotransmitter-induced glycogen metabolism in cultured cortical astrocytes. *J. Neurochem.*, 88: 900–908.

Arnulf, I., Sastre, J.P., Buda, C., and Jouvet, M. (1998). Hyperoxia increases paradoxical sleep rhythm in the pontine cat. *Brain Res.*, 807: 160–166.

Baker, T.L. and McGinty, D.J. (1979). Sleep–waking patterns in hypoxic kittens. *Dev. Psychobiol.*, 12: 377–389.

Benington, J.H. and Heller, C. (1995). Restoration of brain energy metabolism as the function of sleep. *Prog. Neurobiol.*, 45: 347–360.

Berger, R.J. and Phillips, N.H. (1993). Sleep and energy conservation. *NIPS*, 8: 276–281.

Brown, A.M. (2004). Brain glycogen re-awakened. *J. Neurochem.*, 89: 537–552.

Brown, A.M., Tekkök, S.B., and Ransom, B.R. (2003). Glycogen regulation and functional role in mouse white matter. *J. Physiol.*, 549: 501–512.

Campbell, S.S. and Tobler, I. (1984). Animal sleep: a review of sleep duration across phylogeny. *Neurosci. Biochem. Rev.*, 8: 269–300.

Chastrette, N., Cespuglio, R., and Jouvet, M. (1990). POMC-derived peptides and sleep in the rat. Part 1: hypnogenic properties of ACTH derivatives. *Neuropeptides*, 15: 61–74.

Denoyer, M., Sallanon, M., Kitahama, K., Aubert, C., and Jouvet, M. (1989). Reversibility of para-chlorophenylalanine-induced insomnia by intrahypothalamic microinjection of L-5-hydroxytryptophan. *Neuroscience*, 28: 83–94.

Dringen, R. and Hamprecht, B. (1992). Glucose, insulin, and insulin-like growth factor I regulate the glycogen content of astroglia-rich primary cultures. *J. Neurochem.*, 58: 511–517.

Dringen, R., Gebhardt, R., and Hamprecht, B. (1993). Glycogen in astrocytes: possible function as lactate supply for neighboring cells. *Brain Res.*, 623: 208–214.

Everson, C.A. and Crowley, W.R. (2004). Reductions in circulating anabolic hormones induced by sustained sleep deprivation in rats. *Am. J. Physiol. Endocrinol. Metab.*, 286: E1060–E1070.

Franck, G., Salmon, E., Poirier, R., Sadzot, B., and Franco, G. (1987). Etude du métabolisme glucidique cérébral régional chez l'homme au cours de l'éveil et du sommeil, par tomographie à emission de positons. *Rev. Electroenceph. Neurophysiol. Clin.*, 17: 71–77.

Franken, P., Gip, P., Hagiwara, G., Ruby, N.F., and Heller, H.C. (2003). Changes in brain glycogen after sleep deprivation vary with genotype. *Am. J. Physiol. Regul. Integr. Comp. Physiol.*, 285: 413–419.

Gibson, G.E. and Shimada, M. (1980). Studies on the metabolic pathways of the acetyl group for acetylcholine synthesis. *Biochem. Pharmacol.*, 29: 167–174.

Gip, P., Hagiwara, G., Sapolsky, R.M., Cao, V.H., Heller, H.C., and Ruby, N.F. (2004). Glucocorticoids influence brain glycogen levels during sleep deprivation. *Am. J. Physiol. Regul. Integr. Comp. Physiol.*, 286: 1057–1062.

Giuditta, A., Capano, C.P., and Zucconi, G.G. (1984). The Neurochemical approach to the study of sleep. In: Lajtha, A. (Ed.). *Handbook of Neurochemistry*. New York: Plenum Press, pp. 443–476.

Gruetter, R. (2003). Glycogen: the forgotten cerebral energy store. *J. Neurosci. Res.*, 74: 179–183.

Guppy, M., Bradshaw, S.D., Fergusson, B., Hansen, I.A., and Atwood, C. (1987). Metabolism in lizards: low lactate turnover and advantages of heterothermy. *Am. J. Physiol.*, 253: 77–82.

Heiss, W.D., Pawlik, G., Herlolz, K., Wagner, R., and Wienhard, K. (1985). Regional cerebral metabolism in man during wakefulness, sleep and dreaming. *Brain Res.*, 327: 362–366.

Heller, H.C., Musacchia, X.J., and Wang, L.C.H. (1988). *Living in the Cold*. New York: Elsevier.

Himms-Haggen, J. (1976). Cellular thermogenesis. *Annu. Rev. Physiol.*, 38: 315–351.

Horne, J.A. (1985). Mammalian sleep function with particular reference to man. In: Mayes, A.R. (Ed.). *Sleep Mechanisms and Functions in Humans and Animals — An Evolutionary Perspective*. Wokingham, England: Van Nostrand, pp. 262–311.

Horvath, T.L., Diano, S., Sotonyi, P., Heiman, M., and Tschop, M. (2001). Minireview: ghrelin and the regulation of energy balance — a hypothalamic perspective. *Endocrinology*, 142: 4163–4169.

Huertas, J. and McMillin, J.K. (1968). Paradoxical sleep: effect of low partial pressures of atmospheric oxygen. *Science*, 159: 745–746.

Hungs, M. and Mignot, E. (2001). Hypocretin/orexin, sleep and narcolepsy. *Bioessays*, 23: 397–408.

Jouvet, M. (1994). Phylogeny of the states of sleep. *Acta Psychiat. Belg.*, 94: 256–267.

Kalinchuk, A.V., Urrila, A.S., Alanko, L., Heiskanen, S., Wigren, H.K., Suomela, M., Stenberg, D., and Porkka-Heiskanen, T. (2003). Local energy depletion in the basal forebrain increases sleep. *Eur. J. Neurosci.*, 17: 863–869.

Karadzic, Y. and Mrsulja, B. (1969). Deprivation of paradoxical sleep and brain glycogen. *J. Neurochem.*, 16: 29–34.

Karmanova, I.G. (1982). Evolution of sleep. In: Koella, W.P. (Ed.). *Evolution of Sleep*. New York: Karger Press, pp. 1–147.

Karnovsky, M.L., Reich, P., Anchors, J.M., and Burrow, B.L. (1983). Changes in brain glycogen during slow-wave sleep in the rat. *J. Neurochem.*, 41: 1498–1501.

Kennedy, C., Gillin, J.C., Mendelson, W., Suda, S., Miyaoka, M., Ito, M., Nakamura, R.K., Storch, F.I., Pettigrew, K., Mishkin, M., and Sokolov, L. (1982). Local cerebral glucose utilization in non-rapid eye movement sleep. *Nature*, 297: 325–327.

Kong, J., Shepel, P.N., Holden, C.P., Mackiewicz, M., Pack, A.I., and Geiger, J.D. (2002). Brain glycogen decreases with increased periods of wakefulness: implications for homeostatic drive to sleep. *J. Neurosci.*, 22: 5581–5587.

Konings, W.N. and Michels, P.A.M. (1980). Electron-transfer-driven solute translocation across bacterial membranes. In: Knowles, C.J. (Ed.). *Diversity of Bacterial Respiratory Systems*. Boca Raton: CRC Press, pp. 33–86.

Laughton, J.D., Charnay, Y., Belloir, B., Pellerin, L., Magistretti, P.J., and Bouras, C. (2000). Differential messenger RNA distribution of lactate dehydrogenase LDH-1 and LDH-5 isoforms in the rat brain. *Neuroscience*, 96: 619–625.

Lefresne, P., Beaujouan, J.C., and Glowinski, J. (1978). Origin of the acetyl moiety of acetylcholine in rat striatal synaptosomes: a specific pyruvate dehydrogenase involved in Ach synthesis? *Biochimie*, 60: 479–487.

Lydic, R., Baghdoyan, H.A., Hibbard, L., Bonyak, E.V., De Joseph, M.R., and Hawkins, R.A. (1991). Regional brain glucose metabolism is altered during rapid eye movements in cat: a preliminary study. *J. Comp. Neurol.*, 304: 517–529.

Magistretti, P.J. and Pellerin, L. (1997). Regulation by neurotransmitters of glial energy metabolism. *Adv. Exp. Med. Biol.*, 429: 137–143.

Magistretti, P.J. and Pellerin, L. (1999). Cellular mechanisms of brain energy metabolism and their relevance to functional brain imaging. *Philos. Trans. R. Soc. Lond. B.*, 354: 1155–1163.

Magistretti, P.J., Sorg, O., Naichen, Y., Pellerin, L., De Rham, S., and Martin, J.-L. (1994). Regulation of astrocyte energy metabolism by neurotransmitters. *Renal Physiol. Biochem.*, 17: 168–171.

Magistretti, P.J., Pellerin, L., Rothman, D.L., and Shulman R.G. (1999). Energy on demand. *Science*, 283: 496–497.

Maquet, P., Dive, D., Salmon, E., Sadzot, B., Franco, G., Poirier, R., Von Frenckell, R., and Franck, G. (1990). Cerebral glucose utilization during sleep–wake cycle in man determined by positron emission tomography and 2-fluoro-2-deoxy-D-glucose method. *Brain Res.*, 513: 136–143.

Marsden, P.L. and Wildschiodtz, G. (1994). Cerebral oxygen metabolism during the sleep–wake cycle in man. *J. Sleep Res.*, 3: 154–158.

McGinty, D. and Szymusiak, R. (2000). The sleep–wake switch: a neuronal alarm clock. *Nat. Med.*, 6: 510–511.

Meister, B. (2000). Control of food intake via leptin receptors in the hypothalamus. *Vitam. Horm.*, 59: 265–304.

Mottin, S., Laporte, P., Jouvet, M., and Cespuglio, R. (1997). Determination of NADH in the rat brain during sleep–wake states with an optic fibre sensor and time-resolved fluorescence procedures. *Neuroscience*, 79: 683–693.

Muroya, S., Funahashi, H., Yamanaka, A., Kohno, D., Uramura, K., Nambu, T., Shibahara, M., Kuramochi, M., Takigawa, M., Yanagisawa, M., Sakurai, T., Shioda, S., and Yada, T. (2004). Orexins (hypocretins) directly interact with neuropeptide Y, POMC and glucose-responsive neurons to regulate Ca^{2+} signaling in a reciprocal manner to leptin: orexigenic neuronal pathways in the mediobasal hypothalamus. *Eur. J. Neurosci.*, 19: 1524–1534.

Netchiporouk, L.I., Shram, N.F., Jaffrezic-Renault, N., Martelet, C., and Cespuglio, R. (1996). *In vivo* brain glucose measurements: differential normal pulse voltammetry with enzyme-modified carbon fiber microelectrodes. *Anal. Chem.*, 68: 4358–4364.

Netchiporouk, L., Shram, N., Salvert, D., and Cespuglio, R. (2001). Brain extracellular glucose assessed by voltammetry throughout the rat sleep–wake cycle. *Eur. J. Neurosci.*, 13: 1429–1434.

Nicholls, D.G. (1976). Brown fat mitochondria. *Trends Biochem. Sci.*, 1: 128–130.

Parmeggiani, P.L. (1985). Interactions between temperature and sleep regulations. In: Heller, H.C., Musacchia, J., and Wang, L.C.U. (Eds.). *Living in the Cold.* New York: Elsevier, pp. 177–184.

Pellegri, G., Rossier, C., Magistretti, P.J., and Martin, J.L. (1996). Cloning, localization and induction of mouse brain glycogen synthase. *Mol. Brain Res.*, 38: 191–199.

Pellerin, L. and Magistretti, P.J. (2004). Neuroenergetics: calling upon astrocytes to satisfy hungry neurons. *Neuroscientist*, 10: 53–62.

Pelleymounter, M.A., Cullen, M.J., Baker, M.B., Hecht, R., Winters, D., Boone, T., and Collins, F. (1995). Effects of the obese gene product on body weight regulation in ob/ob mice. *Science*, 269: 540–543.

Petit, J.M., Tobler, I., Allaman, I., Borbély, A.A., and Magistretti, P.J. (2002). Sleep deprivation modulates brain mRNAs encoding genes of glycogen metabolism. *Eur. J. Neurosci.*, 16: 1163–1167.

Petitjean, F., Buda, C., Janin, M., David, M., and Jouvet, M. (1979). Effets du chloramphenicol sur le sommeil du chat, comparaison avec le thiamphénicol, l'erythromycine et l'oxytétracycline. *Psychopharmacology*, 66: 147–153.

Pfeiffer, B., Elmer, K., Roggendorf, W., Reinhart, P.H., and Hamprecht, B. (1990). Immunohistochemical demonstration of glycogen phosphorylase in rat brain slices. *Histochemistry*, 94: 73–80.

Pfeiffer-Guglielmi, B., Fleckenstein, B., Jung, G., and Hamprecht, B. (2003). Immunocytochemical localization of glycogen phosphorylase isoenzymes in rat nervous tissues by using isozyme-specific antibodies. *J. Neurochem.*, 85: 73–81.

Phelps, C.H. (1972). Barbiturate-induced glycogen accumulation in brain. *Brain Res.*, 39: 225–234.

Porkka-Heiskanen, T., Strecker, R.E., Thakkar, M., Bjorkum, A.A., Greene, R.W., and McCarley, R.W. (1997). Adenosine: a mediator of the sleep-inducing effects of prolonged wakefulness. *Science*, 276: 1265–1268.

Porkka-Heiskanen, T., Strecker, R.E., and McCarley, R.W. (2000). Brain site-specificity of extracellular adenosine concentration changes during sleep deprivation and spontaneous sleep: an *in vivo* microdialysis study. *J. Neurosci.*, 99: 507–517.

Porkka-Heiskanen, T., Alanko, L., Kalinchuk, A., and Stenberg, D. (2002). Adenosine and sleep. *Sleep Med. Rev.*, 6: 321–332.

Purves, W.K., Orians, G.H., Heller, H.C., and London, J. (1992). Physiologie, homéostasie et regulation de la température corporelle. In: Flammarion, E. (Ed.). *Le Monde du Vivant*. Paris: Editions Flammarion, pp. 741–764.

Ramm, P. and Frost, B.J. (1983). Regional metabolic activity in the brain during sleep–wake activity. *Sleep*, 6: 196–216.

Ramm, P. and Frost, B.J. (1986). Cerebral and local cerebral metabolism in the cat during slow wave and REM sleep. *Brain Res.*, 365: 112–124.

Reich, P., Geyer, S.J., and Karnovsky, M.L. (1972). Metabolism of brain during sleep and wakefulness. *J. Neurochem.*, 19: 487–497.

Rechtschaffen, A., Bergmann, B.M., Everson, C.A., Kushida, C.A., and Gilliland, M.A. (1989). Sleep deprivation in the rat: X. Integration and discussion of the findings. *Sleep*, 12: 68–87.

Reivich, M., Isaacs, G., Evarts, E., and Kety, S. (1968). The effect of slow wave sleep and REM sleep on regional cerebral blood flow in cats. *J. Neurochem.*, 15: 301–306.

Richter, D. and Dawson, R.M.C. (1948). Brain metabolism in emotional excitement and in sleep. *Am. J. Physiol.*, 154: 73–79.

Riou, F., Cespuglio, R., and Jouvet, M. (1982). Endogenous peptides and sleep in the rat. III. The hypnogenic properties of vasoactive intestinal polypeptide. *Neuropeptides*, 2: 265–277.

Rough, V.H. (2002). Glucose sensing neurons: are they physiologically relevant? *Physiol. Behav.*, 76: 403–413.

Sakai, K. (1988). Executive mechanisms of paradoxical sleep. *Arch. Ital. Biol.*, 479: 225–240.

Sakurai, T. (2003). Orexin: a link between energy homeostasis and adaptive behaviour. *Curr. Opin. Clin. Nutr. Metab. Care*, 6: 353–360.

Sakurai, T., Amemiya, A., Ishii, M., Matsuzaki, I., Chemelli, R.M., Tanaka, H., Williams, S.C., Richardson, J.A., Kozlowski, G.P., Wilson, S., Arch, J.R., Buckingham, R.E., Haynes, A.C., Carr, S.A., Annan, R.S., McNulty, D.E., Liu, W.S., Terrett, J.A., Elshourbagy, N.A., Bergsma, D.J., and Yanagisawa, M. (1998). Orexins and orexin receptors: a family of hypothalamic neuropeptides and G protein-coupled receptors that regulate feeding behavior. *Cell*, 92: 573–585.

Sallanon, M., Denoyer, M., Kitahama, K., Aubert, C., Gay N., and Jouvet, M. (1989). Long-lasting insomnia induced by preoptic neuron lesions and its transient reversal by muscimol injection into the posterior hypothalamus in the cat. *Neuroscience*, 32: 669–683.

Saper, C.B., Chou, T.C., and Scammell, T.E. (2001). The sleep switch: hypothalamic control of sleep and wakefulness. *Trends Neurosci.*, 24: 726–731.

Sawaya, R. and Ingvar, D.H. (1989). Cerebral blood flow and metabolism in sleep. *Acta Neurol. Scand.*, 80: 481–491.

Serres, S., Bouyer, J.J., Bezancon, E., Canioni, P., and Merle, M. (2003). Involvement of brain lactate in neuronal metabolism. *NMR Biomed.*, 16: 430–439.

Shimizu, H., Tabushi, K., Hishikawa, Y., Kakimoto, Y., and Kaneko, Z. (1966). Concentration of lactic acid in rat during natural sleep. *Nature*, 26: 936–937.

Shram, N.F., Netchiporouk, L.I., Martelet, C., Jaffrezic-Renault, N., and Cespuglio, R. (1998). *In vivo* voltammetric detection of rat brain lactate with carbon fibre microelectrodes coated with lactate oxidase. *Anal. Chem.*, 70: 2618–2622.

Shram, N., Netchiporouk, L., and Cespuglio, R. (2002). Lactate in the brain of the freely moving rat: voltametric monitoring of the changes related to the sleep–wake states. *Eur. J. Neurosci.*, 16, 461–466.

Simon, E., Pierau, F.K., and Taylor, D.C. (1986). Central and peripheral thermal control of effectors in homeothermic temperature regulation. *Physiol. Rev.*, 66: 235–300.

Siesjö, B.K. (1978). *Brain Energy Metabolism.* New York: John Wiley & Sons, Interscience Publication, pp. 151–379.

Sorg, O. and Magistretti, P.J. (1992). Vasoactive intestinal peptide and noradrenaline exert long-term control on glycogen levels in astrocytes: blockade by protein synthesis inhibition. *J. Neurosci.*, 12: 4923–4931.

Taheri, S., Zeitzer, J.M., and Mignot, E. (2002). The role of hypocretins (orexins) in sleep regulation and narcolepsy. *Annu. Rev. Neurosci.*, 25: 283–313.

Townsend, R.E., Prinz, P.N., and Obrist, W.D. (1973). Human cerebral blood flow during sleep and waking. *J. Appl. Physiol.*, 35: 620–625.

Tsacopoulos, M. and Magistretti, P.J. (1996). Metabolic coupling between glia and neurons. *J. Neuroscience*, 16: 877–885.

Tschop, M., Smiley, D.L., and Heiman, M.L. (2000). Ghrelin induces adiposity in rodents. *Nature*, 407: 908–913.

Tucek, S. (1984). Problems in the organization and control of acetylcholine synthesis in brain neurons. *Prog. Biophys. Mol. Biol.*, 44: 1–46.

Walker, J.M. and Berger, R.J. (1980). Sleep as an adaptation for energy conservation functionally related to hibernation and shallow torpor. *Prog. Brain Res.*, 53: 255–278.

Weber, J.M. and Haman, M. (1996). Pathways for metabolic fuels and oxygen in high performance fish. *Comp. Biochem. Physiol.*, 113: 33–38.

Wren, A.M., Seal, L.J., Cohen, M.A., Brynes, A.E., Frost, G.S., Murphy, K.G., Dhillo, W.S., Ghatei, M.A., and Bloom, S.R. (2001). Ghrelin enhances appetite and increases food intake in humans. *J. Clin. Endocrinol. Metab.*, 86: 5992.

Wu, M.F., John, J., Maidment, N., Lam, H.A., and Siegel, J.M. (2002). Hypocretin release in normal and narcoleptic dogs after food and sleep deprivation, eating, and movement. *Am. J. Physiol. Regul. Integr. Comp. Physiol.*, 283: 1079–1086.

Yamanaka, A., Beuckmann, C.T., Willie, J.T., Hara, J., Tsujino, N., Mieda, M., Tominaga, M., Yagami, K., Sugiyama, F., Goto, K., Yanagisawa, M., and Sakurai, T. (2003). Hypothalamic orexin neurons regulate arousal according to energy balance in mice. *Neuron*, 38: 701–713.

Chapter 2

HUMORAL MECHANISMS OF SLEEP

Ferenc Obal Jr. and James M. Krueger[1]

The concept of humoral regulation of sleep stems from classical endocrinology. Hormones were identified by means of transfer experiments. Thus, after stimulation of a donor animal, tissue fluids were transferred to recipient animals, which, in turn, responded to the injectant. Ischimori (reviewed by Inoué, 1989) and Legendre and Piéron (1913) reported that brain extracts and cerebrospinal fluid (CSF) samples obtained from sleep-deprived dogs elicited sleep in recipient dogs. Several successful replications of these transfer experiments were subsequently reported but there were only three studies that resulted in the isolation of a sleep-promoting substance. The three studies produced four candidate sleep regulatory substances.

Monnier and Hösli (1964) used thalamic stimulation to promote sleep in rabbits, and the sleep-promoting factor was dialysated from the venous blood leaving the brain. The substance is a nonapeptide, named delta sleep-inducing peptide (DSIP) (Schoenenberger *et al.*, 1978). DSIP, however, did not prove to be a reliable sleep-inducing substance. The other three substances were isolated from tissue fluids of sleep-deprived animals. Uchizono *et al.* (1978) extracted two somnogenic substances from brain stems of sleep-deprived rats. Processing of these extracts resulted in the identification of a pyrimidine nucleoside, uridine (Komoda *et al.*, 1983), and a small peptide, oxidized glutathione (Komoda *et al.*, 1990), as sleep factors. Finally,

---

[1] krueger@vetmed.wsu.edu

Table 1. Criteria for sleep regulatory substances

The SRS should induce or maintain physiological sleep and, within limits, should induce sleep that mimics that observed after sleep loss

The concentration or turnover of the SRS or its receptors should vary with sleep propensity

Inhibition of the SRS should inhibit spontaneous sleep

The SRS should promote sleep via one or more of the known sleep regulatory networks

Conditions that promote (e.g., mild increases in ambient temperature) or inhibit (e.g., sleep apnea) sleep should alter the amount or metabolism of the SRS

Sleep induced by the SRS should be readily reversible and other behaviors normal after somnogenic doses of the SRS

Pappenheimer obtained CSF containing a transferable sleep-promoting substance, Factor S, from sleep-deprived goats (Miller *et al.*, 1967). A substance with chemical characteristics indistinguishable from Factor S was identified as a muramyl peptide from human urine and rabbit brain (Krueger *et al.*, 1980). The significance of all these findings remains to be determined.

More recently, a variety of additional sleep-promoting substances was characterized. Of these, we discuss the non-rapid eye movement sleep (NREMS) promoting substances, growth hormone releasing hormone (GHRH), interleukin-1β (IL1), tumor necrosis factor α (TNF), adenosine, and prostaglandin D_2 (PGD_2), and the REMS-promoting substances, vasoactive intestinal polypeptide (VIP) and prolactin (PRL), because all of these substances have fulfilled the criteria for sleep regulatory substances (SRSs) (Table 1) (reviewed, Krueger and Obal, 1994). We also briefly mention three other substances, oleamide, cholecystokinin (CCK), and insulin, although insufficient information exists to classify them as SRSs.

NREMS Regulatory Substances

Growth hormone releasing hormone

GHRH is a peptide containing 40–44 amino acid residues and is a member of the secretin-glucagon family. As a neurohormone of the somatotropic axis, GHRH is produced in hypothalamic arcuate nucleus (ARC) neurons and is released from terminals at the median eminence. The blood carries GHRH to the anterior pituitary where GHRH stimulates the synthesis and release of growth hormone (GH) from somatotroph cells. GH is a major anabolic hormone of the body. The effects of GH are, in part, direct actions and, in part, mediated by insulin-like growth factor-1 (IGF-1). The somatotropic axis also includes an inhibitory neurohormone, somatostatin, which suppresses the release of both GHRH in the hypothalamus and GH in the pituitary. As a neurotransmitter, GHRH is released from neurons in the ARC, neurons in the area around the ventral rim of the ventromedial nucleus, and neurons in the paraventricular nucleus, which project predominantly to the anterior hypothalamus/preoptic region (AH/PO). Stimulation of GH secretion and promotion of NREMS are regarded as two parallel and independent outputs of the hypothalamic GHRHergic network. The two outputs are normally synchronized, which appear as NREMS-coupled GH secretion but desynchronization is also possible. The NREMS-associated GH secretion has been confirmed in a number of species, and it is best documented in human subjects (Van Cauter and Plat, 1998).

GHRH mRNA levels and GHRH peptide contents in the hypothalamus display diurnal variation that correlate with sleep–wake activity, and respond to sleep deprivation (Obal and Krueger, 2003). GHRH receptors in the hypothalamus are also responsive to sleep deprivation (Gardi *et al.*, 2002). These changes suggest enhanced GHRH release during the period of deep NREMS, i.e., during the first portion of the diurnal rest period and during recovery sleep after sleep deprivation. Intense GHRH release, however, starts already during sleep deprivation.

Administration of GHRH increases the duration of NREMS and enhances electroencephalographic (EEG) slow-wave activity during NREMS in rats, rabbits, mice, and humans (reviewed, Steiger *et al.*, 1998; Obal and Krueger, 2003, 2004). It is effective after systemic, intracerebroventricular, and intrapreoptic injections. The REMS response to GHRH is inconsistent; no changes and increases in REMS have been reported. Experiments in hypophysectomized rats and other observations suggest that stimulation of REMS by GHRH is mediated by GH. Inhibition of GHRH by means of antagonists or immunoneutralization is followed by decreases in NREMS and REMS. The somatotropic axis includes several negative feedback mechanisms, which inhibit GHRHergic neurons. Both IGF-1 and GH inhibit GHRH release. These actions are mediated at least in part via somatostatin. Somatostatin is a strong suppressor of GHRHergic activity. Octreotide, a somatostatin analog with longer half-life than somatostatin, high doses of IGF-1, or GH elicit simultaneous suppression of GH secretion and sleep in animals and human subjects (Hajdu *et al.*, 2003; Obal and Krueger, 2003, 2004).

Chronic diminution in GHRHergic activity is associated with decreases in NREMS and REMS as shown in transgenic and mutant animal models (Obal *et al.*, 2003; Obal and Krueger, 2003, 2004). Sleep decreases in *dw/dw* rats and *lit/lit* mice bearing non-functional GHRH receptors, and in TH-hGH transgenic mice in which GHRH production is suppressed by human GH released from tyrosine hydroxylase-positive neurons in the brain. Deficiency in GHRHergic activity is associated with GH and IGF-1 deficiencies, the animals are dwarfs, and it is important to differentiate among the consequences of these defects. First, GH replacement fails to correct the NREMS loss while it normalizes REMS in the *lit/lit* mice. Second, "spontaneous dwarf rats" (SDRs) with a point mutation in the GH gene resulting in GH deficiency display decreases in REMS. NREMS time is not reduced in the SDRs; on the contrary, duration of NREMS is increased possibly due to enhanced GHRHergic activity. Mice bearing transgenes fusing the coding region of rat GH gene with the promoter region of the metallothionein gene produce huge amounts of GH and are giants. These mice not only exhibit greatly increased REMS time but their NREMS time is also modestly enhanced though the high GH is predicted to suppress GHRH production. It is believed that the increases in NREMS might be related to some metabolic actions of GH in these animals.

Experiments with microinjection of GHRH and its antagonist suggest that the AH/PO is the site of action for NREMS promotion by GHRH (Zhang *et al.*, 1999). GHRH elicits rises in intracellular calcium in a population of GABAergic neurons (De *et al.*, 2002). These GABAergic neurons are the likely candidate for mediating the effects on sleep. Interestingly, IL1 also stimulates most of the GHRH-responsive neurons. IL1 upregulates GHRH receptors (Taishi *et al.*, 2004). That IL1 makes sleep-promoting neurons more responsive to GHRH might play a role in the increases in NREMS elicited by IL1, and it may contribute to somnolence associated with the acute-phase response to infections.

Cytokines

Cytokines are regulatory proteins signaling via juxtacrine, autocrine, paracrine, and endocrine mechanisms. The names of individual cytokines often reflect the type of biological activity used to isolate them, e.g., TNF and nerve growth factor (NGF) or the fields within which those who discovered them worked, e.g., IL1 and brain-derived neurotrophic factor (BDNF).

Cytokines form complex networks characterized by much redundancy and biphasic actions that depend upon the signaling context and ligand concentration. For instance, TNF can be either neuroprotective or induce neurodegeneration; specific effects depend upon the array of intracellular adaptor proteins that bind to the intracellular domain of the TNF receptors. The brain cytokine network is only just beginning to be understood. The action of cytokines in brain injury is better understood than their physiological roles. Regardless, there is now much evidence that cytokines have many physiological roles within the brain ranging from neural plasticity to sleep (Krueger *et al.*, 2001). Many cytokines have sleep-promoting activity; the list includes IL1α, IL1β, TNFα, TNFβ, IL2, IL6, IL8, IL15, IL18, acidic fibroblast growth factor, NGF, BDNF, neurotrophins 3 and 4, glia-derived neurotrophic factor, several interferons, epidermal growth factor, and granulocyte-macrophage colony-stimulating factor. Other cytokines have the ability to inhibit the production or actions of the pro-somnogenic cytokines and inhibit sleep; the list includes, IL4, IL10, IL13, IGF-1, the soluble TNF receptor, the soluble IL1 receptor, and transforming growth factor β (Obal and Krueger, 2003). Here, we focus on two cytokines, IL1β and TNFα, since their involvement in physiological sleep regulation is well established and sleep regulation was one of the first physiological roles defined for brain cytokines (Vitkovic *et al.*, 2000).

Systemic or intracerebroventricular administration of either TNF or IL1 enhances NREMS in all the species thus far tested: mice, rats, rabbits, cats, sheep, monkeys, and humans (Obal and Krueger, 2003). IL1 or TNF also enhances EEG slow-wave activity during NREMS; such activity is indicative of greater sleep intensity. Low doses of IL1 or TNF promote NREMS, while after high doses sleep is often inhibited. Low somnogenic doses can promote NREMS without affecting REMS although slightly higher doses that promote NREMS often inhibit REMS. There is also a time-of-day dependency of the effect of IL1 on sleep; thus, after intracerebral injection of a moderate dose (10 ng human IL1β) into rats, sleep is promoted if injected at the onset of dark hours. In contrast, if the same dose is injected at the onset of daylight hours, sleep is inhibited (Opp *et al.*, 1991). Although the reasons for these dose and time-dependent effects remain unknown, it seems likely that they are related to the multiple molecular feedback networks stimulated by these cytokines. For instance, both upregulate glucocorticoids and they in turn can inhibit sleep. Both IL1 and TNF, in sufficient amounts, also induce fever. However, their pyrogenic actions are not directly related to their somnogenic actions. Thus, antipyretics block IL1-induced fevers but not IL1-induced sleep responses (Krueger *et al.*, 1984). Further, low doses of IL1 or TNF are somnogenic but not pyrogenic.

Inhibition of IL1 or TNF inhibits spontaneous NREMS, thereby suggesting that these cytokines are involved in physiological sleep regulation (reviewed, Krueger *et al.*, 2001). Injection of either antibodies to either IL1 or TNF, the soluble IL1 receptor, the soluble TNF receptor, active fragments of either soluble receptor, or the IL1 receptor antagonist inhibits spontaneous sleep. These inhibitors also inhibit the NREMS rebound that occurs after sleep deprivation. Further, as mentioned above, substances that inhibit the actions or production of IL1 or TNF also inhibit spontaneous sleep, e.g., alpha melanocyte stimulating hormone, corticotrophin releasing hormone, glucocorticoids, and anti-inflammatory cytokines like IL4, 10, and 13. Mice that lack the IL1 type I receptor (Fang *et al.*, 1997) or the TNF 55-kD receptor (Fang *et al.*, 1998) sleep less than control mice although the sleep deficits are small and confined to specific times of the day.

Both IL1 and TNF are produced in the brain. Although neurons, glia, and endothelial cells all produce these cytokines, the cellular source of cytokines involved in physiological actions remains unknown. Regardless, hypothalamic levels of IL1β mRNA and TNFα mRNA vary with sleep propensity (Krueger *et al.*, 2001; Taishi *et al.*, 1999). They are highest at the beginning of the light cycle in rats when sleep propensity is highest. Protein levels of both IL1 and TNF also are highest at this time (Floyd and Krueger, 1997; Nguyen *et al.*, 1998). IL1-like activity varies with the sleep–wake cycle in CSF of cats (Lue *et al.*, 1988). TNF plasma levels in humans correlate with EEG slow-wave activity (Darko *et al.*, 2002).

Under several conditions that induce excess sleep, the sleep responses may be mediated via the brain cytokine network. For example, sleep loss is associated with increases in brain levels of IL1 and TNF mRNAs and excess sleep upon recovery (Mackiewicz *et al.*, 1996; Taishi *et al.*, 1997, 1999). Rats put on a cafeteria diet sleep more; their hypothalamic IL1 mRNA levels are also upregulated (Hansen *et al.*, 1998a). A mild increase in ambient temperature is also associated with increases in sleep and this effect is blocked by TNF inhibition (Takahashi and Krueger, 1997). Infectious challenge enhances both sleep and cytokine production (reviewed, Majde and Krueger, 2002). Other pathologies are also associated with altered circulating cytokine levels and changes in sleep. For instance, TNF is elevated in patients with chronic fatigue (Moss *et al.*, 1999), sleep apnea (Liu *et al.*, 2000), chronic insomnia (Vgontzas *et al.*, 2002), and post-dialysis fatigue

(Dreisbach *et al.*, 1998). In contrast, rheumatoid arthritic patients receiving the TNF-soluble receptor report reduced fatigue (Franklin, 1999).

Systemic cytokines can reach the brain via several routes. They enter the brain via the circumventricular organs where the blood–brain barrier is absent, they may be transported into the brain, they can elicit transcription of IL1 or other signaling molecules in endothelial cells (e.g., NO), and they may act via sensory neurons in the vagus nerve (Hansen *et al.*, 1998b). For example, the sleep-promoting activity of systemic TNF or IL1 is attenuated after vagotomy (Kubota *et al.*, 2001). Systemic IL1 induces increases in hypothalamic IL1 mRNA and this effect is blocked after subdiaphragmatic vagotomy (Hansen *et al.*, 1998b). The contributions of systemic versus central cytokines to physiological sleep regulation remains unknown.

The mechanisms by which IL1 and TNF affect sleep have been investigated at the molecular, cellular, and network levels. Both substances activate the transcription factor nuclear factor kappa B (NFκB). The translocation of NFκB into the nuclei of cortical (Chen *et al.*, 1999) and basal forebrain neurons (Basheer *et al.*, 2001) is stimulated by sleep loss and an inhibitor of NFκB translocation suppresses sleep (Kubota *et al.*, 2000). Activation of lateral hypothalamic NFκB also occurs after sleep loss (Brandt *et al.*, 2004). In addition, NFκB seems to be involved in enhanced production of IL1, TNF, NGF, adenosine A1 receptors, cyclooxygenase-2, and several prosomnogenic cytokines (Figure 1). Other downstream molecular mechanisms are shared by IL1 and TNF. For instance, both can enhance NO and NO is involved in sleep regulation (reviewed, Obal and Krueger, 2003). NFκB is related to this action to the extent that it promotes inducible NO synthase production. As already mentioned, hypothalamic GABAergic cells are receptive for both IL1 and GHRH and anti-GHRH antibodies attenuate IL1-induced sleep responses thereby suggesting that GHRH and IL1 share a common pathway within the hypothalamus. IL1 and TNF also induce a variety of feedback signals inhibitory to both their production and somnogenic actions (see above).

IL1 and TNF promote NREMS via multiple CNS sites. Thus, IL1 upregulates hypothalamic GHRH receptors (Taishi *et al.*, 2004) and may also stimulate GHRH synthesis. IL1 also stimulates sleep-active anterior hypothalamic neurons while inhibiting wake-active neurons in this area (Alam *et al.*, 2001). Whether these cells are the IL1- and GHRH-receptive GABAergic neurons described earlier remains unknown. IL1 microinjected into the locus ceruleus (DeSarro *et al.*, 1997) or dorsal rahpe (Imeri *et al.*, 2002) also enhances sleep. TNF also enhances NREMS after injection into

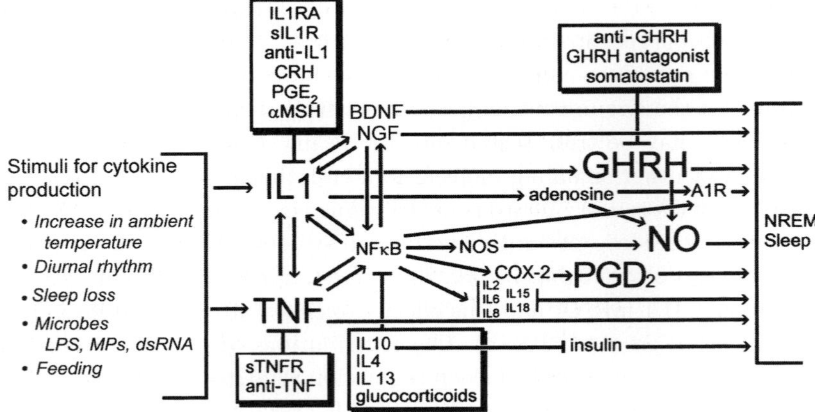

Figure 1. Molecular networks are involved in sleep regulation. Substances in boxes inhibit sleep and inhibit the production or actions of the sleep-promoting substances illustrated via feedback mechanisms. Inhibition of one step does not completely block sleep, since parallel sleep-promoting pathways exist. These redundant pathways provide stability to sleep regulation. Our knowledge of the biochemical events involved in sleep regulation is more extensive than that illustrated. A major goal of sleep research is to associate specific molecular steps to the neural networks involved in sleep regulation. Abbreviations: IL1RA, IL1 receptor antagonist; sIL1R, soluble IL1 receptor; anti-IL1, anti-IL1 antibodies; CRH, corticotrophin releasing hormone; PGD2, prostaglandin D2; αMSH, α melanocyte stimulating hormone; sTNFR, soluble TNF receptor; anti-TNF, anti-TNF antibodies; TGFβ, transforming growth factor beta; IGF1, insulin-like growth factor; A1R, adenosine A1 receptor; COX-2, cyclooxygenase-2 (see text for other abbreviations).

the anterior hypothalamus (Kubota *et al.*, 2002) or the locus ceruleus (DeSarro *et al.*, 1997). Such findings suggest that cytokines promote sleep, in part, via multiple known sleep regulatory circuits.

New findings suggest an additional site of cytokine action on sleep. Injection of either TNF (Yoshida *et al.*, 2004) or IL1 (Yasuda *et al.*, 2004) onto the surface of the somatosensory cortex unilaterally induces state-dependent enhancements of EEG slow-wave activity on the ipsilateral side but not on the contralateral side. Further, inhibition of TNF unilaterally inhibits the enhanced EEG slow-wave activity occurring during NREMS induced by sleep loss on the side the soluble receptor was injected. These data suggest a local action of cytokines and this is consistent with their actions in other tissues. Such results are also consistent with the view that sleep is a fundamental property of small groups of highly interconnected neurons (neuronal groups) (Krueger and Obal, 2003). In this view, local sleep results from activity-induced production of cytokines and other sleep regulatory substances that act via autocrine, juxtacrine, and paracrine pathways to alter the input–output relationships of the nearby neuronal groups. Such localized altered functional states have been described (Carter *et al.*, 2003). The activity-dependent production of several cytokines has been reported (reviewed, Krueger and Obal, 2003) and their ability to alter input–output relationships are known, e.g., as described above IL1 alters the activity of wake-active neurons. The pathways by which cortical cytokines interact with the known sleep regulatory circuits are not yet fully characterized. Recent preliminary evidence, however, suggests that IL1 applied unilaterally to the somatosensory cortex activates reticular thalamic neurons as well as medial preoptic and ventrolateral preoptic neurons (Churchill *et al.*, in press). These findings suggest a mechanism by which local sleep-like states of neuronal groups are coordinated into whole animal sleep.

Adenosine

The purine nucleoside adenosine is a compound ideally suited for cellular autoregulation, including the regulation neuronal discharge as a function of previous activity. Adenosine is a component of ATP, the compound that stores and provides energy for biochemical processes. Neurons use ATP extensively for the maintenance and recovery of resting ion balance after action potentials and, therefore, prolonged activity is associated with significant hydrolysis of ATP and adenosine release. Adenosine is also released from the second messenger cAMP. Excess adenosine is transported out of the cell. ATP is also found extracellularly because some neurotransmitter vesicles release ATP along with their neurotransmitters. Extracellular ATP is metabolized to adenosine by ectoenzymes. Adenosine modulates neuronal activity via adenosine receptors. The A2 receptors are excitatory whereas the A1 receptors are inhibitory, they elicit hyperpolarization through opening of potassium channels. Hence, intense neuronal activity results in significant adenosine release, and adenosine acting on A1 receptors diminishes further neuronal activity.

Microdialysis experiments detected rises in extracellular adenosine during wakefulness and decreases in adenosine in NREMS and REMS in various brain sites. The basal forebrain and cortex were the areas where sustained adenosine release was found during sleep deprivation (Porkka-Heiskanen *et al.*, 1997). Systemic administration of adenosine antagonists in the form of caffeine is widely practiced in various cultures to stimulate arousal. Intracerebral or systemic injection of adenosine or adenosine agonists increases sleep duration and/or enhances EEG slow-wave activity during NREMS. The basal forebrain is the area that mediates the effects of adenosine on sleep: rises in extracellular concentration of adenosine in this area increase NREMS and REMS whereas adenosine antagonists decrease sleep (reviewed, Strecker *et al.*, 2000).

It seems that cholinergic neurons in the basal forebrain are both the major source and the primary target of adenosine. These cholinergic neurons project to the cortex and promote arousal (Zaborszky and Duque, 2003). Adenosine inhibits them via A1 receptors (reviewed, Strecker *et al.*, 2000). In addition, A1 receptors might be expressed presynaptically on terminals stimulating the cholinergic neurons. Inhibition of transmitter release from these terminals decreases the activation of cholinergic neurons. Finally, via A1 receptors, adenosine may cause presynaption inhibition of GABAergic neurons suppressing sleep-active neurons thereby causing disinhibition of sleep-promoting neurons. A1 receptors also activate a transcription factor, NFκB, which can induce the production of other sleep-promoting substances and can induce upregulation of A1 receptors (Basheer *et al.*, 2001). Adenosine may, however, directly stimulate sleep-active neurons acting on A2 receptors. GABA/galaninergic sleep-active neurons in the ventrolateral preoptic area may be stimulated by adenosine (Scammel *et al.*, 2001). These neurons might also be activated through disinhibition by adenosine (Chamberlin *et al.*, 2003).

In the A1 receptor knockout mouse, reduced sleep and altered recovery after sleep deprivation were observed (Kaushal *et al.*, 2002). However, in another study normal sleep was found in the mice suggesting an adaptation to the loss of the A1 receptor (Stenberg *et al.*, 2003). Spontaneous sleep did not change in A2a receptor knockout mice but the NREMS rebound was attenuated after sleep deprivation (Urade *et al.*, 2003).

Prostaglandin D_2 (PGD$_2$)

Prostaglandins are unsaturated fatty acids containing a cyclopentane ring. They are eicosanoids produced from arachidonic acid through the cyclooxygenase pathway (COX-1 and COX-2), which results in PGH$_2$. PGH$_2$ is converted by specific enzymes into various eicosanoids including PGD$_2$. Lipocalin-type glutathione-independent PGD synthase is responsible for PGD$_2$ production in the brain and it differs from the hematopoetic glutathion-dependent PGD synthase in peripheral tissue (Urade *et al.*, 1996).

PGD$_2$ concentrations in the CSF display sleep-related variations that are higher during the rest period than in the active period, and higher during NREMS than in wakefulness in the rat. Sleep deprivation enhances PGD$_2$ contents in the CSF (Ram *et al.*, 1997). Intracerebroventricular or intrapreoptic administration of PGD$_2$ increases the time spent in NREMS and REMS in the rat and rhesus monkey (Ueno *et al.*, 1982; Onoe *et al.*, 1988). Inhibition of PGD$_2$ synthesis decreases sleep in the rat and increases the incidence of arousal-like behavior in fetal sheep (Lee *et al.*, 2002). Spontaneous sleep is not altered in transgenic mice expressing excess human PGD synthase but sleep can be stimulated by clipping their tail, which induces significant rises in brain PGD$_2$ production (Pinzar *et al.*, 2000).

PGD synthase is expressed in the leptomeninges, the epithelial cells of the choroid plexus, and, weakly, in oligodendrocytes. Both PGD$_2$ and the enzyme are secreted into the CSF, and the enzyme appears as β-trace protein in the CSF of humans (Blödorn *et al.*, 1996). The prostanoid receptors are also predominantly expressed in the leptomeninges. The receptors mediating promotion of NREMS reside in arachnoid cells near the ventrolateral preoptic area on the surface of the basal forebrain. It is assumed that in response to PGD$_2$, the arachnoid cells release adenosine that stimulates the sleep-active neurons in the ventrolateral preoptic area via A2 receptors (Mizoguchi *et al.*, 2001; Urade *et al.*, 2003). PGD$_2$ is posited to act as an amplifier mechanism in sleep regulation. The stimuli that elicit PGD$_2$ production in the leptomeninges are believed to arise from the brain, and they might be cytokines, like IL1 or TNF produced locally. The role of PGD$_2$ would be to integrate and convey sleep need to the basal forebrain via volume conduction in the CSF.

REMS Regulatory Substances

Vasoactive intestinal peptide

VIP is a peptide composed of 28 amino acid residues. It is a member of the secretin-glucagon family, and thus exhibits homology to GHRH. In rats, intracerebral GHRH receptors display strong affinity for VIP (Gardi *et al.*, 2002). Intracerebral administration of VIP stimulates NREMS but inhibition of endogenous VIP does not alter NREMS in the rat suggesting that the NREMS-promoting activity is mediated by an alien receptor, perhaps the GHRH receptor. Exogenous VIP does not stimulate NREMS in cats and rabbits (reviewed, Obal and Krueger, 2003).

VIP promotes REMS in rats, cats, and rabbits after intracerebral administration (Riou *et al.*, 1982; Drucker-Colin *et al.*, 1984; Obal *et al.*, 1989). Antagonists of, or antibodies to, VIP selectively inhibit REMS. CSF samples obtained from REMS-deprived cats contain a REMS-promoting material, which can be immunoneutralized by means of antibodies to VIP (Drucker-Colin *et al.*, 1988). In fact, VIP accumulates during REMS deprivation in the CSF of cats and VIP concentration in the CSF declines during recovery (Jimenez-Anguiano *et al.*, 1993).

VIP is an ubiquitous neurotransmitter in the brain. It might be relevant for sleep regulation that VIP is a neurotransmitter displaying a circadian rhythm in the suprachiasmatic and paraventricular nuclei and may modulate sleep through the diurnal rhythm. Stimulation of REMS is the most likely function of VIP residing in brain stem neurons implicated in triggering REMS. Microinjection of VIP into the oral pontine reticular nucleus or pontine reticular formation induces prolonged increases in REMS in rats (Bourgin *et al.*, 1997; Kohlmeier and Reiner, 1999). REMS deprivation upregulates VIP receptors in brain stem areas involved in the generation of REMS (Jimenez-Anguiano *et al.*, 1996). Finally, VIP in the hypothalamus stimulates expression of PRL mRNA (Bredow *et al.*, 1994), and VIP is also secreted into the pituitary portal circulation as a neurohormone and stimulates PRL secretion in the anterior pituitary. Hence, PRL may contribute to REMS promotion by VIP.

Prolactin (PRL)

PRL is a protein hormone closely related to GH. Circulating PRL is secreted from the anterior pituitary. In small quantities, PRL is also synthesized in neurons in the hypothalamus. Systemic or intracerebroventricular administration of PRL elicits selective increases in REMS in cats with the brain stem transected at midpontine level, and in rabbits and rats (reviewed, Roky *et al.*, 1995). The REMS response occurs only during the rest phase (light period) in the rat. Large enhancements in REMS and small increases in NREMS time are observed during the light period in rats rendered hyperprolactinemic by pituitary grafts (Obal *et al.*, 1997). Patients with PRL-producing adenoma, however, fail to display changes in REMS; instead, their NREMS is increased (Frieboes *et al.*, 1998). Immunoneutralization of systemic PRL causes slight decreases in REMS in rats. The duration of

REMS decreases and the diurnal rhythm of REMS is abolished in hypoprolactinemic rats but normalizes in constant light or dark (Lobo *et al.*, 1999). Recently, we observed permanent and selective decreases in REMS during the rest phase in PRL knockout mice, and infusion of PRL was capable of increasing REMS in these animals. Finally, stimulation of pituitary secretion of PRL by means of systemic VIP or ether stress is followed by increases in REMS in the rat (Bodosi *et al.*, 2000); PRL might also be involved in the REMS response to restraint stress (Meerlo *et al.*, 2001). These REMS responses are blocked after hypophysectomy or immunoneutralization of PRL in rats, and in PRL knockout mice.

The mechanism through which PRL increases REMS is currently unclear. PRL may modulate the circadian regulation of REMS at the level of the hypothalamus or it may act in the brain stem structures generating REMS. The long (2–3 hr) latency of the REMS response to exogenous PRL suggests that some metabolic actions mediate the sleep effects. It is noted that GH also stimulates REMS. Human GH, which has a high affinity to PRL receptors, promotes REMS in both humans and rats (reviewed, Obal and Krueger, 2003).

Sleep Factor Candidates

Oleamide

Oleamide is an unsaturated fatty acid amide, structurally related to the endogenous cannabinoid anandamide. Oleamide was isolated from the CSF of sleep-deprived cats (Cravatt *et al.*, 1995). It has a weak NREMS-promoting activity in rats and mice after systemic or intracerebral injections (Mendelson and Basile, 2001). Oleamide interacts with a number of receptors and membrane processes all of which may mediate its actions. The sleep response to oleamide is similar to that elicited by anandamide (Murillo-Rodríguez *et al.*, 1998). Some observations suggest that oleamide acts via the central cannabinoid receptor, CB1. Alternatively, oleamide interferes with the metabolism of anadamide, and the high concentration of anadamide is responsible for the sleep effects (Mechoulam *et al.*, 1997). Sleep promotion by anandamide might result from accumulation of extracellular adenosine in the basal forebrain (Murillo-Rodríguez *et al.*, 2003).

Cholecystokinin

CCK is a peptide hormone with strong homology to gastrin. The major form contains eight amino acid residues. CCK is secreted from the upper intestines, predominantly from the duodenum, in response to fat and proteins/peptides. Exogenous administration of CCK elicits a satiety syndrome including drowsiness and sleep, and thus CCK has been implicated in the mechanism of postprandial sleep (reviewed, Obal and Krueger, 2003). CCK binds to CCK-A receptors at the periphery and to CCK-B receptors in the brain. The CCK-A receptors expressed in sensory vagal fibers are the candidates for mediating the sleep promoting action of CCK (Shemiyakin and Kapas, 2001). Sleep is, however, not altered in mutant rats with a defect of the CCK-A receptor gene suggesting that the loss of CCK action is fully compensated (Sei *et al.*, 1999).

Insulin

Insulin is a peptide hormone secreted by the endocrine pancreas in response to rises in blood glucose concentration. Robust increases and decreases in NREMS were reported in response to insulin and in experimental diabetes mellitus, respectively, in rats (Danguir, 1984). However, subsequent experiments detected only minor NREMS loss in diabetic rats, and the sleep response to insulin was also small. IGF-1 receptors in the brain were suggested to mediate the effects of insulin on sleep (reviewed, Obal and Krueger, 2003).

Conclusion

We now recognize that neurons, like all living cells, constantly produce and respond to large numbers of molecules. Further, at least some of this production and sensitivity to stimuli is dependent upon changes in cellular membrane potentials. However, different techniques are used to electrically characterize cells than are used to chemically characterize cells. This has led to separate sleep literatures with the consequence that, until recently, there has been little attempt to match the networks of sleep regulatory substances (e.g., Figure 1) to the sleep regulatory neural networks. Each methodology has limitations. Thus, for example, it is not possible to know if a single cell whose action potentials correlate with sleep/wake cycles is in a causative pathway leading to or maintaining sleep. Although biochemical studies can directly demonstrate causality, i.e., their administration induces sleep, they are greatly limited in temporal resolution. Further, an assumption underlining much of past sleep regulatory work was that there are neurons or substances whose actions are specific to sleep. However, this concept of one neuron–one function now seems naïve. Thus, any cells involved in sleep regulation must be responsive to one or more of the wide array of stimuli that affect sleep and, conversely, they must signal one or more cells within the effector networks that manifest the consequences of sleep. Humoral signals seem to play a major role in such signaling although we have much to learn.

Acknowledgments

This work was supported by the National Institutes of Health, grant numbers NS25378, NS27250, NS31453, and HD36520, to Dr James Krueger and by the Hungarian National Science Foundation (OTKA-T-043156) and Ministry of Health (ETT 103 04/2003) to Dr Ferenc Obal, Jr.

References

Alam, N., McGinty, D., Imeri, L., Opp, M., and Szymusiak, R. (2001). Effects of interleukin-1 beta on sleep- and wake-related preoptic anterior hypothalamic neurons in unrestrained rats. *Sleep*, 24: A59.

Basheer, R., Rainnie, D.G., Porkka-Heiskanen, T., Ramesh, V., and McCarley, R.W. (2001). Adenosine, prolonged wakefulness, and A1-activated NF-κB DNA binding in the basal forebrain of the rat. *Neuroscience*, 104: 731–739.

Blödorn, B., Mäder, M., Urade, Y., Hayaishi, O., Felgenhauer, K., and Bruck, W. (1996). Choroid plexus: the major site of mRNA expression for the beta-trace protein (prostaglandin D synthase) in human brain. *Neurosci. Lett.*, 209: 117–120.

Bodosi, B., Obal, F. Jr., Gardi, J., Komlódi, J., Fang, J., and Krueger, J.M. (2000). An ether stressor increases REM sleep in rats: possible role of prolactin. *Am. J. Physiol.*, 279: 1590–1598.

Bourgin, P., Lebrand, C., Escourrou, P., Gaultier, C., Franc, B., Hamon, M., and Adrien, J. (1997). Vasoactive intestinal polypeptide microinjections into the oral pontine tegmentum enhance rapid eye movement sleep in the rat. *Neuroscience*, 77: 351–360.

Brandt, J.A., Churchill, L., Rehman, A., Ellis, A., Mémet, S., Israël, A., and Krueger, J.M. (2004). Sleep-deprivation increases activation of nuclear factor kappa B in lateral hypothalamic cells. *Brain Res.*, 1004: 91–97.

Bredow, S., Kacsoh, B., Obal, F. Jr., Fang, J., and Krueger, J.M. (1994). Increase of prolactin mRNA in the rat hypothalamus after intracerebroventricular injection of VIP or PACAP. *Brain Res.*, 660: 301–308.

Carter, K.M., Dansereau, R.P., and Rector, D.M. (2003). Sleep dependence of auditory evoked potentials in rat somatosensory cortex. *Sleep*, 26: A14.

Chamberlin, N.L., Arrigoni, E., Chou, T.C., Scammell, T.E., Greene, R.W., and Saper, C.B. (2003). Effects of adenosine on gabaergic synaptic inputs to identified ventrolateral preoptic neurons. *Neuroscience*, 119: 913–918.

Chen, Z., Gardi, J., Kushikata, T., Fang, J., and Krueger, J.M. (1999). Nuclear factor-kappa B-like activity increases in murine cerebral cortex after sleep deprivation. *Am. J. Physiol.*, 276: 1812–1818.

Churchill, L., Yasuda, K., Blindheim, K., Falter, M., Yasuda, T., Krueger, J.M. (2004). Asymmetry in Fos- and IL1β-immunoreactivity induced by IL1β microinjection into the cortex implicates the cortical/thalamic circuitry involved in EEG asymmetry. *J. Sleep Res.*, 13: Sl.

Cravatt, B.F., Próspero-García, O., Siuzdak, G., Gilula, N.B., Henriksen, S.J., Boger, D.L., and Lerner, R.A. (1995). Chemical characterization of a family of brain lipids that induce sleep. *Science*, 268: 1506–1509.

Danguir, J. (1984). Sleep deficits in diabetic rats: restoration following chronic intravenous or intracerebroventricular infusions of insulin. *Brain Res. Bull.*, 12: 641–645.

Darko, D.F., Miller, J.C., Gallen, C., White, J., Koziol, J., Brown, S.J., Hayduk, R., Atkinson, J.H., Assmus, J., Munnel, D.T., Naitotl, P., McCutchen, A., and Mitler, M.M. (2002). Sleep electroencephalogram delta-frequency amplitude, night plasma levels of tumor necrosis factor alpha, and human immunodeficiency virus infection. *Proc. Natl. Acad. Sci. USA*, 92: 12080–12084.

De, A., Churchill, L., Obal, F. Jr., Simasko, S., and Krueger, J.M. (2002). GHRH and IL1β increase cytoplasmic Ca^{2+} levels in cultured hypothalamic GABAergic neurons. *Brain Res.*, 949: 209–212.

DeSarro, G., Gareri, P., Sinopoli, V.A., David, E., and Rotiroti, D. (1997). Comparative, behavioural and electrocortical effects of tumor necrosis factor-alpha and interleukin-1 microinjected into the locus cereuleus of rat. *Life Sci.*, 60: 555–564.

Dreisbach, A.W., Hendrickson, T., Beezhold, D., Riesenberg, L.A., and Sklar, A.H. (1998). Elevated levels of tumor necrosis factor alpha in postdialysis fatigue. *Int. J. Artif. Organs*, 21: 83–86.

Drucker-Colin, R., Bernal-Pedraza, J., Fernández-Cancino, F., and Oksenberg, A. (1984). Is vasoactive intestinal polypeptide (VIP) a sleep factor? *Peptides*, 5: 837–840.

Drucker-Colin, R., Próspero-García, O., Arankowsky-Sandoval, G., and Pérez-Monfort, R. (1988). Gastropancreatic peptides and sensory stimuli as REM factors. In: Inoué, S., and Schneider-Helmert, D. (Eds.). *Sleep Peptides: Basic and Clinical Approaches*. Berlin: Springer, pp. 73–94.

Fang, J., Wang, Y., and Krueger, J.M. (1997). Mice lacking the TNF 55 kD receptor fail to sleep more after TNF alpha treatment. *J. Neurosci.*, 17: 5949–5955.

Fang, J., Wang, Y., and Krueger, J.M. (1998). The effects of interleukin-1 beta on sleep are mediated by the type I receptor. *Am. J. Physiol.*, 274: 655–660.

Floyd, R.A. and Krueger, J.M. (1997). Diurnal variations of TNF alpha in the rat brain. *Neuroreport*, 8: 915–918.

Franklin, C.M. (1999). Clinical experience with soluble TNF p75 receptor in rheumatoid arthritis. *Sem. Arthritis Rheum.*, 29: 171–181.

Frieboes, R.-M., Murck, H., Stalla, G.K., Antonijevic, I.A., and Steiger, A. (1998). Enhanced slow wave sleep in patients with prolactinoma. *J. Clin. Endocrinol. Metab.*, 83: 2706–2710.

Gardi, J., Taishi, P., Speth, R., Obal, F. Jr., and Krueger, J.M. (2002). Sleep deprivation alters hypothalamic growth hormone-releasing hormone mRNA and binding sites. *Neurosci. Lett.*, 329: 69–72.

Hajdu, I., Szentirmai, E., Obal, F. Jr., and Krueger, J.M. (2003). Different brain structures mediate drinking and sleep suppression elicited by the somatostatin analog, octreotide, in rats. *Brain Res.*, 994: 115–123.

Hansen, M.K., Taishi, P., Chen, Z., and Krueger, J.M. (1998a). Cafeteria-feeding induces interleukin-1β mRNA expression in rat liver and brain. *Am. J. Physiol.*, 43: 1734–1739.

Hansen, M.K., Taishi, P., Chen, Z., and Krueger, J.M. (1998b). Vagotomy blocks the induction of interleukin-1 beta mRNA in the brain of rats in response to systemic interleukin-1 beta. *J. Neurosci.*, 18: 2247–2253.

Imeri, L., Bianchi, S., Mariotti, M., and Opp, M.R. (2002). Interleukin-1 microinjected into the dorsal raphe nucleus enhances NREM sleep in rats. *J. Sleep Res.*, 11: 107.

Inoué, S. (1989). *Biology of Sleep Substances.* Boca Raton, FL: CRC Press, Inc.

Jimenez-Anguiano, A., Baez-Saldana, A., and Drucker-Colin, R. (1993). Cerebrospinal fluid (CSF) extracted immediately after REM sleep deprivation prevents REM rebound and contains vasoactive intestinal peptide (VIP). *Brain Res.*, 631: 345–348.

Jimenez-Anguiano, A., García-García, F., Mendoza-Ramírez, J.L., Durán-Vázquez, A., and Drucker-Colin, R. (1996). Brain distribution of vasoactive intestinal peptide receptors following REM sleep deprivation. *Brain Res.*, 728: 37–46.

Kaushal, N., Johansson, B., Halldner, L., Fredholm, B., and Greene, R.W. (2002). Reduced slow wave activity in the adenosine A1 receptor knockout mice. *Soc. Neurosci. Abst.*, 27: 2378.

Kohlmeier, K.A. and Reiner, P.B. (1999). Vasoactive intestinal polypeptide excites medial pontine reticular formation neurons in the brainstem rapid eye movement sleep-induction zone. *J. Neurosci.*, 19: 4073–4081.

Komoda, Y., Ishikawa, M., Nagasaki, H., Iriki, M., Honda, K., Inoué, S., Higashi, A., and Uchizono, K. (1983). Uridine, a sleep-promoting substance from brainstem of sleep-deprived rats. *Biomed. Res.*, 4: 223–227.

Komoda, Y., Honda, K., and Inoué, S. (1990). SPS-B, a physiological sleep regulator from the brainstems of sleep-deprived rats, identified as oxidized glutathione. *Chem. Pharm. Bull.*, 28: 2057–2059.

Krueger, J.M. and Obal, F. Jr., (1994). Sleep factors. In: Saunders, N.A., and Sullivan, C.E. (Eds.). *Sleep and Breathing.* New York, NY: Marcel Dekker, Inc., pp. 79–112.

Krueger, J.M. and Obal, F. Jr. (2003). Sleep Function. *Front. Biosci.*, 8: 511–519.

Krueger, J.M., Bacsik, J., and García-Arraras, J. (1980). Sleep-promoting material from human urine and its relation to Factor S from brain. *Am. J. Physiol.*, 238: 116–123.

Krueger, J.M., Walter, J., Dinarello, C.A., Wolff, S.M., and Chedid, L. (1984). Sleep-promoting effects of endogenous pyrogen (interleukin-1). *Am. J. Physiol.*, 246: 994–999.

Krueger, J.M., Obal, F. Jr., Fang, J., Kubota, T., and Taishi, P. (2001). The role of cytokines in physiological sleep regulation. *Ann. N.Y. Acad. Sci.*, 933: 211–221.

Kubota, T., Kushikata, T., Fang, J., and Krueger, J.M. (2000). Nuclear factor-kappaB inhibitor peptide inhibits spontaneous and interleukin-1 beta-induced sleep. *Am. J. Physiol. Regul. Integr. Comp. Physiol.*, 279: 404–413.

Kubota, T., Fang, J., Guan, Z., Brown, R.A., and Krueger, J.M. (2001). Vagotomy attenuates tumor necrosis factor-alpha-induced sleep and EEG delta-activity in rats. *Am. J. Physiol.*, 280: 1213–1220.

Kubota, T., Li, N., Guan, Z., Brown, R.A., and Krueger, J.M. (2002). Intrapreoptic microinjection of TNF-alpha enhances non-REMS in rats. *Brain Res.*, 932: 37–44.

Lee, B., Hirst, J.J., and Walker, D.W. (2002). Prostaglandin D synthase in the prenatal ovine brain and effects of its inhibition with selenium chloride on fetal sleep/wake activity *in utero. J. Neurosci.*, 22: 5679–5686.

Legendre, R. and Piéron, H. (1913). Recherches sur le besoin de sommeil consécutif á une veille prlongée. *Z. Allg. Physiol.*, 14: 235–262.

Liu, H., Kiu, J., Xiong, S., Sgen, G., Zhang, Z., and Xu, Y. (2000). The change in interleukin-6 and tumor necrosis factor in patients with obstructive sleep apnea syndrome. *J. Tongji Med. Univ.*, 20: 200–202.

Lue, F.A., Bail, F.A., Jephtha-Ocholo, J., Carayanniotis, K., Gorczynski, R., and Moldofsky, H. (1988). Sleep and cerebrospinal fluid interleukin-1 like activity in the cat. *Int. J. Neurosci.*, 42: 179–183.

Lobo, L.L., Claustrat, B., Debilly, G., Paut-Pagano, L., Jouvet, M., and Valatx, J.-L. (1999). Hypoprolactinemic rats under conditions of constant darkness or constant light. Effects on the sleep-wake cycle, cerebral temperature and sulfatoxymelatonin levels. *Brain Res.*, 835: 282–289.

Mackiewicz, M., Sollars, P.J., Ogilvie, M.D., and Pack, A.I. (1996). Modulation of IL-1 beta gene expression in the rat CNS during sleep deprivation. *Neuroreport*, 7: 529–533.

Majde, J.A. and Krueger, J.M. (2002). Neuroimmunology of sleep. In: D'Haenen, H., DeBoer, J.A., Westernberg, H., and Willner, P. (Eds.). *Textbook of Biological Psychiatry.* London: John Wiley & Sons.

Mechoulam, R., Fride, E., Hanus, L., Sheskin, T., Bisogno, T., Di Marzo, V., Bayewitch, M., and Vogel, Z. (1997). Anandamide may mediate sleep induction. *Nature*, 389: 25–26.

Meerlo, P., Easton, A., Bergmann, B.M., and Turek, F.W. (2001). Restraint increases prolactin and REM sleep in C57BL/6J but not in BALB/cJ mice. *Am. J. Physiol.*, 281: R846–R854.

Mendelson, W.B. and Basile, A. (2001). The hypnotic actions of the fatty acid amide, oleamide. *Neuropsychopharmacology*, 25: S36–S39.

Miller, T.B., Goodrich, C.A., and Pappenheimer, J.R. (1967). Sleep-promoting effects of cerebrospinal fluid from sleep deprived goats. *Proc. Natl. Acad. Sci. USA*, 58: 513–517.

Mizoguchi, A., Eguchi, N., Kimura, K., Kiyohara, Y., Qu, W.-M., Huang, Z.-L., Mochizuki, T., Lazarus, M., Kobayashi, T., Kaneko, T., Narumiya, S.,

Urade, Y., and Hayaishi, O. (2001). Dominant localization of prostaglandin D receptors on arachnoid trabecular cells in mouse basal forebrain and their involvement in the regulation of non-rapid eye movement sleep. *Proc. Natl. Acad. Sci. USA*, 98: 11674–11679.

Monnier, M. and Hösli, L. (1964). Dialysis of sleep and waking factor in blood of the rabbit. *Science*, 146: 796–798.

Moss, R.B., Mercandetti, A., and Vohdani, A. (1999). TNF alpha and chronic fatigue syndrome. *J. Clin. Immunol.*, 19: 314–316.

Murillo-Rodríguez, E., Sánchez-Alvarez, M., Navarro, L., Martínez-González, D., Drucker-Colin, R., and Próspero-García, O. (1998). Anandamide modulates sleep and memory in rats. *Brain Res.*, 812: 270–274.

Murillo-Rodríguez, E., Blanco-Centurión, C., Sánchez, C., Piomelli, D., and Shiromani, P.J. (2003). Anandamide enhances extracellular levels of adenosine and induces sleep: an *in vivo* microdialysis study. *Sleep*, 26: 943–947.

Nguyen, K.T., Deak, T., Owens, S.M., Kohno, T., Fleshner, M., Watkins, L.R., and Maier, S.F. (1998). Exposure to acute stress induces brain interleukin-1 beta protein in the rat. *J. Neurosci.*, 18: 2239–2246.

Obal, F. Jr. and Krueger, J.M. (2003). Biochemical regulation of non-rapid-eye-movement sleep. *Front. Biosci.*, 8: 520–550.

Obal, F. Jr. and Krueger, J.M. (2004). GHRH and sleep. *Sleep Med. Rev.* 8: 367–377.

Obal, F. Jr., Opp, M., Cady, A.B., Johannsen, L., and Krueger, J.M. (1989). Prolactin, vasoactive intestinal peptide, and peptide-histidine-methionine elicit selective increases in REM sleep in rabbit. *Brain Res.*, 490: 292–300.

Obal, F. Jr., Kacsoh, B., Bredow, S., Guha-Thakurta, N., and Krueger, J.M. (1997). Sleep in rats rendered chronically hyperprolactinemic with anterior pituitary grafts. *Brain Res.*, 755: 130–136.

Obal, F. Jr., Alt, J., Taishi, P., Gardi, J., and Krueger, J.M. (2003). Sleep in mice with non-functional growth hormone-releasing hormone receptors. *Am. J. Physiol.*, 284: 131–139.

Onoe, H., Ueno, R., Fujita, I., Nishino, H., Oomura, Y., and Hayaishi, O. (1988). Prostaglandin D2, a cerebral sleep-inducing substance in monkeys. *Proc. Natl. Acad. Sci. USA*, 85: 4082–4086.

Opp, M.R., Obál, F. Jr., and Krueger, J.M. (1991). Interleukin-1 alters rat sleep: temporal and dose-related effects. *Am. J. Physiol.*, 260: 52–58.

Pinzar, E., Kanaoka, Y., Inui, T., Eguchi, N., Urade, Y., and Hayaishi, O. (2000). Prostaglandin D synthase gene is involved in the regulation of non-rapid eye movement sleep. *Proc. Natl. Acad. Sci. USA*, 97: 4903–4907.

Porkka-Heiskanen, T., Strecker, R.E., Thakkar, M., Bjorkum, A.A., Greene, R.W., and McCarley, R.W. (1997). Adenosine: a mediator of the sleep-inducing effects of prolonged wakefulness. *Science*, 276: 1265–1268.

Ram, A., Pandey, H.P., Matsumura, H., Kasahara-Orita, K., Nakajima, T., Takahata, R., Satoh, S., Terao, A., and Hayaishi, O. (1997). CSF levels of prostaglandins, especially the level of prostaglandin D2, are correlated with increasing propensity towards sleep in rats. *Brain Res.*, 751: 81–89.

Riou, F., Cespuglio, R., and Jouvet, M. (1982). Endogenous peptides and sleep in the rat III the hypnogenic properties of vasoactive intestinal polypeptide. *Neuropeptides*, 2: 265–277.

Roky, R., Obal, F. Jr., Valatx, J.-L., Bredow, S., Fang, J., Pagano, L.-P., and Krueger, J.M. (1995). Prolactin and rapid eye movement sleep regulation. *Sleep*, 18: 536–542.

Scammel, T.E., Gerashchenko, D.Y., Mochizuki, T., McCarthy, M.T., Estabrooke, I.V., Sears, C.B., Urade, Y., and Hayaishi, O. (2001). An adenosine A2a agonist increases sleep and induces Fos in ventrolateral preoptic neurons. *Neuroscience*, 107: 653–663.

Schoenenberger, G.A., Maier, P.F., Tobler, H.J., Wilson, K., and Monnier, M. (1978). The delta (EEG) sleep inducing peptide (DSIP) XI. Amino acid analysis, sequence, synthesis and activity of the nonapeptide. *Pflügers Arch.*, 376: 119–129.

Sei, M., Sei, H. and Shima, K. (1999). Spontaneous activity, sleep, and body temperature in rats lacking the CCK-A receptor. *Physiol. Behav.*, 68: 25–29.

Shemiyakin, A. and Kapas, L. (2001). L-364,718, a cholecystokinin-A receptor antagonist, suppresses feeding-induced sleep in rat. *Am. J. Physiol.*, 280: 1420–1426.

Steiger, A., Antonijevic, I.A., Bohlhalter, S., Frieboes, R.M., Friess, E., and Murck, H. (1998). Effects of hormones on sleep. *Hormone Res.*, 49: 125–130.

Stenberg, D., Litonius, E., Halldner, L., Johansson, B., Fredholm, B.B., and Porkka-Heiskanen, T. (2003). Sleep and its homeostatic regulation in mice lacking the adenosine A1 receptor. *J. Sleep Res.*, 12: 283–290.

Strecker, R.E., Morairty, S., Thakkar, M.M., Porkka-Heiskanen, T., Basheer, R., Dauphin, L.J., Rainnie, D.G., Portas, C.M., Greene, R.W., and McCarley, R.W. (2000). Adenosinergic modulation of basal forebrain and preoptic/anterior hypothalamic neuronal activity in the control of behavioral state. *Behav. Brain Res.*, 115: 183–204.

Taishi, P., Bredow, S., Guha-Thakurta, N., Obal, F. Jr., and Krueger, J.M. (1997). Diurnal variations of interleukin-1 beta mRNA and beta-actin mRNA in rat brain. *J. Neuroimmunol.*, 75: 69–74.

Taishi, P., Gardi, J., Chen, Z., Fang, J., and Krueger, J.M. (1999). Sleep deprivation increases the expression of TNF alpha mRNA and TNF 55 kD receptor mRNA in rat brain. *The Physiologist*, 42: A4.

Taishi, P., De, A., Alt, J., Gardi, J., Obal, F. Jr., and Krueger, J.M. (2004). Interleukin-1β stimulates growth hormone-releasing hormone receptor mRNA expression in the rat hypothalamus *in vitro* and *in vivo*. *J. Neuroendocrinol.*, 16: 1–6.

Takahashi, S. and Krueger, J.M. (1997). Inhibition of tumor necrosis factor prevents warming-induced sleep responses in rabbits. *Am. J. Physiol.*, 272: 1325–1329.

Uchizono, K., Higashi, A., Iriki, M., Nagasaki, H., Ishikawa, M., Komoda, Y., Inoué, S., and Honda, K. (1978). Sleep-promoting fractions obtained from the brain-stem of sleep-deprived rats. In: Ito, M., Kubota, K.,

Tsukahara, N., and Yagi, K. (Eds.). *Integrative Control Functions of the Brain*. Amsterdam: Elsevier/North-Holland Biomedical Press, pp. 392–396.

Ueno, R., Ishikawa, Y., Nakayama, T., and Hayaishi, O. (1982). Prostaglandin D2 induces sleep when microinjected into the preoptic area conscious rats. Biochem. *Biophys. Res. Commun.*, 109: 575–582.

Urade, Y., Hayaishi, O., and Matsumura, H. (1996). Molecular mechanism of sleep regulation by prostaglandin D2. *J. Lipid Mediat. Cell Signal.*, 14: 71–82.

Urade, Z., Eguchi, N., Qu, W.-M., Sakata, M., Huang, Z.-L., Chen, J.-F., Schwarzschild, M.A., Fink, J.S., and Hayaishi, O. (2003). Minireview: Sleep regulation in adenosine A_{2A} receptor-deficient mice. *Neurology*, 61: S94–S96.

Van Cauter, E. and Plat, L. (1998). Interrelations between sleep and the somatotropic axis. *Sleep*, 21: 553–565.

Vitkovic, L., Bockaert, J., and Jacque, C. (2000). Inflammatory cytokines: neuromodulators in normal brain? *J. Neurochem.*, 74: 457–471.

Vgontzas, A.N., Zoumakis, M., Papanicolaou, D.A., Bixler, E.O., Prolo, P., Lin, H.M., Vella-Bueno, A., Kales, A., and Chrousos, G.P. (2002). Chronic insomnia is associated with a shift of interleukin-6 and tumor necrosis factor secretion from nighttime to daytime. *Metabolism*, 51: 887–892.

Yasuda, T., Yoshida, H., García, F., and Krueger, J.M. (2004). Local application of IL-1β induces asymmetry in the slow wave sleep EEG. *Sleep*, 27: A2–A3.

Yoshida, H., Peterfi, Z., García-García, F., Kirkpatrick, R., Yasuda, T., and Krueger, J.M. (2004). Asymmetrics in slow wave sleep EEG induced by local application of TNFα. *Brain Res.* 1009: 129–136.

Zaborszky, L. and Duque, A. (2003). Sleep-wake mechanisms and basal forebrain circuitry. *Front. Biosci.*, 8: 1146–1168.

Zhang, J., Obal, F. Jr., Zheng, T., Fang, J., Taishi, P., and Krueger, J.M. (1999). Intrapreoptic microinjection of GHRH or its antagonist alters sleep in rats. *J. Neurosci.*, 19: 2187–2194.

Chapter 3

NEUROTRANSMITTERS, NEUROMODULATORS, AND SLEEP

Ritchie E. Brown and Robert W. McCarley[1]

This chapter is intended as a general introduction for medical-PhD students to the topic of how neurotransmitters and neuromodulators regulate the sleep–wake cycle. For more detailed information the interested reader should consult recent reviews for an overview (Jones, 1991; McCormick, 1992; Mignot *et al.*, 2002; Pace-Schott and Hobson, 2002; Jones, 2003; Steriade and McCarley, 2004) or references in individual sections for specific information on particular neurotransmitters/neuromodulators. We will begin by considering the classical neurotransmitters glutamate, gamma aminobutyric acid (GABA), and glycine. Subsequently, we will examine the central role of the neurotransmitter/neuromodulator acetylcholine and the "global" neuromodulators noradrenaline, serotonin, histamine, dopamine, and the orexins/hypocretins. We will conclude by looking at the "local" neuromodulators, in particular adenosine.

The changes in physiology that occur across the sleep–wake cycle involve practically the whole central nervous system (CNS). Thus, it is not surprising that many different signaling molecules are involved; neurotransmitters and neuromodulators play different roles in these changes. Classical neurotransmitters are responsible for point-to-point communication between neurons or between the periphery and the nervous system (Figure 1). They are stored in vesicles and released at well-defined points of contact

---

[1] robert_mccarley@hms.harvard.edu

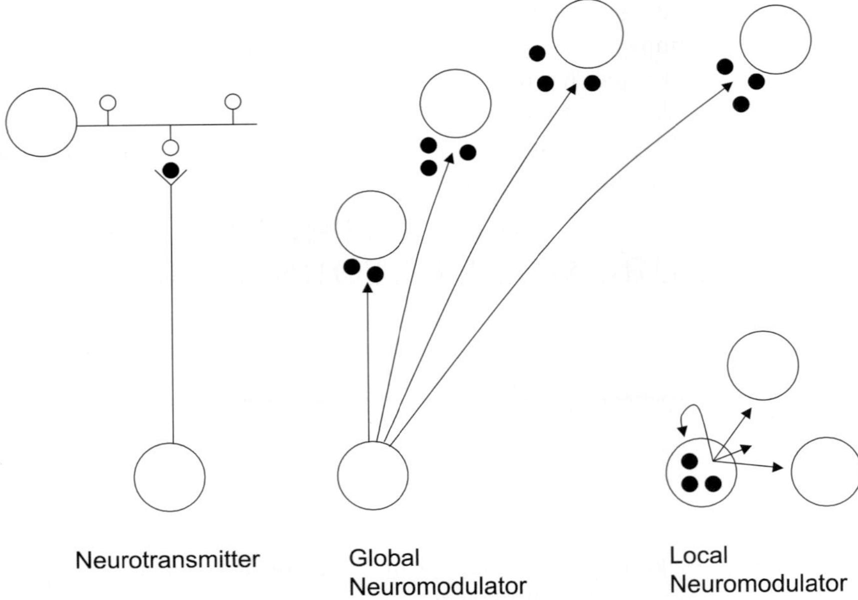

Figure 1. Differing modes of action of neurotransmitters, global neuromodulators, and local neuromodulators. Classical neurotransmitters are responsible for point-to-point communication between neurons or between the periphery and the nervous system. Global neuromodulators are contained within small, discrete populations of neurons with long and widespread axonal projections to large areas of the CNS. Local neuromodulators are produced and released in the same region, affecting the activity of neurons only within those areas.

between neurons or between neurons and effector systems, i.e., at synapses. Neurotransmitters are released by the influx of calcium that occurs when an action potential depolarizes presynaptic terminals and opens voltage-gated calcium channels in those terminals. Once released, the neurotransmitter binds to receptor proteins on the postsynaptic cell, leading to the opening (or occasionally to the closing) of ion channels and thereby affecting the excitability of that cell, i.e., the likelihood that it will fire an action potential. The sphere of action of a neurotransmitter is largely restricted to the synapse where it is released. Examples of classical neurotransmitters are acetylcholine, the neurotransmitter released at mammalian neuromuscular junctions, and the amino acids glutamate, GABA and glycine.

In contrast to classical neurotransmitters, neuromodulators are not normally released at well-defined synapses but instead are released in a more diffuse fashion, affecting many neurons as well as glia and blood vessels in the immediate vicinity of the point where they are released (Figure 1). Many neuromodulators are contained within small, discrete populations of neurons with long and widespread axonal projections to large areas of the CNS. Thus, they are able to modulate CNS function in a global fashion and are ideally designed to play a crucial role in the sleep–wake cycle. Examples of these types of neuromodulators are the biogenic amines noradrenaline, serotonin, and histamine as well as the newly discovered peptides, the orexins/hypocretins. Also to be included in this class is acetylcholine, which acts as a classical neurotransmitter at the neuromuscular junction, but acts in a more neuromodulatory fashion in the CNS and plays a pivotal role in the control of wakefulness and sleep. Other neuromodulators are produced and released locally, affecting the activity of neurons only within those areas. Examples of neuromodulators in this class are the purine adenosine, the gas nitric oxide, and many peptides.

Neurotransmitters and neuromodulators exert their effects by binding to specific receptor proteins on neurons and thereby leading to the opening or closing of ion channels (Figure 2). These receptors can either be ionotropic, i.e., they are themselves ion channels, or metabotropic, meaning that they are coupled to GTP-hydrolyzing proteins (G-proteins) and affect ion channels indirectly. When ion channels in the membrane are opened, the membrane potential of the cell shifts in the direction of the equilibrium potential of the ion or ions for which the channel is permeable. This equilibrium potential is in turn determined by the concentrations of the ion or ions inside and outside the cell (and can be calculated using the Nernst or Goldman–Hodgkin–Katz equations).

Excitatory neurotransmitters/neuromodulators (e.g., glutamate) act to increase the probability of a neuron firing an action potential and normally activate ionotropic receptors that are mixed cation channels or metabotropic receptors that are coupled to the G_q family of G-proteins. In contrast, inhibitory neurotransmitters/neuromodulators (e.g., GABA, glycine) decrease the probability of a neuron firing an action potential and activate ionotropic receptors permeable to chloride or metabotropic receptors coupled to the $G_{i/o}$ family of G-proteins (Figure 2). In addition to affecting cellular excitability, neurotransmitters and neuromodulators can often affect the probability of release of other neurotransmitters/neuromodulators by acting on presynaptic receptors and have longer-lasting actions on synaptic plasticity and gene expression.

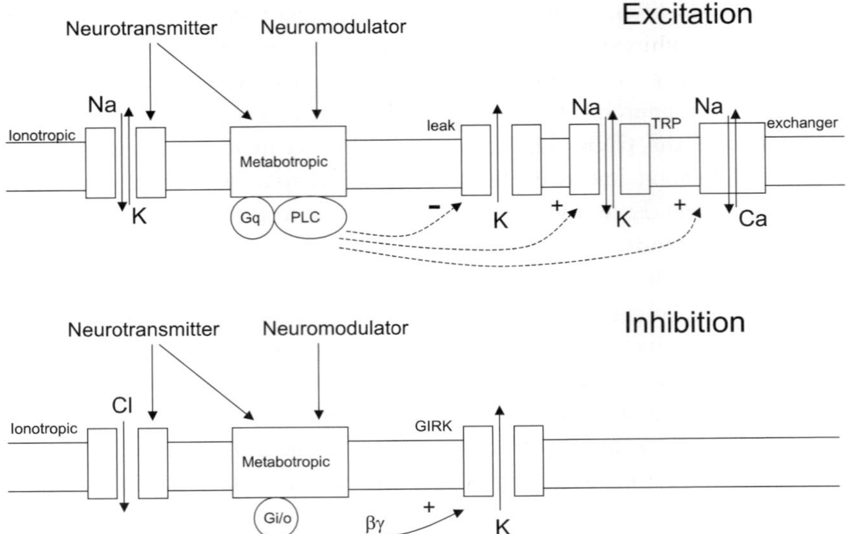

Figure 2. Mechanisms by which neurotransmitters and neuromodulators modulate neuronal excitability. Neurotransmitters and neuromodulators excite neurons via activation of ionotropic receptors permeable to cations (glutamate AMPA and NMDA receptors, nicotinic acetylcholine receptors, and serotonin 5-HT$_3$ receptors) and metabotropic receptors coupled to G$_q$ G-proteins and phospholipase C-β (Class I metabotropic glutamate receptors, muscarinic M$_1$, M$_3$, and M$_5$ acetylcholine receptors, noradrenaline α1 receptors, histamine H$_1$ receptors, serotonin 5-HT$_2$ receptors, dopamine D$_1$/D$_5$ receptors, and orexin OX$_1$ and OX$_2$ receptors). These metabotropic receptors cause excitation by (i) blockade of leak potassium channels; (ii) activation of mixed cation channels, most likely those of the transient receptor potential (TRP) family; and (iii) activation of sodium/calcium exchange. One or more of these mechanisms may be active in individual neurons. The intracellular effectors for these pathways are still largely unresolved. All of these mechanisms increase excitability by moving the membrane potential of the cell closer to the threshold for action potential generation. Neurotransmitters and neuromodulators inhibit neurons via activation of ionotropic receptors permeable to chloride (GABA$_A$ receptors and glycine receptors) and metabotropic receptors coupled to G$_{i/o}$ (G-proteins that inhibit adenylyl cyclase) (GABA$_B$ receptors, noradrenaline α2 receptors, serotonin 5-HT$_1$, histamine H$_3$ receptors, dopamine D$_2$, D$_3$, and D$_4$ receptors, and adenosine A$_1$ receptors). The gb subunits stimulate G-protein activated inwardly rectifying potassium (GIRK) channels. These receptors inhibit action potential generation by hyperpolarizing the membrane and decreasing the input resistance of the neurons.

Glutamate

One of the main tools used for the characterization of the behavioral state is the electroencephalogram (EEG), which essentially reflects the discharges of pyramidal neurons in the neocortex. Pyramidal neurons in the cortex use glutamate as their main neurotransmitter, as do projection neurons in the thalamus, which convey information to the cortex from most sensory modalities (Figure 3). Firing of neurons in the cortex, either in concert with or independently of the thalamus, generates the different types of rhythms observed in the EEG during different sleep–wake states (Steriade *et al.*, 1993; Steriade and McCarley, 2004). Stimulation of the brainstem reticular core leads to low-voltage fast activity in the EEG through excitation of nonspecific thalamic neurons, which have widespread projections to the cortex. The majority of reticular neurons are also glutamatergic so that all the main components of the reticular activating system (reticular formation → nonspecific thalamic nuclei → cortex) use glutamate as neurotransmitter. For many years it was thought that this reticular activating system was the main or exclusive pathway that the brain uses to achieve cortical low-voltage fast activity [observed in the EEG during wake or rapid-eye-movement (REM) sleep]. More recently, it has become apparent that other extrathalamic pathways originating from neurons located close to the reticular neurons and utilizing other neurotransmitters in addition to glutamate (see acetylcholine and the biogenic amines below) play a crucial role (Dringenberg and Vanderwolf, 1998; Jones, 2003). Furthermore, it is apparent that multiple overlapping and partially redundant systems are present. Glutamatergic neurons in the reticular formation with descending projections to the medulla and spinal cord are important in the control of muscle atonia during REM sleep (Figure 3).

Glutamate is the major excitatory neurotransmitter in the CNS. In addition to the reticular formation, thalamus and cortex, glutamatergic neurons are present in other regions important in regulating the sleep–wake cycle, for instance, in the basal forebrain and hypothalamus. In most cases though, their role in these regions has not been as well elaborated. One pathway which should also be mentioned is that from retinal ganglion cells to the suprachiasmatic nuclei (SCN) of the hypothalamus, which has an important function in resetting circadian phase according to photic cues (Shirakawa and Moore, 1994).

Glutamate acts on three main types of receptors (Figure 2), AMPA/kainate, NMDA, and metabotropic (mGluR) receptors (Pin and Duvoisin, 1995; Dingledine *et al.*, 1999). The AMPA/kainate and NMDA receptors are ionotropic receptors permeable to sodium and potassium and, to a lesser extent, calcium, whereas mGluRs are coupled to G-proteins. Glutamate receptors are not major targets of drugs that modulate behavioral state but the anesthetic ketamine and the hallucinogen/drug

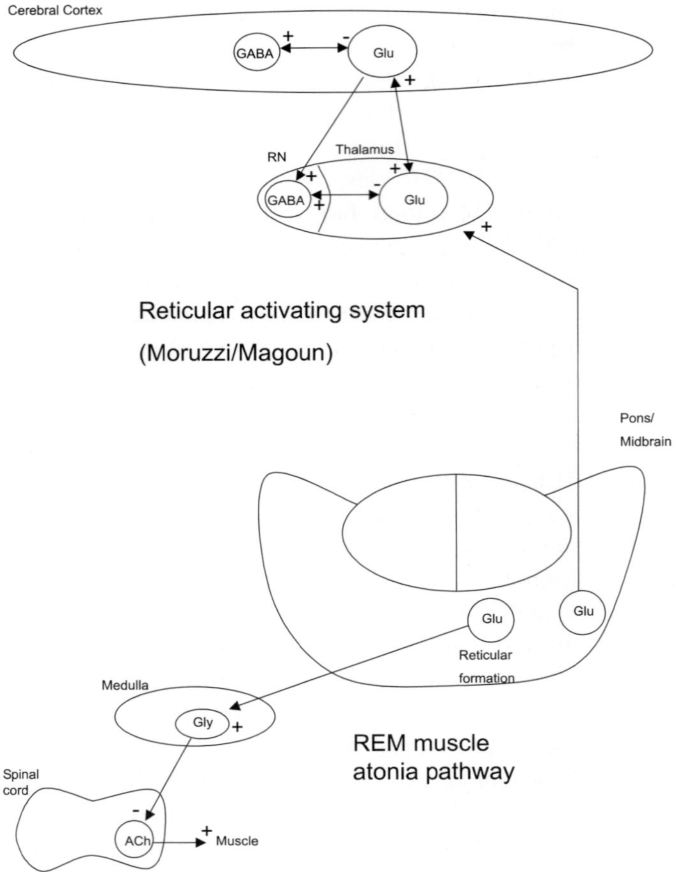

Figure 3. Selected amino acid neurotransmitter systems involved in control of EEG activation and muscle atonia. Midbrain reticular neurons excite thalamic neurons projecting to the cortex. The thalamic neurons are themselves glutamatergic and excite cortical pyramidal neurons leading to desynchronization of the cortex. This pathway together with brainstem pathways utilizing the neurotransmitters acetylcholine, noradrenaline, and serotonin (see Figures 5 and 6) make up the reticular activating system of Moruzzi and Magoun. Interactions of glutamatergic neurons in the thalamus and cortex with GABAergic neurons in the cortex and reticular nucleus (RN) of the thalamus generate the different rhythms recorded in the EEG during sleep and waking. Glutamatergic neurons in the pontine reticular formation are active during rapid-eye-movement (REM) sleep and are important in the control of muscle atonia. They project to and excite glycinergic neurons in the ventral medulla, which in turn inhibit motoneurons. Abbreviations: Glu, glutamate; GABA, gamma-amino butyric acid, Gly, glycine. In this and subsequent figures a plus sign indicates an excitatory action on the target area and a minus sign an inhibitory action.

of abuse phencyclidine (PCP) both act on NMDA receptors. The NMDA receptor is also one molecular target of ethanol but it is not the main one responsible for its sedative effects.

Gamma-Aminobutyric Acid

GABA is the major inhibitory neurotransmitter in the brain. Locally projecting inhibitory GABAergic interneurons in most brain areas provide a continuous and variable inhibitory tone upon projection neurons and shape their firing patterns. In particular, the GABAergic neurons of the reticular nucleus of the thalamus and interneurons of the neocortex and hippocampus play a critical role in the generation of EEG rhythms (Figure 3; McCormick, 1992; Steriade *et al.*, 1993; Steriade and McCarley, 2004).

Recently, much attention has been directed toward GABAergic long-projection neurons (Figure 4) and their role in the control of sleep and wakefulness (Gallopin *et al.*, 2000; Saper *et al.*, 2001; Szymusiak *et al.*, 2001). Particular emphasis has been placed on a small group of GABAergic (and galaninergic) neurons in the anterior hypothalamus, termed the ventral lateral preoptic nucleus (VLPO). Already at the beginning of the 20th century, the Viennese neurologist von Economo discovered that patients suffering from incurable insomnia following the flu pandemic of 1918 had damage to the anterior hypothalamus (Von Economo, 1926). More recent experiments identified neurons in this area that have increased firing rates during slow-wave sleep (SWS) as compared to wakefulness or (REM) sleep (Szymusiak and McGinty, 1986). The increase in firing of these neurons precedes the transition to SWS. Anatomical experiments showed that VLPO neurons project densely to wake-active neurons located in the tuberomammillary (TM) nucleus, the dorsal raphe (DR), and the locus coeruleus (Sherin *et al.*, 1996, 1998; Steininger *et al.*, 2001). Thus, it is thought that increased firing of VLPO neurons shuts off these wake-active neurons and promotes the transition from wakefulness to slow wave sleep (SWS). In addition to this role in the normal sleep–wake cycle, this area or a closely related area appears to mediate the increase in sleepiness associated with viral or bacterial infection (Elmquist *et al.*, 1997; Scammell *et al.*, 1998). This increase is likely mediated through the action of cytokines although the precise cellular mechanisms are still under investigation (Figure 4).

In addition to the VLPO neurons, long-projection GABAergic neurons in the basal forebrain, medial septum, and ventral tegmental area all appear to modulate the higher-frequency EEG rhythms observed during

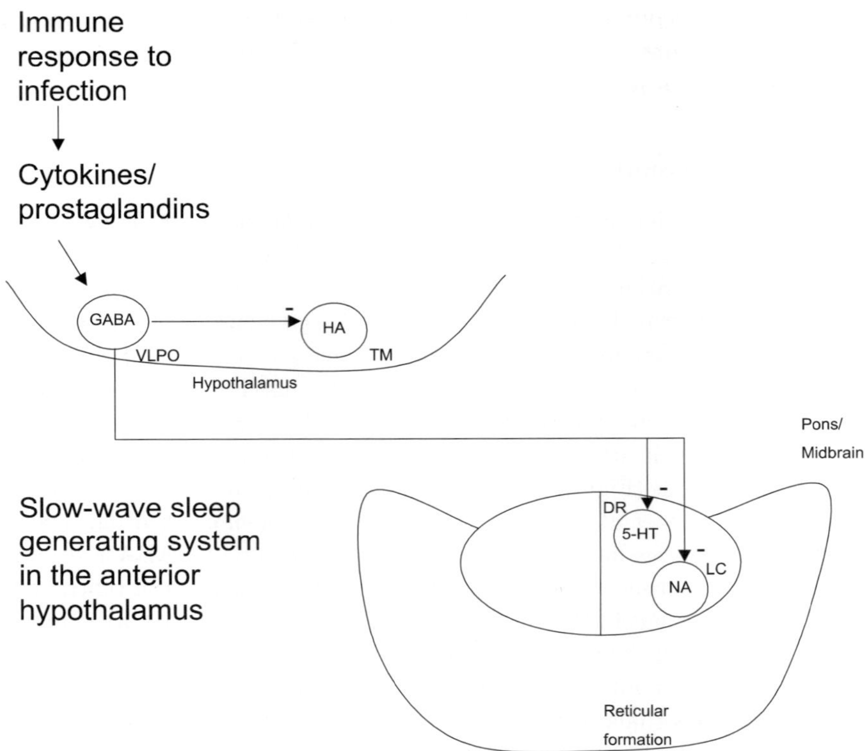

Figure 4. SWS generating system in the anterior hypothalamus/basal forebrain. GABAergic neurons in the anterior hypothalamus/basal forebrain, in particular those in the ventrolateral preoptic area (VLPO) project to and inhibit wake-promoting aminergic systems in the tuberomammillary nucleus [TM; histamine (HA)], dorsal raphe [DR; serotonin (5-HT)] and locus coeruleus [LC; noradrenaline (NA)]. Preoptic area neurons are thought to be activated (directly or indirectly) during the immune response to infection by the action of cytokines and prostaglandins. In addition, cytokines may promote sleep by inhibiting basal forebrain cholinergic neurons. VLPO neurons are also disinhibited (i.e., activated) by the sleep-promoting factor adenosine (not shown).

waking (theta, beta, alpha, gamma) (Manns *et al.*, 2000; Lee *et al.*, 2001). The primary neurotransmitter of projection neurons in the suprachiasmatic nucleus, the major generator of circadian rhythms, is also GABA (Moore *et al.*, 2002).

GABA acts on three types of receptors — $GABA_A$, $GABA_B$, and $GABA_C$. $GABA_A$ and $GABA_B$ receptors are widespread in the CNS, whereas $GABA_C$ receptors are limited mainly to the retina. Both $GABA_A$

and $GABA_C$ receptors are ionotropic receptors permeable to chloride ions, whereas $GABA_B$ receptors are metabotropic receptors coupled to inwardly rectifying potassium channels via the $\beta\gamma$ subunits of G_i/G_o G-proteins (Figure 2).

$GABA_A$ receptors are important clinically since they are the major target of sedative and anxiolytic compounds which act allosterically to potentiate the effect of GABA (by blocking desensitization) and increase neuronal inhibition (McKernan *et al.*, 2000). $GABA_A$ receptors also mediate the depressant action of ethanol (McKernan and Whiting, 1996).

$GABA_A$ receptors are pentamers made up from a large number of alternative subunits (McKernan and Whiting, 1996). Currently, six α, three β, three γ, as well as δ, ε, θ, and π subunits are known. Studies in expression systems have shown that coexpression of α and β subunits produces functional GABA-gated channels, but that inclusion of a γ subunit is essential to produce modulation by benzodiazepines. The most common subunit composition *in vivo* is thought to be the combination of two α subunits with two β subunits and one γ subunit. Very recently, the tools of modern neuroscience have been applied to determine the subunits and neuronal loci responsible for the sedative action of benzodiazepines and general anesthetics. The high-affinity binding of benzodiazepines such as diazepam is conferred by the γ_2 subunit and adjacent α_1, α_2, α_3, or α_5 subunits. A particular amino acid (histidine 101) in the $\alpha_{1,2,3,5}$ subunits is necessary for diazepam binding and generation of transgenic mice that have that histidine exchanged for arginine (normally present in α_4 and α_6) and abolishes the sedative effect of diazepam in α_1 mutant mice but not in the other subunits (Rudolph *et al.*, 1999; McKernan *et al.*, 2000). One site where benzodiazepines and other sedatives act to cause sleepiness may be the histaminergic tuberomammillary (TM) nucleus. Histamine neurons express the γ_2 $GABA_A$ subunit (Sergeeva *et al.*, 2002) and injection of GABAergic antagonists into the TM attenuate the sedative response to GABAergic agents (Nelson *et al.*, 2002).

$GABA_B$ receptors are one major target of the sedative and drug of abuse, gamma hydroxybutyric acid (GHB), which is used in the treatment of narcolepsy (Wong *et al.*, 2004).

Glycine

Glycine is the major inhibitory neurotransmitter in the spinal cord and in parts of the brainstem. Glycine acts upon an ionotropic receptor permeable to chloride and similar in structure to $GABA_A$ receptors. Glycine is involved in the regulation of muscle tone and in particular the loss of muscle tone that occurs during REM sleep (REM muscle atonia). Intracellular recordings from spinal cord motoneurons in the cat by Chase and Morales (1990) demonstrated that motoneurons receive a barrage of inhibitory postsynaptic potentials (IPSPs) which inhibit them during REM sleep. Furthermore, they showed that these potentials can be abolished by administration of the relatively selective glycine receptor antagonist, strychnine (Chase *et al.*, 1989). The main source of the glycine responsible for REM muscle atonia appears to be a group of neurons in the ventral medulla termed the nucleus magnocellularis in the cat which are in turn activated by glutamatergic neurons of the subcoerulear reticular formation in the pons (Figure 3; Chase *et al.*, 1986; Lai and Siegel, 1988; Lai *et al.*, 1999). However, local glycinergic interneurons in the spinal cord are also likely to be involved.

Acetylcholine

Acetylcholine plays a central role in the control of sleep–wake states and conscious awareness (Jones, 1991; Perry *et al.*, 1999). Acetylcholine levels are at their highest in the cortex during states when consciousness is present, i.e., during wakefulness and REM sleep (when most dreaming occurs) (Jasper and Tessier, 1971). Release of acetylcholine in the cortex causes low-voltage fast activity to be recorded in the EEG via its effects on pyramidal neurons and GABAergic interneurons while acetylcholine release in the thalamus switches the firing of thalamic relay neurons from the burst firing mode observed during SWS to the single-spike tonic firing seen during wakefulness or REM sleep (McCormick, 1992). In the reticular formation, acetylcholine release is highest during REM sleep (Leonard and Lydic, 1997) and infusion of cholinergic agonists into the pons triggers an REM-sleep like state (Baghdoyan *et al.*, 1984).

Two main groups of cholinergic neurons are important in the context of the sleep–wake cycle (Figure 5; Jones, 1993; Steriade, 2004). Neurons in the medial septum/basal forebrain (diagonal band, nucleus magnocellularis, substantia inominata) provide the cholinergic innervation of the hippocampus and cortex, respectively, whereas neurons in the laterodorsal tegmentum (LDT) and pedunculopontine nucleus (PPT) are responsible for acetylcholine release in the thalamus and brainstem. In both of these regions, presumed cholinergic neurons which are primarily wake-active and

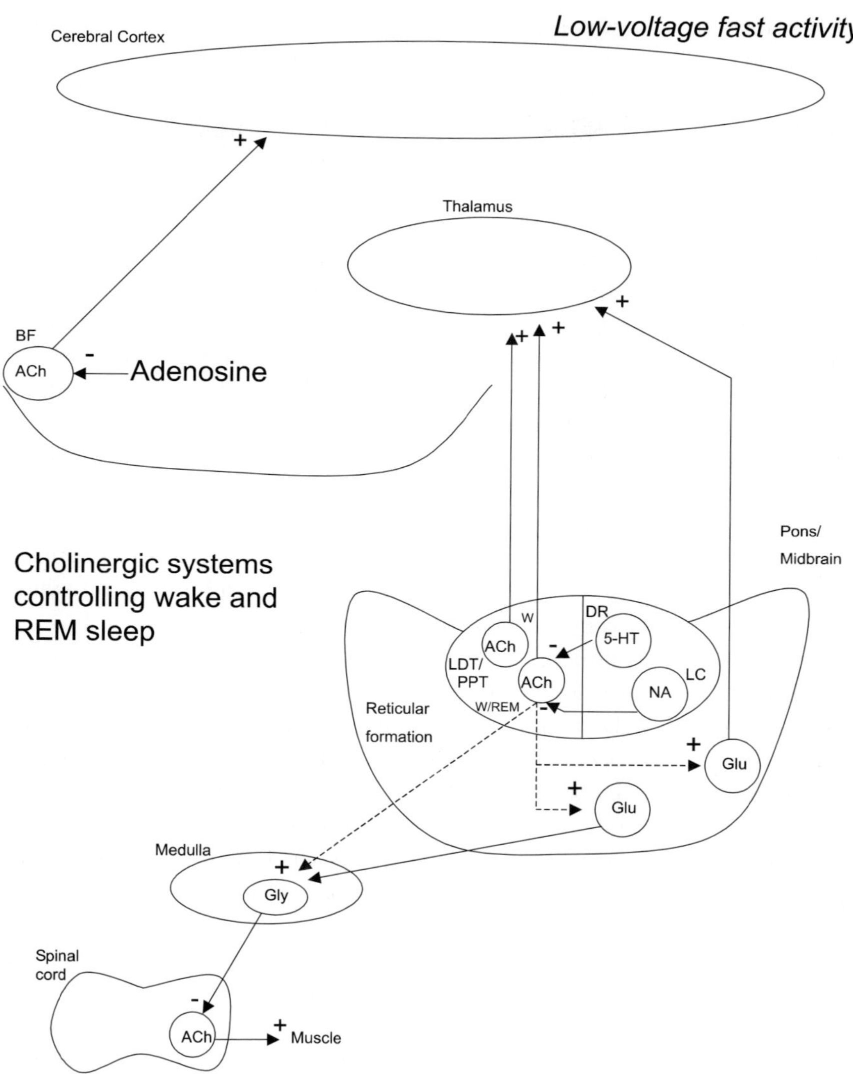

Figure 5. Cholinergic systems controlling wake and REM sleep. Two main groups of cholinergic neurons are important in the context of the sleep–wake cycle. Neurons in the basal forebrain (BF) provide the cholinergic innervation of the cortex, whereas neurons in the laterodorsal tegmentum (LDT) and pedunculopontine nucleus (PPT) are responsible for acetylcholine release in the thalamus and brainstem. In both of these regions, presumed cholinergic neurons which are primarily wake-active (W) and those which have a wake-REM on (W/REM) profile have been observed. Cholinergic basal forebrain neurons are excited by noradrenaline, histamine, and orexin during the waking state.

those which have a wake-REM on profile have been observed (Steriade *et al.*, 1990a; Thakkar *et al.*, 1998; Manns *et al.*, 2000). The cholinergic neurons also have the ability to fire in bursts (in contrast to most aminergic neurons), which will lead to an enhanced release of neurotransmitter in target areas and may be important in the context of certain features of wakefulness and REM sleep [e.g., ponto-geniculo-occipital (PGO) spikes] (El Mansari *et al.*, 1989; Steriade *et al.*, 1990b).

Many neurotransmitters involved in the sleep–wake cycle converge upon the basal forebrain cholinergic neurons (Jones, 2003). These cells are excited by wake-active neurons releasing the neurotransmitters noradrenaline, histamine, and the orexins/hypocretins but are inhibited by serotonin released from wake-active neurons in the raphe nuclei (Khateb *et al.*, 1993, 1995; Fort *et al.*, 1995; Eggermann *et al.*, 2001). Injection of noradrenaline into the basal forebrain leads to an increase in fast gamma EEG activity, reduction of slow delta activity and promotion of waking at the expense of slow-wave sleep (Cape and Jones, 1998). The basal forebrain cholinergic neurons appear to play a unique role in the mediation of the sleepiness associated with prolonged wakefulness through their inhibition by adenosine (Strecker *et al.*, 2000; see below).

Lesion studies conducted primarily in cats by Jouvet and co-workers established that the cellular machinery responsible for generating REM sleep is located at the ponto-mesencephalic junction (Jones, 1991). Subsequent immunohistochemical studies showed that two major groups of cholinergic cells are located in this area within the LDT and PPT. These cholinergic neurons play a role in all components of REM sleep including REMs, muscle atonia, and PGO spikes through their projections to reticular neurons and to the thalamus. REM-active cholinergic neurons are inhibited by serotonin (Luebke *et al.*, 1992; Leonard and Llinás, 1994; Thakkar *et al.*, 1998) and likely also noradrenaline during the waking state and SWS but

---

Figure 5. (*Continued*) They are a key site mediating the effects of the sleep-promoting factor adenosine, which directly inhibits them via A_1 receptors. W/REM neurons in the LDT/PPT are inhibited during W and SWS by serotonin [from dorsal raphe (DR)] and noradrenaline [from locus coeruleus (LC)] but are released from this inhibition during REM (reciprocal interaction model). Currently, it is hypothesized that these neurons trigger muscle atonia via excitation (most likely disinhibition) of glutamatergic pontine reticular neurons and excitation of ventral medullary glycinergic neurons. They also trigger PGO waves via excitation of thalamic neurons and EEG low-voltage fast activity via excitation of glutamatergic midbrain reticular neurons. For interactions between thalamus and cortex see Figure 3.

are released from this inhibition during REM sleep when the serotonin and noradrenaline neurons fall silent (modified reciprocal-interaction model of REM sleep) (McCarley and Massaquoi, 1992).

Acetylcholine activates both ionotropic (nicotinic mixed cation channels) and metabotropic (muscarinic) receptors (Figure 2). Activation of nicotinic acetylcholine receptors leads to excitation of dopaminergic ventral tegmental area neurons, to the excitation of many interneurons in the hippocampus and neocortex and to the release of neurotransmitters (in particular glutamate) via depolarization of presynaptic terminals (Dani, 2001). Stimulation of excitatory muscarinic receptors (G_q-coupled, M_1, M_3, M_5) also excites dopaminergic ventral tegmental area neurons and more importantly in the context of the sleep–wake cycle leads to a depolarization of thalamic and cortical principal cells along with a blockade of the slow after-hyperpolarizations which follow action potentials (McCormick, 1992). These excitatory actions of acetylcholine are the primary mediators of low-voltage fast activity in the cortex. Inhibitory muscarinic receptors ($G_{i/o}$ coupled, M_2, M_4) are autoreceptors negatively regulating the excitability of cholinergic cell bodies and acetylcholine release but are also present postsynaptically on many neurons. In particular, they are prevalent in the reticular formation where they appear to be involved in the generation of REM (Baghdoyan and Lydic, 1999).

Nicotinic receptors appear to be one target of volatile general anesthetics such as halothane and isofluorane (Downie *et al.*, 2002). Muscarinic antagonists such as atropine and scopolamine also potently decrease cortical low-voltage fast activity and wakefulness and are potent hallucinogens (Perry *et al.*, 1999).

Noradrenaline

Noradrenaline neurons are clustered in a number of different nuclei scattered throughout the brainstem. The largest of these nuclei is the locus coeruleus (LC) which provides most of the noradrenergic input to the forebrain, as well as sending projections to the brainstem and spinal cord (Figure 6; Jones, 1991). Noradrenaline neurons in the LC fire at low rates (2–10 Hz) in a tonic, pacemaker-like fashion during waking, and increase their firing during stress or when the animal is in a potentially dangerous situation (Rasmussen *et al.*, 1986). Their firing slows down during SWS and ceases completely during REM sleep (Hobson *et al.*, 1975; Rasmussen *et al.*, 1986). This cessation of firing contributes to the initiation of REM

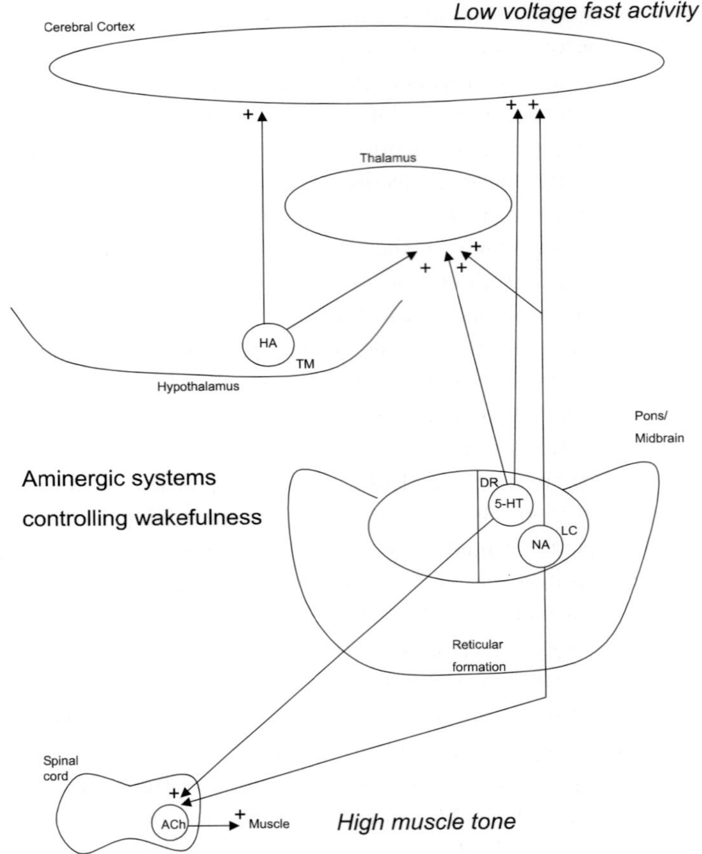

Figure 6. Aminergic systems controlling wakefulness. Wake-active, REM-off aminergic neurons in the tuberomammillary nucleus [TM; histamine (HA)], dorsal raphe [DR; serotonin (5-HT)], and locus coeruleus [LC; noradrenaline (NA)] converge on common effector systems in the thalamus and cortex to promote wakefulness and EEG low-voltage fast activity. Serotonin and noradrenaline neurons also project to the spinal cord and directly excite motoneurons, promoting high muscle tone during waking. Interactions (mainly excitatory) also exist between the different arousal promoting systems (not shown). Noradrenaline and histamine have excitatory, while serotonin has inhibitory actions on basal forebrain cholinergic neurons (Figure 5). For interactions between thalamus and cortex see Figure 3.

sleep and in particular to REM muscle atonia (Hobson *et al.*, 1975; Nishino and Mignot, 1997; Wu *et al.*, 1999). Noradrenaline depolarizes motoneurons and thus facilitates muscle tone (Figure 6). Removal of this input during REM, together with the increase in glycinergic IPSPs leads to hyperpolarization of motoneurons and muscle atonia (Lai *et al.*, 2001). In addition to direct effects on motoneurons, noradrenaline modulates REM sleep and muscle atonia through hyperpolarization of cholinergic brainstem neurons (Williams and Reiner, 1993) and through effects upon subcoerulear reticular neurons (Tononi *et al.*, 1988). Inappropriate activation of REM muscle atonia circuits occurs during attacks of cataplexy (reduction or loss of muscle tone triggered by emotionally arousing stimuli) in the disease narcolepsy (Nishino and Mignot, 1997). The efficacy of antidepressants in treating cataplexy is correlated with their efficacy in inhibiting the uptake of noradrenaline (Nishino and Mignot, 1997). Furthermore, LC neurons have been shown to cease firing in close temporal association with cataplectic attacks in narcoleptic dogs (Wu *et al.*, 1999).

Noradrenaline facilitates waking via excitation of basal forebrain cholinergic neurons and DR serotonergic neurons and inhibition of sleep-promoting GABAergic VLPO neurons (Jones, 2003). Furthermore, noradrenaline acts upon similar effector mechanisms as described for muscarinic receptors in the thalamus and neocortex, leading to depolarization of thalamic relay neurons and cortical pyramidal neurons and block of their slow after-hyperpolarizations (McCormick, 1992). During stress situations noradrenergic neurons contribute to emotional arousal through effects in the amygdala and other parts of the limbic system (Cahill *et al.*, 1994). Activity of noradrenaline neurons during wakefulness may be necessary for learning-related changes in gene expression (Cirelli and Tononi, 2004).

Noradrenaline acts upon three types of receptors (Figure 2), all of which are metabotropic receptors (McCormick, 1992). Activation of α_1 receptors leads to stimulation of G_q G-proteins and is responsible for large depolarizations mediated by noradrenaline (e.g., in the dorsal raphe serotonin neurons and cortical pyramidal neurons). Activation of β-receptors leads to small depolarizations and block of slow after-hyperpolarizations in cortical cells (Haas and Konnerth, 1983). Binding of noradrenaline to α_2 receptors leads to hyperpolarizations (e.g., in noradrenaline neurons themselves) as well as to inhibition of neurotransmitter release.

Histamine

In addition to describing an anterior hypothalamic sleep-promoting center (see above), von Economo (1926) also identified a posterior hypothalamic waking center. Located within this region are wake-promoting neurons

releasing the neurotransmitters histamine and the orexins/hypocretins. Histamine neurons are located in the TM and send projections to all parts of
the CNS (Brown *et al.*, 2001; Haas and Panula, 2003). Histamine neurons
are similar in many respects to the noradrenergic LC neurons, although
their role in modulating muscle tone does not appear to be as prominent.
Like noradrenaline neurons, they discharge slowly and tonically during waking, less during SWS, and cease firing during REM sleep (Lin, 2000; John
et al., 2004). Similar to LC cells their activity is increased by stress. Histamine neurons promote waking via excitatory actions in the basal forebrain, thalamus, and cortex (Figure 6; same effectors as those activated
by muscarinic and noradrenaline receptors) (Brown *et al.*, 2001). They do
not, however, have a direct action upon VLPO neurons (Gallopin *et al.*,
2000). Functional knockout of the histamine system (in histamine decarboxylase knockout mice) does not lead to prominent changes in the normal
sleep–wake cycle but compromises the enhanced arousal normally seen in
novel or stressful environments (Parmentier *et al.*, 2002).

Histamine activates three types of receptors (Brown *et al.*, 2001). Histamine H_1 receptors are coupled to G_q/phospholipase C and mediate most
of the strong excitatory actions of histamine as well as the strongest
wake-promoting actions. Antihistamines used in the treatment of inflammation are mild sedatives if they cross the blood–brain barrier and block central H_1 receptors. Histamine H_2 receptors are coupled to Gs G-proteins and
mediate blockade of sAHPs in cortical pyramidal cells (Haas and Konnerth,
1983). Histamine H_3 receptors are autoreceptors that modulate the activity
of histamine neurons and histamine release.

Very recent experiments in narcoleptic dogs revealed that while the
activity of noradrenaline LC neurons ceases and that of serotonergic DR
neurons is reduced during cataplexy, the firing rate of histamine neurons
is maintained or even enhanced. Thus, histamine neurons are likely to be
important for the preservation of consciousness that accompanies the loss
of muscle tone seen during cataplexy (John *et al.*, 2004).

Serotonin

Serotonin neurons are located within the raphe nuclei of the brainstem.
The largest collection of these neurons is located in the DR, which innervate
most of the forebrain and parts of the brainstem and spinal cord (Figure 6).
Serotonin neurons are similar in some respects to noradrenaline LC neurons and histamine TM neurons but there are also important differences.

Like histamine and noradrenaline neurons, serotonin neurons fire slowly in a wake-active, REM-off pattern (McGinty and Harper, 1976; Trulson and Jacobs, 1979). Unlike histamine and noradrenaline neurons, most serotonin neurons maintained *in vitro* are not spontaneously active or fire at lower levels than seen *in vivo* during waking (Vandermaelen and Aghajanian, 1983). Application of noradrenaline, histamine, or orexins activates a long-lasting inward current, which causes depolarization and tonic firing at a rate similar to that seen during the waking state (2–3 Hz), i.e., afferent inputs from other wake-active systems are necessary to maintain the firing of serotonin neurons during waking (Vandermaelen and Aghajanian, 1983; Levine and Jacobs, 1992; Brown *et al.*, 2002). Serotonin activates similar effector mechanisms in the thalamus and cortex as the other amines (McCormick, 1992) and inhibits sleep-active VLPO neurons (Gallopin *et al.*, 2000), but interestingly blockade of serotonin synthesis leads to a profound and long-lasting insomnia (Mouret *et al.*, 1968). The mechanism of this apparently paradoxical sleep-promoting action of serotonin may involve the basal forebrain where serotonin, in contrast to noradrenaline and histamine, inhibits basal forebrain cholinergic neurons (Cape and Jones, 1998; Jouvet, 1999).

Serotonin, like noradrenergic LC neurons, plays a crucial role in the alternation of SWS and REM sleep and in particular in the control of PGO spikes (Jacobs *et al.*, 1973; Lydic *et al.*, 1987a,b). Serotonin inhibits wake/REM-active cholinergic LDT neurons (Thakkar *et al.*, 1998) and inhibits the pontine component of PGO waves (P-waves) when injected into the subcoerulear P-wave generator region (Datta *et al.*, 2003). The modified reciprocal interaction theory of REM sleep (McCarley/Hobson) proposes that REM sleep is generated when serotonin and noradrenaline neurons cease firing, thus releasing REM-active cholinergic neurons from inhibition and allowing them to activate effector neurons in the reticular formation (McCarley and Massaquoi, 1992). Antidepressants such as the selective serotonin re-uptake inhibitors (e.g., Prozac^{TM}) or monoamine oxidase inhibitors cause a complete and long-lasting suppression of REM sleep (Jouvet *et al.*, 1965). Interestingly, individuals suffering from unipolar depression, in which the serotonin system is strongly implicated, have sleep–wake abnormalities including disruption of the timing of REM sleep (McCarley and Massaquoi, 1986).

The pharmacology and physiology of serotonin are extremely complex but in the context of the sleep–wake cycle the most important serotonin receptors are the 5-HT$_{1A}$ receptor (G$_{i/o}$ coupled), the 5-HT$_{2A/B/C}$ receptor (G$_q$-coupled), and the 5-HT$_3$ receptor (mixed cation channel) (Figure 2;

Portas *et al.*, 2000). The 5-HT$_{1A}$ receptor acts as an inhibitory autoreceptor on serotonin neuron cell bodies and as an inhibitory heteroreceptor on postsynaptic neurons, e.g., cholinergic LDT wake/REM-on neurons (Thakkar *et al.*, 1998). The 5-HT$_2$ receptor mediates strong excitations of TM, thalamic, and cortical neurons (McCormick, 1992; Eriksson *et al.*, 2001) and can also act presynaptically on thalamocortical afferents (Marek and Aghajanian, 1998). Activation of the 5-HT$_3$ receptor leads to a direct depolarization of select neuronal subpopulations, in particular certain inhibitory interneurons in the hippocampus and cortex (Kawa, 1994).

Dopamine

The largest groups of dopamine neurons are present in the substantia nigra (projecting to the dorsal striatum) and ventral tegmental area (projecting to the cortex and limbic system). The intrinsic electrophysiological properties of dopamine neurons in these areas are similar to those of other aminergic neurons. However, unlike other aminergic neurons the average firing rate of dopamine neurons does not vary across the sleep–wake cycle (Miller *et al.*, 1983). In contrast to the other aminergic neurons dopamine neurons have the ability to fire bursts of action potentials, which enhance neurotransmitter release in target areas and are normally triggered in the presence of external cues signaling unexpected rewards (e.g., food) (Schultz, 1998). Whether the number of bursts of dopamine neurons changes across the sleep–wake cycle or not has not been investigated in detail.

The dopamine system is interesting in the context of the sleep–wake cycle in that the most potent CNS stimulants known, the amphetamine-like compounds, work by inhibiting the dopamine transporter (DAT) and thereby increase dopaminergic tone in target regions (Wisor *et al.*, 2001). The mechanisms by which these compounds act to increase wakefulness are still under investigation.

Orexins/Hypocretins

The peptides orexin A/hypocretin 1 and orexin B/hypocretin 2 were discovered simultaneously by two groups in the late 1990s (hence the two names) (de Lecea *et al.*, 1998; Sakurai *et al.*, 1998). They were found to be produced selectively by a small group of neurons located in the perifornical area of the lateral hypothalamus. They project to large areas of the CNS and particularly densely to areas involved in sleep–wake control such as the aminergic nuclei and basal forebrain. Although discovered only relatively recently, already a considerable amount is known about this system. This can be attributed largely to the link between this system and the disease narcolepsy (Taheri *et al.*, 2002).

Narcolepsy is a debilitating disease affecting humans and other mammals (Nishino and Mignot, 1997). It is characterized by a tetrad of symptoms: excessive daytime sleepiness (EDS), cataplexy, sleep-associated hallucinations, and sleep paralysis. Primarily, it is a disease in which the timing and synchrony of sleep–wake states is disrupted. Patients cannot maintain prolonged periods of waking during the day or prolonged periods of sleep during the night and elements of sleep intrude into normal wakefulness, e.g., muscle paralysis.

A large body of evidence now suggests that degeneration of orexin/hypocretin neurons is responsible for the majority of narcolepsy cases (Taheri *et al.*, 2002). Initial evidence for the involvement of this system in narcolepsy came in two classic papers, which showed that mice lacking the preproorexin gene have a narcoleptic phenotype and that genetically narcoleptic Doberman Pinschers have a defect in the orexin receptor 2 gene (Chemelli *et al.*, 1999; Lin *et al.*, 1999). Subsequently, it has been shown that there is a massive loss of orexin/hypocretin neurons in the brains of narcoleptic humans examined postmortem as well as a dramatic reduction in the levels of orexin/hypocretin in the cerebrospinal fluid of living narcolepsy patients (Peyron *et al.*, 2000; Thannickal *et al.*, 2000; Taheri *et al.*, 2002). Gene defects in the orexin type II receptor have been found in a small number of early-onset narcolepsy cases (Taheri *et al.*, 2002). The insult that results in the destruction of orexin/hypocretin neurons has not so far been discovered but an auto-immune reaction is suspected (Lin *et al.*, 2001).

The mechanisms by which orexins/hypocretins control sleep–wake states are under intense investigation (Brown, 2003). Orexins/hypocretins promote wakefulness by exciting many other wake-active systems such as histamine TM neurons, basal forebrain and brainstem acetylcholine neurons, noradrenergic LC neurons, and serotonergic DR neurons as well as intralaminar thalamic neurons (Figures 3, 5, and 6). Injection of orexins into many of these sites leads to enhanced wakefulness. Orexins do not however, directly affect SWS-active GABAergic VLPO neurons (Figure 4). The mechanism by which orexins prevent cataplexy are still to be resolved but effects on the LC subcoerulear reticular formation are likely to be involved (Brown, 2003).

Orexin neurons were so named because of their location within the lateral hypothalamic feeding center and because orexin A infusion leads to a mild increase in food intake (Sakurai *et al.*, 1998). Inhibition of orexin neurons by the hormones leptin and glucose may be involved in the coupling of arousal to availability of food and in postprandial sleepiness (Willie *et al.*, 2001; Yamanaka *et al.*, 2003).

Orexins activate two receptors, OX_1 (hcrtr1) and OX_2 (hcrtr2), both of which are coupled to G_q G-proteins, activation of which leads mainly to excitatory effects, e.g., (Brown *et al.*, 2002). Currently, the main symptoms of narcolepsy are treated with amphetamine-like stimulants (to counteract the EDS) and antidepressants (to counteract the cataplexy) but in the future it is to be expected that drugs selectively targeting orexin receptors will be available (Nishino and Mignot, 1997; Mignot *et al.*, 2002).

Adenosine

The purine adenosine differs from all the neurotransmitters and neuromodulators described above in several ways (Dunwiddie and Masino, 2001). It is present and released from many, if not all, neurons since it is a by-product of cellular metabolism and is formed by the breakdown of the ubiquitous energy molecule ATP. As such its concentration is closely coupled to energy consumption. Adenosine is not released from synaptic vesicles (although ATP may be) but instead is conveyed to the extracellular space by plasma membrane transporters or is formed there locally from ATP by the action of ectonucleotidases.

Evidence from our laboratory and others over the past decade has implicated adenosine as a sleep-promoting factor (Porkka–Heiskanen *et al.*, 1997; Basheer *et al.*, 2000; Strecker *et al.*, 2000). In rats and cats in many areas of the brain, adenosine levels rise during waking and drop substantially during SWS. In particular, in the basal forebrain adenosine levels rise during waking and importantly they continue to rise during the wakefulness induced by sleep deprivation, produced by gentle handling (Porkka–Heiskanen *et al.*, 2000). Adenosine inhibits identified cholinergic neurons *in vitro* whereas *in vivo*, adenosine inhibits wake-active neurons (Thakkar *et al.*, 2003a). Inactivation of the A_1 receptor in the basal forebrain using antisense technology reduces the increase of EEG delta power seen during recovery sleep following sleep deprivation (Thakkar *et al.*, 2003b). Furthermore, in the neighboring VLPO, adenosine disinhibits presumed sleep-active GABA/galaninergic neurons (Chamberlin *et al.*, 2003). Thus, adenosine appears to act via a dual mechanism — inhibition of wake-active neurons (Figure 5) and excitation (indirect) of sleep-active neurons (Figure 6).

Four receptors for adenosine are known — A_1, A_{2a}, A_{2b}, and A_3 (Figure 2). All are metabotropic receptors (Fredholm *et al.*, 2001). Of these, the A_1 receptor seems to be the most important for sleep–wake regulation. A_1 receptors are coupled to $G_{i/o}$ G-proteins and inhibit neurons (e.g., basal forebrain cholinergic neurons) via activation of G-protein regulated inwardly rectifying potassium channels as well as inhibition of voltage-gated calcium channels (Greene and Haas, 1991). They also inhibit neurotransmitter release when present presynaptically, e.g., on GABAergic inputs to VLPO neurons (Chamberlin *et al.*, 2003). The primary pharmacological action of the widely used mild stimulants theophylline (present in tea) and caffeine (present in tea, coffee, colas, and other soft drinks) is antagonism of the adenosine A_1 receptor (Fredholm *et al.*, 1999).

Miscellaneous Neuromodulators

In addition to the orexins/hypocretins a number of other peptide neurotransmitters play a role in the control of the sleep–wake cycle. Galanin is colocalized with GABA in VLPO neurons and exerts weak but long-lasting inhibitory effects on histamine, noradrenaline, and serotonin neurons (Sherin *et al.*, 1998). Cholecystokinin (CCK), neurotensin, and somatostatin are colocalized with other neurotransmitters and locally regulate the firing patterns of wake- or sleep-active neurons. In particular, neurotensin seems to be important in regulating the burst firing of basal forebrain cholinergic neurons (Cape *et al.*, 2000). A related peptide to somatostatin, cortistatin, seems to antagonize the effects of acetylcholine and promote the induction of SWS (de Lecea *et al.*, 1996).

The gas nitric oxide, which was recently found to act as a local hormone/neuromodulator, may play an important role in the sleep–wake cycle since cholinergic neurons in the basal forebrain and brainstem express the synthesizing enzyme, nitric oxide synthase (Vázquez *et al.*, 2002).

Summary

(I) *Which neurotransmitter systems are involved in generation and maintenance of wakefulness?*

Noradrenaline neurons in the (LC), serotonin neurons in the (DR) nucleus, histamine neurons in the nucleus (TM), orexin/hypocretin neurons in the perifornical area, glutamatergic neurons in the reticular formation, and acetylcholine neurons in the basal forebrain and LDT/PPT are all wake-active and contribute to the generation of the waking state. These systems mutually reinforce each other and converge to a large extent upon common effector mechanisms in the thalamus and cortex although they also have individual roles to play in particular behaviors present during waking.

(II) *What turns off the wake-active neurons and generates SWS?*

The most important contributor to the initiation of SWS seems to be an increase in the activity of neurons in the VLPO area of the anterior hypothalamus, which inhibit wake-active neurons in the TM, DR, and LC via the release of GABA and galanin.

(III) *Which substances mediate the sleepiness associated with prolonged wakefulness?*

One of the main contributors to the sleepiness associated with prolonged wakefulness is an inhibition of basal forebrain cholinergic neurons by the purine adenosine, acting on A_1 receptors. Adenosine builds up in the basal forebrain as a function of prior wakefulness. Other mediators are likely to be involved, in particular serotonin, which also inhibits these neurons.

(IV) *How is REM sleep and the cycle of SWS/REM sleep periods generated?*

The cycle of REM and SWS sleep appears to be generated through the interaction of brainstem cholinergic REM-on cells and monoaminergic (serotonin, noradrenaline) REM-off cells. When the cholinergic cells are released from the inhibition of the monoamines, they excite effector neurons in the reticular formation leading to the signs of REM sleep.

(V) *How does the circadian oscillator in the SCN interact with sleep–wake systems?*

The GABAergic output neurons of the SCN do not appear to directly influence the major sleep–wake nuclei described above but instead act upon the preoptic area and posterior/lateral hypothalamus through local circuits in the anterior hypothalamus. The details of these circuits are still under investigation.

(VI) *Which neurotransmitter systems are involved in sleep disorders?*

To date, the only neurotransmitter system that has been closely linked to a particular sleep disorder is the orexin/hypocretin system, which degenerates or is otherwise dysfunctional in the disease narcolepsy.

(VII) *What are the major targets of sedatives/anesthetics?*

Strong sedatives and anesthetics interact with multiple neurotransmitter systems. However, their major common target appears to be the

$GABA_A$ receptor. Other targets which may be important in their action are nicotinic acetylcholine receptors and leak potassium channels. Mild over-the-counter sedatives usually act upon histamine H_1 receptors.

(VIII) *What are the major targets of stimulants?*

The strongest stimulants known, amphetamine-like substances, have as a common target the dopamine transporter and, thus, potentiate the action of dopamine. In addition, they lead to enhanced release and concentrations of noradrenaline and serotonin. The novel stimulant modafinil (Provigil^{TM}) also acts upon this target but is likely to also have other actions since it does not cause a sleep rebound and is not addictive. Mild stimulants theophylline and caffeine act by blocking adenosine A_1 receptors.

References

Baghdoyan, H.A. and Lydic, R. (1999). M2 muscarinic receptor subtype in the feline medial pontine reticular formation modulates the amount of rapid eye movement sleep. *Sleep*, 22: 835–847.

Baghdoyan, H.A., Rodrigo-Angulo, M.L., McCarley, R.W., and Hobson, J.A. (1984). Site-specific enhancement and suppression of desynchronized sleep signs following cholinergic stimulation of three brainstem regions. *Brain Res.*, 306: 39–52.

Basheer, R., Porkka-Heiskanen, T., Strecker, R.E., Thakkar, M.M., and McCarley, R.W. (2000). Adenosine as a biological signal mediating sleepiness following prolonged wakefulness. *Biol. Signals Recept.*, 9: 319–327.

Brown, R.E. (2003). Involvement of hypocretins/orexins in sleep disorders and narcolepsy. *Drug News Perspect.*, 16: 75–79.

Brown, R.E., Sergeeva, O.A., Eriksson, K.S., and Haas, H.L. (2002). Convergent excitation of dorsal raphe serotonin neurons by multiple arousal systems (orexin/hypocretin, histamine and noradrenaline). *J. Neurosci.*, 22: 8850–8859.

Brown, R.E., Stevens, D.R., and Haas, H.L. (2001). The physiology of brain histamine. *Prog. Neurobiol.*, 63: 637–672.

Cahill, L., Prins, B., Weber, M., and McGaugh, J.L. (1994). Beta-adrenergic activation and memory for emotional events. *Nature*, 371: 702–704.

Cape, E.G. and Jones, B.E. (1998). Differential modulation of high-frequency gamma-electroencephalogram activity and sleep-wake state by noradrenaline and serotonin microinjections into the region of cholinergic basalis neurons. *J. Neurosci.*, 18: 2653–2666.

Cape, E.G., Manns, I.D., Alonso, A., Beaudet, A., and Jones, B.E. (2000). Neurotensin-induced bursting of cholinergic basal forebrain neurons promotes gamma and theta cortical activity together with waking and paradoxical sleep. *J. Neurosci.*, 20: 8452–8461.

Chamberlin, N.L., Arrigoni, E., Chou, T.C., Scammell, T.E., Greene, R.W., and Saper, C.B. (2003). Effects of adenosine on gabaergic synaptic inputs to identified ventrolateral preoptic neurons. *Neuroscience*, 119: 913–918.

Chase, M.H. and Morales, F.R. (1990). The atonia and myoclonia of active (REM) sleep. *Annu. Rev. Psychol.*, 41: 557–584.

Chase, M.H., Morales, F.R., Boxer, P.A., Fung, S.J., and Soja, P.J. (1986). Effect of stimulation of the nucleus reticularis gigantocellularis on the membrane potential of cat lumbar motoneurons during sleep and wakefulness. *Brain Res.*, 386: 237–244.

Chase, M.H., Soja, P.J., and Morales, F.R. (1989). Evidence that glycine mediates the postsynaptic potentials that inhibit lumbar motoneurons during the atonia of active sleep. *J. Neurosci.*, 9: 743–751.

Chemelli, R.M., Willie, J.T., Sinton, C.M., Elmquist, J.K., Scammell, T., Lee, C., Richardson, J.A., Williams, S.C., Xiong, Y., Kisanuki, Y., Fitch, T.E., Nakazato, M., Hammer, R.E., Saper, C.B., and Yanagisawa, M. (1999). Narcolepsy in orexin knockout mice: molecular genetics of sleep regulation. *Cell*, 98: 437–451.

Cirelli, C. and Tononi, G. (2004). Locus ceruleus control of state-dependent gene expression. *J. Neurosci.*, 24: 5410–5419.

Dani, J.A. (2001). Overview of nicotinic receptors and their roles in the central nervous system. *Biol. Psychiatry*, 49: 166–174.

Datta, S., Mavanji, V., Patterson, E.H., and Ulloor, J. (2003). Regulation of rapid eye movement sleep in the freely moving rat: local microinjection of serotonin, norepinephrine, and adenosine into the brainstem. *Sleep*, 26: 513–520.

de Lecea, L., Criado, J.R., Prospero-Garcia, O., Gautvik, K.M., Schweitzer, P., Danielson, P.E., Dunlop, C.L., Siggins, G.R., Henriksen, S.J., and Sutcliffe, J.G. (1996). A cortical neuropeptide with neuronal depressant and sleep-modulating properties. *Nature*, 381: 242–245.

de Lecea, L., Kilduff, T.S., Peyron, C., Gao, X., Foye, P.E., Danielson, P.E., Fukuhara, C., Battenberg, E.L., Gautvik, V.T., Bartlett, F S., Frankel, W.N., van den Pol, A.N., Bloom, F.E., Gautvik, K.M., and Sutcliffe, J.G. (1998). The hypocretins: hypothalamus-specific peptides with neuroexcitatory activity. *Proc. Natl. Acad. Sci. USA*, 95: 322–327.

Dingledine, R., Borges, K., Bowie, D., Traynelis, S.F. (1999). The glutamate receptor ion channels. *Pharmacol. Rev.*, 51: 7–61.

Downie, D.L., Vicente-Agullo, F., Campos-Caro, A., Bushell, T.J., Lieb, W.R., and Franks, N.P. (2002). Determinants of the anesthetic sensitivity of neuronal nicotinic acetylcholine receptors. *J. Biol. Chem.*, 277: 10367–10373.

Dringenberg, H.C. and Vanderwolf, C.H. (1998). Involvement of direct and indirect pathways in electrocorticographic activation. *Neurosci. Biobehav. Rev.*, 22: 243–257.

Dunwiddie, T.V. and Masino, S.A. (2001). The role and regulation of adenosine in the central nervous system. *Annu. Rev. Neurosci.*, 24: 31–55.

Eggermann, E., Serafin, M., Bayer, L., Machard, D., Saint-Mleux, B., Jones, B.E., and Muhlethaler, M. (2001). Orexins/hypocretins excite basal forebrain cholinergic neurons. *Neuroscience*, 108: 177–181.

El Mansari, M., Sakai, K., and Jouvet, M. (1989). Unitary characteristics of presumptive cholinergic tegmental neurons during the sleep-waking cycle in freely moving cats. *Exp. Brain Res.*, 76: 519–529.

Elmquist, J.K., Scammell, T.E., and Saper, C.B. (1997). Mechanisms of CNS response to systemic immune challenge: the febrile response. *Trends Neurosci.*, 20: 565–570.

Eriksson, K.S., Stevens, D.R., and Haas, H.L. (2001). Serotonin excites tuberomammillary neurons by activation of Na(+)/Ca(2+)-exchange. *Neuropharmacology*, 40: 345–351.

Fort, P., Khateb, A., Pegna, A., Muhlethaler, M., and Jones, B.E. (1995). Noradrenergic modulation of cholinergic nucleus basalis neurons demonstrated by *in vitro* pharmacological and immunohistochemical evidence in the guinea-pig brain. *Eur. J. Neurosci.*, 7: 1502–1511.

Fredholm, B.B., Battig, K., Holmen, J., Nehlig, A., and Zvartau, E.E. (1999). Actions of caffeine in the brain with special reference to factors that contribute to its widespread use. *Pharmacol. Rev.*, 51: 83–133.

Fredholm, B.B., IJzerman, A.P., Jacobson, K.A., Klotz, K.N., and Linden, J. (2001). International Union of Pharmacology. XXV. Nomenclature and classification of adenosine receptors. *Pharmacol. Rev.*, 53: 527–552.

Gallopin, T., Fort, P., Eggermann, E., Cauli, B., Luppi, P.H., Rossier, J., Audinat, E., Muhlethaler, M., and Serafin, M. (2000). Identification of sleep-promoting neurons *in vitro*. *Nature*, 404: 992–995.

Greene, R.W. and Haas, H.L. (1991). The electrophysiology of adenosine in the mammalian central nervous system. *Prog. Neurobiol.*, 36: 329–341.

Haas, H. and Panula, P. (2003). The role of histamine and the tuberomamillary nucleus in the nervous system. *Nat. Rev. Neurosci.*, 4: 121–130.

Haas, H.L. and Konnerth, A. (1983). Histamine and noradrenaline decrease calcium-activated potassium conductance in hippocampal pyramidal cells. *Nature*, 302: 432–434.

Hobson, J.A., McCarley, R.W., and Wyzinski, P.W. (1975). Sleep cycle oscillation: reciprocal discharge by two brainstem neuronal groups. *Science*, 189: 55–58.

Jacobs, B.L., Asher, R., and Dement, W.C. (1973). Electrophysiological and behavioral effects of electrical stimulation of the raphe nuclei in cats. *Physiol. Behav.*, 11: 489–495.

Jasper, H.H. and Tessier, J. (1971). Acetylcholine liberation from cerebral cortex during paradoxical (REM) sleep. *Science*, 172: 601–602.

John, J., Wu, M.F., Boehmer, L.N., and Siegel, J.M. (2004). Cataplexy-active neurons in the hypothalamus; implications for the role of histamine in sleep and waking behavior. *Neuron*, 42: 619–634.

Jones, B.E. (1991). Paradoxical sleep and its chemical/structural substrates in the brain. *Neuroscience*, 40: 637–656.

Jones, B.E. (1993). The organization of central cholinergic systems and their functional importance in sleep-waking states. *Prog. Brain Res.*, 98: 61–71.

Jones, B.E. (2003). Arousal systems. *Front. Biosci.*, 8: s438–s451.

Jouvet, M. (1999). Sleep and serotonin: an unfinished story. *Neuropsychopharmacology*, 21: 24S–27S.

Jouvet, M., Vimont, P., and Delorme, F. (1965). Elective suppression of paradoxal sleep in the cat by monoamine oxidase inhibitors. *C. R. Seances Soc. Biol. Fil.*, 159: 1595–1599.

Kawa, K. (1994). Distribution and functional properties of 5-HT3 receptors in the rat hippocampal dentate gyrus: a patch-clamp study. *J. Neurophysiol.*, 71: 1935–1947.

Khateb, A., Fort, P., Alonso, A., Jones, B.E., and Muhlethaler, M. (1993). Pharmacological and immunohistochemical evidence for serotonergic modulation of cholinergic nucleus basalis neurons. *Eur. J. Neurosci.*, 5: 541–547.

Khateb, A., Fort, P., Pegna, A., Jones, B.E., and Muhlethaler, M. (1995). Cholinergic nucleus basalis neurons are excited by histamine *in vitro*. *Neuroscience*, 69: 495–506.

Lai, Y.Y. and Siegel, J.M. (1988). Medullary regions mediating atonia. *J. Neurosci.*, 8: 4790–4796.

Lai, Y.Y., Clements, J.R., Wu, X.Y., Shalita, T., Wu, J.P., Kuo, J.S., and Siegel, J.M. (1999). Brainstem projections to the ventromedial medulla in cat: retrograde transport horseradish peroxidase and immunohistochemical studies. *J. Comp. Neurol.*, 408: 419–436.

Lai, Y.Y., Kodama, T., and Siegel, J.M. (2001). Changes in monoamine release in the ventral horn and hypoglossal nucleus linked to pontine inhibition of muscle tone: an *in vivo* microdialysis study. *J. Neurosci.*, 21: 7384–7391.

Lee, R.S., Steffensen, S.C., and Henriksen, S.J. (2001). Discharge profiles of ventral tegmental area GABA neurons during movement, anesthesia, and the sleep–wake cycle. *J. Neurosci.*, 21: 1757–1766.

Leonard, C.S. and Llinas, R. (1994). Serotonergic and cholinergic inhibition of mesopontine cholinergic neurons controlling REM sleep: an *in vitro* electrophysiological study. *Neuroscience*, 59: 309–330.

Leonard, T.O. and Lydic, R. (1997). Pontine nitric oxide modulates acetylcholine release, rapid eye movement sleep generation, and respiratory rate. *J. Neurosci.*, 17: 774–785.

Levine, E.S. and Jacobs, B.L. (1992). Neurochemical afferents controlling the activity of serotonergic neurons in the dorsal raphe nucleus: microiontophoretic studies in the awake cat. *J. Neurosci.*, 12: 4037–4044.

Lin, J.S. (2000). Brain structures and mechanisms involved in the control of cortical activation and wakefulness, with emphasis on the posterior hypothalamus and histaminergic neurons. *Sleep Med. Rev.*, 4: 471–503.

Lin, L., Hungs, M., and Mignot, E. (2001). Narcolepsy and the HLA region. *J. Neuroimmunol.*, 117: 9–20.

Lin, L., Faraco, J., Li, R., Kadotani, H., Rogers, W., Lin, X., Qiu, X., de JP, Nishino, S., and Mignot, E. (1999). The sleep disorder canine narcolepsy is caused by a mutation in the hypocretin (orexin) receptor 2 gene. *Cell*, 98: 365–376.

Luebke, J.I., Greene, R.W., Semba, K., Kamondi, A., McCarley, R.W., and Reiner, P.B. (1992). Serotonin hyperpolarizes cholinergic low-threshold burst neurons in the rat laterodorsal tegmental nucleus *in vitro*. *Proc. Natl. Acad. Sci. USA*, 89: 743–747.

Lydic, R., McCarley, R.W., and Hobson, J.A. (1987a). Serotonin neurons and sleep. I. Long term recordings of dorsal raphe discharge frequency and PGO waves. *Arch. Ital. Biol.*, 125: 317–343.

Lydic, R., McCarley, R.W., and Hobson, J.A. (1987b). Serotonin neurons and sleep. II. Time course of dorsal raphe discharge, PGO waves, and behavioral states. *Arch. Ital. Biol.*, 126: 1–28.

Manns, I.D., Alonso, A., and Jones, B.E. (2000). Discharge profiles of juxtacellularly labeled and immunohistochemically identified GABAergic basal forebrain neurons recorded in association with the electroencephalogram in anesthetized rats. *J. Neurosci.*, 20: 9252–9263.

Marek, G.J. and Aghajanian, G.K. (1998). The electrophysiology of prefrontal serotonin systems: therapeutic implications for mood and psychosis. *Biol. Psychiatry*, 44: 1118–1127.

McCarley, R.W. and Massaquoi, S.G. (1986). A limit cycle mathematical model of the REM sleep oscillator system. *Am. J. Physiol.*, 251: R1011–R1029.

McCarley, R.W. and Massaquoi, S.G. (1992). Neurobiological structure of the revised limit cycle reciprocal interaction model of REM cycle control. *J. Sleep Res.*, 1: 132–137.

McCormick, D.A. (1992). Neurotransmitter actions in the thalamus and cerebral cortex and their role in neuromodulation of thalamocortical activity. *Prog. Neurobiol.*, 39: 337–388.

McGinty, D.J. and Harper, R.M. (1976). Dorsal raphe neurons: depression of firing during sleep in cats. *Brain Res.*, 101: 569–575.

McKernan, R.M., Rosahl, T.W., Reynolds, D.S., Sur, C., Wafford, K.A., Atack, J.R., Farrar, S., Myers, J., Cook, G., Ferris, P., Garrett, L., Bristow, L., Marshall, G., Macaulay, A., Brown, N., Howell, O., Moore, K.W., Carling, R.W., Street, L.J., Castro, J.L., Ragan, C.I., Dawson, G.R., and Whiting, P.J. (2000). Sedative but not anxiolytic properties of benzodiazepines are mediated by the GABA(A) receptor alpha1 subtype. *Nat. Neurosci.*, 3: 587–592.

McKernan, R.M. and Whiting, P.J. (1996). Which GABAA-receptor subtypes really occur in the brain? Trends Neurosci., 19: 139–143.

Mignot, E., Taheri, S., and Nishino, S. (2002). Sleeping with the hypothalamus: emerging therapeutic targets for sleep disorders. *Nat. Neurosci.*, 5 (suppl.): 1071–1075.

Miller, J.D., Farber, J., Gatz, P., Roffwarg, H., and German, D.C. (1983). Activity of mesencephalic dopamine and non-dopamine neurons across stages of sleep and walking in the rat. *Brain Res.*, 273: 133–141.

Moore, R.Y., Speh, J.C., and Leak, R.K. (2002). Suprachiasmatic nucleus organization. *Cell Tissue Res.*, 309: 89–98.

Moruzzi, G. and Magoun, H.W. (1995). Brain stem reticular formation and activation of the EEG. 1949. *J. psychiatry Clin. Neurosci.*, 7: 251–267.

Mouret, J., Bobillier, P., and Jouvet, M. (1968). Insomnia following parachlorophenylalanine in the rat. *Eur. J. Pharmacol.*, 5: 17–22.

Nelson, L.E., Guo, T.Z., Lu, J., Saper, C.B., Franks, N.P., and Maze, M. (2002). The sedative component of anesthesia is mediated by GABA(A) receptors in an endogenous sleep pathway. *Nat. Neurosci.*, 5: 979–984.

Nishino, S. and Mignot, E. (1997). Pharmacological aspects of human and canine narcolepsy. *Prog. Neurobiol.*, 52: 27–78.

Pace-Schott, E.F. and Hobson, J.A. (2002). The neurobiology of sleep: genetics, cellular physiology and subcortical networks. *Nat. Rev. Neurosci.*, 3: 591–605.

Parmentier, R., Ohtsu, H., Djebbara-Hannas, Z., Valatx, J.L., Watanabe, T., and Lin, J.S. (2002). Anatomical, physiological, and pharmacological characteristics of histidine decarboxylase knock-out mice: evidence for the role of brain histamine in behavioral and sleep-wake control. *J. Neurosci.*, 22: 7695–7711.

Perry, E., Walker, M., Grace, J., and Perry, R. (1999). Acetylcholine in mind: a neurotransmitter correlate of consciousness? *Trends Neurosci.*, 22: 273–280.

Peyron, C., Faraco, J., Rogers, W., Ripley, B., Overeem, S., Charnay, Y., Nevsimalova, S., Aldrich, M., Reynolds, D., Albin, R., Li, R., Hungs, M., Pedrazzoli, M., Padigaru, M., Kucherlapati, M., Fan, J., Maki, R., Lammers, G.J., Bouras, C., Kucherlapati, R., Nishino, S., and Mignot, E. (2000). A mutation in a case of early onset narcolepsy and a generalized absence of hypocretin peptides in human narcoleptic brains. *Nat. Med.*, 6: 991–997.

Pin, J.P. and Duvoisin, R. (1995). The metabotropic glutamate receptors: structure and functions. *Neuropharmacology*, 34: 1–26.

Porkka-Heiskanen, T., Strecker, R.E., Thakkar, M., Bjorkum, A.A., Greene, R.W., and McCarley, R.W. (1997). Adenosine: a mediator of the sleep-inducing effects of prolonged wakefulness. *Science*, 276: 1265–1268.

Porkka-Heiskanen, T., Strecker, R.E., and McCarley, R.W. (2000). Brain site-specificity of extracellular adenosine concentration changes during sleep deprivation and spontaneous sleep: an *in vivo* microdialysis study. *Neuroscience*, 99: 507–517.

Portas, C.M., Bjorvatn, B., and Ursin, R. (2000). Serotonin and the sleep/wake cycle: special emphasis on microdialysis studies. *Prog. Neurobiol.*, 60: 13–35.

Rasmussen, K., Morilak, D.A., and Jacobs, B.L. (1986). Single unit activity of locus coeruleus neurons in the freely moving cat. I. During naturalistic behaviors and in response to simple and complex stimuli. *Brain Res.*, 371: 324–334.

Rudolph, U., Crestani, F., Benke, D., Brunig, I., Benson, J.A., Fritschy, J.M., Martin, J.R., Bluethmann, H., and Mohler, H. (1999). Benzodiazepine actions mediated by specific gamma-aminobutyric acid(A) receptor subtypes. *Nature*, 401: 796–800.

Sakurai, T., Amemiya, A., Ishii, M., Matsuzaki, I., Chemelli, R.M., Tanaka, H., Williams, S.C., Richarson, J.A., Kozlowski, G.P., Wilson, S., Arch, J.R.,

Buckingham, R.E., Haynes, A.C., Carr, S.A., Annan, R.S., McNulty, D.E., Liu, W.S., Terrett, J.A., Elshourbagy, N.A., Bergsma, D.J., and Yanagisawa, M. (1998). Orexins and orexin receptors: a family of hypothalamic neuropeptides and G protein-coupled receptors that regulate feeding behavior. *Cell*, 92: 573–585.

Saper, C.B., Chou, T.C., and Scammell, T.E. (2001). The sleep switch: hypothalamic control of sleep and wakefulness. *Trends Neurosci.*, 24: 726–731.

Scammell, T., Gerashchenko, D., Urade, Y., Onoe, H., Saper, C., and Hayaishi, O. (1998). Activation of ventrolateral preoptic neurons by the somnogen prostaglandin D2. *Proc. Natl. Acad. Sci. USA*, 95: 7754–7759.

Schultz, W. (1998). Predictive reward signal of dopamine neurons. *J. Neurophysiol.*, 80: 1–27.

Sergeeva, O.A., Eriksson, K.S., Sharonova, I.N., Vorobjev, V.S., and Haas, H.L. (2002). GABA(A) receptor heterogeneity in histaminergic neurons. *Eur. J. Neurosci.*, 16: 1472–1482.

Sherin, J.E., Shiromani, P.J., McCarley, R.W., and Saper, C.B. (1996). Activation of ventrolateral preoptic neurons during sleep. *Science*, 271: 216–219.

Sherin, J.E., Elmquist, J.K., Torrealba, F., and Saper, C.B. (1998). Innervation of histaminergic tuberomammillary neurons by GABAergic and galaninergic neurons in the ventrolateral preoptic nucleus of the rat. *J. Neurosci.*, 18: 4705–4721.

Shirakawa, T. and Moore, R.Y. (1994). Glutamate shifts the phase of the circadian neuronal firing rhythm in the rat suprachiasmatic nucleus *in vitro*. *Neurosci. Lett.*, 178: 47–50.

Steininger, T.L., Gong, H., McGinty, D., and Szymusiak, R. (2001). Subregional organization of preoptic area/anterior hypothalamic projections to arousal-related monoaminergic cell groups. *J. Comp. Neurol.*, 429: 638–653.

Steriade, M. (2004). Acetylcholine systems and rhythmic activities during the waking-sleep cycle. *Prog. Brain Res.*, 145: 179–196.

Steriade, M. and McCarley, R.W. (2005). *Brain Control of Wakefulness and Sleep*. New York: Kluwer Academic/Plenum.

Steriade, M., Datta, S., Pare, D., Oakson, G., and Curro Dossi, R.C. (1990a). Neuronal activities in brain-stem cholinergic nuclei related to tonic activation processes in thalamocortical systems. *J. Neurosci.*, 10: 2541–2559.

Steriade, M., Pare, D., Datta, S., Oakson, G., and Curro, D.R. (1990b). Different cellular types in mesopontine cholinergic nuclei related to ponto-geniculo-occipital waves. *J. Neurosci.*, 10: 2560–2579.

Steriade, M., McCormick, D.A., and Sejnowski, T.J. (1993). Thalamocortical oscillations in the sleeping and aroused brain. *Science*, 262: 679–685.

Strecker, R.E., Morairty, S., Thakkar, M.M., Porkka-Heiskanen, T., Basheer, R., Dauphin, L.J., Rainnie, D.G., Portas, C.M., Greene, R.W., and McCarley, R.W. (2000). Adenosinergic modulation of basal forebrain and preoptic/anterior hypothalamic neuronal activity in the control of behavioral state. *Behav. Brain Res.*, 115: 183–204.

Szymusiak, R. and McGinty, D. (1986). Sleep-related neuronal discharge in the basal forebrain of cats. *Brain Res.*, 370: 82–92.

Szymusiak, R., Steininger, T., Alam, N., and McGinty, D. (2001). Preoptic area sleep-regulating mechanisms. *Arch. Ital. Biol.*, 139: 77–92.

Taheri, S., Zeitzer, J.M., and Mignot, E. (2002). The role of hypocretins (orexins) in sleep regulation and narcolepsy. *Annu. Rev. Neurosci.*, 25: 283–313.

Thakkar, M.M., Strecker, R.E., and McCarley, R.W. (1998). Behavioral state control through differential serotonergic inhibition in the mesopontine cholinergic nuclei: a simultaneous unit recording and microdialysis study. *J. Neurosci.*, 18: 5490–5497.

Thakkar, M.M., Delgiacco, R.A., Strecker, R.E., and McCarley, R.W. (2003a). Adenosinergic inhibition of basal forebrain wakefulness-active neurons: a simultaneous unit recording and microdialysis study in freely behaving cats. *Neuroscience*, 122: 1107–1113.

Thakkar, M.M., Winston, S., and McCarley, R.W. (2003b). A1 receptor and adenosinergic homeostatic regulation of sleep-wakefulness: effects of antisense to the A1 receptor in the cholinergic basal forebrain. *J. Neurosci.*, 23: 4278–4287.

Thannickal, T.C., Moore, R.Y., Nienhuis, R., Ramanathan, L., Gulyani, S., Aldrich, M., Cornford, M., and Siegel, J.M. (2000). Reduced number of hypocretin neurons in human narcolepsy. *Neuron*, 27: 469–474.

Tononi, G., Pompeiano, M., and Pompeiano, O. (1988). Desynchronized sleep suppression after microinjection of the beta-adrenergic agonist isoproterenol in the dorsal pontine tegmentum. *Arch. Ital. Biol.*, 126: 125–128.

Trulson, M.E. and Jacobs, B.L. (1979). Raphe unit activity in freely moving cats: correlation with level of behavioral arousal. *Brain Res.*, 163: 135–150.

Vandermaelen, C.P. and Aghajanian, G.K. (1983). Electrophysiological and pharmacological characterization of serotonergic dorsal raphe neurons recorded extracellularly and intracellularly in rat brain slices. *Brain Res.*, 289: 109–119.

Vázquez, J., Lydic, R., and Baghdoyan, H.A. (2002). The nitric oxide synthase inhibitor NG-Nitro-L-arginine increases basal forebrain acetylcholine release during sleep and wakefulness. *J. Neurosci.*, 22: 5597–5605.

Von Economo, C. (1926). Die Pathologie des Schlafes. In: Von Bethe, A., Von Bergmann, G., Embden, G., and Ellinger, A. (Eds.). *Handbuch des Normalen und Pathologischen Physiologie*. Berlin: Springer, pp. 591–610.

Williams, J.A. and Reiner, P.B. (1993). Noradrenaline hyperpolarizes identified rat mesopontine cholinergic neurons *in vitro*. *J. Neurosci.*, 13: 3878–3883.

Willie, J.T., Chemelli, R.M., Sinton, C.M., and Yanagisawa, M. (2001). To eat or to sleep? Orexin in the regulation of feeding and wakefulness. *Annu. Rev. Neurosci.*, 24: 429–458.

Wisor, J.P., Nishino, S., Sora, I., Uhl, G.H., Mignot, E., and Edgar, D.M. (2001). Dopaminergic role in stimulant-induced wakefulness. *J. Neurosci.*, 21: 1787–1794.

Wong, C.G., Gibson, K.M., and Snead, O.C. III (2004). From the street to the brain: neurobiology of the recreational drug gamma-hydroxybutyric acid. *Trends Pharmacol. Sci.*, 25: 29–34.

Wu, M.F., Gulyani, S.A., Yau, E., Mignot, E., Phan, B., and Siegel, J.M. (1999). Locus coeruleus neurons: cessation of activity during cataplexy. *Neuroscience*, 91: 1389–1399.

Yamanaka, A., Beuckmann, C.T., Willie, J.T., Hara, J., Tsujino, N., Mieda, M., Tominaga, M., Yagami, K., Sugiyama, F., Goto, K., Yanagisawa, M., and Sakurai, T. (2003). Hypothalamic orexin neurons regulate arousal according to energy balance in mice. *Neuron*, 38: 701–713.

Chapter 4

A POSSIBLE ROLE FOR SLEEP IN SYNAPTIC HOMEOSTASIS

Giulio Tononi[1] and Chiara Cirelli

This paper discusses a novel hypothesis — the synaptic homeostasis hypothesis — which claims that sleep plays a role in the regulation of synaptic weight in the brain. As we shall see, the synaptic homeostasis hypothesis can account for several aspects of sleep and its regulation, and makes several specific predictions. In brief, the hypothesis is as follows: (1) wakefulness is associated with synaptic potentiation in several cortical circuits; (2) synaptic potentiation is tied to the homeostatic regulation of slow-wave activity; (3) slow-wave activity is associated with synaptic down-scaling; and (4) synaptic downscaling is tied to the beneficial effects of sleep on neural function and, indirectly, on performance. In its bare bones, the hypothesis concerns mainly non-rapid eye movement (NREM) sleep and the cerebral cortex, but it is not difficult to see how it could be extended to account for rapid-eye-movement (REM) sleep and to apply to other brain structures, such as the hippocampus.

A useful way of introducing the synaptic homeostasis hypothesis is to relate it to one of the best-established models of sleep regulation — the two-process model of sleep regulation developed by A. Borbély (Borbély, 1982; Borbély and Ackermann, 2000). This model distinguishes between the circadian regulation of sleep propensity (process C) and its homeostatic regulation (process S). The circadian component describes the distribution

---

[1]gtononi@wisc.edu

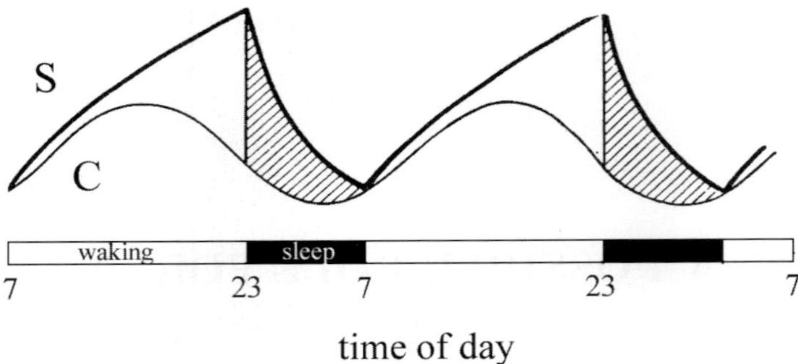

Figure 1. The two process models of sleep regulation. Time course of homeostatic process S and circadian process C. (Modified from Borbély and Achermann, 2000.)

of sleep during the 24 h. It is well understood, both in its mechanisms, centred in the suprachiasmatic nucleus, and in its function, which is to restrict sleep to a time of day that is ecologically appropriate. The homeostatic component describes what one might call the essence of sleep: how the need for sleep accumulates the longer an animal stays awake, and how such a need is discharged. As elegantly demonstrated in a long series of studies (Borbély, 2001), the homeostatic component can be modelled as a slower exponential increase of process S during wakefulness, and a faster exponential decrease during sleep (Figure 1). However, in this case mechanisms and functions are not known: the challenge is to establish what biological process, if any, corresponds to process S.

According to the hypothesis, process S describes the process of synaptic homeostasis. Specifically, the curve in Figure 1 can be interpreted as reflecting how the net amount of synaptic strength in the cerebral cortex (and possibly other brain structures) changes as a function of wakefulness and sleep. Thus, the hypothesis claims that, under normal conditions, the net amount of synaptic strength increases during wakefulness and reaches a maximum just before going to sleep. Then, as soon as sleep ensues, total synaptic strength begins to decrease and reaches a baseline level by the time sleep ends.

In addition to claiming the correspondence between process S, or sleep need, and total synaptic strength, the hypothesis proposes specific mechanisms whereby synaptic strength would increase during wakefulness and decrease during sleep, and suggests why the tight regulation of net synaptic strength would be of great importance to the brain.

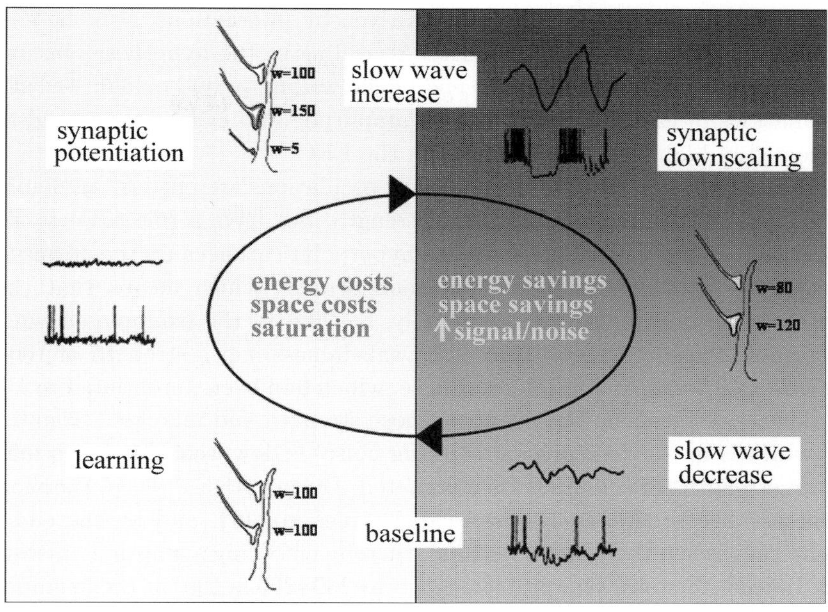

Figure 2. The synaptic homeostasis hypothesis (Tononi and Cirelli, 2003) (see text for details).

Synaptic Homeostasis: A Schematic Diagram

The diagram in Figure 2 presents a simplified version of the main points of the hypothesis. During wakefulness (yellow background), the electroencephalogram (EEG) is activated, the animal interacts with its environment, and it acquires information about it. Information is stored in distributed cortical circuits largely through long-term synaptic potentiation. This potentiation occurs when the firing of a pre-synaptic neuron is followed by the firing of a post-synaptic neuron, and the neuromodulatory milieu signals that it is an appropriate time for learning, which is the case during alert wakefulness. Strengthened synapses are indicated in red, with their strength indicated by a number.

When the animal goes to sleep (blue background), it becomes virtually disconnected from the environment, and neural activity is generated internally. Changes in the neuromodulatory milieu trigger the occurrence of slow oscillations, comprising depolarised and hyperpolarised phases, which affect every neuron in the cortex. The changed neuromodulatory milieu also ensures that synaptic activity is not followed by synaptic potentiation. Since synaptic activity during sleep is not driven by interactions with the environment, this makes adaptive sense. According to the hypothesis, because average synaptic strength at the end of the waking period is high, the slow oscillations of early sleep are of high amplitude and synchronous, and are reflected in high slow-wave activity in the EEG.

The hypothesis also claims that slow oscillations are not just an epiphenomenon of the increased synaptic strength, but have a role to play. The repeated sequences of depolarisation–hyperpolarisation cause the downscaling of the synapses impinging on each neuron, which means that they all decrease in strength proportionally, by 20% in the example shown in Figure 2. Thus, a synapse that after wakefulness had a strength of 100 is downscaled to 80, and another synapse, which had been potentiated to 150, is downscaled to 120. The synapse whose strength had increased from 0 to 5 (which is meant to represent learning noise) is downscaled below a minimum strength threshold and is eliminated. During NREM sleep, therefore, synapses are progressively downscaled (green colour), and by the end of sleep they reach their baseline value, thereby enforcing synaptic homeostasis. Indeed, the total synaptic strength was 200 (100 + 100) at the beginning of wakefulness and 200 (120 + 80) at the end of sleep.

The reduced synaptic strength reduces the amplitude and synchronisation of the slow oscillations, which is reflected in a reduced slow-wave activity in the EEG. Because of the dampening of the slow oscillation, downscaling is progressively reduced, making the process self-limiting when synaptic strength reaches an appropriate baseline level. Finally, the animal wakes up, neural circuits preserve a trace of the previous experiences (minus the noise), but are kept efficient at an appropriate level of synaptic strength, and the cycle can begin again.

After this brief and schematic depiction of the hypothesis, we now turn to describing its main points in more detail, and to discussing some of the evidence that supports it, as well as some potential objections.

Wakefulness and Synaptic Potentiation

During wakefulness, when animals explore novel situations, attend to their surroundings, react to sensory stimuli, perform motor tasks, think, make associations, and are punished or rewarded, they learn about their environment. Underlying learning are long-lasting changes in the strength or number of synaptic connections between neurons, which are mediated by complicated cascades of cellular events. The best characterised forms of long-term change in synaptic weight are known as long-term potentiation (LTP) and long-term depression (LTD).

The synaptic homeostasis hypothesis states that wakefulness is accompanied by LTP-like changes in a large fraction of cortical circuits, resulting in a net increase in synaptic weight. Synaptic potentiation would occur through much of waking life, whenever the animal is alert and making behavioural choices, whether or not it is specifically engaged in experimental learning paradigms. After all, synapses and neurons do not know whether they are engaged in a learning paradigm, but only whether strong pre-synaptic firing is accompanied by post-synaptic depolarisation in the presence of appropriate levels of neuromodulators. Note that, according to the hypothesis, waking plasticity would produce a net increase in synaptic weight impinging onto cortical neurons, that is, much more LTP than LTD (at least in the adult). This is not so unlikely if one considers that, on a background of low spontaneous activity, the cerebral cortex engages in sensory, motor, or cognitive tasks by having select groups of neurons strongly increase, rather than decrease, their firing rate. It has been calculated, based on energy constraints, that background firing rates in the cerebral cortex are likely to be between 0.1 and 1 Hz, and that, at any given time (say 1 s), only about 0.3% of neurons can afford to fire at 50 Hz or more (Lennie, 2003). Synapses among these strongly firing neurons are the ones more likely to be potentiated and to store information about the day's experiences.

Direct evidence supporting this part of the hypothesis comes from anatomical work reporting a net and diffuse increase in synaptic density in animals exposed to enriched environments likely to induce LTP-like molecular changes (Klintsova and Greenough, 1999). Another study has demonstrated that stimulating a whisker for 24 h produces a selective net increase of synaptic density (by 35%) on cortical neurons in the corresponding barrel field (Knott *et al.*, 2002). Less direct, but strongly suggestive evidence comes from the finding that spontaneous wakefulness is regularly associated with the diffuse induction of molecular changes generally associated with LTP (Cirelli and Tononi, 2000), including the phosphorylation of CRE-binding protein (CREB) and the induction of plasticity-related genes such as *Arc*, *BDNF*, and *NGFI-A* (e.g., Wallace *et al.*, 1995; Ying *et al.*, 2002; Silva, 2003). This spontaneous induction of LTP-related genes can increase further if the environment is more stimulating and rich in novel objects. During sleep, by contrast, the expression of LTP-related genes is severely reduced or abolished (Cirelli and Tononi, 2000).

Support for this part of the hypothesis also comes from positron emission tomography (PET) experiments in humans (Braun *et al.*, 1997) and deoxyglucose studies in rats (Vyazovskiy *et al.*, 2004b). In the human study, which aimed at evaluating regional blood flow changes in sleep, Braun *et al.* (1997) reported a remarkable difference in the absolute value of cerebral oxygen utilisation during the same control condition (awake at rest) in the morning versus in the evening. Quite unexpectedly, oxygen utilisation was 18% higher at the end of the waking day than after a night of sleep, and this was the case almost everywhere in the brain. A change of this magnitude is not usually seen in PET studies, even less so when comparing two identical "resting" conditions. An intriguing possibility is that the increased oxygen utilisation at the end of the waking day may be due to a net increase in synaptic strength in a large fraction of neural circuits. Indeed, nearly 80% of cortical grey matter metabolism is related to neural activity (Attwell and Laughlin, 2001; Rothman *et al.*, 2003), half of it to support action potentials and half to support post-synaptic potentials. Since synaptic strength controls $\approx$40% of the cortex energy needs directly, and potentially more because of indirect effects on firing rates (Pavlides and Winson, 1989; Hirase *et al.*, 2001), the results of Braun *et al.* (1997) could be explained in terms of a net increase in synaptic strength between morning and evening. The deoxyglucose study is also consistent with this picture, in that glucose utilisation appears to be considerably higher in waking before sleep than in waking after sleep (Vyazovskiy *et al.*, 2004b).

From an evolutionary perspective, it makes sense that the potentiation of neural circuits should occur during wakefulness, when an animal is active and exposed to the environment, and not during sleep, when neural activity is unrelated to external events (Tononi and Cirelli, 2001). However, given that spontaneous mean firing rates of cortical neurons in wakefulness and sleep are comparable (Steriade, 2003), how is the induction of LTP-related genes restricted to wakefulness? One reason may be that sensory, motor, or cognitive activities that occur during active wakefulness are often associated, in a small sub-set of neurons, with high peak firing rates that are likely to give rise to LTP-related plastic changes (Sjostrom *et al.*, 2001). Another reason is that the firing of the noradrenergic system is high during wakefulness, especially during salient events, while it is very low or absent during sleep (Hobson *et al.*, 1975; Aston-Jones and Blomm, 1981). If the noradrenergic innervation of the cerebral cortex is destroyed, P-CREB, Arc, BDNF, and NGFI-A are down to the levels seen in sleep even when the animal is awake and behaving, and even if the waking EEG is essentially unchanged (Cirelli *et al.*, 1996). Consistent with these observations, norepinephrine is important for the induction of LTP (Gu, 2002; Walling and Harley, 2004), and noradrenergic lesions impair at least some forms of learning (Robbins and Everitt, 1995).

Synaptic Potentiation and Slow-Wave Homeostasis

During much of sleep, neurons in the cerebral cortex fire and stop firing together in waves of activity having frequencies of less than 4.5 Hz. Such slow-wave activity, which is the most pronounced EEG feature of NREM sleep, is also a reliable predictor of sleep intensity. An important feature of slow-wave activity during sleep is that it increases as a function of previous wakefulness, and it gradually decreases in the course of sleep (Borbély and Ackermann, 2000). This homeostatic regulation suggests that slow-wave activity may be linked to some restorative aspect of sleep. The present hypothesis states that the homeostatic regulation of slow-wave activity is tied to the amount of synaptic potentiation that has occurred during previous wakefulness. Specifically, the higher the amount of synaptic potentiation in cortical circuits during wakefulness, the higher the increase in slow-wave activity during subsequent sleep.

This portion of the hypothesis relies on the evidence from both animals and humans. For example, a direct prediction of the hypothesis is that, if wakefulness is not accompanied by LTP-like changes in synaptic strength, the homeostatic increase in slow-wave activity after wakefulness should be eliminated. This prediction was tested by examining animals with a lesioned noradrenergic system, which have a greatly reduced expression of LTP-related molecules in the cerebral cortex after periods of wakefulness (Cirelli *et al.*, 1996; Cirelli and Tononi, 2000, 2004). Although in these animals the amount and timing of sleep are unchanged, results from our laboratory indicate the blunting of the peak in slow-wave activity that is normally seen in the morning hours after the nocturnal activity phase (Cirelli *et al.*, 2005). Thus, it may be that it is not wakefulness as such, but the induction of LTP-related molecules normally associated with wakefulness, that is responsible for driving the homeostatic increase in slow-wave activity. Further studies indicate that norepinephrine lesioned animals have a blunted slow-wave response to sleep deprivation (Cirelli *et al.*, 2005). A related prediction of the hypothesis is that there should be a relationship between the kinds of activities that animals are engaged in during wakefulness, the corresponding level of induction of LTP-related genes (Kelly and Deadwyler, 2003), and the amount of slow-wave activity during subsequent sleep (Meerlo *et al.*, 2001).

Molecular correlates of LTP or of learning in humans are, of course, not available. Nevertheless, it is likely that when we actively engage in various waking tasks, strong synaptic activation is accompanied by cellular and molecular changes similar to those occurring in other mammals. A key prediction of the hypothesis is that, to the extent that synaptic potentiation is particularly strong in specific brain areas, slow-wave activity during subsequent sleep should increase disproportionately in that area, a kind of local intensification of sleep. Local differences in slow-wave homeostasis have been described in both humans and rodents, with frontal regions showing an especially strong response to sleep deprivation (Finelli *et al.*, 2000; Huber *et al.*, 2000; Vyazovskiy *et al.*, 2002). Since anterior cortical regions are especially susceptible to the effects of sleep deprivation, perhaps working harder than other brain areas during wakefulness (Horne, 1992), and perhaps more plastic than posterior ones (Grutzendler *et al.*, 2002; Trachtenberg *et al.*, 2002), a possible relationship to synaptic potentiation is at least conceivable. Direct evidence linking brain activation with local sleep homeostasis has been sought in two studies employing a lateralised task, one in humans (Kattler *et al.*, 1994) and one in rats (Vyazovskiy *et al.*, 2000). Both studies found a slight asymmetry in power between the two sides after the lateralised task, but the magnitude of the effect was fairly small. In the human study, this may have been due to the use of passive vibration of the hand, which is probably a much less potent stimulus for circuit potentiation than an active task.

Most recently, we have searched for signs of local slow-wave homeostasis using high definition EEG and a visuomotor task (Ghilardi *et al.*, 2000) that actively engages a subject's attention (Huber *et al.*, 2004). In this task, performed shortly before bedtime, subjects reach for visual targets using a hand-held cursor while unconsciously adapting to systematic rotations imposed to the perceived cursor trajectory (Ghilardi *et al.*, 2000). One week earlier or later, subjects performed a control task that was subjectively indistinguishable and kinematically identical, but in which the cursor trajectory was not rotated. Thus, the only difference between the two tasks was that the rotation adaptation task involved (implicit) learning and thus, presumably, LTP-like changes in the brain, whereas the control task did not. Previous PET work had shown that such learning involves a circumscribed region in right parietal cortex (Ghilardi *et al.*, 2000).

We predicted that, if such strong activation is associated with the induction of LTP-related molecular changes, and if these are tied to slow-wave homeostasis, there should be an increase in slow waves during the sleep

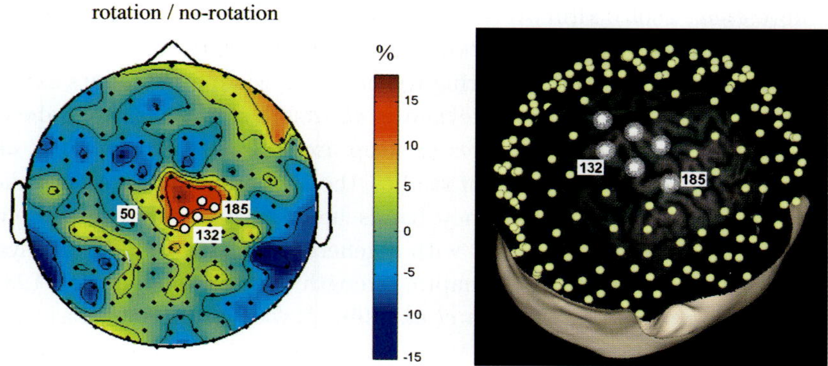

Figure 3. Local slow-wave activity homeostasis after the acquisition of a rotation task. Left panel: Topographic distribution of the percentage change in slow-wave activity during NREM sleep between the rotation and the no-rotation condition. White dots indicate the six electrodes showing increased slow-wave activity after rotation adaptation. Right panel: Anatomical localisation of the six electrodes (large white dots) showing increased slow-wave activity after rotation adaptation. All 256 electrodes (yellow dots) were digitised and co-registered with the subject's magnetic resonance images. Electrode 185 projects onto area 40, electrode 132 onto area 7. (Modified from Huber *et al.*, 2004.)

episode subsequent to the learning task compared to the control task. Furthermore, such increase should be localised to the appropriate brain region. We tested this prediction by recording the sleep EEG using a 256-channel system (Figure 3). When we compared the rotation and no-rotation condition, we found a local increase of slow-wave activity (27%) extending over a small cluster of electrodes. The increase in power was largely selective for the slow-wave frequency range, and it declined over time, just like the global homeostatic response of slow-wave activity. Finally, using an infrared system, we found that the increase of slow-wave activity was localised exactly at the predicted spot in the right parietal cortex. Thus, the presumed induction of local plastic changes associated with practising a visuomotor task is associated with a local induction of slow-wave activity in subsequent sleep.

What could be the mechanism linking local synaptic potentiation during wakefulness with increased slow waves during sleep? A straightforward explanation could be that the amount of slow waves recordable via EEG reflects the overall strength of cortico-cortical synapses, and thereby represents a direct reflection of the amount of potentiation. Evidence that the amplitude of synchronised activity is heavily influenced by the amount and efficacy of synaptic transmission comes both from experimental (Amzica and Steriade, 1995) and from modelling work (Bazhenov *et al.*, 2002;

Compte *et al.*, 2003). Moreover, slow-wave activity changes during the lifespan in a way that seems to follow cortical synaptic density (Feinberg, 1982). Also, after visual deprivation during the critical period, a procedure associated with synaptic depression (Heynen *et al.*, 2003), slow waves are reduced by 40% in the absence of changes in sleep architecture (Miyamoto *et al.*, 2003). Finally, according to recent studies, the increase in power after wakefulness extends to other frequency bands besides the slow-wave or delta band, which would be consistent with a generalised increase in neural synchronisation due to increased synaptic strength (Borbély and Tobler, 1984; Cajochen *et al.*, 1995; Aeschbach *et al.*, 1997; Huber *et al.*, 2000; Cajochen *et al.*, 2001).

Other local mechanisms could also contribute to tying the amplitude of slow oscillations to the extent of synaptic potentiation during wakefulness. Underlying slow-wave activity in the EEG is a slow oscillation of the membrane potential of cortical cells (Steriade, 2003). The slow oscillation comprises a depolarised up-phase, during which neurons fire at relatively high rates, followed by a hyperpolarised down-phase, during which neurons are silent. The down-phase is probably brought about by a sodium-dependent potassium current that is activated as a function of neuronal firing. According to modelling studies, a net potentiation of synaptic inputs causes a stronger activation of the sodium-dependent potassium current, which leads in turn to a longer and more hyperpolarised down-phase, and thus to slow oscillations of increased amplitude (Hill and Tononi, unpublished results).

Slow-Wave Homeostasis and Synaptic Downscaling

We have assumed that LTP-related changes occurring in the cortex during wakefulness lead to a net increase in synaptic weight onto neurons, and that such increase is reflected in an increased slow-wave activity. Is such slow-wave activity a mere epiphenomenon, or does it have some functional significance? According to the hypothesis, slow waves occurring in the cortex during sleep would actively promote a generalised depression or downscaling of synapses. In this way, the total synaptic weight to neurons would progressively return to a baseline level, thus effecting a kind of synaptic homeostasis. Correspondingly, since the amplitude of slow waves would be tied to total synaptic weight, power in the delta band would progressively return to a baseline level, consistent with slow-wave homeostasis.

A need to rescale synaptic weight after learning, in order to preserve a constant level of synaptic input without obliterating memory traces, confer stability to neuronal firing, maintain unused synapses, and prevent runaway potentiation or depression, has long been recognised in computational models of synaptic plasticity (e.g., Miller and MacKay, 1994). Mathematically, rescaling of the synapses impinging on the same neuron can be achieved by subtracting an amount proportional to the strength of each synapse, i.e., dividing each weight by the same factor. Recently, a process of this kind has been shown to occur *in vitro* and *in vivo* in neocortical cells (Turrigiano, 1999; Desai *et al.*, 2002). In these experiments, blocking or reducing neural activity induces a proportional increase in the strength of all synapses impinging on a neuron, while increasing neural activity does the opposite. Since the net effect is to make silent cells more excitable and hyperactive cells less excitable, the process has been called activity-dependent synaptic scaling, and it is assumed to serve neuronal homeostasis.

According to the hypothesis, sleep would serve primarily to scale synapses down, rather than up. This is because, from a functional point of view, sleep would counteract the net increase in synaptic strength occurring during wakefulness. Moreover, as we shall see below, the mode of brain activity during sleep seems to be ideally suited to promote downscaling rather than upscaling. The direct goal of downscaling during sleep would be the control of synaptic weight, although downscaling would also help, indirectly, to regulate firing levels. Like activity-dependent synaptic scaling, downscaling during slow-wave activity would affect most or all of a neuron's synapses. In this respect, downscaling is conceptually different from LTD, which affects select groups of synapses, or depotentiation, which affects only recently potentiated ones (Kemp and Bashir, 2001). Since downscaling would affect all synapses in a similar manner, it would not require any fine-tuning at the level of the individual synapse. By contrast, selective potentiation or depression of specific synapses would require carefully titrated synaptic activations, which would not be easy to achieve considering that neural activity during sleep is, by and large, intrinsically generated. Despite these differences, we hypothesise that downscaling is likely to use many of the same molecular mechanisms involved in depression/depotentiation and activity-dependent scaling. Substantial evidence indicates that these forms of plasticity depend on the dephosphorylation and subsequent internalisation of α-amino-3-hydroxy-5-methylisoxazole-4-propionic acid (AMPA) receptors, which ultimately leads to a reduction in synaptic efficacy (Turrigiano, 2000; Malinow and Malenka, 2002). Whichever the specific mechanism, the hypothesis is that a generalised synaptic downscaling during sleep ensures the maintenance of balanced synaptic input to cortical neurons. Thus, the homeostasis of sleep and slow waves would both effect and reflect the homeostasis of synapses (Tononi and Cirelli, 2003).

This part of the hypothesis relies on several considerations. As we have seen, the fundamental cellular phenomenon underlying NREM sleep is the slow oscillation, which is thought to organise slow-wave activity in the cortex, and which is seen in virtually every cortical cell recorded intracellularly (Steriade, 2003). The slow oscillation occurs at a frequency that is ideally suited to induce depotentiation/depression in stimulation paradigms, namely, less than 1 Hz (Kemp and Bashir, 2001). Thus, from a frequency perspective alone, slow-wave sleep would be a good candidate for promoting depotentiation/depression.

Several factors could explain why low-frequency activity during sleep might promote depression. For example, changes in calcium dynamics, which are crucial for depression (Kemp and Bashir, 2001), are likely to occur during slow waves. The unique neuromodulatory milieu of NREM sleep — low acetylcholine, norepinephrine, serotonin, and histamine — may also be important, as well as the fact that depression (Sheng and Hyoung, 2003) is prevented by BDNF, which is low in sleep (Cirelli and Tononi, 2000, 2004). The most significant factor promoting downscaling, however, could be the very sequence of depolarisation (up-phase) and hyperpolarisation (down-phase) that characterises slow oscillations at the cellular level (Steriade, 2003). The close temporal pairing between generalised spiking (or depolarisation) at the end of the up-phase and generalised hyperpolarisation at the beginning of the down-phase may indicate to synapses that pre-synaptic input was not effective in driving post-synaptic activity, a key requirement for depression (Kemp and Bashir, 2001). Note that, for downscaling to work properly based on pre-synaptic firing followed by post-synaptic hyperpolarisation, average firing rates during sleep should be reasonably uniform across cortical neurons. Otherwise, the amount of downscaling would be excessively dependent on pre-synaptic firing rates, and it would be difficult to obtain a proportional decrease in the strength of all synapses impinging on a post-synaptic neuron. It is likely that firing rates in the cortex are kept uniform by the existence of several mechanisms of firing homeostasis. Alternatively, depolarisation–hyperpolarisation sequences might be sufficient to trigger downscaling, in which case all synapses impinging on the same post-synaptic neuron would be guaranteed to have an equal opportunity of downscaling. Yet another possibility is that depression may be powerfully triggered by the temporal paring between generalised hyperpolarisation at the end of the down-phase and generalised spiking at the beginning of the up-phase.

Whatever the precise mechanism, an appealing feature of this entire process is that it could be self-limiting. This would be the case if the reduction of slow-wave activity observed macroscopically in the EEG were to correspond to a reduction of slow oscillations at the single-cell level, and thus to a reduction of downscaling. For example, the progressive reduction of synaptic strength due to downscaling would reduce post-synaptic depolarisation, an effect further amplified by the reduced synchronisation of slow oscillations among different cells. As a consequence, sodium-dependent potassium currents that bring about the hyperpolarised phase would be progressively less activated. Eventually, cortical cells would stop alternating between crisp up- and down-phases, and hover instead around an intermediate membrane potential inadequate for downscaling.

A role for NREM sleep in downscaling is compatible with recent molecular evidence. We have seen that during NREM sleep the expression of LTP-related molecules reaches a low level (Cirelli and Tononi, 2000). A nearly exhaustive screening of gene expression in sleeping and awake rats indicates that NREM sleep may be a time during which molecules implicated in depotentiation/depression are selectively upregulated (Cirelli *et al.*, 2004; Cirelli and Tononi, 2004). Such molecules include calcineurin, a phosphatase that dephosphorylates AMPA receptors potentiated during LTP, protein phosphatase I, calmodulin-dependent kinase IV, glutamate receptor δ_2 subunit, FK506 binding protein 12, inositol 1,4,5-trisphosphate receptor, amphiphysin II, and several proteins involved in vesicle recycling. Also, NREM sleep is associated with higher levels of insulin (Simon *et al.*, 1994), which promotes the internalisation of AMPA receptors and LTD (Man *et al.*, 2000). Thus, at least at the molecular level, sleep may not just be unfavourable to synaptic potentiation, but specifically conducive to generalised synaptic depotentiation/depression. More direct tests of this prediction can be envisaged. It is already known that sleep altogether favours dephosphorylation in the brain (Cirelli and Tononi, 1998). One could further measure phosphorylation levels in sleep and wakefulness of residues of the AMPA channel involved in potentiation/depotentiation and depression/dedepression, as well as indices of AMPA receptor internalisation.

Another intriguing indication that NREM sleep may be associated with synaptic downscaling comes from studies of monocular visual deprivation in kittens, a well-known model of cortical plasticity. During a critical period of brain development, occluding one eye when the animal is awake in the light for 6 h greatly reduces the ability of cortical cells to respond to the occluded eye. It is now thought that such plastic reduction is due to LTD of cortical connections related to the deprived eye (Heynen *et al.*, 2003). The plastic depression of responses to the occluded eye can be increased if the animal remains awake in the light, but not in the dark, for six more hours. Remarkably, an equivalent increase in depression can be seen if the animal is allowed to sleep for 6 h in the dark (Frank *et al.*, 2001). This result has been interpreted in terms of sleep-mediated "consolidation," but it could as well be due to sleep-related downscaling.

Further evidence for possible downscaling during sleep comes from multi-unit recordings. Consider, for example, the so-called "reactivation" of hippocampal firing patterns (Wilson and McNaughton, 1994) during large-amplitude irregular activity sleep states (corresponding to slow-wave activity states in the cerebral cortex). Increases in correlated firing patterns during sleep are presumably the consequence of increased synaptic strength between neurons co-activated in familiar waking environments. Such reactivation of correlated firing patterns is often taken as suggestive of sleep-related consolidation (Wilson and McNaughton, 1994). However, the strength of the correlation, and presumably the strength of underlying synapses, actually decays rapidly during sleep (within 30 min; Kudrimoti *et al.*, 1999), in line with the synaptic homeostasis hypothesis (see also Colgin *et al.*, 2004). And of course, to the extent that slow-wave activity in the cerebral cortex reflects the strength of synaptic coupling between neuronal populations, as is postulated by the hypothesis, the exponential decrease of slow-wave activity during sleep at both a global (Borbély and Ackermann, 2000; Vyazovskiy *et al.*, 2004a) and a local level (Huber *et al.*, 2004) would be a strong indication that downscaling is indeed occurring rapidly soon after we enter sleep.

Why should downscaling require sleep? If it is so essential to the energetic budget of neurons, could it not take place during wakefulness, thereby eliminating the need for sleep? While downscaling during wakefulness cannot be ruled out *a priori*, there are several reasons why sleep might be necessary. Perhaps the most important reason is that, in order to determine how much downscaling is needed to maintain synaptic homeostasis, a neuron should be able to assess its total synaptic input in an unbiased manner, which is to say off-line, independent of behavioural requirements. This is difficult to do during wakefulness, as the waking day might be spent in reiterating certain behavioural tasks, so that certain neural circuits are strongly and repeatedly activated. Based on high average synaptic input, neurons partaking in such circuits would have to conclude that they need a much heavier dose of downscaling that they actually do. During sleep, by contrast, neural activity occurs spontaneously and off-line, virtually disconnected from behavioural requirements. This spontaneous activity is likely to reflect synaptic strength rather than outside influences. In this way, a neuron's synaptic input would represent an unbiased estimate of the synaptic strength impinging on it, and could downscale appropriately. Another reason why downscaling might best occur during sleep is that, at the molecular level, generalised changes in synaptic strength may be incompatible with the need to selectively increase the strength of certain synapses, as is the case during learning. And of course, to the extent that downscaling is promoted by repetitive depolarisation–hyperpolarisation sequences, these are perfectly compatible with sleep but would seriously interfere with behaviour if they were to occur during wakefulness.

The Functional Advantages of Synaptic Downscaling during Sleep

According to the hypothesis, synaptic downscaling during sleep would offer several benefits. Perhaps the most important one is in terms of energy expenditure. As mentioned above, about 40% of energy requirements of the grey matter of the cerebral cortex — by far the most metabolically expensive tissue in the body — are due to neuronal repolarisation following post-synaptic potentials. The higher the synaptic weight impinging on a neuron, the higher this portion of the energy budget. Moreover, increased synaptic weight is thought to lead to increased average firing rates (Pavlides and Winson, 1989; Hirase *et al.*, 2001), and spikes in turn are responsible for another 40% of the grey matter energy budget. Therefore, it would seem energetically prohibitive for the brain to let synaptic weight grow without checks as a result of waking plasticity. Indeed, if the PET data of Braun *et al.* (1997) offer any indication, it would seem that after just one waking day energy expenditure grows by as much as 18%. Sleep, and the accompanying downscaling of synapses, would then be needed to interrupt the growth of synaptic strength associated with waking and prevent synaptic overload. Moreover, downscaling during sleep would recalibrate cortical circuits, yielding a brain that would still keep trace of previous waking experiences while being energetically efficient. In this sense, sleep would be the price we have to pay for plasticity during wakefulness.

Another benefit of synaptic downscaling during sleep would be in terms of space requirements. Synaptic strengthening is thought to be accompanied by morphological changes, including increased size of terminal boutons and spines, and synapses may even grow in number (Knott *et al.*, 2002; Trachtenberg *et al.*, 2002). But space is a precious commodity in the brain, and even minuscule increases in volume are extremely dangerous. Thus, the limitations of the brain's real estate require tools to keep synaptic weight in check.

It is also likely that, due to the combined energy and space costs of uninterrupted synaptic plasticity, the ability of the brain to acquire new information would rapidly grind to a halt in the absence of downscaling. In this sense, sleep would not only be the price we have to pay for plasticity the previous day, but also an investment to be able to learn afresh the next day. Indeed, in certain brain areas, such as the hippocampus, radical synaptic downscaling may be necessary to clean the slate and rapidly adapt to a new environment. Another benefit of downscaling with a threshold would be to promote synaptic competition, which may be especially important during development, when exuberant synaptic growth is known to occur. For example, connections between strongly correlated neurons would survive, while others may be eliminated (Cohen-Cory, 2002). In the adult, downscaling could benefit learning in yet another way by increasing signal-to-noise ratios in the relevant brain circuits. To illustrate, consider again the visuomotor task discussed in connection with local slow-wave homeostasis. The neural substrates of many forms of visuomotor learning are thought to be changes in synaptic strength within circuits in motor and parietal areas. PET studies indicate that, during visuomotor learning, brain activation is at first diffuse and bilateral, and only after further practice does it converge upon more restricted foci of cortical activation (Ghilardi *et al.*, 2000). This pattern is not surprising, since visuomotor learning is an incremental process, during which early executions are tentative and inaccurate, and only slowly converge upon smooth, correct trajectories. What is noteworthy is that at any given execution, local circuits have no way of knowing which synapses and neurons were contributing to correct or incorrect aspects of the movement. Thus, while synapses contributing to a correct movement will become progressively more efficacious (signal), other synapses contributing to erroneous or imperfect movements will also be potentiated (noise; in Figure 2, this is indicated by the appearance, in addition to the appropriately strengthened red synapse with a weight of 150, of a small red synapse with a weight of 5).

It is here that synaptic downscaling during sleep can play a role. According to the hypothesis, during sleep the strength of each synapse would decrease by a proportional amount, until the total amount of synaptic weight impinging on each neuron returns to a baseline level. Provided there is a threshold below which synapses become ineffective or silent, synapses contributing to the noise, being on average weaker than those contributing to the signal, would cease to interfere in the execution, and the signal-to-noise ratios would increase (in Figure 2, this is indicated by the disappearance during sleep of the red synapse with a weight of 5). Indeed, just as predicted, when subjects were tested after sleep following the rotation adaptation task, they showed a significant enhancement of their performance, which was absent in subjects who were trained in the morning and were re-tested after 8 h of wakefulness. Moreover, performance enhancement after sleep was strongly correlated with the increase in slow-wave activity in the right parietal areas involved in the task. Finally, the strongest correlation (0.9) was with the increase of signal-to-noise ratios during learning.

Other groups have recently found that sleep can indeed enhance performance in certain tasks (Karni *et al.*, 1994; Stickgold *et al.*, 2000; Fisher *et al.*, 2002; Mednick *et al.*, 2002; Walker *et al.*, 2002; Fenn *et al.*, 2003; Maquet *et al.*, 2003). These studies generally assume that sleep may enhance performance by "replaying" patterns of neural activity obtained during training in wakefulness. It is frequently suggested that such replay may actually potentiate synapses (e.g., Sejnowsky and Destexhe, 2000; Steriade and Timofeev, 2003). The synaptic homeostasis hypothesis, by contrast, predicts that sleep may enhance performance by global downscaling, thanks to the postulated increase in signal-to-noise ratios. This possibility is not only more economical (and energy efficient), but it also has the important advantage of not requiring great fidelity in sleep replays. Indeed, the fidelity of such replays appears to be so low (Ribeiro *et al.*, 2004) that, if LTP-like changes were not turned off during sleep, the brain would run a serious risk of "learning" correlations that are not present in the real world, but only in its dreams (Cirelli *et al.*, 1996; Tononi and Cirelli, 2001). Of course, some kind of consolidation of recently strengthened synapses, yielding a competitive advantage, is not mutually exclusive with the occurrence of overall downscaling.

REM Sleep

To the extent that the synaptic homeostasis hypothesis applies to NREM sleep, it is inevitable to ask what it might suggest concerning REM sleep. Indeed, for a long time REM sleep has been the privileged target of new ideas about the functions of sleep, especially of ideas related to memory or synaptic plasticity. Thus, it has been suggested that REM sleep might serve to develop, consolidate, maintain, or even erase synaptic traces.

Nevertheless, with the exception of a role in neuronal maturation during development, the evidence is not strong (Rechtschaffen, 1998; Siegel, 2001). An intriguing possibility is that REM sleep could be achieving, by different means, an effect partly similar to the one postulated here for NREM sleep. This is suggested by the fact that NREM and REM sleep to some extent can substitute for each other (Borbély and Ackermann, 2000). Moreover, an increase in NREM often produces a decrease in REM sleep, and vice versa (Borbély and Ackermann, 2000). This inverse relationship is often considered to represent a reciprocal inhibition or antagonism between the two different kinds of sleep, but it could also mean that they tend to satisfy the same need. An extreme example may be offered by long-term sleep deprivation in rats (Rechtschaffen *et al.*, 1999). After days of total sleep deprivation, the initial sleep rebound is constituted predominantly by REM sleep, and it is followed only later by periods of NREM sleep. The episodes of rebound REM sleep are extraordinarily long, lasting occasionally even 30–40 min, against a normal average of 2 min. This massive REM sleep rebound after long-term sleep deprivation is a puzzling phenomenon: why should an animal, exhausted and on the brink of death, enter a long-lasting state of cerebral hyperactivity? REM sleep rebound after forced wakefulness is also problematic for models of sleep regulation according to which process S can only decrease during NREM sleep. Indeed, when the rebound of REM abates and NREM sleep becomes more prevalent, slow-wave activity is much lower than one would expect. One could of course suggest some kind of "inhibitory" action of REM sleep on process S, but it seems more parsimonious to suggest that REM sleep may be performing a similar function as NREM sleep with respect to process S, i.e., according to the hypothesis, synaptic downscaling. It may even be that REM sleep may be more efficient than NREM sleep at producing downscaling, albeit less precise. This would account for the predominance of REM sleep in sleep rebound after sleep deprivation, and for the high proportion of REM sleep in very young animals, where presumably synaptic homeostasis needs to counteract bulk synaptic growth and imbalances, and be less concerned with preserving acquired memories. Indeed, a role of REM sleep in synaptic downscaling would be consistent with its prominence *in utero*, whereas such prominence would be hard to explain if REM sleep were promoting memory consolidation, at a time when there is still little, if anything, to remember.

What are the mechanisms by which REM sleep could produce synaptic downscaling? Little is known about molecular changes or synaptic modifications that may be specific to REM sleep. We know, however, that as in NREM sleep, the brain is virtually disconnected from the environment, and the noradrenergic (and serotonergic) system is silent. This suggests that, like NREM sleep, REM sleep may be a time during which synaptic activation may be dissociated from the acquisition of new information. On the other hand, the neuromodulatory milieu is not identical to that of NREM sleep; the cholinergic system, for example, is strongly activated, and spontaneous firing levels are at least as high, if not higher than, in quiet wakefulness. Finally, in several species there are phasic, random bursts of neural activity such as ponto-genito-occipital (PGO) waves. An interesting possibility is that, in the appropriate neuromodulatory milieu of REM sleep, spontaneous activity may produce a net downscaling effect. Support for this possibility comes from work in the developing *Xenopus* retinotectal system (Cohen-Cory, 2002; Zhou *et al.*, 2003), where activity-dependent synaptic modifications induced by patterned neural activity and visual stimuli are rapidly reversed by subsequent exposure to spontaneous or random activity. This reversal depends on the burst spiking and activation of N-methyl-D-aspartate (NMDA) glutamate receptors. Further support for this possibility comes from studies of spike-timing-dependent synaptic plasticity (Song *et al.*, 2000; Song and Abbott, 2001). In spike-timing-dependent synaptic plasticity, pre-synaptic spikes arriving slightly before post-synaptic firing produce synaptic potentiation, whereas random pre- and post-synaptic action potentials result in net synaptic depression. Thus, random firing during REM sleep could produce results similar to a net downscaling, with associated metabolic and other benefits similar to those produced by NREM sleep. Moreover, if synapses among strongly correlated neurons were at a competitive advantage because of reduced depression (or increased potentiation), REM sleep could be especially effective at promoting synaptic competition and at increasing signal-to-noise ratios. This possibility would agree well with the regular alternation between NREM and REM sleep (cf., Giuditta *et al.*, 1995) and the reported cooperativeness between the two stages of sleep in certain procedural tasks (Stickgold *et al.*, 2001). Moreover, it would agree with the important role played by spontaneous activity in the development of neural connectivity (Cohen-Cory, 2002).

Acknowledgment

This work was supported by the National Institute of Mental Health (RO1-MH65135).

References

Aeschbach, D., Matthews, J.R., Postolache, T.T., Jackson, M.A., Giesen, H.A., and Wehr, T.A. (1997). Dynamics of the human EEG during prolonged wakefulness: evidence for frequency-specific circadian and homeostatic influences. *Neurosci. Lett.*, 239: 121–124.

Amzica, F. and Steriade, M. (1995). Disconnection of intracortical synaptic linkages disrupts synchronization of a slow oscillation. *J. Neurosci.*, 15: 4658–4677.

Aston-Jones, G. and Bloom, F. (1981). Activity of norepinephrine-containing locus coeruleus neurons in behaving rats anticipates fluctuations in the sleep-waking cycle. *J. Neurosci.*, 1: 876–886.

Attwell, D. and Laughlin, S.B. (2001). An energy budget for signaling in the grey matter of the brain. *J. Cereb. Blood Flow Metab.*, 21: 1133–1145.

Bazhenov, M., Timofeev, I., Steriade, M., and Sejnowski, T.J. (2002). Model of thalamocortical slow-wave sleep oscillations and transitions to activated states. *J. Neurosci.*, 22: 8691–8704.

Borbély, A.A. (1982). A two process model of sleep regulation. *Hum. Neurobiol.*, 1: 195–204.

Borbély, A.A. (2001). From slow-waves to sleep homeostasis: new perspectives. *Arch. Ital. Biol.*, 139: 53–61.

Borbély, A.A. and Ackermann, P. (2000). Sleep homeostasis and models of sleep regulation. In: Kryger, M.H., Roth, T., and Dement, W.C. (Eds.). *Principles and Practice of Sleep Medicine*. New York: Raven Press, pp. 377–390.

Borbély, A.A., Tobler, I., and Hanagasioglu, M. (1984). Effect of sleep deprivation on sleep and EEG power spectra in the rat. *Behav. Brain Res.*, 14: 171–182.

Braun, A.R., Balkin, T.J., Wesenten, N.J., Carson, R.E., Varga, M., Baldwin, P., Selbie, S., Belenky, G., and Herscovitch, P. (1997). Regional cerebral blood flow throughout the sleep-wake cycle. An H2(15)O PET study. *Brain*, 120: 1173–1197.

Cajochen, C., Foy, R., and Dijk, D.J. (1999). Frontal predominance of a relative increase in sleep delta and theta EEG activity after sleep loss in humans. *Sleep Res.*, 2: 65–69 (on-line).

Cajochen, C., Knoblauch, V., Krauchi, K., Renz, C., and Wirz-Justice, A. (2001). Dynamics of frontal EEG activity, sleepiness and body temperature under high and low sleep pressure. *Neuroreport*, 12: 2277–2281.

Cirelli, C., Huber, R., Gopalakrishnan, A., Southard, T.L., and Tononi, G. (2005). Locus ceruleus control of slow-wave homeostasis. *J. Neurosci.*, 25(18): 4503–4511.

Cirelli, C. and Tononi, G. (2000). Differential expression of plasticity-related genes in waking and sleep and their regulation by the noradrenergic system. *J. Neurosci.*, 20: 9187–9194.

Cirelli, C. and Tononi, G. (2004). Locus ceruleus control of state-dependent gene expression. *J. Neurosci.*, 24: 5410–5419.

Cirelli, C., Pompeiano, M., and Tononi, G. (1996). Neuronal gene expression in the waking state: a role for the locus coeruleus. *Science*, 274: 1211–1215.

Cirelli, C., Gutierrez, C.M., and Tononi, G. (2004). Extensive and divergent effects of sleep and wakefulness on brain gene expression. *Neuron*, 41: 35–43.

Cohen-Cory, S. (2002). The developing synapse: construction and modulation of synaptic structures and circuits. *Science*, 298: 770–776.

Colgin, L.L., Kubota, D., Jia, Y., Rex, C.S., and Lynch, G. (2004). Long-term potentiation is impaired in rat hippocampal slices that produce spontaneous sharp waves. *J. Physiol.*, 558: 953–961.

Compte, A., Sanchez-Vives, M.V., McCormick, D.A., and Wang, X.J. (2003). Cellular and network mechanisms of slow oscillatory activity (<1 Hz) and wave propagations in a cortical network model. *J. Neurophysiol.*, 89: 2707–2725.

Desai, N.S., Cudmore, R.H., Nelson, S.B., and Turrigiano, G.G. (2002). Critical periods for experience-dependent synaptic scaling in visual cortex. *Nat. Neurosci.*, 5: 783–789.

Feinberg, I. (1982). Schizophrenia: caused by a fault in programmed synaptic elimination during adolescence? *J. Psychiatr. Res.*, 17: 319–334.

Fenn, K.M., Nusbaum, H.C., and Margoliash, D. (2003). Consolidation during sleep of perceptual learning of spoken language. *Nature*, 425: 614–616.

Finelli, L.A., Baumann, H., Borbély, A.A., and Ackermann, P. (2000). Dual electroencephalogram markers of human sleep homeostasis: correlation between theta activity in waking and slow-wave activity in sleep. *Neuroscience*, 101: 523–529.

Fischer, S., Hallschmid, M., Elsner, A.L., and Born, J. (2002). Sleep forms memory for finger skills. *Proc. Natl. Acad. Sci. USA*, 99: 11987–11991.

Frank, M.G., Issa, N.P., and Stryker, M.P. (2001). Sleep enhances plasticity in the developing visual cortex. *Neuron*, 30: 275–287.

Gais, S., Plihal, W., Wagner, U., and Born, J. (2000). Early sleep triggers memory for early visual discrimination skills. *Nat. Neurosci.*, 3: 1335–1339.

Ghilardi, M., Ghez, C., Dhawan, V., Moeller, J., Mentis, M., Nakamura, T., Antonini, A., and Eidelberg, D. (2000). Patterns of regional brain activation associated with different forms of motor learning. *Brain Res.*, 871: 127–145.

Giuditta, A., Ambrosini, M.V., Montagnese, P., Mandile, P., Cotugno, M., Grassi, Z.G., and Vescia, S. (1995). The sequential hypothesis of the function of sleep. *Behav. Brain Res.*, 69: 157–166.

Grutzendler, J., Kasthuri, N., and Gan, W.B. (2002). Long-term dendritic spine stability in the adult cortex. *Nature*, 420: 812–816.

Gu, Q. (2002). Neuromodulatory transmitter systems in the cortex and their role in cortical plasticity. *Neuroscience*, 111: 815–835.

Heynen, A.J., Yoon, B.J., Liu, C.H., Chung, H.J., Huganir, R.L., and Bear, M.F. (2003). Molecular mechanism for loss of visual cortical responsiveness following brief monocular deprivation. *Nat. Neurosci.*, 6: 854–862.

Hirase, H., Leinekugel, X., Czurko, A., Csicsvari, J., and Buzsaki, G. (2001). Firing rates of hippocampal neurons are preserved during subsequent sleep episodes and modified by novel awake experience. *Proc. Natl. Acad. Sci. USA*, 98: 9386–9390.

Hobson, J.A., McCarley, R.W., and Wyzinski, P.W. (1975). Sleep cycle oscillation: reciprocal discharge by two brainstem neuronal groups. *Science*, 189: 55–58.

Horne, J. (1992). Human slow-wave sleep and the cerebral cortex. *J. Sleep Res.*, 1: 122–124.

Huber, R., Deboer, T., and Tobler, I. (2000). Effects of sleep deprivation on sleep and sleep EEG in three mouse strains: empirical data and simulations. *Brain Res.*, 857: 8–19.

Huber, R., Ghilardi, M.F., Massimini, M., and Tononi, G. (2004). Local sleep and learning. *Nature*, 430: 78–81.

Karni, A., Tanne, D., Rubenstein, B.S., Askenasy, J.J., and Sagi, D. (1994). Dependence on REM sleep of overnight improvement of a perceptual skill. *Science*, 265: 679–682.

Kattler, H., Dijk, D.J., and Borbély, A.A. (1994). Effect of unilateral somatosensory stimulation prior to sleep on the sleep EEG in humans. *J. Sleep Res.*, 3: 159–164.

Kelly, M.P. and Deadwyler, S.A. (2003). Experience-dependent regulation of the immediate-early gene arc differs across brain regions. *J. Neurosci.*, 23: 6443–6451.

Kemp, N. and Bashir, Z.I. (2001). Long-term depression: a cascade of induction and expression mechanisms. *Prog. Neurobiol.*, 65: 339–365.

Klintsova, A.Y. and Greenough, W.T. (1999). Synaptic plasticity in cortical systems. *Curr. Opin. Neurobiol.*, 9: 203–208.

Knott, G.W., Quairiaux, C., Genoud, C., and Welker, E. (2002). Formation of dendritic spines with GABAergic synapses induced by whisker stimulation in adult mice. *Neuron*, 34: 265–273.

Kudrimoti, H.S., Barnes, C.A., and McNaughton, B.L. (1999). Reactivation of hippocampal cell assemblies: effects of behavioral state, experience, and EEG dynamics. *J. Neurosci.*, 19: 4090–4101.

Lennie, P. (2003). The cost of cortical computation. *Curr. Biol.*, 13: 493–497.

Malinow, R. and Malenka, R.C. (2002). AMPA receptor trafficking and synaptic plasticity. *Annu. Rev. Neurosci.*, 25: 103–126.

Man, H.Y., Lin, J.W., Ju, W.H., Ahmadian, G., Liu, L., Becker, L.E., Sheng, M., and Wang, Y.T. (2000). Regulation of AMPA receptor-mediated synaptic transmission by clathrin-dependent receptor internalization. *Neuron*, 25: 649–662.

Maquet, P., Schwartz, S., Passingham, R., and Frith, C. (2003). Sleep-related consolidation of a visuomotor skill: brain mechanisms as assessed by functional magnetic resonance imaging. *J. Neurosci.*, 23: 1432–1440.

Mednick, S.C., Nakayama, K., Cantero, J.L., Atienza, M., Levin, A.A., Pathak, N., and Stickgold, R. (2002). The restorative effect of naps on perceptual deterioration. *Nat. Neurosci.*, 5: 677–681.

Meerlo, P., de Bruin, E.A., Strijkstra, A.M., and Daan, S. (2001). A social conflict increases EEG slow-wave activity during subsequent sleep. *Physiol. Behav.*, 73: 331–335.

Miller, K.D. and MacKay, D.J.C. (1994). The role of constraints in Hebbian learning. *Neural Comput.*, 6: 100–126.

Miyamoto, H., Katagiri, H., and Hensch, T. (2003). Experience-dependent slow-wave sleep development. *Nat. Neurosci.*, 6: 553–554.

Pavlides, C. and Winson, J. (1989). Influences of hippocampal place cell firing in the awake state on the activity of these cells during subsequent sleep episodes. *J. Neurosci.*, 9: 2907–2918.

Rechtschaffen, A. (1998). Current perspectives on the function of sleep. *Perspect. Biol. Med.*, 41: 359–390.

Rechtschaffen, A., Bergmann, B.M., Gilliland, M.A., and Bauer, K. (1999). Effects of method, duration, and sleep stage on rebounds from sleep deprivation in the rat. *Sleep*, 22: 11–31.

Ribeiro, S., Gervasoni, D., Soares, E.S., Zhou, Y., Lin, S.C., Pantoja, J., Lavine, M., and Nicolelis, M.A. (2004). Long-lasting novelty-induced neuronal reverberation during slow-wave sleep in multiple forebrain areas. *PLoS. Biol.*, 2: E24.

Robbins, T.W. and Everitt, B.J. (1995). Central norepinephrine neurons and behaviour. In: Bloom, F.E. and Kupfer, D.J. (Eds.). *Psychopharmacology: The Fourth Generation of Progress.* New York: Raven Press, pp. 363–372.

Rothman, D.L., Behar, K.L., Hyder, F., and Shulman, R.G. (2003). *In vivo* NMR studies of the glutamate neurotransmitter flux and neuroenergetics: implications for brain function. *Annu. Rev. Physiol.*, 65: 401–427.

Sejnowski, T.J. and Destexhe, A. (2000). Why do we sleep? *Brain Res.*, 886: 208–223.

Siegel, J.M. (2001). The REM sleep-memory consolidation hypothesis. *Science*, 294: 1058–1063.

Silva, A.J. (2003). Molecular and cellular cognitive studies of the role of synaptic plasticity in memory. *J. Neurobiol.*, 54: 224–237.

Simon, C., Brandenberger, G., Saini, J., Ehrhart, J., and Follenius, M. (1994). Slow oscillations of plasma glucose and insulin secretion rate are amplified during sleep in humans under continuous enteral nutrition. *Sleep*, 17: 333–338.

Sjostrom, P.J., Turrigiano, G.G., and Nelson, S.B. (2001). Rate, timing, and cooperativity jointly determine cortical synaptic plasticity. *Neuron*, 32: 1149–1164.

Song, S. and Abbott, L.F. (2001). Cortical development and remapping through spike timing-dependent plasticity. *Neuron*, 32: 339–350.

Song, S., Miller, K.D., and Abbott, L.F. (2000). Competitive Hebbian learning through spike-timing-dependent synaptic plasticity. *Nat. Neurosci.*, 3: 919–926.

Steriade, M. (2003). The corticothalamic system in sleep. *Front. Biosci.*, 8: 878–899.

Steriade, M. and Timofeev, I. (2003). Neuronal plasticity in thalamocortical networks during sleep and waking oscillations. *Neuron*, 37: 563–576.

Stickgold, R., Hobson, J.A., Fosse, R., and Fosse, M. (2001). Sleep, learning, and dreams: off-line memory reprocessing. *Science*, 294: 1052–1057.

Stickgold, R., Whidbee, D., Schirmer, B., Patel, V., and Hobson, J.A. (2000). Visual discrimination task improvement: a multi-step process occurring during sleep. *J. Cogn. Neurosci.*, 12: 246–254.

Tononi, G. and Cirelli, C. (2001). Some considerations on sleep and neural plasticity. *Arch. Ital. Biol.*, 139: 221–241.

Tononi, G. and Cirelli, C. (2003). Sleep and synaptic homeostasis: a hypothesis. *Brain Res. Bull.*, 62: 143–150.

Trachtenberg, J.T., Chen, B.E., Knott, G.W., Feng, G., Sanes, J.R., Welker, E., and Svoboda, K. (2002). Long-term *in vivo* imaging of experience-dependent synaptic plasticity in adult cortex. *Nature*, 420: 788–794.

Turrigiano, G.G. (1999). Homeostatic plasticity in neuronal networks: the more things change, the more they stay the same. *Trends Neurosci.*, 22: 221–227.

Turrigiáno, G.G. (2000). AMPA receptors unbound: membrane cycling and synaptic plasticity. *Neuron*, 26: 5–8.

Vyazovskiy, V., Borbély, A.A., and Tobler, I. (2000). Unilateral vibrissae stimulation during waking induces interhemispheric EEG asymmetry during subsequent sleep in the rat. *J. Sleep Res.*, 9: 367–371.

Vyazovskiy, V.V., Borbély, A.A., and Tobler, I. (2002). Interhemispheric sleep EEG asymmetry in the rat is enhanced by sleep deprivation. *J. Neurophysiol.*, 88: 2280–2286.

Vyazovskiy, V., Ackermann, P., Borbély, A.A., and Tobler, I. (2004a). Interhemispheric coherence of the sleep electroencephalogram in mice with congenital callosal dysgenesis. *Neuroscience*, 124: 481–488.

Vyazovskiy, V., Welker, E., Fritschy, J., and Tobler, I. (2004b). Regional pattern of metabolic activation is reflected in the sleep EEG after sleep deprivation combined with unilateral whisker stimulation in mice. *Eur. J. Neurosci.*, 20: 1363–1370.

Walker, M.P., Brakefield, T., Morgan, A., Hobson, J.A., and Stickgold, R. (2002). Practice with sleep makes perfect: sleep-dependent motor skill learning. *Neuron*, 35: 205–211.

Wallace, C.S., Withers, G.S., Weiler, I.J., George, J.M., Clayton, D.F., and Greenough, W.T. (1995). Correspondence between sites of NGFI-A induction and sites of morphological plasticity following exposure to environmental complexity. *Mol. Brain Res.*, 32: 211–220.

Walling, S.G. and Harley, C.W. (2004). Locus ceruleus activation initiates delayed synaptic potentiation of perforant path input to the dentate gyrus in awake rats: a novel beta-adrenergic- and protein synthesis-dependent mammalian plasticity mechanism. *J. Neurosci.*, 24: 598–604.

Wilson, M.A. and McNaughton, B.L. (1994). Reactivation of hippocampal ensemble memories during sleep. *Science*, 265: 676–679.

Ying, S.W., Futter, M., Rosenblum, K., Webber, M.J., Hunt, S.P., Bliss, T.V., and Bramham, C.R. (2002). Brain-derived neurotrophic factor induces long-term potentiation in intact adult hippocampus: requirement for ERK activation coupled to CREB and upregulation of arc synthesis. *J. Neurosci.*, 22: 1532–1540.

Zhou, Q., Tao, H.W., and Poo, M.M. (2003). Reversal and stabilization of synaptic modifications in a developing visual system. *Science*, 300: 1953–1957.

Chapter 5

ELECTROENCEPHALOGRAPHY, POLYSOMNOGRAPHY, AND OTHER SLEEP RECORDING SYSTEMS

Rosa Peraita-Adrados[1]

Sleep recording in the laboratory is performed by polygraphic recording, or polysomnogram, which involves simultaneous recording of different physiological signals and enables us to evaluate sleep-related disorders. The technique is referred to as polysomnography (PSG) or by a more simple term such as sleep study. Today, it is part of the routine work-up and is standardised in all sleep laboratories. PSG is the gold standard in different sleep conditions although it should be limited to those patients with a suitable clinical indication.

In this chapter, we shall look first at the classic electroencephalography (EEG), which is the basic method for studying sleep, then at the PSG recording technique, its analysis, and interpretation. Furthermore, we shall examine other types of ambulatory recording systems based on the use of simplified methods.

Other space–time descriptions of sleep states are being carried out with the development of new techniques such as magneto-encephalography or imaging: cerebral mapping, PET, or functional MRI, which will not be examined in this chapter.

---

[1]mperaita.hgugm@salud.madrid.org

Classic EEG

The development of the electroencephalographic technique by Hans Berger
in the 1930s enables us to record the electrical activity of the brain on the
surface of the scalp (Berger, 1929).

The activity of the neurons of the cerebral cortex generates sufficient
electrical fields to be captured by electrodes placed on the scalp and connected
to a polygraph, that is, to an amplifier connected to a paper recorder or to a
digital PC. These amplified and filtered signals make up the EEG recording.

Electrodes and derivations

When the EEG is recorded, the electrodes are positioned on the scalp
according to Jasper's (1958) "10–20" system of electrode placement
recommended by the International Federation of Societies for Electroencephalography and Clinical Neurophysiology (1983) (Figure 1). Using
this standardised system, a total of 21 electrodes are fixed to the
scalp on the left and right hemispheres: Fp (pre-frontal), F (frontal),
C (central), P (parietal), T (temporal: anterior, mid-temporal, posterior),
and O (occipital); in addition, three electrodes are placed on the mid-line

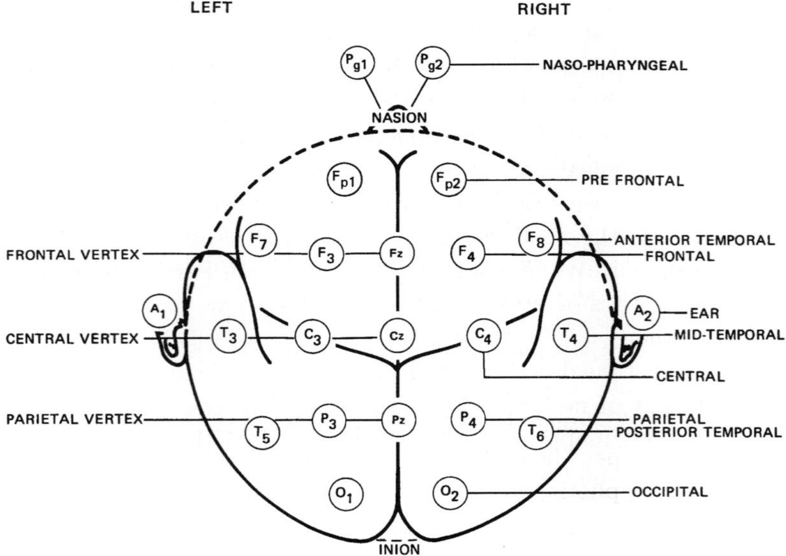

Figure 1. The international 10–20 system indicates the positions of the electrodes to be
ascertained by accurate measurement of the head. P_{g1} and P_{g2} are optional electrodes
to record mild-temporal lobe activity in epileptic patients.

F_Z (frontal), C_Z (vertex), and P_Z (parietal) and two electrodes are placed on the ear lobe or contralateral mastoid (A1 and A2), which are used as referential electrodes. This setting enables us to carry out a detailed exploration of the activity of all the regions of the brain.

Two types of electrodes are used for EEG recording: active electrodes, which detect the neuronal activity of the underlying cerebral area, and reference electrodes, which serve as a reference point allowing variations in the potential of an active electrode to be observed. A lead that records the difference in potential between two electrodes is a bipolar lead; one which records the difference in potential between an active electrode and a reference electrode is a referential lead. Each group of leads recorded simultaneously is known as a montage. A montage formed by bipolar leads is a bipolar montage, which can follow the anterior–posterior or transversal line of the head. A referential montage is composed of referential leads.

Brain rhythms

Brain activity is classified into four bands of frequencies corresponding to different brain rhythms, defined by their frequency in hertz and by their amplitude in microvolts:

- *Alpha rhythm*: frequency between 8 and 14 Hz and amplitude <50 mV, starting in the posterior regions of the brain and associated with the state of rest or quiet wakefulness with the eyes closed
- *Beta rhythm*: frequency >13 Hz and amplitude <30 mV, mainly in the anterior regions of the brain, present in several sleep phases
- *Theta rhythm*: frequency from 4 to 8 Hz and low amplitude, which appears in states of brain activation
- *Delta rhythm*: frequency <4 Hz and wide amplitude, which is observed in all the regions of the brain during slow-wave sleep.

This basal brain activity, which changes during sleep stages, is superimposed by different transient grapho-elements, as we shall see below.

The baseline EEG should contain at least 20 min of artefact-free recording and periods when the eyes are opened and closed. Other stimuli such as hyperventilation, photic, and sleep should be recorded whenever possible.

Sleep stages

In the last century, Bremer (1935) was the first to show changes in the electrical activity of the brain during sleep. Loomis *et al.* (1937) observed that this activity shows typical changes during sleep and classified five stages of sleep. Moruzzi and Magoun (1949) show that sleep is an active physiological process with modifications of the electrical activity of the brain dependent on specific mechanisms and from the brainstem nuclei and areas extending from the medulla to the posterior diencephalon. The discovery of rapid eye movements (REM) by Aserinsky and Kleitman (1953) marked a new stage in sleep research. These authors observed rapid and binocular eye movements every 90 min under the eyelids of sleeping children. In later studies, Dement and Kleitman (1957) showed that this stage was associated with dreamings. Jouvet and Michel (1959) realised that the EEG of an animal which seemed to be sleeping deeply showed low-voltage fast activity, and tonic activity of the neck muscles had completely disappeared. Two types of sleep were thus distinguished: paradoxical or with REM, muscular atonia and oniric mental activity and non-REM.

Polysomnography

Polysomnographic sleep monitoring demands a rigorous and complex methodology which simultaneously uses techniques as varied as neurophysiology or respiratory physiology. This type of examination provides indispensable information for diagnosing sleep disorders (Besset, 2003).

A sleep recording is obtained in a suitable laboratory. The bedroom of the laboratory is a standard bedroom which should be soundproofed and with well-regulated lighting, temperature, and humidity. It has a video camera and a closed-circuit television. This audio/video monitoring is mandatory for assessment of the patient's body position, breathing noises, body and limb movements, for characterisation of arousal disorders and suspected nocturnal seizures. Audio/video and PSG should be synchronised (VPSG) (Ramos Platón, 1996).

In order to define the phases of sleep, it is necessary to obtain a recording of the electrical activity in the EEG, muscle tone (EMG), and electro-oculography (EOG) according to the guidelines of the manual published by Rechtschaffen and Kales (1968).

Electroencephalography

In order to understand the maturation of the stages of sleep and establish their differences, it is necessary to record the electrical activity of the brain by electroencephalogram. The electrode types, methods of application, and other recommendations stated in the American EEG Society (1994) guidelines in EEG, should be followed.

According to Rechtschaffen and Kales' recommendation, the EEG is usually recorded with only two electrodes situated on the central regions of both hemispheres using the lobe of the contralateral ear as a reference (C3–A2 and C4–A1). However, we would recommend additional channels (5–13), which are required to permit adequate assessment of other EEG characteristics (focal or generalised interictal and/or ictal paroxysmal activity; background asymmetries, drugs effects, etc.).

Recordings can be performed using amplifiers with a sensitivity of 7.5–10 mm for a 50-mV signal with a time constant setting at 0.3 s (high-pass). It comprises a high-frequency (low-pass) 0.5-Hz filter. Filters of 60–75 Hz are recommended as well as 50- to 60-Hz rejecter active filters.

Electrooculography

The EOG recording is essential for the identification of the REM stage. The electrodes, preferably self-adhesive, are situated at the external canthus of each eye or above and below each eye in order to record the horizontal or vertical movements. Changes in voltage are thus detected when the eye rotates since the polarity of the retina is negative with respect to the cornea. Each of the electrodes is connected to the same referential electrode in such a way that the eye movements appear on the trace as an out-of-phase voltage deflection and can easily be distinguished from electrical brain activity (slow waves and K complexes).

When the patient is falling asleep, slow and oscillating eye movements are observed. During the REM stage there are rapid and conjugate eye movements in very characteristic bursts. Recordings can be performed using standard EEG amplifiers with a time constant setting at 0.3 s and minimum gain of 7.5 μV/mm. The high-frequency filter must be limited to 15 Hz.

Muscle Tone

The EMG of the antigravitory muscles is essential for identifying REM characterised by muscular atonia. In humans, two surface electrodes separated by 2 cm are applied to the submental or chin muscles for determining the level of muscle tone. Since tonic EMG activity decreases even during slow-wave sleep, high gains should be used, 20 mm for a 50-mV signal or higher to provide an adequate baseline EMG level during wakefulness. The recording is obtained through standard EEG amplifiers with an adjusted time constant of at least 0.03 s and a low-pass filter set at 120 Hz to record all the muscular signals.

Sleep Stages

From a functional perspective, sleep and wakefulness are distinguished on the continuum of wakefulness levels. The visual identification of sleep stages is based on the changes observed at EEG, EOG, and EMG levels during each epoch. The epoch, an arbitrarily chosen interval of time, is the standard 30 s of the polysomnogram. This is a simplified description of sleep, based on criteria established in adults by Rechtschaffen and Kales, and in children by Anders *et al.* (1971). Automatic sleep analysis methods, which are constantly being developed and evaluated, have not yet replaced visual analysis, and much work will be needed before a new, more complex classification emerges, based on the principles of signal analysis.

Sleep stages are routinely scored from 0 to 5. Stages 0 and 5 are generally referred to as wakefulness and REM sleep, respectively. The progressive numbering of stages from 1 to 4 corresponds to the relative depth of sleep, that is, stage 4 is considered to be deeper than stage 1.

Wakefulness

EEG: It is taken during active wakefulness, with the eyes open, and is characterised by low-voltage, mixed frequency activity. Quiet wakefulness, with the eyes closed, corresponds to alpha activity, mainly in the parieto-occipital regions. Its reactivity is characteristic and disappears with visual external sensory stimuli or with intense mental activity.

EOG: The control of eye movements is voluntary and involves rapid deflections and eye blinks.

EMG: Characterised by a variable-amplitude tonic activity depending on the level of muscular relaxation, interspersed with phasic increases in association with voluntary movements.

Stage 1

The transition from wakefulness to sleep. This stage can also be observed during the night after transitory awakenings.

EEG: This slows down gradually and the alpha rhythm spreads to anterior regions; afterwards it is fragmented and substituted by a theta activity of 4–7 Hz. Vertex sharp waves (negative short waves, isolated or in bursts) appear.

EOG: Slow eye movements appear. These are wide and mainly horizontal and asynchronous.

EMG: A low-voltage tonic activity is observed. This is interrupted by abrupt muscular contractions of the extremities (myoclonic hypnagogic jerks), which may wake the patient. Sometimes the patient experiences hypnagogic hallucinations (visual, tactile, or auditory) associated with these jerks.

Stage 2

The first appearance of phase 2 is considered the real onset of sleep.

EEG: The grapho-elements which are typical of this phase are spindles, rhythmic waves of between 12 and 14 Hz and 20–30 μV in amplitude. These are short and intermittent and usually join to K complexes (preceding, overlapping, or succeeding them). K complexes involve a rapid negative wave followed by a positive wave, which is slower and higher in amplitude. These appear spontaneously or are provoked by sensory, mainly acoustic, stimuli. Spindles and K complexes are found in the vertex leads and superimpose theta activity, which slows down and whose amplitude increases progressively.

EOG: At the onset of the phase, some slow eye movements can be observed. These gradually disappear.

EMG: Tonic activity may be attenuated and body movements rarely appear.

Stage 3

EEG: Slow-wave activity increases progressively in such a way that the delta waves take up between 20 and 50% of the epoch until a synchronised pattern gradually appears. Spindles and K complexes are still visible during this stage.

EOG: No activity is recorded.

EMG: There are no modifications with respect to stage 2.

Stage 4

EEG: High-voltage delta activity takes up more than 50% of the epoch recording. Both stages 3 and 4 make up slow-wave sleep (SWS) and mental activity is scarce.

EOG: No activity is recorded.

EMG: Very low-amplitude tonic activity may persist.

REM stage (paradoxical sleep)

The EEG shows a low-voltage desynchronised activity, similar to that of stage 1. "Sawtooth waves" can be observed over the vertex or frontal regions, with a frequency in the theta range and with an amplitude of between 40 and 50 μV.

EOG: REMs appear. These may be horizontal, vertical, and oblique, binocularly symmetrical, isolated, or in bursts.

EMG: Suppression of muscle tone may appear with the exception of some twitches in the facial muscles and the distal muscles of the extremities. In this stage, we must distinguish between tonic events (muscular atonia and EEG), which persist throughout the stage, and phasic events, which appear at random (REMs or twitches).

Movement time

According to the Rechtschaffen and Kales' Manual, movement time (MT) refers to the epochs preceding and following sleep stages, but in which the EEG and EOG tracings are obscure in more than half the epoch due to muscle tension and/or amplifier blocking artefacts associated with movement of the subject. MT is interpreted as a separate category, and is neither wakefulness nor sleep.

Sleep cycle and percentage of sleep stages

Adult normal sleep starts with a brief stage 1 followed by stages 2, 3, 4, and REM. This sequence of stages is defined as a sleep cycle with a duration of between 70 and 100 min. Depending on the duration of night-time sleep, four to six cycles per night can be observed with a mean duration of 90 min. There is a greater percentage of SWS during the first half of the night and a greater percentage of REM sleep during the second half. According to Williams *et al.* (1964), the percentage of sleep stages can vary in normal subjects: stage 1 (0.36–16.7%), stage 2 (34.6–60.2%), stage 3 (2.5–15.3%), stage 4 (4.5–23.5%), and REM stage (14.4–29.9%).

Sleep states in infants

Spontaneous foetal movements can be identified at approximately 10 weeks of gestation, and behavioural states can be distinguished in the foetus using ultrasound monitoring techniques (Mulder *et al.*, 1987). Behavioural states should be considered not only as a basis for descriptive behavioural classification, but also as distinct modes of brain activity.

In the newborn and infant, sleep stages are not differentiated in the same way as in the adult. Different criteria and rules for classification must be applied. Wakefulness, quiet sleep (QS), and active sleep (AS), equivalent to REM sleep in the adult, are distinguished in premature babies from the 26th week of gestational age. Wakefulness is characterised by abundant muscular activity and artefacts which are often difficult to distinguish from AS, therefore the observation of behaviour is fundamental, since sleep onset will always be through AS during the first weeks of life. QS and AS differ, in EEG terms, in that there is a contrast between a relatively continuous pattern during AS (Figure 2) and a relatively

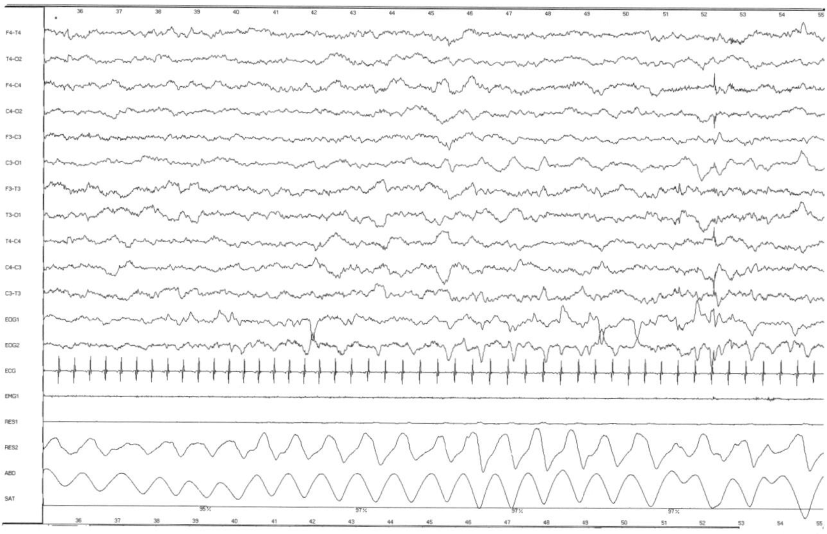

Figure 2. Polysomnographic recording of a premature baby born at 34 weeks gestational age, taken when 3 weeks old. In AS, the EEG shows a continuous EEG rhythmic theta activity of moderate amplitude, bursts of REMs, inactive chin EMG, and irregular respiration with a SaO_2 of between 95 and 97%. Montage: 11 EEG channels (bipolar derivations), right and left EOG, ECG, chin EMG, Res1 (sound), Res2 (airflow), Res3 (abdominal effort), Sat (SaO_2). Epoch = 30 s; EEG sensitivity = 10 μV.

                            R. Peraita-Adrados

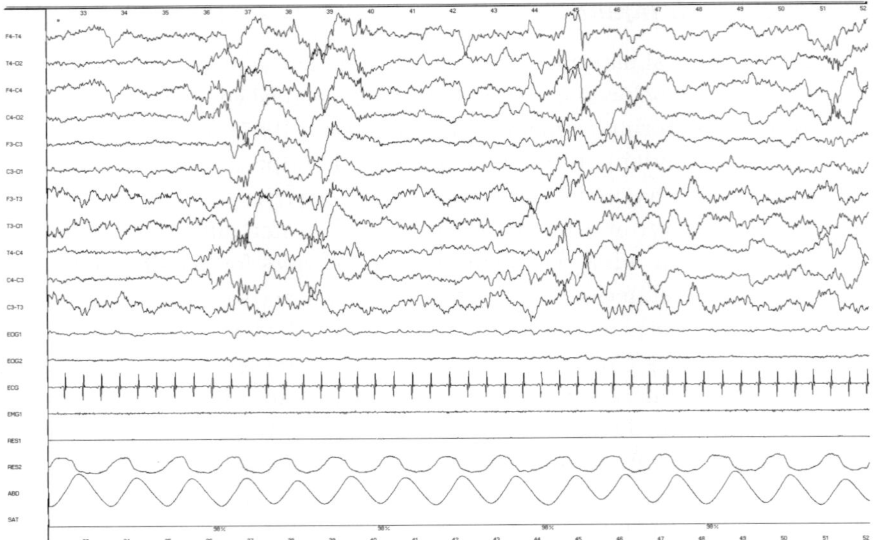

Figure 3. QS in the baby from Figure 2. The EEG shows a discontinuous EEG activity pattern with bursts of delta waves, EOG inactivity, low voltage in EMG, and regular respiration.

discontinuous pattern during QS (Figure 3). AS is characterised by continuous background activity concomitant with atonia and REMs. In QS, high-voltage bursts of slow waves with fast superimposed rhythm lasting several seconds are separated by periods of very low-voltage activity of a longer duration. The interburst periods tend to shorten with maturation, assuming the alternating pattern "tracé alternant," typical of full-term infants, described by Dreyfus-Brisac (1964) and Dreyfus-Brisac and Monod (1975). During QS, no REMs are observed and in the EMG tonic activity is not permanent. The transitional or indeterminate sleep (IS), corresponds to a stage in which the characteristics of the two stages previously referred to are incomplete (Anders *et al.*, 1971; Curzi-Dascalova *et al.*, 1988; Curzi-Dascalova and Mirmiran, 1996). With the appearance of the first spindles and continuous delta rhythms between the sixth and eighth weeks of life, two stages of NREM sleep appear, stages 1+2 and stages 3+4, as well as REM (Guilleminault and Souquet, 1979) (Figures 4 and 5). From the eighth month of life, the adult classification is used with slight modifications (Samson-Dolfus, 2003).

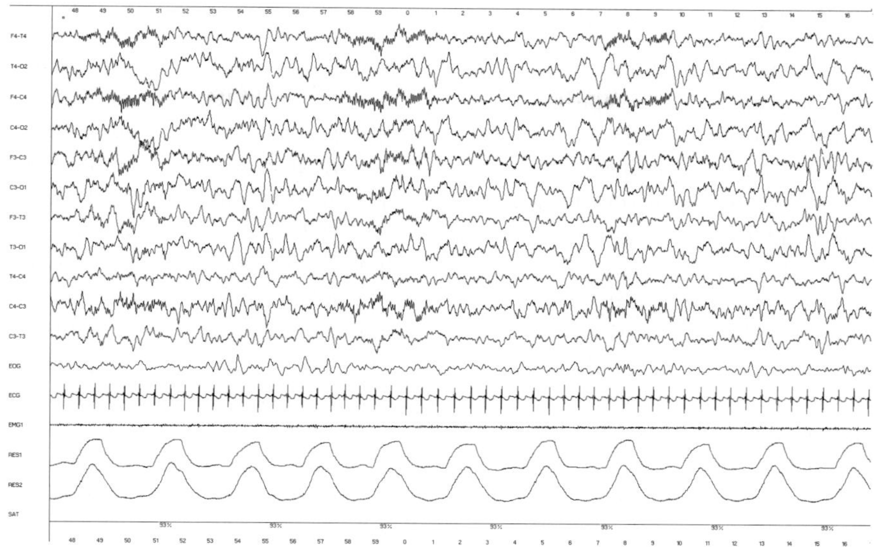

Figure 4. Infant 2 months old: SWS with spindles.

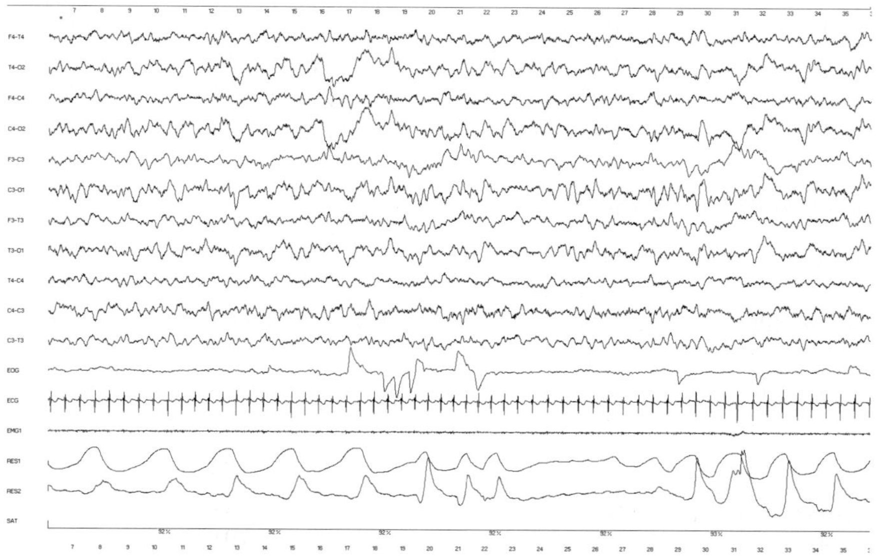

Figure 5. Active-REM sleep. Same infant as in Figure 4.

Indications for PSG in Infants

PSG in neonates and infants allows concurrent identification of events such as bradycardia and tachycardia, laryngeal stridor, inadequate cephalic posture, unusual crying or moans, excessive sweating, changes in colouring, regurgitation, abnormal movements, seizures, etc. Synchronised video/audio PSG recordings are used routinely in apnea of prematurity and also in the evaluation of an apparent life-threatening event (ALTE) in infants. We want to stress the fact that this recording does not have a predictive value for the sudden infant death syndrome (SIDS), either in future victims or among their siblings. The information obtained is important, both from the development viewpoint (maturational criteria) and for the detection of cardiorespiratory events, and alterations of sleep structure and architecture are of an undeniable prognostic value (Guilleminault *et al.*, 1975).

Other indications include congenital central hypoventilation syndrome, sleep-related hypoxemia, gastro-oesophageal reflux (GER), congenital malformations of mid-face, head, neck, and chest, etc.

Cardiac and Respiratory Variables

When a study of sleep-related breathing disorders is made, basic polygraphy must be implemented by the electrocardiographic (ECG) recording, oro-nasal respiratory airflow, thoracic and abdominal effort, EMG of both tibialis anterior muscles, snoring, oxyhaemoglobin saturation, and posture.

Electrocardiography

This is recorded in one channel using two surface electrodes: one in the sternal area and the other at a lateral chest location. However, the type of amplification and the speed used for PSG do not permit an accurate determination of cardiac rhythm disturbances. If a precise diagnosis appears to be necessary, a Holter-ECG monitoring system should be used simultaneously.

Respiratory Signals

Airflow

Monitoring of the air exchange may be accomplished by a variety of transducers, but the use of thermistors has been widely accepted. Thermistors and thermocouples are sensitive to temperature variations. They detect properly the different types of apneas, but are not reliable in the recording of hypopneas, and they do not detect the inspiratory flow limitations or snoring in the case of upper airway resistance.

The flow pressure sensor is of interest in diagnosis and has replaced oro-nasal airflow using thermistors. Technically, the sensor is a pressure transducer, which detects changes in respiratory flow and nasal snoring. It uses disposable airflow cannulas (nasal or oro-nasal) of different sizes for children and adults. Both the cannula and the nasal tubes, similar to those used in oxygen therapy, are inserted in the nostrils and above the upper lip in the mouth. Patency of the nares must always be checked. The transducer has two outlets: one for the nasal pressure airflow and the other for snoring. Both outlets are connected to the digital polygraph headbox.

Respiratory effort

Monitoring of the thoracic and abdominal movements associated with breathing may be accomplished by several methods: intercostal EMG, thoracic and abdominal impedance, or by using strain gauges.

The use of a single strain gauge, whether thoracic or abdominal, should be avoided because during REM sleep a dissociation of thoracic and abdominal movements or even paradoxical respiration may occur, and these variations in respiratory effort could not be recognised using a single belt. This method does not allow quantification of respiratory effort.

Oesophageal balloons permit the measurement of endothoracic pressure swings during respiration. The balloon is placed in the oesophagus at about 35 cm from the nares and connected to a pressure transducer. This method allows accurate assessments of respiratory efforts, which can be perfectly quantified. Nevertheless, paradoxical respiration cannot be detected.

Inductance plethysmography appears to be more precise than strain gauges for assessing all types of apneas. The high cost is a limitation for the device.

Both respiratory effort and airflow can be monitored by AC amplifiers. As respiratory movements are very slow, a time constant of 1-sec high-pass filter associated with a 15-Hz low-pass filter gives an adequate reproduction of the responses. The sensitivity settings are usually set to provide the desired amplitude of the respiratory movements.

Blood oxygenation

Saturation O_2 (SaO_2) continuous monitoring is mandatory to provide information regarding the severity of the respiratory dysfunction. Pulse oximetry, a non-invasive technique, provides the most convenient method for evaluating arterial oxygenation during sleep. It is recommended because of its low price and widely used in most laboratories. The technique is based on the principle of the differences in infrared wavelength absorption for oxy-haemoglobin and reduced haemoglobin. The sensors can be placed on the finger or earlobe and connected to the DC amplifier of the polygraph.

Transcutaneous PO_2 and PCO_2 are widely used in the neonatal intensive care unit and should be monitored in specific circumstances.

PSG with ECG and respiratory variables are mandatory in the study of sleep-related breathing disorders: sleep apnea syndrome; upper airway resistance syndrome; hypoventilation syndromes (congenital alveolar hypoventilation, primary alveolar hypoventilation, hypoventilation–obesity, chronic hypoventilation due to rib cage involvement); overlap syndromes; neuromuscular diseases with respiratory involvement; and SIDS. In addition, titration of continuous positive airway pressure (CPAP) or bilevel positive airway pressure (BiPAP) in patients with these conditions and follow-up studies where an adjustment of therapy is necessary.

Body or Limb Movements

Periodic leg movements (Coleman, 1982) are recorded using surface EMG electrodes, a piezoelectric acceleration transducer or other form of actigraph applied to the anterior tibialis muscles. The gain should be adapted to the sensitivity of the sensors. The recording can be extended to the soleus and quadriceps muscles. If the movements also involve the arms, the deltoid, triceps and biceps muscles must also be recorded. The installation and setting is similar to that of submental EMG.

Synchronised video/audio PSG is crucial in the analysis of the recording.

Optional Variables

Oesophageal pH

This is measured using a pH meter which is placed 5 cm above the gastro-oesophageal sphincter via a catheter inserted in the nose. The pH meter is connected to a DC pre-amplifier in the polygraph. In principle, oesophageal pH should not be performed together with the PSG recording, since the cannula could prevent the superior respiratory airway from collapsing (Groswasser *et al.*, 2000)

Temperature

The measurement of core temperature via a rectal temperature probe may be necessary in case of circadian sleep–wake disorders.

Nocturnal penile tumescence

This is recorded via two ring transducers which are placed at the base of the penis and the balano-preputial sulcus. This measurement is used in the evaluation of male impotence in order to differentiate between organic and psychogenic causes.

Other Sleep Recording Systems

In the sleep laboratory, the PSG provides complete information but it does have its limitations: high cost, restriction of patient movements, restrictions due to other studies being performed simultaneously on the same patient or epidemiological studies in a large series of patients. Other limitations include patients whose management is complicated or who are unable to come to the laboratory, like children, etc.

Technological advances have made it possible to develop alternative ambulatory recording systems. These are compact and adapted to the patient, who can carry them comfortably or connect them at home. Furthermore, technical assistance can be minimised and a computerised and compressed whole-night record needs less time for scoring than the visual analysis of PSG.

Actigraphy

This technique involves recording motor activity and indirectly measures some characteristics of sleep such as timetables, duration and level of the activation (power) of movements. Current systems are similar to a wrist-watch and can be worn comfortably. They record, process, and store movements over prolonged periods of time (days or weeks) depending on the condition studied. The sensor is a piezoelectric beam with capability of detection in all three axes of movement.

The actigraph includes a timer, which makes it possible to identify the time corresponding to a specific level of activity. It also includes an event marker, which the subject can activate at any time, e.g., lights-off/lights-on, and which enables sleep latency to be evaluated. Actimetry overestimates

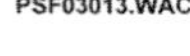

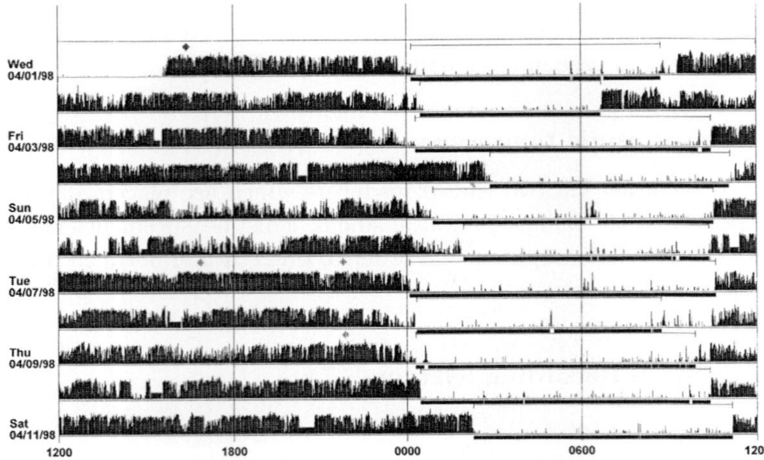

Figure 6. Actigraphic 11-day recording in a patient who sleeps regularly during the week. On saturday and sunday nights, the sleep period is delayed due to the patient's going out.

the duration of sleep latency and underestimates total sleep time as well as wake after sleep onset (WASO) (Sadeh *et al.*, 1989, 1994; Cole *et al.*, 1992). The actigraph is connected to a PC via an interface with software for the visualisation, analysis, and printing of the recording (Figure 6). There are several programs for the analysis of data, based on different algorithms which have previously been validated by a simultaneous PSG recording in a series of patients with different conditions. The actigraph recording must be correlated with a sleep log in which patients note the time they go to bed and get up in the morning, night awakenings, and diurnal naps, etc. The actigraphy does not have an indication to evaluate a single night of sleep, regardless of the pathology. It is mainly applied in the study of sleep–wake rhythm disorders, since the rest–activity cycle is closely linked to the sleep–wakefulness cycle. The modern models include a sensor, which makes it possible to measure skin temperature or core body temperature via a remote probe in chronobiological research studies.

Holter-EEG and ambulatory monitoring systems

Long-term EEG recording (Oxford Medilog 9200 recorder) has been used on a standard audiocassette using analogue tape recording.

It has 24-h autonomy and makes it possible to record the subject carrying out everyday activities. It has been used for the differential diagnosis of nocturnal epileptic seizures and parasomnias by Broughton (1989). Today, analogue tape recorders have been completely replaced by digital systems, which are cheaper and have a larger storage capacity.

With the increasing interest of other signals in the differential diagnosis of sleep disorders, these systems become more complex and provide information about respiration, SaO_2, body movements, and posture, etc., at the cost of reducing the number of EEG channels. New and increasingly sophisticated recording systems appear every day, but they are not always rigorously validated (Coccagna, 2000) before their use.

One of the most widely used systems is MESAM IV (Penzel *et al.*, 1990), which includes a recording of snoring, heart rate, oximetry, and posture. This has been validated for the early recognition of sleep-related breathing disorders (Guilleminault *et al.*, 1990). The Vitalog system includes respiratory effort, airflow, oximetry, body movements, and posture (Miles, 1990).

Ambulatory PSG is currently being developed in two directions. One is in the field of neurophysiology with long-term EEG recordings, and the other is for the diagnosis of sleep-related breathing disorders.

PSG versus sleep simplified systems

When comparisons between PSG and simplified methods were made it was assumed that PSG was the "gold standard." These simplified studies are referred to as screening, pre-selection, ambulatory, or limited studies (Stradling, 1995).

According to the American Academy of Sleep Medicine (Position Statement 2000), it appears to be cost advantageous to include sleep-monitoring procedures in the diagnosis of sleep-disordered breathing (SDB). The cost of using PSG in detecting SDB compares favourably with other ambulatory diagnostic tests.

The diagnosis of SDB should be made in a sleep laboratory using cardiorespiratory PSG and a qualified technician in accordance with ASDA (1994). Annual follow-up of these patients can be by ambulatory recording, except in the case of a suspected associated pathology or when the CPAP pressure must be modified (Besset, 2003).

The main indications of ambulatory monitoring include screening of sleep-related breathing disorders, therapy control in patients diagnosed with sleep-related breathing disorders via PSG in the sleep laboratory and in research studies.

References

AASM Position Statement. Cost justification for diagnosis and treatment of obstructive sleep apnea. (2000). *Sleep*, 3: 1017–1018.

Anders, T., Emde, R., and Parmelee, A. (1971). A Manual of Standardized Terminology, Techniques and Criteria for Scoring of States of Sleep and Wakefulness in Newborn Infants. Los Angeles: UCLA Brain Information Service/BRI Publications Office.

American Electroencephalographic Society. (1994). Guideline fifteen: guideline for polysomnographic assessment of sleep related disorders (polysomnography). *J. Clin. Neurophysiol.*, 11: 116–124.

American Electroencephalographic Society Guidelines in EEG and Evoked Potentials and Polysomnography. (1994). Guideline one: minimum technical requirements for performing clinical electroencephalography. *J. Clin. Neurophysiol.*, 11: 1–5.

ASDA. (1994). Standards of Practice Committee of the American Sleep Disorders Association: Practice parameters for the use of portable recording in the assessment of obstructive sleep apnea. *Sleep*, 17: 372–377.

Aserinsky, E. and Kleitman, N. (1953). Regularly occurring periods of eye motility and concomitant phenomena during sleep. *Science*, 118: 273–274.

Berger, H. (1929). Über das Elektrenkephalogramm des Menschen. Arch. Psychiat. Nervenkr., 87: 527.

Besset, A. (2003). Polysomnography. In: Billiard, M. (Ed.). *Sleep. Physiology Investigations and Medicine.* New York: Kluwer Academic/Plenum Publishers, pp. 127–138.

Bremer, F. (1935). Cerveau "isolé" et physiologie du sommeil. *C.R. Soc. Biol.*, 118: 1235–1241.

Broughton, R.J. (1989). Ambulant home monitoring of sleep and its disorders. In: Kryger, M.H., Roth, T., and Dement, W.C. (Eds.). *Principles and Practice of Sleep Medicine.* Philadelphia: W.B. Saunders Co, pp. 696–701.

Coccagna, G. (2000). Fisiologia del sonno. In: Coccagna, G. (Ed.). *Il sonno e i suoi disturbi.* Padova: Piccin Nuova Libraria, pp. 1–84.

Cole, R.J., Fripke, D.F., Green, W., Mullaney, D.J., and Gillin, J.C. (1992). Automatic sleep/wake identification from wrist activity. *Sleep*, 15: 461–469.

Coleman, R.M. (1982). Periodic movements in sleep (nocturnal myoclonus) and restless legs syndrome. In: Guilleminault, C. (Ed.). *Sleeping and Walking Disorders (Indications and Techniques).* Menlo Park, CA: Addison-Wesley, pp. 265–295.

Curzi-Dascalova, L. and Mirmiran, M. (1996). Scoring of behavioural status. In: Curzi-Dascalova, L. and Mirmiran, M. (Eds.). *Manual of Methods for Recording and Analyzing Sleep-Wakefulness Status in Preterm and Full-Term Infant.* Paris: Les Editions INSERM, pp. 39–54.

Curzi-Dascalova, L., Peirano, P., and Morel-Kahn, F. (1988). Development of sleep status in normal premature and full-term newborns. *Dev. Psychobiol.*, 21: 431–444.

Dement, W.C. and Kleitman, N. (1957). Cyclical variations in EEG during sleep and their relation to eye movements, body motility and dreaming. *Electroencephalogr. Clin. Neurophysiol.*, 9: 673–690.

Dreyfus-Brisac, C. (1964). The electroencephalogram of the premature infant and full-term new-born. Normal and abnormal development of waking and sleeping patterns. In: Kellaway, P. and Petersen, I. (Eds.). *Neurological and Electroencephalographic Correlative Studies in Infancy.* New York: Grune and Sratton, pp. 186–207.

Dreyfus-Brisac, C. and Monod, N. (1975). The EEG of full-term newborns and premature infants. In: Lairy, R. (Ed.). *Handbook of EEG and Clinical Neurophysiology.* Amsterdam: Elsevier, pp. 6–23.

Groswasser, J., Scaillon, M., Rebuffat, E., Simon, T., De Groote, A., Sottiaux, M., and Kahn, A. (2000). Naso-oesophageal probes decrease the frequency of sleep apnoeas in infants. *J. Sleep Res.*, 9: 193–196.

Guilleminault, C. and Souquet, M. (1979). Sleep states and related pathology. In: Korobkin, R. and Guilleminault, C. (Eds.). *Advances in Perinatal Neurology.* New York: Spectrum Publications, pp. 225–247.

Guilleminault, C., Peraita-Adrados, R., Souquet, M., and Dement, W.C. (1975). Apneas during sleep in infants. Possible relation with the sudden infant death syndrome: facts and hypotheses. *Science*, 190: 659–677.

Guilleminault, C., Penzel, T., Stoohs, R., Masterson, M.B., and Peter, J.H. (1990). Cyclical variation of heart rate and snoring: an ambulatory device. In: Miles, L.E. and Broughton, R.J. (Eds.). *Medical Monitoring in the Home and Work Environment.* New York: Raven Press, pp. 265–273.

Jaspers, H.H. (1958). The ten-twenty electrode system of the International Federation. *Electroencephalogr. Clin. Neurophysiol.*, 10: 371–375.

Jaspers, H.H. (1983). The ten-twenty electrode system of the International Federation. In: *The International Federation of Societies for Electroencephalography and Clinical Neurophysiology. Recommendations for the Practice of Clinical Neurophysiology.* Amsterdam: Elsevier, pp. 3–9.

Jouvet, M. and Michel, F. (1959). Corrélations électromyographiques du sommeil chez le chat decortiqué et mésencéphalique chronique. *C.R. Soc. Biol.*, 153: 422–425.

Loomis, A.L., Harvey, E.N., and Hobart, G.A. (1937). Cerebral states during sleep as studied by human brain potentials. *J. Exp. Psychol.*, 21: 127–144.

Miles, L.E. (1990). A portable microcomputer for long-term physiological monitoring in the home and work environment. In: Miles, L.E. and Broughton, R.J. (Eds.). *Medical Monitoring in the Home and Work Environment.* New York: Raven Press, pp. 47–58.

Moruzzi, G. and Magoun, H.W. (1949). Brain stem reticular formation and activation of the EEG. *Electroencephalogr. Clin. Neurophysiol.*, 1: 455–473.

Mulder, E.J.H., Visser, G.H., Bekedam, D.J., and Prechtl, H.F. (1987). Emergence of behavioural status in fetuses of type 1 diabetic women. *Early Human Dev.*, 15: 231–251.

Penzel, T., Amend, G., Meinzer, K., Peter, J.H., and Von Wichert, P. (1990). MESAM: a heart rate and snoring recorder for detection of obstructive sleep apnea. *Sleep*, 13: 175–182.

Ramos Platón, M.J. (1996). El sueño normal. In: Ramos Platón, M.J. (Ed.). *Sueño y Procesos cognitivos*. Madrid: Síntesis Psicológica, pp. 21–55.

Rechtschaffen, A. and Kales, A. (1968). A Manual of Standardized Terminology, Techniques and Scoring System for Sleep Stages in Human Subjects. Public Health Service Publication No. 204. Washington, DC: US Government Printing Office.

Sadeh, A., Alster, J., Urbach, D., and Lavie, L. (1989). Actigraphycally based automatic bedtime sleep-wake scoring. *J. Ambulat. Monit.*, 2: 209–216.

Sadeh, A., Sharkey, K.M., and Carskadon, M.A. (1994). Activity-based sleep wake identification: an empirical test of methodological issues. *Sleep*, 17: 201–207.

Samson-Dolfus, D. (2003). Normal sleep in children. In: Billiard, M. (Ed.). *Sleep, Physiology and Pathology*. New York: Kluwer Academic/Plenum Publishers, pp. 11–30.

Stradling, J.R. (1995). The sleep study, recording and analysis. In: Stradling, J.R. (Ed.). *Handbook of Sleep-Related Breathing Disorders*. New York: Oxford University Press, pp. 87–116.

Williams, H.L., Agnew, H.W., and Webb, W.B. (1964). Sleep patterns in young adults: an EEG study. *Electroencephalogr. Clin. Neurophysiol.*, 17: 376.

Chapter 6

BRAIN IMAGING ON PASSING TO SLEEP

Pierre A.A. Maquet[1], Virginie Sterpenich, Geneviève Albouy,
Thanh Dang-Vu, Martin Desseilles, Mélanie Boly,
Perrine Ruby, Steven Laureys, and Philippe Peigneux

Sleep deeply modifies the regulation of most physiological systems (Orem and Keeling, 1980). However, during sleep, no functional changes are more profound than in the central nervous system, for the very reason that the brain generates and maintains sleep and its alternation with wakefulness. The inescapable recurrence of sleep periods suggests that processes beneficial and necessary for normal brain function are taking place during sleep. A large part of sleep research is precisely to investigate these processes at the molecular, cellular, network, and systems levels. Despite this remarkable research effort, a comprehensive understanding of the functions of sleep remains elusive.

In humans, the characterisation of brain function is only possible through neurophysiological [e.g., electro-encephalography (EEG) and magneto-encephalography (MEG)] and hemodynamic [e.g., single-photon emission computed tomography (SPECT) and positron emission tomography (PET), functional magnetic resonance imaging (fMRI)] behavioural measurements. In this chapter, we provide an account of the functional neuroanatomy of non-rapid eye movement (NREM) and rapid-eye-movement (REM) sleep. Early studies showed that the distribution of brain activity is

---

[1]pmaquet@ulg.ac.be

specific for each type of sleep, and differs from the waking pattern of brain activity. While the activity of subcortical structures is easily explained by the mechanisms which generate REM sleep and NREM sleep in animals, the distribution of the activity within the cortex remains harder to explain and its origin remains speculative.

Recently, a more dynamic characterisation of sleep has emerged. For instance, it was shown that cerebral responses in response to external auditory stimulations persist in NREM sleep. Likewise, regional brain function during sleep has been shown to be modulated by new experience acquired during previous wakefulness. The latter findings support the view that plastic brain changes are taking place during sleep. They suggest that sleep has a role in the behavioural adaptation to changing environmental conditions, thereby favouring the survival of the individual.

Regional Brain Activity during Human Sleep

NREM sleep (slow-wave sleep)

In mammals, the neuronal activity observed during NREM sleep oscillations (spindles, delta, and slow rhythms) is characterised by bursting patterns which alternate short bursts of firing with long periods of hyperpolarisation (Steriade and Amzica, 1998). The latter have a major impact on the regional blood flow, which on the average decreases in the areas where these oscillations are expressed. These decreases in blood flow and metabolism reflect more a change in the temporal patterns of neuronal activity (i.e., a bursting pattern) than an actual decrease in average neuronal firing rate. Accordingly, as compared to wakefulness, the average cerebral metabolism and blood flow begin to decrease in light (stage 2) NREM sleep (Madsen *et al.*, 1991a, 1992), and their nadir is observed in deep (stages 3 and 4) NREM sleep or slow-wave sleep (SWS) (Maquet *et al.*, 1990; Madsen *et al.*, 1991b) (Figure 1A).

The cascade of events which underpin the NREM sleep oscillations in the thalamo–neocortical networks is conditional upon a decreased firing in the activating structures of the brainstem tegmentum. In humans, the brainstem blood flow is decreased during light NREM sleep (Kajimura *et al.*, 1999) as during SWS (Braun *et al.*, 1997; Maquet *et al.*, 1997; Kajimura *et al.*, 1999). In light NREM sleep, the pontine tegmentum is specifically deactivated, whereas the mesencephalon seems to retain an activity which is not significantly different from wakefulness (Kajimura *et al.*, 1999). In SWS, both pontine and mesencephalic tegmenta are deactivated.

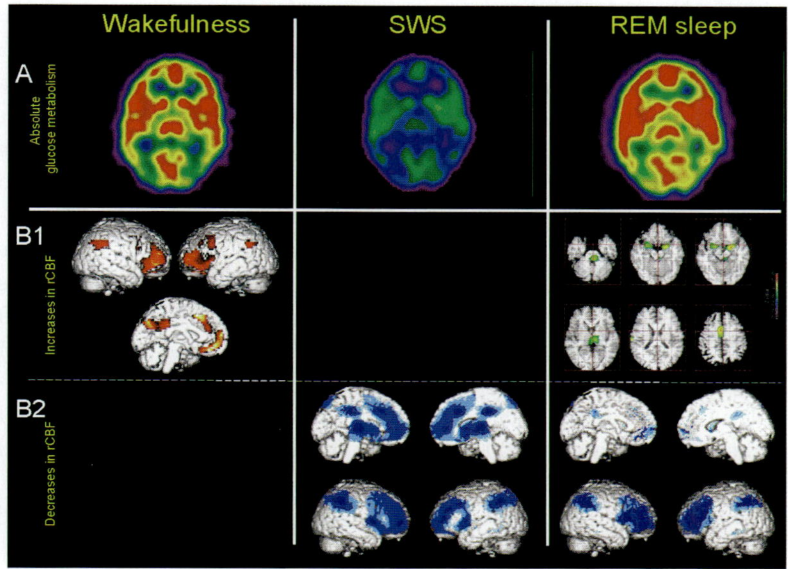

Figure 1. Glucose metabolism and regional cerebral blood flow (rCBF) during wakefulness (first column), deep NREM sleep (second column), and REM sleep (third column). (A) Cerebral glucose metabolism quantified in the same individual at 1-week interval, using fluorodeoxyglucose and PET. The three images are displayed at the same brain level using the same colour scale. There is a significant decrease in the average glucose metabolism during deep NREM sleep as compared to wakefulness. During REM sleep the glucose metabolism is as high as during wakefulness (Maquet *et al.*, 1990). (B1) Distribution of the highest regional brain activity, as assessed by CBF measurement using PET, during wakefulness and REM sleep. The most active regions during wakefulness are located in the polymodal associative cortices in the pre-frontal and parietal lobes (both on the medial wall and convexity) (Maquet, 2000). During REM sleep, the most active areas are located in the pontine tegmentum, the thalami, the amygdaloid complexes, and the anterior cingulate cortex (Maquet *et al.*, 1996). Other data (not shown) have shown a large activity in the occipital cortices, the insula, and the hippocampus (Braun *et al.*, 1997). (B2) Distribution of the lowest regional brain activity, as assessed by CBF measurement using PET, during NREM and REM sleep. In both sleep stages, the least active regions during wakefulness are located in the polymodal associative cortices in the pre-frontal and parietal lobes (convexity). During NREM sleep, the brainstem and thalami are also particularly deactivated.

The thalamus plays a central role in the generation of NREM sleep rhythms, due to the intrinsic properties of its neurons and to the intra-thalamic and thalamo–cortico–thalamic connectivity. Expectedly, in humans, the thalamus is deactivated during both light and deep NREM sleep (Braun *et al.*, 1997; Maquet *et al.*, 1997; Kajimura *et al.*, 1999), in proportion to the power density in the spindle and delta frequency range (Hofle *et al.*, 1997), respectively.

The role of the cortex in the generation of NREM sleep oscillations is equally important and begins to be better understood (Steriade and Amzica, 1998). However, the respective contribution of the different parts of the neocortex in the generation of NREM sleep rhythms is still unknown at the microscopic level. In humans, the deactivation of the cortex is not homogeneous. When compared to wakefulness, the most deactivated areas are located in associative cortices of the frontal, parietal, and to a lesser extent temporal and insular lobes (Braun *et al.*, 1997; Maquet *et al.*, 1997; Andersson *et al.*, 1998; Kajimura *et al.*, 1999), while the primary cortices are the least deactivated.

Polymodal association cortices are the most active cerebral areas during wakefulness (Maquet, 2000). Because of this high waking activity, they might be more profoundly influenced by SWS rhythms than primary cortices (Maquet, 2000), local sleep intensity being homeostatically related to prior waking activity (Kattler *et al.*, 1994).

On the other hand, sleep is not a state of complete unresponsiveness to external stimuli. The first cortical relay areas for exteroceptive stimuli remain relatively active during NREM sleep. In cats involved for some time in an active visual task, neurons in the associative visual cortex can adopt a bursting pattern typical for the sleeping cortex and become less responsive to visual stimulation, while the primary visual areas maintain a normal response to visual inputs (Pigarev *et al.*, 1997). In humans, external stimuli can induce an autonomic or electrophysiological response, in particular after a relevant or meaningful stimulus presentation (Bonnet, 1982). Studies on event-related potentials (ERPs) have demonstrated that external information is efficiently processed during sleep. The brainstem auditory evoked potentials are not modulated by the vigilance state, but rather by the circadian variations of the body temperature, whereas the middle-latency evoked potentials are found to be reduced during deep sleep (Bastuji and García-Larrea, 1999). Long-latency components are also observed during sleep, but are modulated by the sleep stage. During NREM sleep (and especially in stage 2 sleep), ERPs correspond to K-complexes, which are differently affected by the characteristics of the stimulus, the early ones being more connected to the physical attributes of the stimulus and the latter ones to its intrinsic significance (Perrin *et al.*, 2000). Likewise, an fMRI study has shown that the presentation of auditory stimuli activates bilaterally the thalamus and the auditory cortex, during NREM sleep as well as during wakefulness (Portas *et al.*, 2000). Furthermore, hearing one's own name (as compared to hearing a neutral pure tone) additionally activates the left amygdala and prefrontal (associative) cortex. These results suggest that the processing of external stimuli can go beyond the primary cortices during NREM sleep. The mechanisms by which salient stimuli can recruit associative cerebral areas during sleep remain unclear.

REM sleep (paradoxical sleep)

REM sleep is characterised by sustained neuronal activity (Steriade and McCarley, 1990; Jones, 1991) and, correspondingly, by high cerebral energy requirements (Maquet *et al.*, 1990) and blood flow (Madsen *et al.*, 1991c; Franzini, 1992). In this sleeping but working brain, some areas are more active than others; in contrast, other regions have lower than average regional activity.

Neuronal populations in the mesopontine tegmentum are the source of a major activating input to the thalamic nuclei during REM sleep (Steriade and McCarley, 1990). The thalamus forwards this activation to the entire forebrain. Accordingly, in humans, the activation of mesopontine tegmentum and thalamic nuclei has been systematically reported during REM sleep (Maquet *et al.*, 1996; Braun *et al.*, 1997; Nofzinger *et al.*, 1997).

In the forebrain, PET data showed that limbic and paralimbic areas (amygdala, hippocampal formation, anterior cingulate, orbito-frontal, and insular cortices) were among the most active areas in REM sleep (Figure 1B1). Temporal and occipital cortices were also shown to be very active (Braun *et al.*, 1997), although this result is less reproducible (Maquet *et al.*, 1996). In contrast, the prefrontal and parietal areas are relatively quiescent during REM sleep (Maquet *et al.*, 1996; Figure 1B1).

The functional connectivity between brain areas is modified during human REM sleep. The functional relationship between striate and extrastriate cortices, usually excitatory, is inverted during REM sleep (Braun *et al.*, 1998). Likewise, the functional relationship between the amygdala and the temporal and occipital cortices is different during REM sleep than during wakefulness or NREM sleep (Maquet and Phillips, 1998).

The reasons of these changes in the cortical activity patterns remain unclear. A change in neuromodulation might participate to a modification of the forebrain activity and responsiveness during REM sleep, as REM sleep is characterised by a prominent cholinergic tone and a decrease in noradrenergic and serotonergic modulation (Steriade and McCarley, 1990).

Unfortunately, at present, there is no report exploring how changes in the neuromodulation may affect the regional brain function during REM sleep.

The influence of pontine waves or ponto-geniculo-occipital (PGO) waves should also be considered. Several observations suggest that PGO waves also occur during human sleep. In epileptic patients, direct intra-cerebral recordings in the striate cortex showed mono-phasic or di-phasic potentials during REM sleep, isolated or in bursts (Salzarulo *et al.*, 1975). In normal subjects, surface EEG revealed transient occipital and/or parietal potentials time-locked to REMs (McCarley *et al.*, 1983). Source dipoles of MEG signal were localised in the brainstem, thalamus, hippocampus, and occipital cortex during REM sleep (Inoue *et al.*, 1999).

We also tried to get some evidence that activities like pontine or PGO waves exist in humans and result in a hemodynamic signal detectable by PET and cerebral blood flow (CBF) measurements. Since REMs during sleep have been shown to correlate with the occurrence of the so-called PGO waves in cats, we reasoned that the presence of such waves in humans implies that the neural activity of the brain regions from which PGO waves are the most easily recorded in animals (i.e., the dorsal meso-pontine tegmentum, the lateral geniculate bodies, and the occipital cortex) should be more tightly related to spontaneous ocular movements during REM sleep than during wakefulness. We confirmed this hypothesis by showing that the activity in the lateral geniculate body and the occipital cortex is related to REMs more closely during sleep than during wakefulness (Peigneux *et al.*, 2001b). These results support the assumption that pontine or PGO waves do exist in humans. This finding has important functional implications. In rats, the generator of the pontine waves, which has been located in the dorsal part of the subcoeruleus nucleus, projects to a set of brain areas shown to be active in human REM sleep: the occipital cortex, the entorhinal cortex, the hippocampus, the amygdala, as well as brainstem structures participating in the generation of REM sleep (Datta *et al.*, 1998). In cats, although most easily recorded in the pons (Jouvet, 1967), the lateral geniculate bodies (Mikiten *et al.*, 1961), and the occipital cortex (Mouret *et al.*, 1963), PGO waves are observed in many parts of the brain (Hobson, 1964), including limbic areas (amygdala, hippocampus, cingulate gyrus). Taken together, these various experimental elements warrant the hypothesis that activities similar to pontine or PGO waves play a prominent role in shaping the distribution of regional brain activity during REM sleep in humans. This finding is potentially important, for PGO waves have been implicated in various non-exclusive processes such as the alerting reaction to external stimuli or internal signals (Bowker and Morrison, 1976), sensorimotor integration through the transmission of an efferent copy of ocular movements to the visual system (Callaway *et al.*, 1987), and facilitation of brain plasticity (Datta, 1999).

Finally, it is important to stress that these changes in regional brain activity may have a profound impact on other physiological systems. For instance, heart rate is conspicuously more variable during REM sleep than during wakefulness. We were recently able to show that the large variability in heart rate during REM sleep is specifically related to the activity in the amygdaloid complexes (Desseilles *et al.*, in preparation).

Experience-Dependent Changes in Functional Connectivity during Post-Training Sleep

Sleep is believed to participate in the consolidation of memory traces (Maquet, 2001; Peigneux *et al.*, 2001a). Although the processes of this consolidation remain unknown, the reactivation during sleep of neuronal ensembles activated during learning appears as a possible mechanism for the off-line memory processing. Such a reactivation has been reported in at least two experimental situations: in the rat hippocampus and cortex (Pavlides and Winson, 1989; Wilson and McNaughton, 1994; Kudrimoti *et al.*, 1999; Nadasdy *et al.*, 1999; Ribeiro *et al.*, 1999; Louie and Wilson, 2001; Lee and Wilson, 2002) and in the song area of young zebra finches (Dave and Margoliash, 2000). This suggests the generality of the reactivation in the processing of memory traces during sleep. In order to observe the reactivation of brain areas during post-training sleep in humans, we designed a multi-group experiment (Maquet *et al.*, 2000). Normal subjects were trained on a probabilistic serial reaction time (SRT) task. In this task, six permanent position markers are displayed on a computer screen above six spatially compatible response keys. On each trial, a black circle appears below one of the position markers, and the task consists of pressing as fast and as accurately as possible on the corresponding key. The next stimulus is displayed at another location after a 200-ms response–stimulus interval. Unknown to the subjects, the sequential structure of the material is manipulated by generating a series of stimuli based on a probabilistic finite-state grammar that defines legal transitions between successive trials. To assess learning of the probabilistic rules of the grammar, there is a 15% chance, on each trial, that the stimulus generated based on the grammar [grammatical (G) stimuli] is replaced by a non-grammatical (NG), random stimulus.

Assuming that response preparation is facilitated by high predictability, predictable G stimuli should thus elicit faster responses than NG stimuli, but only if the context in which stimuli may occur has been encoded by participants. In this task, contextual sensitivity emerges through practice as a gradually increasing difference between the reaction times (RTs) elicited by G and NG stimuli occurring in specific contexts set by two to three previous trials at most (Cleeremans and McClelland, 1991). A first group of subjects (group 1) were trained on the SRT task in the afternoon, then scanned during the post-training night, both during waking and during various sleep stages (i.e., SWS, stage 2, and REM sleep). A post-sleep training session verified that learning had occurred overnight. The analysis of PET data identified the brain areas that are more active in REM sleep than during resting wakefulness. To ensure that the post-training REM sleep regional CBF (rCBF) distribution differed from the pattern of "typical" REM sleep, a second group of subjects (group 2), not trained to the task, was similarly scanned at night, both when awake and during sleep. The analysis was aimed at detecting the brain areas that would be more active in trained than in non-trained subjects, during REM sleep as compared to resting wakefulness. And finally, to formally test that these brain regions, possibly reactivated during REM sleep, would be among the structures that had been engaged by executing and learning the task, a third group of subjects (group 3) were scanned during wakefulness both while they were performing the SRT task and at rest. The comparison described the brain areas that are activated during the execution of the SRT task. And finally, a conjunction analysis identified the regions that would be both more active during REM sleep in the trained subjects (group 1) compared to the non-trained subjects (group 2) and activated during the execution of the task during waking (group 3), i.e., the regions reactivated in post-training REM sleep. Our results showed that the bilateral cuneus and the adjacent striate cortex, the mesencephalon and the left pre-motor cortex were both activated during the practice of the SRT task and during post-training REM sleep in subjects previously trained on the task, significantly more than in control subjects without prior training, suggesting a reactivation process which may have contributed to overnight performance improvement in the SRT task. In addition, we reasoned that, if the reactivated regions participate in the processing of memory traces during REM sleep, they should establish or reinforce functional connections between parts of the network activated during the task. Consequently, such connections should be stronger, and the synaptic trafficking between network components more intense, during post-training REM sleep than during the typical REM sleep of non-trained subjects. Accordingly, we found that among the reactivated regions, the rCBF in the left pre-motor cortex was significantly more correlated with the activity of the pre-supplementary motor area (SMA) and posterior parietal cortex during post-training REM sleep than during REM sleep in subjects without any prior experience with the task (Laureys *et al.*, 2001). The demonstration of a differential functional connectivity during REM sleep between remote brain areas engaged in the practice of a previously experienced visuo-motor task gave further support to the hypothesis that memory traces are replayed in the cortical network and contribute to the optimisation of the performance. It should be stressed that, in this first experiment, our conclusions were limited by the fact that we could not specify whether the experience-dependent reactivation during REM sleep was related to the simple optimisation of a visuo-motor skill or to the high-order acquisition of the probabilistic structure of the learned material, or both. To test the hypothesis that the cerebral reactivation during post-training REM sleep reflects the reprocessing of high-order information about the sequential structure of the material to be learned, a new group of subjects (group 4) was scanned during sleep after practice on the same SRT task, but using a completely random sequence (Peigneux *et al.*, 2003; Figure 2). The experimental protocol was identical in all respects to the trained group in our original study (Maquet *et al.*, 2000), except for the absence of sequential rules. Therefore, post-training rCBF differences during REM sleep between the subjects trained to the probabilistic SRT or to its random version should be related specifically to the reprocessing of the high-order sequential information.

During post-training REM sleep, blood flow in the left and right cuneus increased more in subjects previously trained to a probabilistic sequence of stimuli than to a random one. Since both groups were exposed prior to sleep to identical SRT practice that differed only in the sequential structure of the stimuli, our result suggests that reactivation of neural activity in the cuneus during post-training REM sleep is not merely due to the acquisition of basic visuo-motor skills, but rather corresponds to the reprocessing of elaborated information about the sequential contingencies contained in the learned material. If the material does not contain any structure, as is the case in the random SRT task, post-training REM sleep reactivation does not occur, or at least to a significantly lesser extent. These results are reminiscent of previous experiments. At the behavioural level, increase in REM sleep duration was observed in rats following aversive

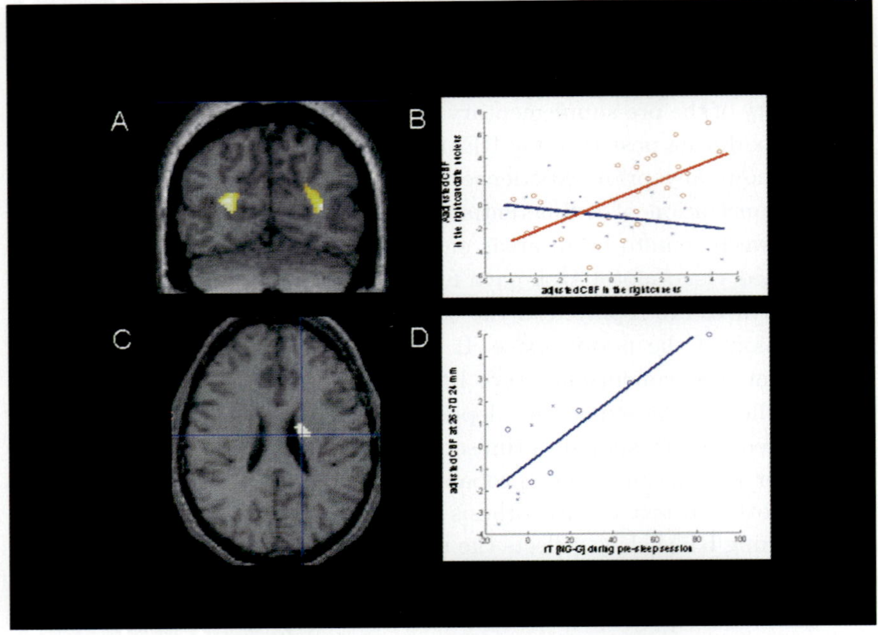

Figure 2. Probabilistic versus random serial reaction time task. (Data from Peigneux *et al.*, 2003.) (A) Statistical parametric maps of the brain regions that both activated during SRT practice (versus rest) and activated more during REM sleep (versus wakefulness) in the probabilistic rather than the random group, superimposed on the coronal section of a subject's normalised MRI at 68 mm behind the anterior commissure. The SPM is displayed at $p < 0.001$, uncorrected. (B) Plot of the regression of centred CBF in the right cuneus (32, −68, 12 mm) and right caudate nucleus (18, −12, 20 mm) during post-training REM sleep in subjects trained to the probabilistic SRT task (red circles) and subjects trained to the random SRT task (blue stars). (C) The right caudate nucleus, with which the right cuneus has a tighter functional connection in subjects trained to the probabilistic SRT task than in subjects trained to the random SRT task. A similar regression is observed between cuneus and caudate nucleus in the left hemisphere. The SPM is displayed at $p < 0.001$, uncorrected. (D) Regression of pre-sleep high-order performance on post-training REM sleep CBF (centred) in the right parieto-occipital fissure (coordinates 26, −70, 24 mm in standard anatomical space), in probabilistic SRT (circles) and random SRT (stars) subjects.

conditioning in which a tone is paired with a footshock, but not after pseudo-conditioning in which the tone and the footshock were not paired (Hennevin and Leconte, 1971).

Using a similar procedure at the systems level, tone-evoked responses were obtained in the medial geniculate nucleus (Hennevin *et al.*, 1993) during REM sleep after a conditioning procedure initiated at wake, but not after pseudo-conditioning. Likewise in humans, REM sleep percentage increased after learning textbook passages, but only when they were meaningful (Verschoor, 1984). A similar situation occurred when the material to learn was so complex that its underlying structure cannot be extracted through practice. Consequently, during REM sleep, functional connections should be reinforced between the reactivated areas and cerebral structures specifically involved in sequence learning only after the practice of the probabilistic version of the task. Indeed, as compared to the practice of the random sequence, we observed that the cuneus establishes or reinforces functional connections with the caudate nucleus during REM sleep following probabilistic SRT practice. The cuneus, which participates in the processing of the probabilistic sequence both during SRT practice and during post-training REM sleep, has been shown to be activated during sequential information processing in the waking state (Schubotz and von Cramon, 2001). On the other hand, the striatum is known to play a main role in implicit sequence learning (Rauch *et al.*, 1995) and specifically in the encoding of the temporal context set by the previous stimulus in the probabilistic SRT task (Peigneux *et al.*, 2000). The finding that the strength of the functional connections between cuneus and striatum is increased during post-training REM sleep suggests the involvement of the basal ganglia in the off-line reprocessing of implicitly acquired high-order sequential information. Finally, a direct relationship between the pre-sleep learning performance and regional blood flow was found in the cuneus. In this region, the regional blood flow during post-training REM sleep is modulated by the level of high-order, but not low-order, learning attained prior to sleep. In other words, the neural activity recorded during REM sleep in brain areas already engaged in the learning process during wakefulness is related to the amount of high-order learning achieved prior to sleep. This latter result further supports the hypothesis that sleep is actively involved in the processing of recent memory traces.

Conclusions

As compared to wakefulness, segregated patterns of regional CBF activity are observed during NREM and REM sleep in humans. The cortical activity is not only influenced by the processes which lead to the generation of specific sleep patterns, but remains responsive to external stimuli. Moreover, the neural populations recently challenged by a new experience are reactivated and increase their functional connectivity during the post-training sleep episodes, suggesting the off-line processing of recent memory traces in sleep.

Acknowledgments

The work summarised in this paper was supported by the Fonds National de la Recherche Scientifique — Belgique (FNRS), the Fondation Médicale Reine Elisabeth, the Research Fund of ULg, PAI/IAP Interuniversity Pole of Attraction P4/22, and the Wellcome Trust. P.A.A.M. and S.L. are supported by the FNRS.

References

Andersson, J.L., Onoe, H., Hetta, J., Lidstrom, K., Valind, S., Lilja, A., Sundin, A., Fasth, K.J., Westerberg, G., Broman, J.E., Watanabe, Y., and Langstrom, B. (1998). Brain networks affected by synchronized sleep visualized by positron emission tomography. *J. Cereb. Blood Flow Metab.*, 18: 701–715.

Bastuji, H. and García-Larrea, L. (1999). Evoked potentials as a tool for the investigation of human sleep. *Sleep Med. Rev.*, 3: 23–45.

Bonnet, M. (1982). Performance during sleep. In: Webb, W. (Ed.). *Biological Rhythms, Sleep and Performance.* Chichester: John Wiley and Sons, pp. 205–237.

Bowker, R.M. and Morrison, A.R. (1976). The startle reflex and PGO spikes. *Brain Res.*, 102: 185–190.

Braun, A.R., Balkin, T.J., Wesenten, N.J., Carson, R.E., Varga, M., Baldwin, P., Selbie, S., Belenky, G., and Herscovitch, P. (1997). Regional cerebral blood flow throughout the sleep-wake cycle. An H2(15)O PET study. *Brain*, 120: 1173–1197.

Braun, A.R., Balkin, T.J., Wesensten, N.J., Gwadry, F., Carson, R.E., Varga, M., Baldwin, P., Belenky, G., and Herscovitch, P. (1998). Dissociated pattern of activity in visual cortices and their projections during human rapid eye movement sleep. *Science*, 279: 91–95.

Callaway, C.W., Lydic, R., Baghdoyan, H.A., and Hobson, J.A. (1987). Pontogeniculooccipital waves: spontaneous visual system activity during rapid eye movement sleep. *Cell. Mol. Neurobiol.*, 7: 105–149.

Cleeremans, A. and McClelland, J.L. (1991). Learning the structure of event sequences. *J. Exp. Psychol. Gen.*, 120: 235–253.

Datta, S. (1999). A physiological substrate for sleep dependent memory processing. *Sleep Res.* 2(suppl. 1): 23 (on-line).

Datta, S., Siwek, D.F., Patterson, E.H., and Cipolloni, P.B. (1998). Localization of pontine PGO wave generation sites and their anatomical projections in the rat. *Synapse*, 30: 409–423.

Dave, A.S. and Margoliash, D. (2000). Song replay during sleep and computational rules for sensorimotor vocal learning. *Science*, 290: 812–816.

Franzini, C. (1992). Brain metabolism and blood flow during sleep. *J. Sleep Res.*, 1: 3–16.

Hennevin, E. and Leconte, P. (1971). The function of paradoxical sleep: facts and theories. *Annee Psychol.*, 71: 489–519.

Hennevin, E., Maho, C., Hars, B., and Dutrieux, G. (1993). Learning-induced plasticity in the medial geniculate nucleus is expressed during paradoxical sleep. *Behav. Neurosci.*, 107: 1018–1030.

Hobson, J.A. (1964). The phasic electrical activity of the cortex and thalamus during desychronized sleep in cats. *C. R. Seances Soc. Biol. Fil.*, 158: 2131–2135.

Hofle, N., Paus, T., Reutens, D., Fiset, P., Gotman, J., Evans, A.C., and Jones, B.E. (1997). Regional cerebral blood flow changes as a function of delta and spindle activity during slow wave sleep in humans. *J. Neurosci.*, 17: 4800–4808.

Inoue, S., Saha, U., and Musha, T. (1999). Spatio-temporal distribution of neuronal activities and REM sleep. In: Mallick, B. and Inoue, S. (Eds.). *Rapid Eye Movement Sleep.* New Delhi: Narosa Publishing House, pp. 214–230.

Jones, B.E. (1991). Paradoxical sleep and its chemical/structural substrates in the brain. *Neuroscience*, 40: 637–656.

Jouvet, M. (1967). Neurophysiology of the states of sleep. *Physiol. Rev.*, 47: 117–177.

Kajimura, N., Uchiyama, M., Takayama, Y., Uchida, S., Uema, T., Kato, M., Sekimoto, M., Watanabe, T., Nakajima, T., Horikoshi, S., Ogawa, K., Nishikawa, M., Hiroki, M., Kudo, Y., Matsuda, H., Okawa, M., and Takahashi, K. (1999). Activity of midbrain reticular formation and neocortex during the progression of human non-rapid eye movement sleep. *J. Neurosci.*, 19: 10065–10073.

Kattler, H., Dijk, D.J., and Borbely, A.A. (1994). Effect of unilateral somatosensory stimulation prior to sleep on the sleep EEG in humans. *J. Sleep Res.*, 3: 159–164.

Kudrimoti, H.S., Barnes, C.A., and McNaughton, B.L. (1999). Reactivation of hippocampal cell assemblies: effects of behavioral state, experience, and EEG dynamics. *J. Neurosci.*, 19: 4090–4101.

Laureys, S., Peigneux, P., Phillips, C., Fuchs, S., Degueldre, C., Aerts, J., Del Fiore, G., Petiau, C., Luxen, A., van der Linden, M., Cleeremans, A., Smith, C., and Maquet, P. (2001). Experience-dependent changes in cerebral functional connectivity during human rapid eye movement sleep. *Neuroscience*, 105: 521–525.

Lee, A.K. and Wilson, M.A. (2002). Memory of sequential experience in the hippocampus during slow wave sleep. *Neuron*, 36: 1183–1194.

Louie, K. and Wilson, M.A. (2001). Temporally structured replay of awake hippocampal ensemble activity during rapid eye movement sleep. *Neuron*, 29: 145–156.

Madsen, P.L., Schmidt, J.F., Holm, S., Vorstrup, S., Lassen, N.A., and Wildschiodtz, G. (1991a). Cerebral oxygen metabolism and cerebral blood flow in man during light sleep (stage 2). *Brain Res.*, 557: 217–220.

Madsen, P.L., Schmidt, J.F., Wildschiodtz, G., Friberg, L., Holm, S., Vorstrup, S., and Lassen, N.A. (1991b). Cerebral O2 metabolism and cerebral blood flow in humans during deep and rapid-eye-movement sleep. *J. Appl. Physiol.*, 70: 2597–2601.

Madsen, P.L., Schmidt, J.F., Wildschiodtz, G., Friberg, L., Holm, S., Vorstrup, S., and Lassen, N.L. (1991c). Cerebral O2 metabolism and cerebral blood flow in humans during deep sleep and rapid-eye-movement sleep. *J. Appl. Physiol.*, 70: 2597–2601.

Maquet, P. (2000). Functional neuroimaging of normal human sleep by positron emission tomography. *J. Sleep Res.*, 9: 207–231.

Maquet, P. (2001). The role of sleep in learning and memory. *Science*, 294: 1048–1052.

Maquet, P. and Phillips, C. (1998). Functional brain imaging of human sleep. *J. Sleep Res.*, 7: 42–47.

Maquet, P., Dive, D., Salmon, E., Sadzot, B., Franco, G., Poirrier, R., von Frenckell, R., and Franck, G. (1990). Cerebral glucose utilization during sleep-wake cycle in man determined by positron emission tomography and [18F]2-fluoro-2-deoxy-D-glucose method. *Brain Res.*, 513: 136–143.

Maquet, P., Dive, D., Salmon, E., Sadzot, B., Franco, G., Poirrier, R., and Franck, G. (1992). Cerebral glucose utilization during stage 2 sleep in man. *Brain Res.*, 571: 149–153.

Maquet, P., Peters, J., Aerts, J., Delfiore, G., Degueldre, C., Luxen, A., and Franck, G. (1996). Functional neuroanatomy of human rapid-eye-movement sleep and dreaming. *Nature*, 383: 163–166.

Maquet, P., Degueldre, C., Delfiore, G., Aerts, J., Peters, J.M., Luxen, A., and Franck, G. (1997). Functional neuroanatomy of human slow wave sleep. *J. Neurosci.*, 17: 2807–2812.

Maquet, P., Laureys, S., Peigneux, P., Fuchs, S., Petiau, C., Phillips, C., Aerts, J., Del Fiore, G., Degueldre, C., Meulemans, T., Luxen, A., Franck, G., Van Der Linden, M., Smith, C., and Cleeremans, A. (2000). Experience-dependent changes in cerebral activation during human REM sleep. *Nat. Neurosci.*, 3: 831–836.

McCarley, R.W., Winkelman, J.W., and Duffy, F.H. (1983). Human cerebral potentials associated with REM sleep rapid eye movements: links to PGO waves and waking potentials. *Brain Res.*, 274: 359–364.

Mikiten, T., Niebyl, P., and Hendley, C. (1961). EEG desynchronization during behavioural sleep associated with spike discharges from the thalamus of the cat. *Fed. Proc.*, 20: 327.

Mouret, J., Jeannerod, M., and Jouvet, M. (1963). L'activité électrique du système visuel au cours de la phase paradoxale du sommeil chez le Chat. *J. Physiol. (Paris)* 55: 305–306.

Nadasdy, Z., Hirase, H., Czurko, A., Csicsvari, J., and Buzsaki, G. (1999). Replay and time compression of recurring spike sequences in the hippocampus. *J. Neurosci.*, 19: 9497–9507.

Nofzinger, E.A., Mintun, M.A., Wiseman, M., Kupfer, D.J., and Moore, R.Y. (1997). Forebrain activation in REM sleep: an FDG PET study. *Brain Res.*, 770: 192–201.

Orem, J. and Keeling, J. (1980). *Physiology in Sleep.* Lubbock: Academic Press.

Pavlides, C. and Winson, J. (1989). Influences of hippocampal place cell firing in the awake state on the activity of these cells during subsequent sleep episodes. *J. Neurosci.*, 9: 2907–2918.

Peigneux, P., Laureys, S., Delbeuck, X., and Maquet, P. (2001a). Sleeping brain, learning brain. The role of sleep for memory systems. *Neuroreport*, 12: 111–124.

Peigneux, P., Laureys, S., Fuchs, S., Delbeuck, X., Degueldre, C., Aerts, J., Delfiore, G., Luxen, A., and Maquet, P. (2001b). Generation of rapid eye movements during paradoxical sleep in humans. *Neuroimage*, 14: 701–708.

Peigneux, P., Maquet, P., Meulemans, T., Destrebecqz, A., Laureys, S., Degueldre, C., Delfiore, G., Aerts, J., Luxen, A., Franck, G., Van der Linden, M., and Cleeremans, A. (2000). Striatum forever, despite sequence learning variability: a random effect analysis of PET data. *Hum. Brain Mapp.*, 10: 179–194.

Peigneux, P., Laureys, S., Fuchs, S., Destrebecqz, A., Collette, F., Delbeuck, X., Phillips, C., Aerts, J., Del Fiore, G., Degueldre, C., Luxen, A., Cleeremans, A., and Maquet, P. (2003). Learned material content and acquisition level modulate cerebral reactivation during posttraining rapid-eye-movements sleep. *Neuroimage*, 20: 125–134.

Perrin, F., Bastuji, H., Mauguiere, F., and García-Larrea, L. (2000). Functional dissociation of the early and late portions of human K-complexes. *Neuroreport*, 11: 1637–1640.

Pigarev, I.N., Nothdurft, H.C., and Kastner, S. (1997). Evidence for asynchronous development of sleep in cortical areas. *Neuroreport*, 8: 2557–2560.

Portas, C.M., Krakow, K., Allen, P., Josephs, O., Armony, J.L., and Frith, C.D. (2000). Auditory processing across the sleep-wake cycle: simultaneous EEG and fMRI monitoring in humans. *Neuron*, 28: 991–999.

Rauch, S., Savage, C., Brown, H., Curran, T., Alpert. N., Kendrick, A., Fischman, A., and Kosslyn, S. (1995). A PET investigation of implicit and explicit sequence learning. *Hum. Brain Mapp.*, 3: 271–286.

Ribeiro, S., Goyal, V., Mello, C.V., and Pavlides, C. (1999). Brain gene expression during REM sleep depends on prior waking experience. *Learn. Mem.*, 6: 500–508.

Salzarulo, P., Liary, G.C., Bancaud, J., Munari, C., Barros Ferreira, J.P., and Stenal, H.Y. (1975). Direct depth recording of the striate cortex during REM sleep in man: are there PGO potentials? *Electroencephalogr. Clin. Neurophysiol.*, 38: 199–202.

Schubotz, R.I. and von Cramon, D.Y. (2001). Interval and ordinal properties of sequences are associated with distinct premotor areas. *Cereb. Cortex*, 11: 210–222.

Steriade, M. and Amzica, F. (1998). Coalescence of sleep rhythms and their chronology in corticothalamic networks. *Sleep Res.*, 1: 1–10. (on-line).

Steriade, M. and McCarley, R.W. (1990). *Brainstem Control of Wakefulness and Sleep*. New York: Plenum Press.

Verschoor, G.T.L.H. (1984). REM bursts and REM sleep following visual and auditory learning. *S. Afr. J. Psychol.*, 14: 69–74.

Wilson, M.A. and McNaughton, B.L. (1994). Reactivation of hippocampal ensemble memories during sleep. *Science*, 265: 676–679.

Chapter 7

HYPOTHALAMIC MECHANISMS OF SLEEP: PERSPECTIVE FROM NEURONAL UNIT RECORDING STUDIES

Dennis McGinty[1], Noor Alam, Natalia Suntsova, Ruben Guzman-Marin, Melvi Methippara, Hui Gong, and Ron Szymusiak

The unraveling of the mystery of the regulation of sleep is a daunting challenge. It appears likely that sleep is controlled by interacting neuronal groups at several levels of the neuroaxis, and is modulated by a host of neurochemical processes. Moreover, the understanding of the functions of sleep remains elusive. It is reasonable to conclude that we will need to apply all of the methods available to us, electrophysiological, fixed and functional anatomy, comparative, molecular, genetic, and physiological, to make progress in this endeavor. In this context, it is important to ask what crucial information is provided by each method.

This chapter will focus on the perspective on hypothalamic sleep mechanisms provided by neuronal unit recording methods in chronic animals. About 35 years ago, we introduced in sleep research the method of microwire unit recording in chronically prepared, freely moving animals (Jacobs *et al.*, 1970). Fixed microwires had been used previously in other disciplines; we combined microwire recordings with a simple mechanical microdrive to permit systematic exploration of a brain site. Initially, the microwire method was questioned by researchers who thought that fine-tipped electrodes

---

[1]dmcginty@mail.ucla.edu

were required to resolve single neuronal units, but this method has gained acceptance and has been adopted in laboratories throughout the world. Nevertheless, it is important to continue to review the issues associated with the method. To complement neuronal unit recording, we now use c-Fos immunostaining to better determine the anatomical features of neurons activated during sleep or waking. Each method has its advantages and limitations, which we will consider. We also summarize recent work that combines microwire recordings with adjacent microdialysis to locally deliver neurochemical agents and assess hypotheses concerning the neurochemical regulation of neuronal activity. The application of chronic unit recording to the functional analysis of brainstem and limbic system sites and details concerning the methodology of microwire recording have been reviewed previously (McGinty and Szymusiak, 1988; McGinty and Siegel, 1992).

The Preoptic Area of the Hypothalamus

More than 70 years ago, von Economo (1930) suggested a role for the preoptic area (POA) of the hypothalamus in sleep facilitation. Patients exhibiting insomnia associated with encephalitis were found postmortem to have lesions in this area. Patients with lesions in the posterior hypothalamus (PH) exhibited hypersomnia, suggesting that this site contained wake-promoting mechanisms. von Economo suggested the concept of opposing sleep-promoting and wake-promoting (arousal) systems. Support for these hypotheses has been provided by many studies using lesions, electrical, chemical, and thermal stimulation, and neuronal unit recording. We will not summarize these data; detailed reviews of the evidence for a POA hypnogenic system are available (McGinty and Szymusiak, 2001, 2003). The functional agreement among methods, including the discovery of POA sleep-activate neurons (SANs), lent strong support for the hypothesis of a POA hypnogenic system. The identification of arousal systems was facilitated by the finding of neuronal phenotypes that correspond to wake-promoting neurochemical agents, norepinephrine (NE), serotonin (5HT), histamine (HA), acetylcholine (ACH), dopamine (DA), and more recently, hypocretin/orexin. In general agreement with von Economo's hypothesis, these neuronal types were found in the posterior hypothalamus, midbrain, and rostral pons (Jones, 1994; Peyron *et al.*, 1998b). Recent work, to be summarized below, shows how the sleep-promoting and arousal systems are interconnected.

Sleep-Active Neurons

Several extracellular recording studies targeting the POA have found SANs, that is, neurons that exhibit increased discharge during NREM and/or REM sleep compared to waking (McGinty and Szymusiak, 2001, 2003). An example from a recent study (Suntsova *et al.*, 2002) of the median preoptic nucleus (MnPN) is shown in Figure 1A. About 75% of MnPN neurons exhibited increased discharge, compared to waking, in NREM, REM, or both. In this example, neuronal discharge increases from less than 5 spikes/s (s/s) during waking to about 10 s/s during NREM and increases further in REM. MnPN SANs also exhibited interesting changes in relation to the sleep cycle. In many neurons, discharge increased during sustained wake episodes 1–3 min before sleep onset. In subsets of SANs within sustained sleep, discharge declined across successive NREM episodes (Figure 1B and C). These sequential changes parallel changes in homeostatic drive for sleep and suggest that MnPN SAN discharge is correlated with sleep propensity or homeostatic drive for sleep.

The identification of the MnPN as a site containing a high concentration of SANs was first achieved using the c-Fos immunoreactive (IR) staining technique. Rapid expression of the proto-oncogene, *c-fos*, has been identified as a marker of neuronal activation in many brain sites (Morgan and Curran, 1991). *c-fos* mRNA was found to be induced within a few minutes after increased neuronal activity, and was characterized as an immediate early gene (IEG). The c-Fos protein dimerizes with protein from another IEG, *c-jun*, and binds to the nuclear AP-1 binding site, to regulate the expression of other genes. The presence of c-Fos IR protein in the nucleus can be readily measured within 30 min of neuronal activation with immunostaining methods. Following the introduction of this method to sleep studies (reviewed in Cirelli and Tononi, 2000), Sherin *et al.*, (1996) described the occurrence of c-Fos IR neurons in the ventrolateral POA (VLPO) following sleep but not following waking. Other POA sites exhibit much c-Fos labeling following waking; the VLPO was thought to be unique because there were few wake-active neurons in this site.

We confirmed the finding of c-Fos IR in the VLPO and found the additional site of segregated SANs in the MnPN (Gong *et al.*, 2000) (Figure 2, upper). The MnPN is a midline nucleus forming a cap above and around the anterior pole of the third ventricle. It extends dorsally in the midline around the anterior border of the decussation of the anterior commmissure and ventrally to the organum vasculosum of the lamina terminalis. Like the

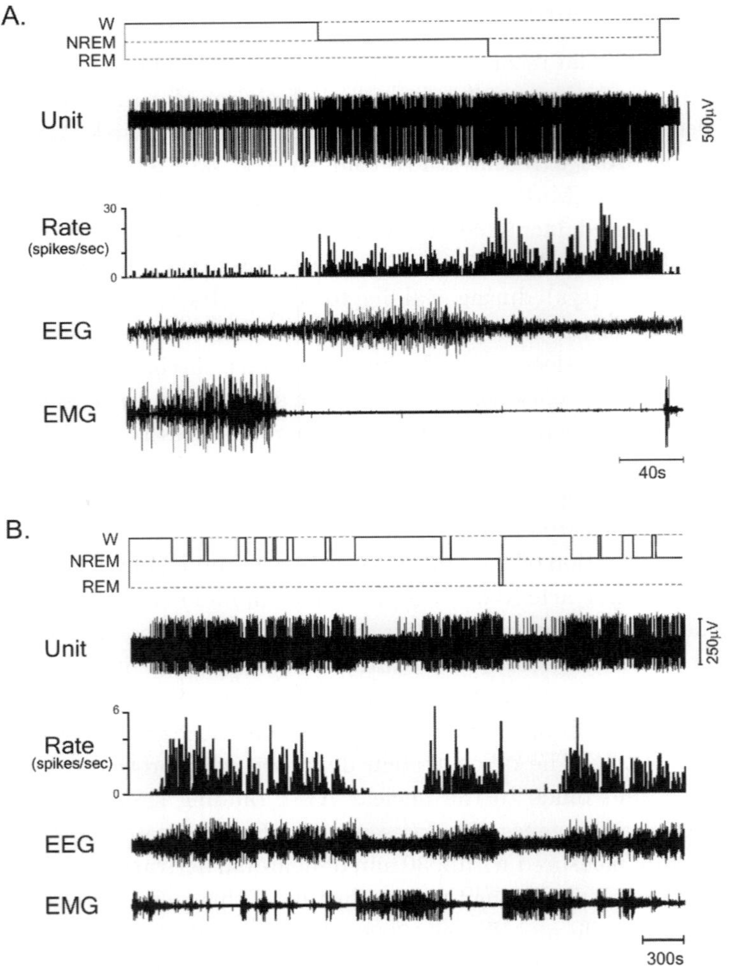

Figure 1. (A) Recording of sleep-active neuron from the MnPN during wake, NREM, and REM in the unrestrained rat (8.6 min). State is indicated by the top line and by EEG and EMG activity. As indicated best by the rate profile, this unit exhibits low discharge during wake, greatly increased discharge at sleep onset and during NREM, and variable but generally higher discharge in REM. (B) Discharge of an MnPN SAN during several successive sleep episodes over 60 min. Note that discharge rate tends to decline within an episode of relatively sustained NREM sleep. (C) Mean discharge rate of a sample of MnPN SANs across eight successive sleep episodes. This analysis confirms that MnPN SANs exhibit declining discharge within successive NREM episodes, suggesting a correlation with sleep drive and a possible role in sleep homeostasis. (All data from Suntsova *et al.*, 2002.)

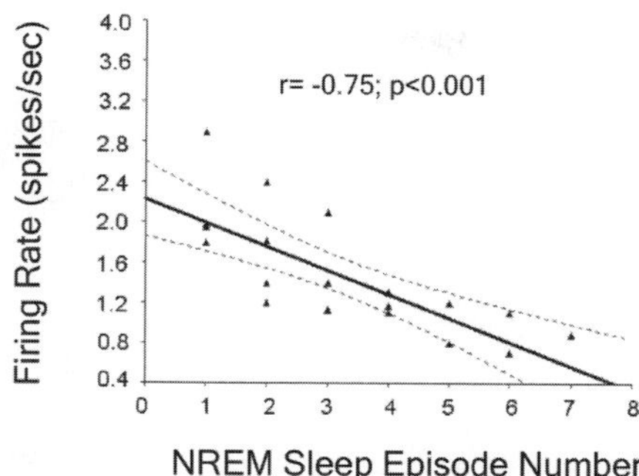

Figure 1. (*Continued*)

VLPO, the MnPN is a site with sleep-related c-Fos IR but only low levels of wake-related c-Fos IR under the conditions of our studies. The number of c-Fos IR neurons in each site was correlated with the amount of sleep during the 2 h preceding the sacrifice of the animals (Figure 2, lower). We also examined c-Fos IR following sleep in animals kept in a mildly elevated ambient temperature that was compatible with sleep. Under these conditions the number of c-Fos IR neurons following sleep, but not waking, was increased in MnPN, but was reduced in VLPO. The role of temperature in sleep control is discussed further below. As noted above, we used electrophysiological methods to confirm a hypothesis that SANs constituted a high proportion of neurons in this site. It should be noted that exposure to osmotic stress (Rowland, 1998) or thermal stress (Scammel *et al.*, 1993) can also increase MnPN c-Fos IR, but these manipulations probably activate different populations of neurons.

We performed a second immunostaining study in which we examined the co-expression of sleep-activated c-Fos IR and glutamic acid decarboxylase (GAD), the marker of GABAergic neurons (Gong *et al.*). In this study, we also examined the effects of sleep deprivation on the numbers of c-Fos IR neurons in VLPO and MnPN as well as the co-expression of GAD and c-Fos. In animals with high levels of spontaneous sleep before sacrifice, in both MnPN and VLPO, more than 75% of c-Fos IR neurons were GABAergic. In MnPN, but not VLPO, following recovery sleep after 24 h of sleep deprivation, by an intermittent treadmill method (Guzmán-Marín *et al.*, 2003), the numbers of c-Fos/GAD double-labeled neurons and the percentage of GAD positive neurons expressing c-Fos were significantly increased compared to the sleep deprivation control group. These findings were congruent with the

 D. McGinty et al.

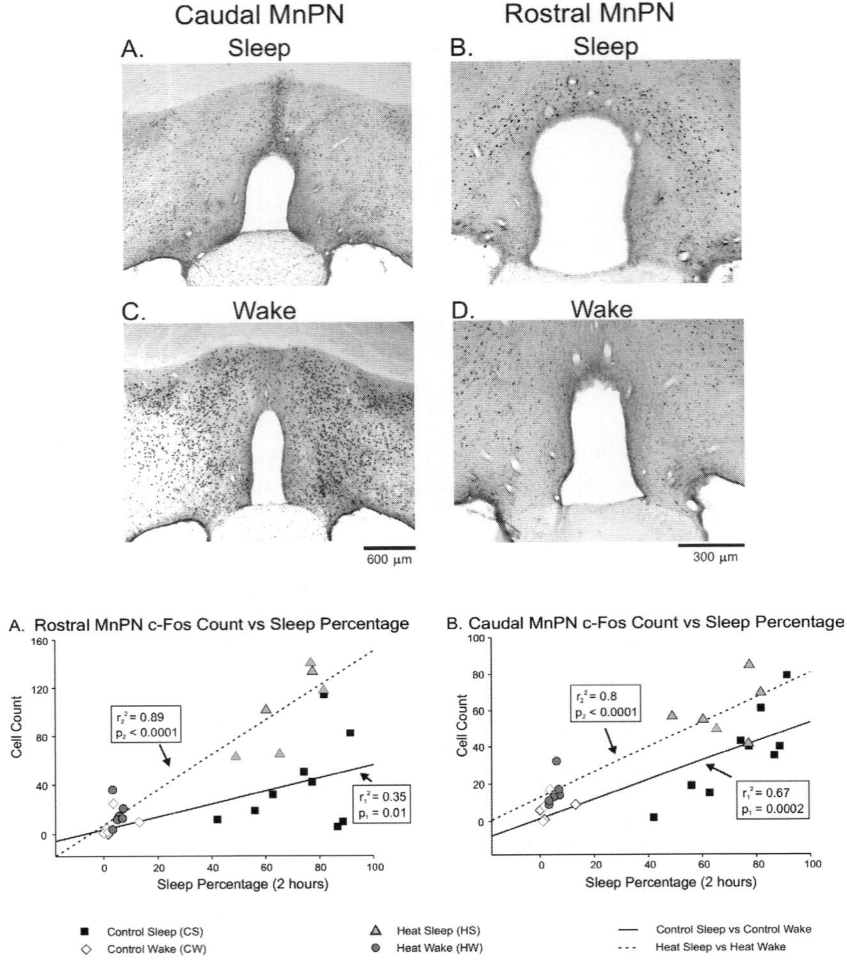

Figure 2. Upper: C-Fos immunostaining in the caudal and rostral MnPN following 2-h periods with at least 70% sleep (A and B), compared to periods with low sleep (C and D). Note the black-stained nuclei in the midline (A) or over the top of the third ventrical (B), which are mostly absent following wake. At the level of the caudal MnPN, there is extensive c-Fos IR in more lateral POA areas following wake. Lower: Correlations between the amount of sleep in the VLPO and in rostral and caudal MnPN and the number of c-Fos IR neurons within standardized grids. Groups were studied at both normal ambient temperatures and an elevated temperature compatible with sleep (31°C). Numbers of c-Fos IR neurons were correlated with the amount of prior sleep. In the heat sleep condition the numbers of labeled neurons and the correlation with sleep were increased in MnPN, but not the VLPO. (From Gong *et al.*, 2000.)

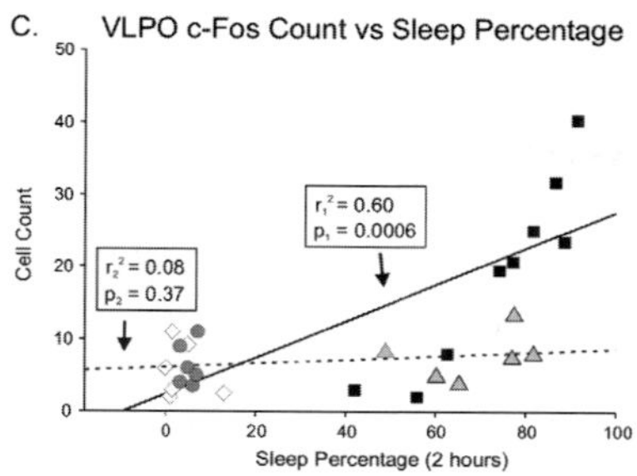

Figure 2. (*Continued*)

electrophysiological data summarized above, suggesting a role of the MnPN in coding sleep propensity or homeostatic drive.

We also confirmed that the VLPO contains a high density of SANs using electrophysiological methods (Szymusiak *et al.*, 1998). Neurons in this site exhibited very low discharge during waking, and progressively increasing discharge during sleep that was correlated with delta power in the EEG. Following 16 h of sleep deprivation, VLPO discharge was increased during sleep, but not during waking. The MnPN and VLPO have been studied in detail because, in these sites, there are few wake-active neurons identified either by c-Fos IR or electrophysiology. However, sleep-related c-Fos IR and SANs identified with electrophysiology are found throughout the lateral POA and adjacent basal forebrain (BF). These findings, and the results of lesion studies, suggest that a POA sleep-promoting neuronal population is diffuse rather than localized exclusively in VLPO or MnPN (McGinty and Szymusiak, 2003).

Arousal Systems

There is extensive evidence for the existence of several putative arousal systems, including the serotonergic dorsal raphe nucleus (DRN), noradrenergic locus coeruleus (LC), histaminergic tuberomammillary nucleus (TMN), hypocretin-neuron containing perifornical lateral hypothalamus (pLH), both brainstem and basal forebrain cholinergic (ACH) systems, as well as unidentified neurons within the posterior hypothalamus (Jones, 1994). This evidence has included recent neuronal unit recording studies carried out in our laboratory (Krilowicz *et al.*, 1994; Steininger *et al.*, 1999; Guzmán-Marín *et al.*, 2000; Alam *et al.*, 2002). With respect to discharge patterns across the sleep–wake cycle, neurons in sites of arousal-related neurons can be classified into two types. Subsets of neurons in the DRN (Guzmán-Marín *et al.*, 2000) (Figure 3) ventral posterior hypothalamus, particularly in the vicinity of the TMN (Steininger *et al.*, 1999), and the pLH (Alam *et al.*, 2002) exhibited a wake-active, REM-off discharge pattern. This sleep–wake discharge profile was described previously in the LC (Hobson *et al.*, 1983). Other neurons within these sites and in other putative wake-promoting sites exhibited a wake-active and REM-active discharge pattern (Krilowicz *et al.*, 1994). It should be noted that both groups of neurons exhibited low discharge in NREM sleep.

As each site contains many neuronal phenotypes, the identification of recorded neurons is a significant issue. Much evidence supports the view that REM-off neurons in the DRN synthesize and release serotonin (Guzmán-Marín *et al.*, 2000), and REM-off neurons in the vicinity of the TMN synthesize and release histamine (Steininger *et al.*, 1999). This evidence includes localization of recorded units with respect to histochemically identified neurons, comparison of spike waveshape and spike train features from *in vitro* and *in vivo* studies (recorded cells can be identified *in vitro*), and responses of neurons to drugs stimulating autoreceptors. Additional evidence may include a comparison of discharge patterns across the sleep–wake cycle and the release of the corresponding transmitter in projection sites. The REM-off neurons in the pLH field have not been identified, evidence that hypocretin neurons are either REM-off (Alam *et al.*, 2002) or REM-active (Kiyashchenko *et al.*, 2002) has been offered.

Neuronal unit recording permits a detailed look at the relationship of neuronal activity to behavior. Wake-related neuronal discharge is associated with motor activity or particular types of movements in wake-active REM-off pLH neurons (Alam *et al.*, 2002), in other PH neurons (Krilowicz *et al.*, 1994), and in DRN neurons (Jacobs and Fornal, 1999). In pLH wake-active neurons, wake discharge was highly correlated with EMG activity. Release of hypocretin is increased during waking with movements (Wu *et al.*, 2002). This finding is congruent with a hypothesis that wake-active, REM-off neurons contain this neuropeptide. These neurons exhibit very low discharge rates during quiet waking without motor activity before sleep onset. This low discharge has made it difficult to determine if changes in discharge precede state changes, as shown for the sleep-activated neurons described above.

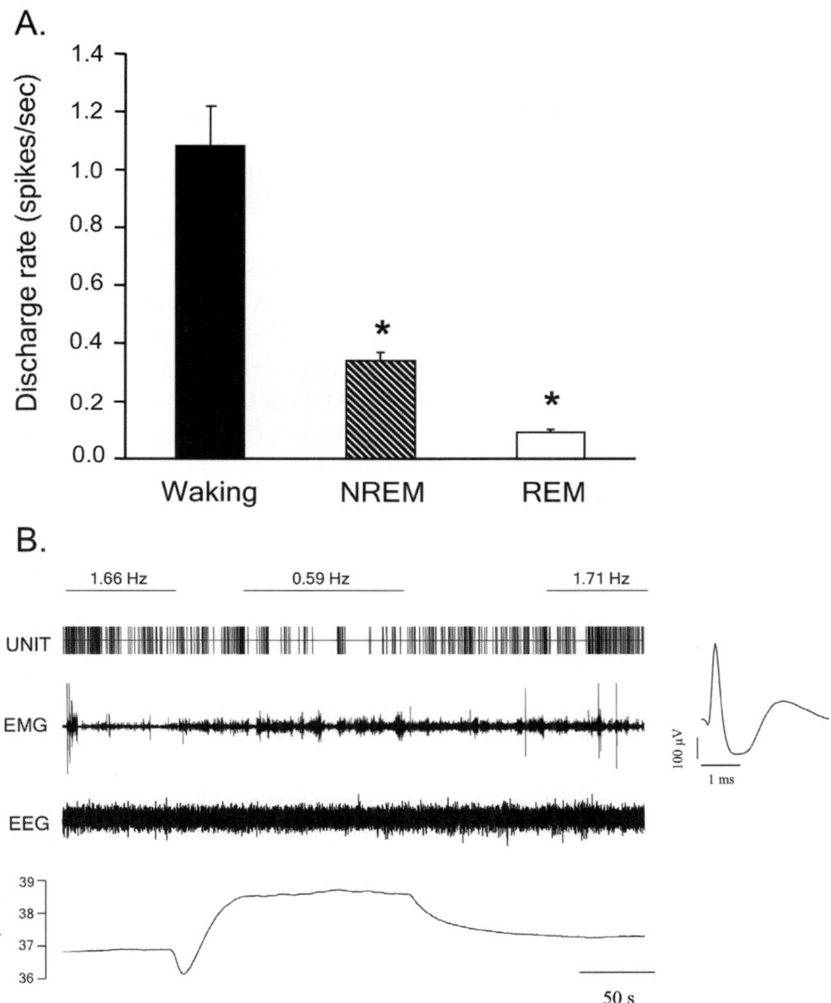

Figure 3. (A) Discharge rates of DRN REM-off neurons in waking, NREM, and REM. This pattern of low but sustained discharge in waking greatly reduced discharge in NREM, and extremely low discharge in REM was found in DRN, TMN, and LC neurons (see text). Some pLH neurons are also "wake-active, REM-off," but these have higher rates in wake with movement. (B) Transient mild local POA warming, indicated by the lower trace, suppresses discharge of a DRN REM-off neuron during waking, inducing a rate typical of NREM sleep in this neuron. EEG analysis showed that waking was sustained during this experiment. (From Guzmán-Marín *et al.*, 2000.) Similar effects of local POA warming have been found on wake-active neurons recorded in the pLH, posterior hypothalamus, and basal forebrain (see text).

Anatomical Connections between POA and Arousal Systems

The POA gives rise to descending pathways that terminate in proximity to the putative arousal systems. Initial studies showed descending projections from the POA and BF to the PH (Yoshimoto *et al.*, 1989; Gritti *et al.*, 1994; Peyron *et al.*, 1998a). Discrete projections from the VLPO and LPO region to the TMN, DRN, and LC sites with terminals in close proximity to monoaminergic neurons have been described (Sherin *et al.*, 1998; Steininger *et al.*, 2001). The MnPN projects of the pLH field and to the DRN (Zardetto-Smith and Johnson, 1995). A recent study shows that MnPN projections to the pLH terminate in proximity to hypocretin neurons (Gong *et al.*, 2002) and originate in GABAergic neurons (Gong *et al.*, 2001). VLPO neurons projecting to the TMN contain the inhibitory neurotransmitter, galanin (Sherin *et al.*, 1998). These studies suggest that MnPN and VLPO neurons have the capacity to release inhibitory neurotransmitters and, consequently, inhibit arousal systems. GABA release is increased during sleep in the posterior hypothalamus (Nitz and Siegel, 1996), DRN (Nitz and Siegel, 1997a), and LC (Nitz and Siegel, 1997b). Physiological evidence for such an inhibitory process is described below.

There is also evidence that arousal systems provide inhibitory input to MnPN and VLPO. *In vitro* studies show that VLPO neurons are inhibited by norepinephrine (NE), serotonin, and acetylcholine (Gallopin *et al.*, 2000), and MnPN neurons are inhibited by NE (Bai and Renaud, 1998). Microinjection of putative wake-promoting neurotransmitters in the POA suppresses sleep.

Reciprocal Changes in Discharge of Sleep-Active and Arousal Systems

The anatomical and physiological studies described above suggest that sleep-active and arousal systems are mutually inhibitory. Support for this hypothesis can be derived from neuronal discharge studies. Figure 4 shows changes in discharge rate across the sleep–wake cycle of MnPN (Suntsova *et al.*, 2002) and VLPO (Szymusiak *et al.*, 1998) sleep-active neurons, on the one hand, and pLH (Alam *et al.*, 2002), DRN (Guzmán-Marín *et al.*, 2000), and TMN (Steininger *et al.*, 1999) wake-active, REM-off neurons, on the other. The reciprocal changes in discharge of SANs and wake-active, REM-off neurons support a suggestion that this network could act like a "flip-flop" circuit. Activation of sleep-active neurons would inhibit wake-promoting neurons, thereby removing inhibition from sleep-active neurons

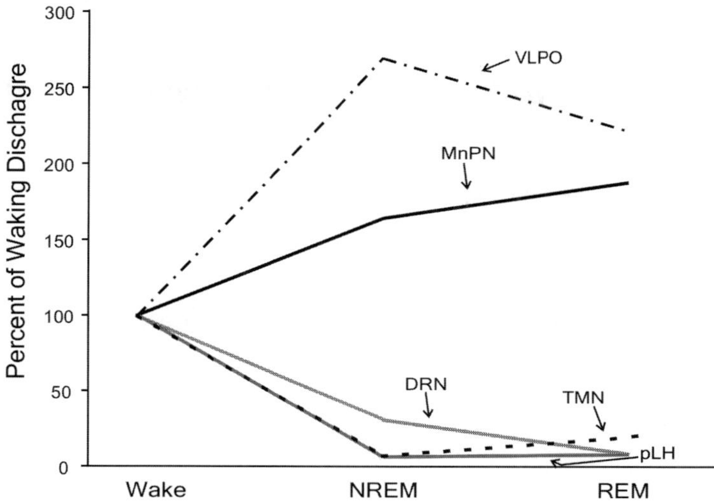

Figure 4. Percent changes in discharge rate compared to wake in NREM and REM sleep. SANs populations in the MnPN and VLPO show contrasting rate changes compared with wake-active, REM-off neurons in the DRN, TMN, and pLH. Changes tend to be "reciprocal," compatible with the hypothesis of inhibitory or mutually inhibitory interactions between SANs and wake-active neurons. (From Szymusiak *et al.*, 1998; Steininger *et al.*, 1999; Guzmán-Marín *et al.*, 2000; Alam *et al.*, 2002; Suntsova *et al.*, 2002.)

with the result of amplifying and stabilizing the state change. Similarly, activation of wake-promoting neurons would inhibit SANs, removing inhibition from arousal systems, and tend to increase and stabilize arousal. It should be emphasized that this is a theoretical model that has not been tested directly.

POA Thermoregulatory Control of Arousal

The POA is an important thermoregulatory control region and contains populations of warm-sensitive and cold-sensitive neurons (WSNs and CSNs). Such neurons exhibit high sensitivity to local warming and cooling over the narrow range of body temperature (Figure 5A). WSNs and CSNs typically constitute 20–30% of POA neurons in the region 1–2 mm from the midline. Local POA warming or cooling elicit counterregulatory thermoregulatory responses (Boulant and Dean, 1986). For example, local POA warming can elicit the heat-loss response, panting. Mild local POA warming also triggers EEG synchrony and NREM onset, tonically facilitates NREM, and increases EEG delta activity within sustained NREM sleep (McGinty

A. Warm-sensitive Neuron

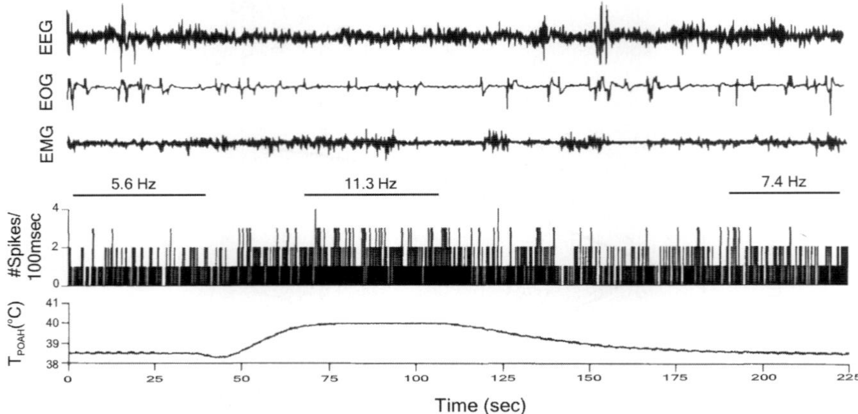

B. Sleep-wake Profile of Thermosensitive Neurons

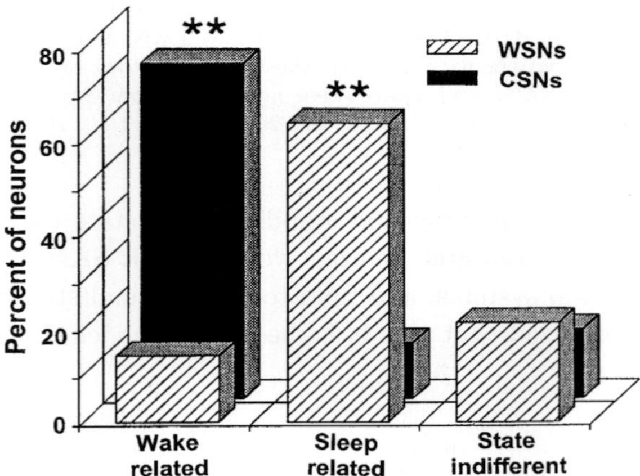

Figure 5. (A) POA WSNs, characterized by consistent discharge rate increase in response to local warming by about 1.5°C during waking. WSNs and CSNs were defined by standard criteria, and constituted about 25% of neurons encountered in the midlateral POA. (B) Based on discharge rates across the sleep–wake cycle, WSNs and CSNs were characterized as sleep-related or wake-related neurons. The analysis showed that about 70% CSNs were wake-related, and about 60% WSNs were sleep-related. (From Alam *et al.*, 1995a.)

and Szymusiak, 2001). These findings suggested that POA WSNs and CSNs participate in sleep control.

We recorded POA thermosensitive neurons during spontaneous sleep–wake (Alam *et al.*, 1995a) and showed that over 60% POA WSNs were sleep-activated, and most CSNs, over 70%, were wake-activated (Figure 5B). The changes in discharge rate occurring at sleep onset were equivalent to those elicited by a strong thermal stimulus, about 2.0°C, while awake. WSNs increased discharge several seconds before the beginning of EEG synchronization at sleep onset. As brain temperature declines at sleep onset, changes in discharge could not be due to changes in local temperature. Since activation of WSNs and/or CSN deactivation by local POA warming is sufficient to elicit, sustain, and "deepen" NREM sleep, and the same neuronal discharge changes occur during spontaneous sleep, it is reasonable to hypothesize that this neuronal process plays a central role in spontaneous NREM sleep.

We showed that local POA warming inhibits discharge of putative wake-promoting neuronal groups. This warming effect was shown in DRN REM-off neurons (Guzmán-Marín *et al.*, 2000), as illustrated in Figure 3, pLH wake-active neurons (Methiparra *et al.*, 2003), and PH (Krilowicz *et al.*, 1994) and basal forebrain (Alam *et al.*, 1995b) wake-active neurons. In these studies, waking was maintained during the warming trials, so changes in discharge reflected direct effects of warming rather than changes in arousal level. These studies show that POA temperature-sensitive neurons participate in the inhibitory regulation of multiple putative wake-promoting systems.

Since sleep, like panting, is a response to POA warming, sleep might have a thermoregulatory function. Sleep onset is associated with lowered body temperature and thermolytic processes. The hypothesis that NREM sleep is tightly coupled to thermoregulatory processes is supported by many additional findings, including the physiological changes accompanying NREM, the coupling of NREM propensity to the circadian temperature rhythm in humans, and the sleep-enhancing effects of body temperature elevations. This evidence is reviewed in detail elsewhere (McGinty and Szymusiak, 2001).

Measuring Neuronal Unit Responses to Neurochemical Processes: Combined Unit Recording and Microdialysis

Many current hypotheses concerning the control of sleep focus on the roles of neurochemical mechanisms (Obal and Krueger, 2003). In order to study the interactions of neurochemical processes with neurophysiological models of sleep control, we have developed the technique of unit recording adjacent to a microdialysis membrane (Figure 6A). The responses of identified sleep-active or wake-active neurons to chemical agents can be assessed. In the example shown in Figure 6B, the application of the putative sleep-promoting agent, adenosine, increased the discharge of a lateral POA/BF SAN, but inhibited a concurrently recorded wake-active neuron (Alam *et al.*, 1999). These findings were consistent with the hypothesis that adenosine can act as a sleep-promoting agent (Porkka-Heiskanen *et al.*, 1997). However, even in the presence of adenosinergic agonists and antagonists, NREM onset and offset were associated with brisk wake-related and SAN neuronal discharge rate changes, suggesting that other modulators also play an essential role in sleep-related neuronal control.

We recently showed that the proposed sleep-promoting substance, Il-1β, delivered by local microdialysis can also inhibit POA/BF wake-active and, in some cases, facilitate sleep-active neurons (Alam *et al.*, 2004). In the same brain area, the putative sleep-promoting substance, PGD2, delivered by micropipette, also facilitates sleep-active neurons (Osaka and Hayaishi, 1995). Thus, multiple sleep-promoting factors can modulate POA/BF SANs and wake-related neurons. The comparative roles of these several substances in the POA/BF during daily sleep and sleep homeostasis is not known.

Using the same method, we have shown that pLH wake-active neurons are inhibited by GABA agonists and facilitated by GABA$_A$ antagonists (Alam *et al.*, 2003), confirming a possible role of GABA in the regulation of these neurons. We extended the analysis of GABAergic effects by examining the immunolabeling of c-Fos and hypocretin adjacent to a microdialysis probe in the same site (Figure 6C). This example shows that administration of the GABA$_A$ antagonist, bicuculline, increased the numbers of hypocretin-expressing neurons that also immunostain for c-Fos. These findings are consistent with the hypothesis that hypocretin-containing neurons are normally inhibited by GABA. We can hypothesize that the sleep-active GABAergic neurons in the MnPN projecting to the pLH are an important source of this inhibition.

Insights Derived from Neuronal Unit Studies

Neuronal unit recording studies showed that both putative sleep-promoting processes concentrated in the POA and putative wake-promoting processes in multiple sites are coded by simple discharge rate changes. SANs increase

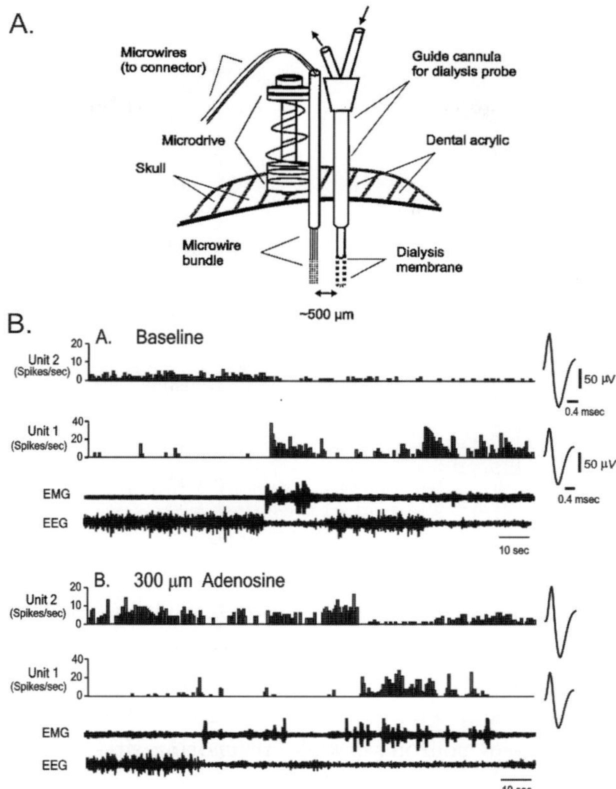

Figure 6. (A) Method for combining microdialysis with adjacent neuronal unit recording. Microwires are advanced by a microdrive mounted on the skull close to the microdialysis probe. The microdialysis membrane is placed at least 12 h before the beginning of the experiment. (B) Experiment showing the effects of local administration of adenosine (300 µM) on a wake-active (unit 1) and a sleep-active neuron (unit 2). Compared to the baseline (upper, with CSF perfusion), during adenosine perfusion, the sleep-active neuron exhibited increased discharge during both sleep and waking, and the wake-active neuron exhibited reduced discharge. Figures on the left are superimposed spike waveforms from samples. (From Alam *et al.*, 1999.) (C) Method of combining microdialysis with immunostaining. On the left (a and c) are horizontally cut sections centered on the longitudinal axis of the probe. On the right (b and d) are higher magnifications showing double-labeling of c-Fos and hypocretin. Bicuculline (20 µM, 60 min) administration (b) greatly increased the c-Fos IR staining of hypocretin-positive neurons compared to aCSF (d). These data demonstrate that activation of hypocretin-containing neurons is under GABAergic control. Filled arrow: hypo+/Fos+; bank arrow: hypo+/Fos−; blank arrowhead: hypo−/Fos+.

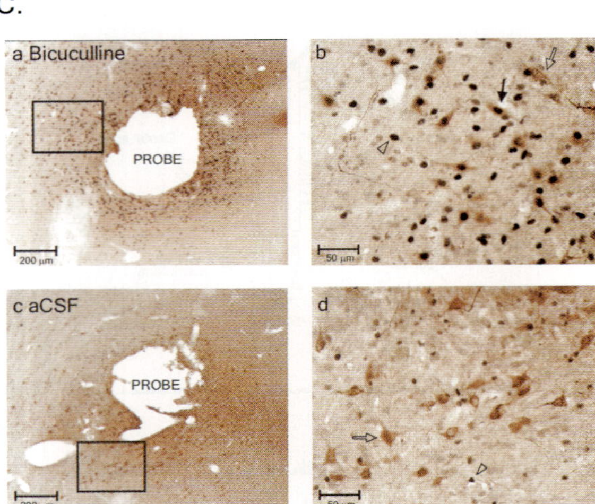

Figure 6. (*Continued*)

discharge directly before sleep onset and, in many cases, sustain these increases in both NREM and REM. Available evidence suggests that some SANs send projections to the sites of wake-promoting neurons and release inhibitory neurotransmitters. Activation of POA WSNs by local warming inhibits activity of neurons in wake-promoting sites. The spontaneous discharge of these WSNs increases during sleep, in fact most WSNs are also SANs.

In both MnPN and VLPO, neuronal discharge is related to measures of homeostatic drive, although not in identical ways. Putative sleep-promoting neurochemical agents, including PGD2, adenosine and IL-1 can directly activate SANs.

Putative wake-promoting neurons are usually of two types, wake-active, REM-off, or wake-active, REM-active. NREM rates are low. Some sets of wake-active neurons exhibit discharge related to motor or EMG activity. Wake-active neurons exhibit low discharge during quiet waking, so discharge changes at sleep-onset transitions cannot be easily assessed.

Since POA lesions suppress sleep, the predominant output of this site is sleep-promoting. Cirelli and Tononi (2000) summarize evidence that POA neurons exhibiting wake-related c-Fos expression may be important in homeostatic sleep regulation. In contrast to most brain sites, POA neurons exhibit persistent wake-associated c-Fos expression with sustained sleep deprivation. POA c-Fos IR is increased by several stimulant drugs, but is lower in old rats, which also show reduced sleep rebound after deprivation. After POA administration of antisense oligonucleotides to *c-fos*, blocking c-Fos IR, rats sleep less the next day, without a compensatory rebound. POA wake-related c-Fos IR does not co-localize with GABA, suggesting that these wake-related neurons are distinct from SANs. Additional work on the interactions of wake-related and sleep-related neurons in the POA is needed.

Comparing Neuronal Unit Recording and Immunostaining Methods

Our summary of findings using chronic unit recording and c-Fos immuno-staining suggests that the two methods provide complementary data, as summarized in Table 1. We emphasize that c-Fos IR is useful in localizing SANs only in sites where SANs are segregated from wake-active neurons. In

Table 1. Comparison of electrophysiological and anatomical (c-Fos) methods

Electrophysiological methods	Anatomical methods
Detailed temporal relation of activity with sleep–wake process, including homeostatic variables	Only gross correlation of activity with state. Some types of neurons do not express c-Fos when activated
Sequential changes in neuronal activity across the sleep cycle	Anatomical distribution of SANs, but only in sites of segregated SANs
Relative changes in activity in NREM and REM sleep	Neuronal phenotype of SANs using double labeling in segregated sites
Change in activity during state transitions	Afferent and efferent connections of SANs
Effects of sleep deprivation on neuronal discharge	Effects of sleep deprivation on specific c-Fos IR in neuronal phenotypes
Time-locked waking behavioral correlates of neuronal discharge	Effects of global behavioral manipulations on c-Fos IR possibly accompanied by potentially confounding correlated processes
Responses to local application of neurochemical agents	Responses to intra-cerebro-ventricular (ICV) or systemic administration of neurochemical agents, usually accompanied by potentially confounding correlated processes
Response to local application of physiological variables such as temperature	Response to whole-body application of physiological variables such as temperature, usually accompanied by potentially confounding correlated processes

much of the POA there is overlap of wake-associated and sleep-associated c-Fos expression, and wake-related c-Fos IR is greater, so one cannot know if labeled cells are functionally specific. However, the c-Fos method provides much critical information concerning the phenotype and connectivity of SANs.

Limitations of Neuronal Unit Recording Methods

Most contemporary unit recording studies in chronic animals utilize the microwire method or other extracellular electrodes. With these methods, it is not possible to determine the specific neuronal phenotype of recorded neurons. As exemplified in the case of serotonin-containing neurons, inferences concerning the phenotype of recorded neurons can sometimes be made on the basis of congruent indirect evidence. Even in this case, the possibility that a particular neuronal phenotype is heterogenous with respect to its behavioral correlates cannot be excluded. More commonly, the phenotype of recorded neurons cannot be determined. The method of juxtacellular recording with pipette electrodes in head-restrained animals can be used to determine neuronal phenotype, but this method is labor-intensive and is used infrequently.

There are several additional limitations to chronic unit recording studies. Many investigators now rely on computerized spike sorting to evaluate sleep–wake related discharge. This method assumes that spike shape is invariant across the sleep–wake cycle, but changes in state may be associated with changes in membrane resistance, so changes in spike shape during state changes could be expected. Changes in local blood flow or slight changes in electrode position due to brain movement can also affect recording properties. It is common to search for cells in awake animals, so neurons selectively active during sleep may be missed. Microelectrode recordings tend to sample larger neurons, so smaller neurons will be undersampled or missed. In sites of tightly packed cells, only multiunit recordings are usually obtained.

Conclusions

We have summarized extensive evidence that activity of POA SANs determines the occurrence of sleep and codes sleep homeostasis. Part of this regulation originates in POA temperature-sensitive neurons. POA SANs regulate the activity of wake-promoting neurons, which, in turn, can regulate EEG, motor, and autonomic features of sleep (Suntsova *et al.*, 2002). The circadian clock sends direct and disynaptic afferents to the sites of SANs in MnPN and VLPO (Deurveilher *et al.*, 2002; Deurveilher and Semba, 2003). Thus, SANs may integrate homeostatic and circadian control of sleep. Given the central role of SANs in the control of sleep, it is important to know what controls SANs activation. SANs respond to several putative sleep-promoting factors, including adenosine, Il-1β, and PGD2, but the proportional role of these factors during spontaneous sleep is not established.

The evidence presented above suggests that, in contrast to whole-animal manipulations, local manipulations in conjunction with chronic unit recording studies may be needed to determine the specificity of effects required to answer critical questions.

Acknowledgments

This research was supported by the Veterans Administration and U.S. Public Health Service grants MH47480, HL60296, MH61354, and MH63323. The authors thank Darya Stewart for assistance.

References

Alam, M.N., McGinty, D., and Szymusiak, R. (1995a). Neuronal discharge of preoptic/anterior hypothalamic thermosensitive neurons: relation to NREM sleep. *Am. J. Physiol.*, 269: 1240–1249.

Alam, M.N., Szymusiak, R., and McGinty, D. (1995b). Local preoptic/anterior hypothalamic warming alters spontaneous and evoked neuronal activity in the magno-cellular basal forebrain. *Brain Res.*, 696: 221–230.

Alam, Md.N., Szymusiak, R., Gong, H., King, J., and McGinty, D. (1999). Adenosinergic modulation of rat basal forebrain neurons during sleep and waking: Neuronal recording with microdialysis. *J. Physiol. (Lond.)*, 521: 679–690.

Alam, M., Gong, H., Alam, T., Jaganath, R., McGinty, D., and Szymusiak, R. (2002). Sleep-waking discharge patterns of neurons recorded in the rat perifornical lateral hypothalamic area. *J. Physiol.*, 538: 619–631.

Alam, Md.N., Kumar, S., Methippara, M.M., Szymusiak, R., and McGinty, D. (2003). GABA-ergic regulation of perifornical-lateral hypothalamic (PF-LHA) neurons during waking and sleep in freely moving rats. *Soc. Neurosci. Abstr.*, 29: 341.5.

Alam, M.N., Kumar, S., Bashir, T., Suntsova, N., Methippara, M.M., Szymusiak, R., and McGinty, D. (2005). GABA-mediated control of hypocretin but not melanin-concentrating hormone-immunoreactive neurones during sleep in rats. *J. Physiol.*, 563: 569–582.

Bai, D. and Renaud, L.P. (1998). Median preoptic nucleus neurons: an *in vitro* patch-clamp analysis of their intrinsic properties and noradrenergic receptors in the rat. *Neuroscience*, 83: 905–916.

Boulant, J.A. and Dean, J.B. (1986). Temperature receptors in the central nervous system. *Ann. Rev. Physiol.*, 48: 639–654.

Cirelli, C. and Tononi, G. (2000). On the functional significance of *c-fos* induction during the sleep-wake cycle. *Sleep*, 23: 453–469.

Deurveilher, S. and Semba, K. (2003). Indirect projections from the suprachiasmatic nucleus to the median preoptic nucleus in rat. *Brain. Res.*, 987: 100–106.

Deurveilher, S., Burns, J., and Semba, K. (2002). Indirect projections from the suprachiasmatic nucleus to the ventrolateral preoptic nucleus: a dual tract tracing study in the rat. *Eur. J. Neurosci.*, 16: 1195–1213.

Gallopin, T., Fort, P., Eggermann, E., Cauli, B., Luppi, P., Rossier, J., Audinat, E., Muhlethaler, M., and Serafin, M. (2000). Identification of sleep-promoting neurons *in vitro*. *Nature*, 404: 992–995.

Gong, H., Szymusiak, R., King, J., Steininger, T., and McGinty, D. (2000). Sleep-related c-Fos expression in the preoptic hypothalamus: effects of ambient warming. *Am. J. Physiol. Regul. Integr. Comp. Physiol.*, 279: 2079–2088.

Gong, H., Szymusiak, R., King, J., Shin, S., and McGinty, D. (2001). Co-localization of c-Fos protein and GABA in preoptic area neurons following sleep. *Sleep*, 24: A155.

Gong, H., McGinty, D., and Szymusiak, R. (2002). Projections from the median preoptic nucleus to hypocretin and forebrain cholinergic systems in rats. *Sleep*, 25: A155.

Gong, H., McGinty, D., Guzmán-Marín, R., Chew, K.-T., Stewart, D., and Szymusiak, R. (2004). Activation of GABAergic neurons in the preoptic area during sleep and in response to sleep deprivation. *J. Physiol.* 556: 935–946.

Gritti, I., Mainville, L., and Jones, B.E. (1994). Projections of GABAergic and cholinergic basal forebrain and GABAergic preoptic-anterior hypothalamic neurons to the posterior lateral hypothalamus of the rat. *J. Comp. Neurol.*, 339: 251–268.

Guzmán-Marín, R., Alam, Md.N., Szymusiak, R., Drucker-Colin, R., Gong, H., and McGinty, D. (2000). Discharge modulation of rat dorsal raphe neurons during sleep and waking: effects of preoptic/basal forebrain warming. *Brain Res.*, 875: 23–34.

Guzmán-Marín, R., Suntsova, N., Stewart, D.R., Gong, H., Szymusiak, R., and McGinty, D. (2003). Sleep deprivation reduces proliferation of cells in the dentate gyrus of the hippocampus in rats. *J. Physiol.*, 549: 563–571.

Hobson, J.A., McCarley, R.W., and Nelson, J.P. (1983). Location and spike-train characteristics of cells in anterodorsal pons having selective decreases in firing rat during desynchronized sleep. *J. Neurophysiol.*, 50: 770–783.

Jacobs, B. and Fornal, C. (1999). 5-HT and motor control: a hypothesis. *Trends Neurosci.*, 16: 346–352.

Jacobs, B.L., Harper, R.M., and McGinty, D.J. (1970). Neuronal coding of motivational level during sleep. *Physiol. Behav.*, 5: 1139–1143.

Jones, B.E. (1994). Basic mechanisms of sleep-wake states. In: Kryger, M.H., Roth, T., and Dement, W.C. (Eds.). *Principles and Practice of Sleep Medicine.* Philadelphia: W.B. Saunders, pp. 145–162.

Kiyashchenko, L.I., Mileykovskiy, B.Y., Maidment, N., Lam, H.A., Wu, M.F., Peever, J.J., and Siegel, J.M. (2002). Release of hypocretin (orexin) during waking and sleep states. *J. Neurosci.*, 22: 5282–5286.

Krilowicz, B.L., Szymusiak, R., and McGinty, D. (1994). Regulation of posterior lateral hypothalamic arousal related neuronal discharge by preoptic anterior hypothalamic warming. *Brain Res.*, 668: 30–38.

McGinty, D. and Siegel, J.M. (1992). Brain neuronal unit discharge in freely moving animals: methods and application in the study of sleep mechanisms. In: Epstein, A.N. and Morrison, A.R. (Eds.). *Progress in Psychobiology and Physiological Psychology.* San Diego: Academic Press, pp. 85–139.

McGinty, D. and Szymusiak, R. (1988). Neuronal unit activity patterns in behaving animals: brainstem and limbic system. *Ann. Rev. Psychol.*, 39: 135–168.

McGinty, D. and Szymusiak, R. (2001). Brain structures and mechanisms involved in the generation of NREM sleep: focus on the preoptic hypothalamus. *Sleep Med. Rev.*, 5: 323–342.

McGinty, D. and Szymusiak, R. (2003). Hypothalamic regulation of sleep and arousal. *Front. Biosci.*, 8: 1074–1083.

Methiparra, M., Alam, Md.N., Szymusiak, R., and McGinty, D. (2003). Preoptic area warming inhibits wake-active neurons in the perifornical lateral hypothalamus. *Brain Res.*, 960: 165–173.

Morgan, J.I. and Curran, T. (1991). Stimulus-transcription coupling in the nervous system: involvement of the inducible proto-oncogenes fos and jun. *Annu. Rev. Neurosci.*, 14: 421–451.

Nitz, D. and Siegel, J.M. (1996). GABA release in posterior hypothalamus across sleep-wake cycle. *Am. J. Physiol.*, 271: 1707–1712.

Nitz, D. and Siegel, J. (1997a). GABA release in the dorsal raphe nucleus: role in the control of REM sleep. *Am. J. Physiol.*, 273: 451–455.

Nitz, D. and Siegel, J.M. (1997b). GABA release in the locus coeruleus as a function of sleep/wake state. *Neuroscience*, 78: 795–801.

Obal, F. Jr. and Krueger, J.M. (2003). Biochemical regulation of non-rapid-eye-movement sleep. *Front. Biosci.*, 8: 520–550.

Osaka, T. and Hayaishi, O. (1995). Prostaglandin D2 modulates sleep-related and noradrenaline-induced activity of preoptic and basal forebrain neurons in the rat. *Neurosci. Res.*, 23: 257–268.

Peyron, C., Petit, J.-M., Rampon, C., Jouvet, M., and Luppi, P.-H. (1998a). Forebrain afferents to the rat dorsal raphe nucleus demonstrated by retrograde and anterograde tracing methods. *Neuroscience*, 82: 443–468.

Peyron, C., Tighe, D.K., van den Pol, A.N., de Lecea, L., Heller, H.C., Sutcliffe, J.G., and Kilduff, T.S. (1998b). Neurons containing hypocretin (orexin) project to multiple neuronal systems. *J. Neurosci.*, 18: 9996–10015.

Porkka-Heiskanen, T., Strecker, R.E., Thakkar, M., Bjorkum, A.A., Greene, R.W., and McCarley, R.W. (1997). Adenosine: a mediator of the sleep-inducing effects of prolonged wakefulness. *Science*, 276: 1265–1268.

Rowland, N.E. (1998). Brain mechanisms of mammalian fluid homeostasis: insights from use of immediate early gene mapping. *Neurosci. Biobehav. Rev.*, 23: 49–63.

Scammel, T., Price, K., and Sagar, S. (1993). Hyperthermia induces *c-fos* expression in the preoptic area. *Brain Res.*, 618: 303–307.

Sherin, J.E., Shiromani, P.J., McCarley, R.W., and Saper, C.B. (1996). Activation of ventrolateral preoptic neurons during sleep. *Science*, 271: 216–219.

Sherin, J.E., Elmquist, J.K., Torrealba, F., and Saper, C.B. (1998). Innervation of histaminergic tuberomammillary neurons by GABAergic and galaninergic neurons in the ventrolateral preoptic nucleus of the rat. *J. Neurosci.* 18: 4705–4721.

Steininger, T.L., Alam, Md.N., Gong, H., Szymusiak, R., and McGinty, D. (1999). Sleep-waking discharge of neurons in the posterior lateral hypothalamus of the albino rat. *Brain Res.*, 840: 138–147.

Steininger, T., Gong, H., McGinty, D., and Szymusiak, R. (2001). Subregional organization of preoptic area/anterior hypothalamic projections to arousal-related monoaminergic cell groups. *J. Comp. Neurol.*, 429: 638–653.

Suntsova, N., Szymusiak, R., Alam, Md.N., Guzmán-Marín, R., and McGinty, D. (2002). Sleep-waking discharge patterns of median preoptic nucleus neurons in rats. *J. Physiol.*, 543: 665–677.

Szymusiak, R., Alam, N., Steininger, T., and McGinty, D. (1998). Sleep-waking discharge patterns of ventrolateral preoptic/anterior hypothalamic neurons in rats. *Brain Res.*, 803: 178–188.

von Economo, C. (1930). Sleep as a problem of localization. *J. Nerv. Ment. Dis.*, 71: 249–259.

Wu, M.F., John, J., Maidment, N., Lam, H.A., and Siegel, J.M. (2002). Hypocretin release in normal and narcoleptic dogs after food and sleep deprivation, eating, and movement. *Am. J. Physiol., Regul. Integr. Comp. Physiol.*, 283: 1079–1086.

Yoshimoto, Y., Sakai, K., Luppi, P.H., Fort, P., Salvert, D., and Jouvet, M. (1989). Forebrain afferents to the cat posterior hypothalamus: a double labeling study. *Brain Res. Bull.*, 23, 83–104.

Zardetto-Smith, A.M. and Johnson, A.K. (1995). Chemical topography of efferent projections from the median preoptic nucleus to pontine monoaminergic cell groups in the rat. *Neuroscience Lett.*, 199: 215–219.

Chapter 8

A PHYSIOLOGICAL VIEW OF REM SLEEP STRUCTURE

Roberto Amici, Christine A. Jones, Emanuele Perez,
and Giovanni Zamboni[1]

In spite of vigorous research, sleep still defies the attempts to understand its mechanisms and function. However, since sleep may be easily defined in behavioural terms, one way to address this difficulty is to describe and analyse processes related to experimentally induced behavioural changes.

The broadest behavioural definition of sleep is to consider that it is related to rest and, likewise, to consider wakefulness as being complementary to activity. Although rest and activity show a rhythm in both vertebrates and invertebrates (Brady, 1974; Rusak and Zucker, 1979), the analogy between rest and sleep, on the one hand, and activity and wakefulness, on the other, is essentially based on criteria derived from sleep behaviour in higher organisms such as mammals: namely, that rest–sleep is characterised by a higher sensory threshold and that a reduction of the time spent in this state is followed by its compensatory increase (cf. Hartse, 1994; Tobler, 2000; Greenspan *et al.*, 2001).

When higher vertebrates (mammals and birds) are considered, the behavioural definition of sleep may also be based on the more restrictive criterion of a rapid reversal to wakefulness from a state in which the behavioural signs of consiousness are absent (Zepelin, 2000). However, the main characteristic of sleep in these classes is that it can be sub-divided into

---

[1]gzamboni@biocfarm.unibo.it

the two basic states of NREM sleep and REM sleep, both of which continue to obey the general rule that a recovery follows deprivation. NREM sleep and REM sleep not only add the ultradian dimension to the sleep cycle, but also add a further degree of organisation, since normally NREM sleep occurs before REM sleep. An unavoidable consequence of this hierarchy in time is that the analysis of the recovery following total sleep deprivation requires that a possible regulatory interplay between the sleep stages is taken into account. The analysis of sleep in terms of the intensification of wake and sleep processes has led to the conceptual framework of sleep homeostasis, derived from classical physiology, in which experimental outcomes can be interpreted. Accordingly, homeostatic sleep regulation rests on the concept that sleep is maintained around an average reference level by counteracting mechanisms and should apply to both NREM sleep and REM sleep (Borbély and Achermann, 2000; Achermann and Borbély, 2003). In the simplest terms, the variable which is regulated is the time spent in a sleep stage, whilst the reference level is the amount of time spent in the same stage of the control or baseline condition. It is evident that with this reasoning the problem of defining the period of time, during which both the amount and the reference level of sleep are measured, remains open.

However, research on sleep has also brought to light other parameters, such as the slow-wave activity during NREM sleep, which is related to the duration of the preceding wake period and is thought to represent the intensity of an underlying process concerning the homeostatic regulation of sleep (Borbély and Achermann, 2000; Achermann and Borbély, 2003).

REM Sleep within the Wake–Sleep Cycle

In contrast, REM sleep appears to resist any analysis based on the intensity of EEG parameters and the description of its processes is still based on the cumulative duration of episodes. This suggests that REM sleep processes do not affect cortical bioelectrical activity in the same way as NREM sleep processes. Thus, although some interaction should exist, as suggested by either the effects of slow-wave activity on the occurrence of REM sleep (Endo *et al.*, 1998) or the possible accumulation of a "drive" for REM sleep during waking and/or NREM sleep (Horne, 2000), it is worth considering the possibility that REM sleep processes are separate from those of NREM sleep. This had been suggested from both the discovery of the suspension of thermoregulation during REM sleep (Parmeggiani, 1977, 1980a) and the analysis of the somatic and vegetative phenomenology of sleep (Parmeggiani, 1980b). These results clearly proved that the progression from wake to sleep is not only characterised by the loss of consciousness, but also by a profound reorganisation of physiological regulations which significantly perturbs vegetative activity during the passage from NREM to REM sleep. The causal explanation for this is most probably in the alteration of hypothalamic integration, which also underlies the loss of the thermoregulatory control (Parmeggiani, 1982).

Studies on the vegetative phenomenology of sleep suggest that the temporal organisation as shown by the occurrence of NREM sleep before REM sleep may be an important characteristic of the ultradian wake–sleep cycle. In fact, in regulatory terms, the course from waking to REM sleep may be seen as the progressive disappearance of integrative physiological regulations, since in the passage from waking to NREM sleep, vegetative functions cease to have the intervention of behavioural adjustments, whilst the transition from NREM sleep to REM sleep entails the lack of both behavioural regulation and a fully operant vegetative activity. It may be noted that, in spite of its regulatory restrictions, REM sleep appears as a fully recognisable state in homeotherms, which are at the top of the evolutionary tree. Both this phylogenetic characteristic and the recovery following deprivation would imply that REM sleep performs an important, albeit unknown, function. However, these theoretical views should be considered carefully, since there are some contradictory experimental findings. For example, whilst in the rat, selective REM sleep deprivation becomes as lethal as total sleep deprivation, due to the induction of a metabolic disorder characterised by an irreversible increase in energy expenditure (Rechtschaffen, *et al.*, 1989; Everson, 1995; Rechtschaffen and Bergmann, 2002), in humans, a much longer pharmacological inhibition of REM sleep shows no physiological consequences (Wyatt *et al.*, 1971; Landolt and Posthuma de Boer, 2001).

Since there are state-dependent changes in physiological regulation, the progress through and the completion of the wake–sleep cycle require that some regulatory adjustments (for example, in a cold environment a posture to minimise heat loss) are mainly performed during the fully regulated stage of waking. The anticipation of physiological regulations has been defined as predictive homeostasis and the term has been introduced with respect to the circadian system (Moore-Ede, 1986). Although it would be tempting to propose an extension of predictive homeostasis to the ultradian aspects of the wake–sleep cycle, it should be mentioned that another two proposals have recently been made to adjourn the concept of homeostasis: the first is rheostasis, the condition in which homeostatic mechanisms are operant, but in which the regulated level is changed within a definite interval of time (Mrosovsky, 1990); the second is allostasis, which describes a condition characterised by anticipatory behavioural and physiological responses, but in which there is the possibility of a physiological overload and breakdown of regulatory capacities (Schulkin, 2003). Since, a discussion on this topic is beyond the limit of this work, we have taken a simpler view by considering homeostasis within its basic physiological meaning as the activity of regulatory processes concerning the whole organism. The full operating capacity of homeostatic regulations during waking and NREM sleep allows us to consider these two states as one type of functional unit, whilst the impairment of homeostatic regulations during REM sleep would imply that it is a separate entity.

It should be stressed that this dual description of the wake–sleep cycle no longer corresponds to the analogy of wake–sleep as activity–rest. With respect to this, the study of processes related to the wake–sleep cycle may be approached by analysing the succession of REM sleep episodes and the period of time intervening between the end of one REM sleep episode and the beginning of the next (REM sleep interval). Moreover, it allows wake–sleep processes and physiological regulations to be simultaneously studied during both the circadian and the ultradian wake–sleep cycles.

A Dichotomy between Intervals Separating Consecutive REM Sleep Episodes

Figure 1 (left) shows the frequency distribution of the duration of REM sleep intervals in the rat kept at normal laboratory temperature (Ta, 23°C). The data shown represent the average frequency distribution during the 12-h L period of the LD cycle, i.e., the period in which the rat produces almost 80% of its daily amount of REM sleep (Borbély and Neuhaus, 1978).

As can be seen, the distribution is clearly bimodal with a minimum at the 3-min class and two maximum values at the 1-min and the 8- to 10-min classes. This type of distribution identifies two populations of intervals, which can be empirically divided into short and long intervals by using the minimal frequency class to set the boundary between them. Thus, for the rat, short intervals last for 3 min or less, while long intervals have a duration longer than 3 min.

The analysis of comparative data shows that the average duration of the ultradian sleep cycle and, consequently, of REM sleep intervals, appears to increase according to both the size and the degree of encephalisation of the species (Dallaire *et al.*, 1974; Zepelin, 2000). Furthermore, a bimodal distribution of REM sleep intervals has been observed in several

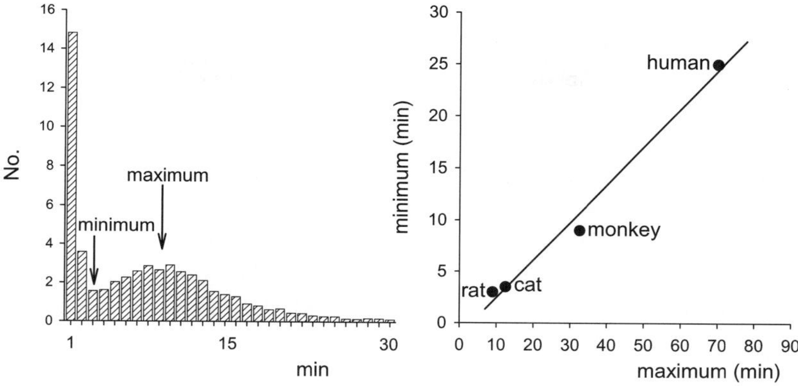

Figure 1. Left: Average frequency distribution of the duration of the interval from the end of one REM sleep episode to the beginning of the subsequent episode (REM sleep interval) under normal laboratory conditions, during the L period of the LD cycle in the rat (74 animals). The frequency class which was taken as the boundary separating short- and long-interval populations (minimum) is at 3 min. The mode for the long-interval population is indicated as maximum. Right: The relationship between the values of the minimum and maximum frequency classes in the rat, cat (Ursin, 1970), monkey (Kripke *et al.*, 1968), and human (Kobayashi *et al.*, 1985; Merica and Gaillard, 1991; Carskadon and Rechtschaffen, 2000).

species, i.e., the cat (Ursin, 1970), Rhesus monkey (Kripke *et al.*, 1968), and humans (Kobayashi *et al.*, 1985; Merica and Gaillard, 1991; Carskadon and Rechtschaffen, 2000). Interestingly, as shown on the right of Figure 1, the duration of the interval belonging to the lowest frequency class (minimum), which sets the boundary between short and long intervals, increases proportionally to that of the mode representing the long REM sleep intervals (maximum). This observation suggests that the occurrence of REM sleep episodes separated by either short or long intervals represents a biological trait which should be under a specific regulation and, therefore, be instrumental to a fine analysis of the regulatory aspects of REM sleep occurrence (Zamboni *et al.*, 1999).

Short versus Long REM Sleep Intervals: Time Course of EEG Power Density, Hypothalamic Temperature and Motor Activity during the Pre-REM Sleep Period

In the rat, cat, and mouse, REM sleep occurrence is usually preceded by specific changes in the EEG pattern, which consist of the appearance of successive short bouts (<10 s) of high-amplitude spindles in the anterior cerebral cortex and are associated with the appearance of a theta rhythm in the dorsal hippocampus (cf. Gottesman, 1996). Such an EEG pattern has been used to define an "intermediate" sleep stage, which is considered to be distinct from both NREM sleep and REM sleep (Gottesman, 1992). In the rat, the analysis of the time course of the EEG power density has shown that delta power progressively decreases, whilst both theta and sigma power progressively rise during the 30- to 60-s period before the onset of a REM sleep episode (Trachsel *et al.*, 1988; Benington *et al.*, 1994). Interestingly, in the rat kept under normal laboratory conditions, such a pattern is not always followed by a consolidated REM sleep episode, but in about 50% of cases, it is followed by a sudden awakening (Mandile *et al.*, 1996; Franken, 2002).

Therefore, it would appear that the passage from NREM sleep to REM sleep is characterised by a period of transition during which it may be supposed that integrative autonomic structures control for the opportunity to leave a behavioural state, during which homeostatic regulations are fully operant (NREM sleep), before entering a state during which they are not (REM sleep). This, together with the fact that REM sleep intervals show a bimodal distribution based on their duration, implies that changes in biological variables within the pre-REM sleep period would be important for REM sleep occurrence.

The time course of the power values in different EEG frequency bands (4-s epochs in the delta, theta, and sigma ranges transformed by using the fast Fourier algorithm), anterior hypothalamic temperature (Thy), and motor activity (MA) during the period preceding a REM sleep episode are shown in Figure 2. The pre-REM sleep periods were separated into six classes according to the duration of REM sleep intervals: three for short REM sleep intervals (30–60 s, 61–120 s, 121–180 s) and three for long REM sleep intervals (181–600 s, 601–900 s, >900 s). The changes shown are within a 90-s window before the start of REM sleep occurrence (0 s) except for intervals falling within the first two classes where the upper limit of the window was set at the lower limit, which defines the class. The data are relative to the L period of the LD cycle and both the power density and MA are expressed as the percentage of their respective average 24-h value.

As can be seen, there are some features which differentiate the pre-REM sleep period which occurs within a short REM sleep interval from that which occurs within a long REM sleep interval:

1. Relative delta power appears much lower within short intervals than within long intervals.

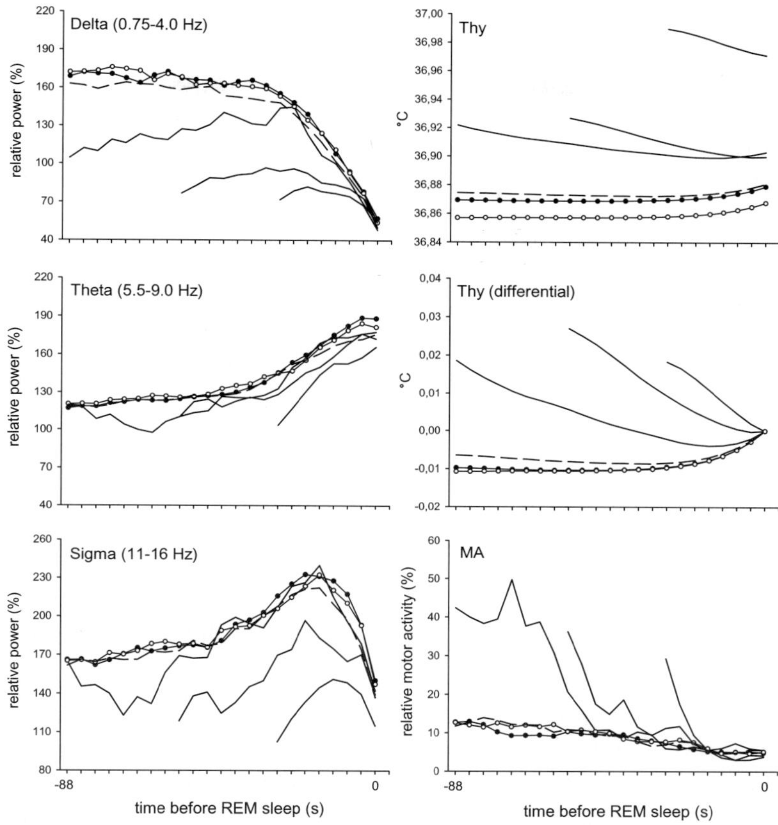

Figure 2. Time course of relative power density values in the delta, theta, and sigma EEG frequency bands, hypothalamic temperature (Thy), and motor activity (MA) during a fixed period, which precedes the start of an REM sleep episode (pre-REM period). The data are shown for six different classes of REM sleep intervals defined according to their duration: three classes include short REM sleep intervals; (31–60 s, 61–120 s, 121–180 s, continuous lines) and three classes include long REM sleep intervals (181–600 s, filled circle; 601–900 s, empty circle; >900 s, dashed line). Changes are shown within a 90 s window before the start of REM sleep occurrence (0 s) except for the first two classes (31–60 s, 61–120 s) for which the upper limit of the window corresponded to the lower limit of the class. Data refer to 31 animals and values for each parameter corresponding to 4 s epochs were first averaged within each class of duration for individual animals, and the average value for all animals used was calculated afterwards. The method for averaging took the onset of an REM sleep episode as 0 s and was carried out backwards along the pre-REM period. Both the power density for each frequency band and the MA are expressed as a percentage of the respective average 24-h value. Thy levels are shown in degrees celsius as either the absolute Thy value or the difference from the value at the beginning of the REM sleep episode. All data shown are relative to the L period of the LD cycle.

2. Relative sigma power appears much lower in the 31- to 60-s class and the 61- to 120-s class than in long intervals for all of the pre-REM period, whilst in the 121- to 180-s class, it attains a level similar to that observed for the long intervals towards the end of the pre-REM period.
3. Absolute Thy levels at the beginning of an REM sleep episode are higher following a short interval than following a long interval. Moreover, as emphasised by the figure showing differential Thy levels with respect to the start of the episode (0 s), Thy appears stable and practically clamped at its lowest level in long intervals, while the higher values of the short intervals decrease rapidly.
4. An intense MA is present in short intervals, whilst long intervals are characterised by its virtual absence.

On the whole, it would appear that the regulatory processes which underlie the transition from a REM sleep interval to a REM sleep episode differ according to discrete subdivisions of the REM sleep interval.

Short versus Long REM Sleep Intervals: Regulatory Aspects within Short-Term REM Sleep Regulation

A short-term regulatory process operating within sleep cycles has been shown in several different species (Ursin, 1970; Benington and Heller, 1994; Vivaldi *et al.*, 1994; Barbato and Wehr, 1998). In fact, the duration of a REM sleep interval appears to be positively correlated to the duration of the preceding REM sleep episode, but not to the episode which follows. However, the relationship between the duration of a REM sleep episode and that of the previous REM sleep interval is not yet apparent. This would imply that the amount of time the animal can spend without REM sleep is controlled for during the preceding REM sleep episode. If this is the case, the subsequent duration of each REM sleep interval is indicative of the functional state relating to this control.

Data relative to the L period of the LD cycle are presented in Figure 3, which shows the duration of the REM sleep interval as the independent variable. Intervals are separated into classes of duration and are on a logarithmic scale (the upper limit of the relevant classes are indicated). The histogram represents the average frequency distribution of interval duration, whilst the circles indicate the average duration of the REM sleep episode which preceded each class of interval (pre-REM sleep episode).

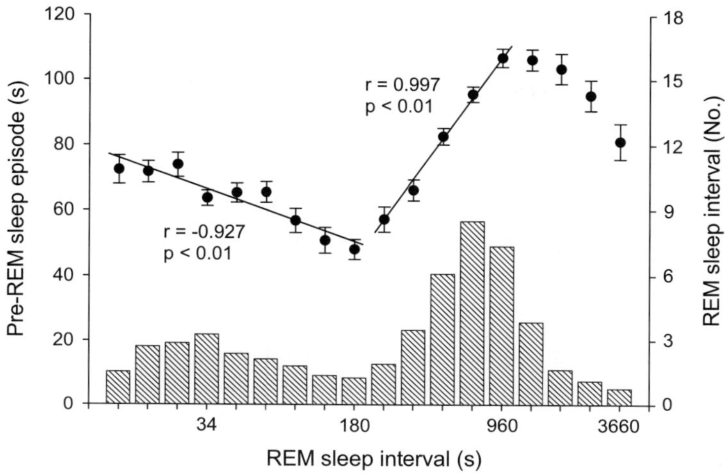

Figure 3. Histogram: Average frequency distribution of the duration of the interval from the end of one REM sleep episode to the beginning of the subsequent episode (REM sleep interval) during the L period of the LD cycle in the rat (74 animals) under normal laboratory conditions. REM sleep intervals are separated into classes based on the duration and are represented as a logarithmic progression. The upper limit of the classes which were relevant to the analysis is shown. Scatter plot: Relationship between the duration of the REM sleep interval and that of the preceding REM sleep episode (pre-REM sleep episode). The duration of the pre-REM sleep episode duration (mean $\pm$ SEM) was calculated by averaging the mean value within each class of duration for individual animals. Linear regression lines for all classes of short intervals ($\leq$180 s) and long intervals within the duration range of 180–960 s, are shown. Pearson's correlation coefficient and p levels are also indicated.

It may be seen that the frequency distribution of the duration of the REM sleep interval, even if it is condensed over a logarithmic scale, has a minimum within the class having an upper limit of 180 s. This value corresponds to a minimum average duration of the pre-REM sleep episode of 50 s (decreasing from a maximum average duration of about 80 s). Beyond this, a steep rise in the duration of the pre-REM sleep episode occurs until it reaches a plateau at 110 s and only begins to decrease when intervals last about 1 h. Both linear regression lines for the relationship between the pre-REM sleep episode and the REM sleep interval are highly significant.

This analysis confirms that there is a positive correlation between the duration of the REM sleep interval and the pre-REM sleep episode in the rat (Benington and Heller, 1994; Vivaldi *et al.*, 1994); however, this only appears to apply to long REM sleep intervals. In contrast, a negative correlation exists for short REM sleep intervals. These data would suggest that the regulatory processes which underlie the relationship between a REM sleep episode (homeostatic regulations not fully operant) and the following REM sleep interval (homeostatic regulations fully operant) are different within the two populations of REM sleep intervals.

Short versus Long REM Sleep Intervals: A Biological Basis for the Classification of REM Sleep Episodes as "Single" or "Sequential"

The boundary which divides REM sleep intervals into two populations appears to be a specific biological trait for each species since it changes in direct proportion to the mode of long REM sleep intervals. From this, and the previous arguments, it may be concluded that the separation of REM sleep intervals into two populations of different duration has a functional meaning. Furthermore, there are relevant differences concerning the processes underlying the regulation of short and long REM sleep intervals which have been observed in the rat. In particular, both the transition from an REM sleep interval to an REM sleep episode and the relationship between an REM sleep episode and the following REM sleep interval appear to be different in the two populations. This would imply that any functional relationship linking two consecutive REM sleep episodes separated by a short interval is different from that between REM sleep episodes separated by a long interval.

On the basis of this, two types of REM sleep episodes can be identified in the rat (Figure 4): "single" REM sleep episodes, which are preceded and followed by long REM sleep intervals (>3 min), and "sequential" REM sleep episodes, which are separated by short REM sleep intervals (≤3 min) and occur in "clusters" (Amici *et al.*, 1994).

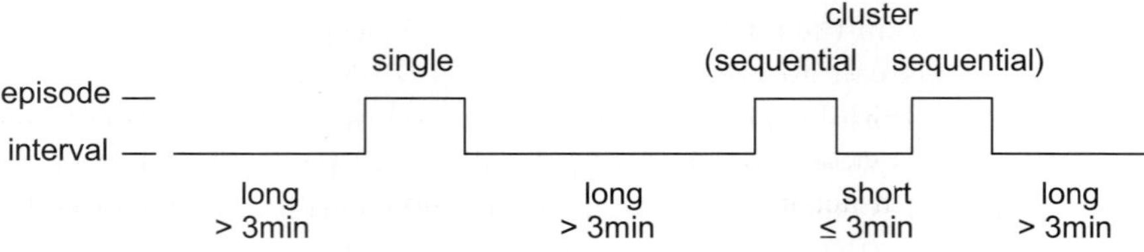

Figure 4. Schematic representation for the classification of REM sleep episodes in the rat (based on the distribution of REM sleep intervals shown in Figure 1).

Clusters form a functional unit of REM sleep, since each cluster consists of a group of sequential REM sleep episodes separated by short intervals, even though the first and the last sequential REM sleep episode of each cluster is preceded and followed, respectively by a long interval. The amount of REM sleep in a cluster can be calculated as the total duration of the constituent sequential REM sleep episodes without taking into account the short intervals within the cluster.

The Biological Relevance of Single and Sequential REM Sleep Episodes within Long-Term REM Sleep Regulation

The biological relevance of short and long REM sleep intervals has been shown in experiments in which the regulation of REM sleep occurrence has been studied within the normal light–dark schedule (Zamboni *et al.*, 2001) and under the influence of different environmental challenges, i.e., changes in ambient temperature (Amici *et al.*, 1994, 1998; Zamboni *et al.*, 2001), administration of rhythmic auditory stimuli (Amici *et al.*, 2000, 2001), and immobilisation stress (Dewasmes *et al.*, 2004).

The time course of REM sleep occurrence in the form of either single or sequential episodes during a 48-h exposure to Ta 0°C and the following 12-h recovery period at normal laboratory Ta (23°C) is shown for the rat in Figure 5.

It may be observed that, in control conditions (Ta 23°C), both single and sequential REM sleep episodes follow a circadian pattern which is altered by the exposure to low Ta due to the immediate depression of REM sleep. However, during the second day of exposure, whilst the occurrence of sequential REM sleep episodes is still depressed, single REM sleep episodes not only recover the circadian pattern of expression, but also have an amount of REM sleep which is close to that observed for single episodes in the control condition. Such a rapid adaptation to the unfavourable ambient condition emphasises the importance of REM sleep for mammals. The recovery period following the exposure is characterised by a rebound of REM sleep which has previously been shown to be quantitatively related to the degree of deprivation in both the cat (Parmeggiani *et al.*, 1980) and the rat (Franken *et al.*, 1993; Amici *et al.*, 1994, 1998, 2002; Zamboni *et al.*, 2001), a result in accordance with a precise homeostatic control of REM sleep. However, as can be seen in Figure 5, such a rebound of REM sleep occurs in the form of sequential episodes whilst the amount of REM sleep in the form of single episodes does not differ from that observed in the

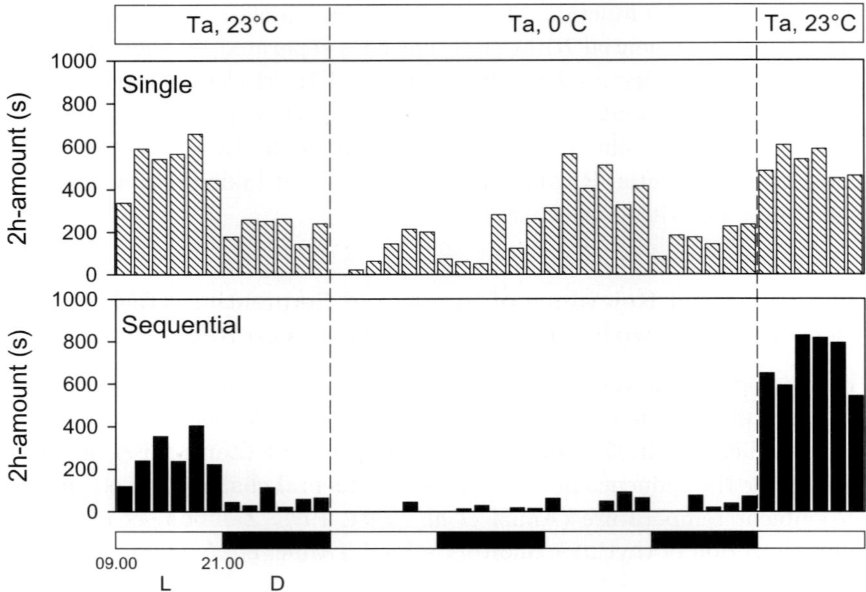

Figure 5. Time course of REM sleep in the rat under the form of either single (upper histogram, shaded) or sequential (lower histogram, filled) REM sleep episodes, in the control condition (Ta, 23°C), during a 48-h period of exposure to Ta 0°C, and during the following 12-h period of recovery at Ta 23°C. Data represent the average amount of REM sleep within 2-h intervals under the form of either single or sequential episodes. (From Amici *et al.*, 1994.)

control condition. Thus, it would appear that REM sleep occurrence in the rat is modulated by either positive or negative changes in the amount of sequential REM sleep episodes.

The analysis of the frequency and the duration of the two types of episodes in the control condition has shown that the average duration of a sequential episode is about 80% that of a single episode, but that the average duration of a REM sleep cluster, i.e., the rapid sequence of sequential episodes, is almost double that of a single episode (Amici *et al.*, 1994, 1998; Zamboni *et al.*, 2001). Moreover, with the exception of the very early period of exposure to low Ta, both the circadian and the ultradian modulation of REM sleep occurrence appear to be due to changes in the frequency and not in the duration of the episodes (Amici *et al.*, 1994, 1998; Zamboni *et al.*, 2001).

The tendency to modulate the amount of REM sleep at different ambient temperatures, by changing the frequency of episodes, has been observed in other mammals of very small size (Sakaguchi *et al.*, 1979; Roussel *et al.*, 1984; Sichieri *et al.*, 1984). Thus, it would appear that in species with an unfavourable surface-to-volume ratio, the tight control on thermoregulation sets an upper limit for the duration of REM sleep, which can only be overridden by adding distinct, but close, episodes. With respect to this, the introduction of short periods of homeostatic control ensures the recovery of an amount of REM sleep (a gap in homeostatic regulation) which is sufficient to recover the amount lost. Interestingly, it has been recently shown that the occurrence of short REM sleep intervals (and consequently that of sequential REM sleep episodes) can be, respectively, depressed or enhanced in the rat by injecting either an agonist (1-(2,5-dimethoxy-4-iodophenyl)-2-aminopropane) or an antagonist (ketanserin) of the $5\text{-}HT_2$ serotonergic receptor into the laterodorsal tegmental nucleus (LDT) (Amici *et al.*, 2004). Since the activity of the serotonergic system appears to be related to the control of different physiological processes (Jacobs and Azmitia, 1992), such as thermoregulation (Myers, 1980) and the response to environmental stressors (Chaouloff *et al.*, 1999), it may be hypothesised that excitation of $5\text{-}HT_2$ receptors in LDT signals an environmental challenge.

The relevance of the separation of REM sleep into single and sequential episodes within the long-term regulatory aspects of REM sleep occurrence has been inferred from experiments in which rats underwent different protocols of exposure to low Tas and recovery at normal laboratory Ta (Amici *et al.*, 1994, 1998; Zamboni *et al.*, 2001). In Figure 6, the relationship between the loss of REM sleep under the influence of different thermal loads (12 h, 24 h, and 48 h at either Ta 0°C or Ta −10°C) and the amount of REM sleep which occurs in the form of either single or sequential REM sleep episodes in the following recovery period at Ta 23°C is shown. Whilst the recovery began at the normal time of light onset for the L period of the LD cycle, in some experiments the light was not switched on and animals recovered in continuous dark. With respect to this, it has been observed that the amount of REM sleep increases when rats, which had been adapted to a 12-h:12-h LD cycle, are kept in the dark during the expected L period (continuous darkness; Fishman and Roffwarg, 1972; Borbély and Neuhaus, 1978).

The results clearly show that a rebound of REM sleep in the form of single episodes does not occur under these conditions. It is the amount of REM sleep in the form of sequential REM sleep episodes, increasing in proportion to the degree of the previous deprivation, that must be related to a process involved in REM sleep homeostasis. However, it would appear

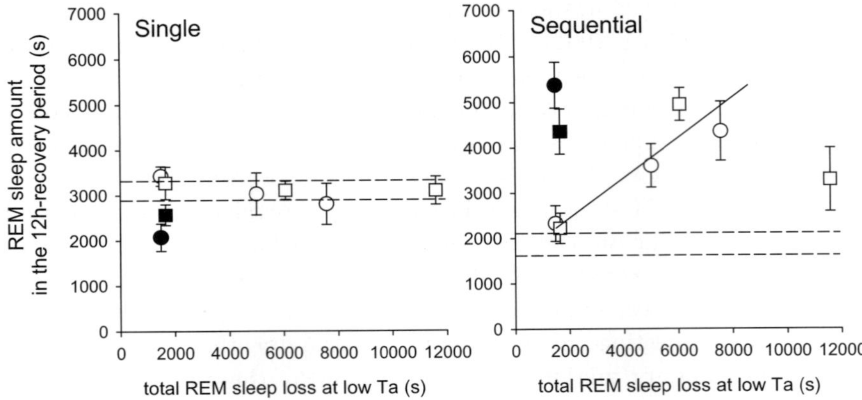

Figure 6. Relationship between the loss of REM sleep under the influence of different thermal loads and the amount of REM sleep which occurs in the form of either single or sequential REM sleep episodes (mean ± SEM) in the 12-h recovery period at Ta 23°C (started at 09:00; L period of the LD cycle) in the rat. Circles and squares indicate animals which had been kept at Ta 0°C and Ta −10°C, respectively (12, 24, and 48 h). The recovery was made in either the light (empty symbols) or the dark (filled symbols). The dashed lines show the range of variation of the control values. The linear regression line, relative to sequential REM sleep episodes, is shown for animals which were allowed to recover in the light, but the value from animals having the highest REM sleep loss (48 h at Ta −10°C) was not included.

that there are two exceptions to this rule, since the amount of sequential REM sleep is greater than expected when the recovery is carried out in the dark, and smaller when the recovery in light follows a 48-h exposure to Ta −10°C. As can be seen, these changes are not proportional to the previous deprivation and, thus, would challenge the hypothesis that REM sleep occurrence is under a homeostatic control.

Changes in Hypothalamic Levels of the Second Messenger 3′,5′-Cyclic Adenosine Monophosphate under Different Ambient Challenges are Related to the Amount of Sequential REM Sleep

In the rat, the interaction between processes related to sleep and thermoregulation have been studied at a biochemical level in brain areas which are known to be relevant for these physiological regulations, in particular, (i) the preoptic area–anterior hypothalamus (PO–AH), since it is well known that it is both the principal structure controlling thermoregulation (Boulant, 2000) and a region involved in the control of the wake–sleep cycle (Parmeggiani, 1980a; Saper *et al.*, 2001); (ii) the ventromedial hypothalamic nucleus (VMH), since it is involved in the control of brown adipose tissue thermogenesis (Perkins *et al.*, 1981; Woods *et al.*, 1996); and (iii) the cerebral cortex (CC) and the hippocampus (HI), since their bioelectrical activity is used to classify behavioural states in the rat (cf. Gottesman, 1992).

In our laboratory, one target of such a biochemical analysis has been the second messenger $3',5'$-cyclic adenosine monophosphate (cAMP), whose intracellular concentration is affected by many neuroactive substances acting on receptors coupled to adenylyl cyclase (for a general review, see Siegel *et al.*, 2000). Since the cAMP signalling cascade leads to the control of protein function by means of phosphorylation (Walaas and Greengard, 1991), it may be expected that changes in cAMP accumulation reflect a change in cellular activity. Furthermore, the maximum accumulation capacity of cAMP in the brain can be evoked by using hypoxia, an unspecific physiological stimulus, which induces an acute increase in cAMP levels in both mice (Gross and Ferrendelli, 1980) and rats (Zamboni *et al.*, 1990).

Basal cAMP levels appear to be closely related to both circadian and ultradian processes in PO–AH and VMH, but not in CC (Zamboni *et al.*, 1982; Perez *et al.*, 1991). Furthermore, these ultradian and circadian changes in basal cAMP levels appear to be affected by the exposure to low Ta in proportion to the thermal load and, in particular, during the exposure to Ta $-10°C$ when cAMP levels are progressively and tonically depressed (Perez *et al.*, 1982, 1995). The biological relevance of these changes may be further supported by the observation that, under the same experimental conditions, the maximum cAMP accumulation capacity is also depressed in these areas, whilst no changes are observed in CC or HI (Zamboni *et al.*, 1996, 2001). The extent of this depression is dependent on the thermal load since the cAMP accumulation capacity of the PO–AH is significantly higher following the exposure to Ta $0°C$ than following the exposure to Ta $-10°C$ (Zamboni *et al.*, 2001). From a behavioural point of view, these biochemical changes are paralleled by a strong depression in REM sleep occurrence in the form of both single and sequential REM sleep episodes (Amici *et al.*, 1998).

Although basal cAMP levels and the maximum cAMP accumulation capacity in PO–AH have been shown to progressively increase when animals are returned to normal laboratory Ta following a 48-h exposure to Ta $-10°C$ (Perez *et al.*, 1982; Zamboni *et al.*, 1996), the maximum cAMP accumulation capacity still remains below control levels 4–5 h into the recovery (Zamboni *et al.*, 1996).

Figure 7 (top) shows the maximum cAMP accumulation capacity at the start of the recovery (0 h) and 4 h and 30 min into the recovery (early recovery period) following the exposure to Ta $-10°$C. Since cAMP concentration

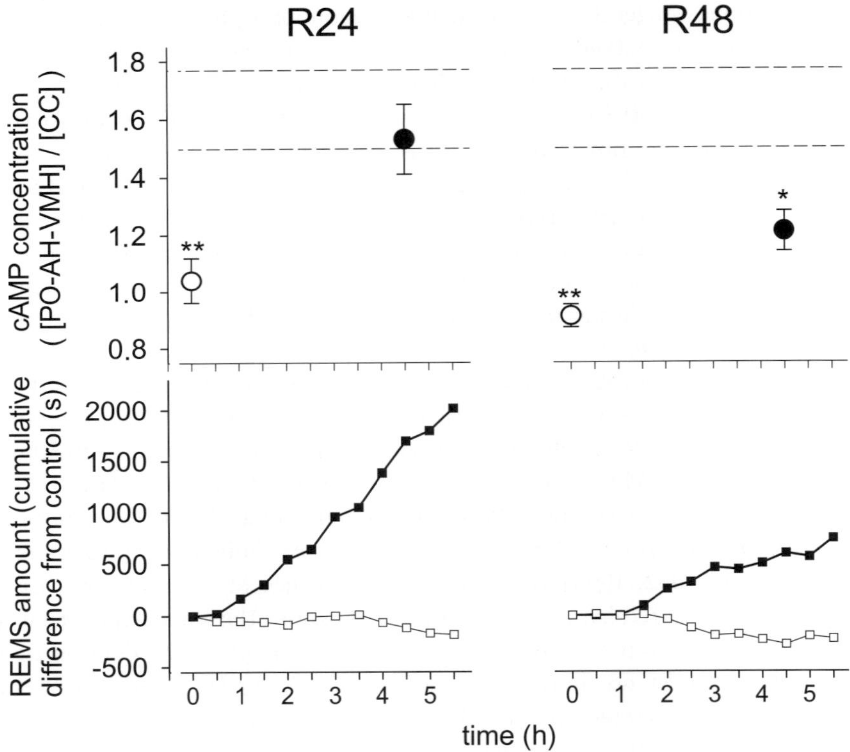

Figure 7. Top: Ratio of maximum cAMP accumulation capacity in PO–AH–VMH to that in CC (pmol/mg protein; bars represent SEM), either at the beginning of (0 h, empty circles) or after 4 h 30 min into (filled circles) the recovery following either a 24-h (R24) or a 48-h (R48) exposure to Ta $-10°$C. Dashed lines indicate the range of values observed in control conditions at normal laboratory Ta. $*p < 0.05$, $**p < 0.01$, with respect to control values. (From Zamboni *et al.*, 2004.) Bottom: Average cumulative differential REM sleep (REMS) amount, in the form of either single (empty squares) or sequential (filled squares) REM sleep episodes during the first 6 h of the recovery period at normal laboratory Ta, following either a 24-h (R24) or a 48-h (R48) exposure to Ta $-10°$C. The amount of REM sleep (s) was calculated every 30 min as the difference from control values at normal laboratory Ta. (From Amici *et al.*, 1998.)

in CC was found to be very stable, the results were expressed as the ratio of the cAMP concentration in PO–AH–VMH to that in CC (relative hypothalamic cAMP concentration). It may be seen that the relative hypothalamic cAMP concentration decreases to approximately the same level following the exposure to Ta $-10°$C, irrespective of the duration. However, it appears that only during the early recovery that follows the 24-h exposure does the capacity to accumulate cAMP attain the control level. In fact, the relative hypothalamic cAMP concentration of the early recovery period that follows the 48-h exposure, although increased with respect to that observed at the end of exposure, still remains significantly below the control level.

The specificity of this response is supported by recent findings concerning the maximal cerebral accumulation of both cAMP and inositol 1,4,5-trisphosphate (IP^3) following either a 24-h or a 48-h exposure to Ta $-10°$C (Zamboni *et al.*, 2004). Whilst the concentration of cAMP decreased in both PO–AH and VMH, but not in CC, IP^3 concentration tended to follow the same pattern of variation in all the brain regions studied, i.e., a slight decrease following a 24-h exposure or an increase following a 48-h exposure.

These biochemical results may be compared with the behavioural findings (Figure 7, bottom) of an experiment in which the pattern of REM sleep occurrence during the exposure to Ta $-10°$C for either 24 h or 48 h and during the following recovery was studied (Amici *et al.*, 1998). The figure shows the cumulative differential amount of REM sleep with respect to control levels, in the form of either single or sequential episodes and calculated for the first 6 h of the recovery. It may be clearly seen that the accumulation of sequential REM sleep episodes during the early recovery from a 48-h exposure is much lower than that observed following a 24-h exposure. Since the amount of REM sleep lost following 48 h of exposure is much greater than that lost following 24 h (Amici *et al.*, 1998), we may conclude that the amount of sequential REM sleep in the early recovery after 48 h of exposure is in conflict with the needs for the maintenance of REM sleep homeostasis.

Further support for the existence of a functional relationship between REM sleep occurrence in the form of sequential episodes and hypothalamic cAMP accumulation is suggested by the observation that basal cAMP concentration in PO–AH of rats kept in continuous darkness (light off during the L period of the LD cycle) is significantly higher (about 20%) than that of animals kept in a normal light-on condition (Perez *et al.*, 1991). Under the same condition, REM sleep in the form of sequential episodes is about 80% higher than the control level observed in the normal light-on L period (Zamboni *et al.*, 2001). Also, when the recovery following a 12-h exposure to either Ta 0°C or −10°C is carried out in continuous darkness, the amount of sequential REM sleep is greatly increased when compared to the recovery in the light, although it is lower following the exposure to Ta −10°C (Figure 6). The latter finding may be related to the fact that the maximal cAMP accumulation capacity, determined in PO–AH at the beginning of the recovery, is significantly higher following the exposure to Ta 0°C than following the exposure to Ta −10°C (Zamboni *et al.*, 2001).

Thus, it appears that a probable reduction in cAMP-dependent protein phosphorylation in a brain region involved in the control of vegetative activity and sleep is concomitant with the inhibition of REM sleep occurrence during the exposure to low Ta and with an impairment in the capacity to generate REM sleep in the form of sequential episodes during the early phase of the recovery. In contrast, the increase in sequential REM sleep episodes observed in continuous darkness is associated with an increase in hypothalamic cAMP concentration. On the basis of this, it may be hypothesised that cAMP-dependent phosphorylation plays an important role in the hypothalamic vegetative control which allows REM sleep to occur in episodes separated by short intervals.

The Structure of REM Sleep as a Regulatory Behavioural Mechanism

The finding that thermoregulation is suspended during REM sleep is almost 40 years old (Parmeggiani and Rabini, 1967) and, in spite of a great deal of work confirming and extending this observation, we do not know as yet why this happens. However, some of the results which we have discussed in this chapter indicate an approach to the problem which has led to two aspects we think may be relevant.

Firstly, the study of the organisation of the wake–sleep cycle based on the regulation of the vegetative system is important. The dual organisation of the wake–sleep cycle emerging from this approach emphasises the relationship between the homeostasis of REM sleep and the homeostasis of the organism. This concept allows sleep to be studied on (i) a short-term basis, by investigating the transition into REM sleep and the changes in physiological regulations induced by the modification of the hypothalamic integrative activity which characterises an REM sleep episode, and (ii) a long-term basis, by determining how REM sleep occurrence is modified according to changes in physiological regulations. An outcome of this approach has been to reduce the temporal order of waking, NREM sleep, and REM sleep into a quantitative relationship between the duration of a REM sleep episode and the duration of the following REM sleep interval, regardless of whether the latter is waking or NREM sleep. From this, it may be inferred that the processes related to wake or NREM sleep influence when the next REM sleep episode will occur, but the duration of the episode itself appears as an intrinsic characteristic.

Secondly, the importance of the role played by the hypothalamus in the interaction between the organisation of the wake–sleep cycle and the regulation of vegetative activity should be emphasised. Although the role of the hypothalamus in the control of wake and sleep has been recently re-evaluated (McGinty and Szymusiak, 2001; Salin-Pascual *et al.*, 2001; Saper *et al.*, 2001), the appraisal of its involvement as a centre for vegetative regulation during sleep is still mainly backed by results concerning thermoregulation (cf. Parmeggiani, 2003). The biochemical signs of plastic changes (cf. Silva *et al.*, 1998) in hypothalamic cellular activity, observed when REM sleep is actively inhibited by very low ambient temperatures, may be taken as the first line of evidence for the occurrence of REM sleep in mammals and birds to be considered as more than a simple correlate of homeothermy (Horne, 2000). With respect to this, a second line of evidence may be given by the observation that a vegetative function, such as the control of the osmolality of extracellular fluid, which is mainly controlled at the hypothalamic level (magnocellular neurons of the paraventricular and supraoptic nuclei) and is phylogenetically much older than thermoregulation (Denton *et al.*, 1996), is not impaired during REM sleep (Zamboni *et al.*, 2003).

These arguments may be extended by returning to the physiological meaning of the behavioural analysis of REM sleep. When we assume that the duration of an episode is an intrinsic characteristic of REM sleep, we should also consider the possibility that the duration of a behavioural state is, in many instances, a tool for physiological regulations (Cabanac, 1996) rather than a regulated variable. In this context, a precise control on the duration of the behaviour suggests the existence of a stereotypical organisation characterising the consummatory phase of instinctive behaviour. The proposal to associate sleep with the consummatory act of instinctive behaviour was advanced by Parmeggiani in 1968 and developed by Moruzzi (1969), the latter considering that both NREM sleep and REM sleep were a chain of consummatory actions preceded by the appetitive phase of drowsiness. However, the compulsory nature of REM sleep occurrence and the existence of a quantitative relationship between the amount lost and recovered has led to the proposal that only this stage is the consummatory phase of the sleep instinct (Parmeggiani, 1973). In our opinion, the close relationship between the duration of an REM sleep interval and that of the preceding REM sleep episode further supports this view, since it is the length of the consummation (REM sleep episode) that determines the duration of the following phase of satiation (REM sleep interval).

It is evident that the behavioural side of a regulation should be related to one or more physiological mechanism(s) and, thus, a behavioural analysis should offer some indications as to the variable(s) under such an integrated regulation. The physiological analysis of REM sleep points to the possibility that this consummatory act is related to the vegetative activity involved in thermoregulation and that, as a consequence, the constant maintenance of homeothermy requires the highest hierarchical control to allow for its tightly regulated suspension during this stage. Thus, naming REM sleep as paradoxical sleep (Jouvet *et al.*, 1959) has been a far-sighted decision, since its enigmatic nature appears to be related more to the functioning of the whole organism than to the EEG pattern.

References

Achermann, P. and Borbély, A.A. (2003). Mathematical models of REM sleep regulation. *Front. Biosci.*, 8: 683–693.

Amici, R., Zamboni, G., Perez, E., Jones, C.A., Toni, I., Culin, F., and Parmeggiani, P.L. (1994). Pattern of desynchronized sleep during deprivation and recovery induced in the rat by changes in ambient temperature. *J. Sleep Res.*, 3: 250–256.

Amici, R., Zamboni, G., Perez, E., Jones, C.A., and Parmeggiani, P.L. (1998). The influence of a heavy thermal load on REM sleep in the rat. *Brain Res.*, 781: 252–258.

Amici, R., Domeniconi, R., Jones, C.A., Morales-Cobas, G., Perez, E., Tavernese, L., Torterolo, P., Zamboni, G., and Parmeggiani, P.L. (2000). Changes in REM sleep occurrence due to rhythmical auditory stimulation in the rat. *Brain Res.*, 868: 241–250.

Amici, R., Morales-Cobas, G., Jones, C.A., Perez, E., Torterolo, P., Zamboni, G., and Parmeggiani, P.L. (2001). REM sleep enhancement due to rhythmical auditory stimulation in the rat. *Behav. Brain Res.*, 123: 155–163.

Amici, R., Cerri, M., Jones, C.A., Luppi, M., Ocampo-Garces, A., Parmeggiani, P.L., Perez, E., Venturi, S., and Zamboni, G. (2002). Sleep regulation in the rat exposed to changes in ambient temperature. *J. Sleep Res.*, 11(suppl. 1): 4.

Amici, R., Sanford, L.D., Kerney, K., McInerney, B., Ross, R.J., Horner, R.L., and Morrison, A.R. (2004). A serotonergic (5-HT2) receptor mechanism in the laterodorsal tegmental nucleus participates in regulating the pattern of rapid-eye-movement sleep occurrence in the rat. *Brain Res.*, 996: 9–18.

Barbato, G. and Wehr, T.A. (1998). Homeostatic regulation of REM sleep in humans during extended sleep. *Sleep*, 21: 267–276.

Benington, J.H. and Heller, H.C. (1994). REM sleep timing is controlled homeostatically by accumulation of REM-sleep propensity in non-REM sleep. *Am. J. Physiol.*, 266: 1992–2000.

Benington, J.H., Kodali, S.K., and Heller, H.C. (1994). Scoring transitions to REM sleep based on the EEG phenomena of pre-REM sleep: an improved analysis of sleep structure. *Sleep*, 17: 28–36.

Borbély, A.A. and Achermann, P. (2000). Sleep homeostasis and models of sleep regulation. In: Kryger, M.H., Roth, T., and Dement, W.C. (Eds.). *Principles and Practice of Sleep Medicine*. Philadelphia: W.B. Saunders, pp. 377–390.

Borbély, A.A. and Neuhaus, H.U. (1978). Daily pattern of sleep, motor activity and feeding in the rat: effects of regular and gradually extended photoperiods. *J. Comp. Physiol.*, 124: 1–14.

Boulant, J.A. (2000). Role of the preoptic-anterior hypothalamus in thermoregulation and fever. *Clin. Infect. Dis.*, 31(suppl. 5): S157–S161.

Brady, J. (1974). The physiology of insect circadian rhythm. *Adv. Insect Physiol.*, 10: 1–115.

Cabanac, M. (1996). The place of behavior in physiology. In: Fregly, M.J. and Blatteis, C.M. (Eds.). *Handbook of Physiology, Section 4: Environmental Physiology*. New York: Oxford University Press, pp. 1523–1536.

Carskadon, M.A. and Rechtschaffen, A. (2000). Monitoring and staging human sleep. In: Kryger, M.H., Roth, T., and Dement, W.C. (Eds.). *Principles and Practice of Sleep Medicine*. Philadelphia: W.B. Saunders, pp. 1197–1215.

Chaouloff, F., Berton, O., and Mormède, P. (1999). Serotonin and stress. *Neuropsychopharmacol.*, 21: 28S–32S.

Dallaire, A., Toutain, P.L., and Ruckebusch, Y. (1974). Sur la périodicité du sommeil paradoxal: faits et hypothèses. *Physiol. Behav.*, 13: 395–400.

Denton, D.A., McKinley, M.J., and Weisinger, R.S. (1996). Hypothalamic integration of body fluid regulation. *Proc. Natl. Acad. Sci. USA*, 93: 7397–7404.

Dewasmes, G., Loos, N., Delanaud, S., Dewasmes, D., and Ramadan, W. (2004). Pattern of rapid-eye movement sleep episode occurrence after an immobilization stress in the rat. *Neurosci Lett.*, 355: 17–20.

Endo, T., Roth, C., Landolt, H.-P., Werth, E., Aeschbach, D., Achermann, P., and Borbély, A.A. (1998). Selective REM sleep deprivation in humans: effects on sleep and sleep EEG. *Am. J. Physiol.*, 274: 1186–1194.

Everson, C.A. (1995). Functional consequences of sustained sleep deprivation in the rat. *Behav. Brain Res.*, 69: 43–54.

Fishman, R. and Roffwarg, H.P. (1972). REM sleep inhibition by light in the albino rat. *Exp. Neurol.*, 36: 166–178.

Franken, P. (2002). Long-term vs. short-term processes regulating REM sleep. *J. Sleep Res.*, 11: 17–28.

Franken, P., Tobler, I., and Borbély, A.A. (1993). Effects of 12-h sleep deprivation and of 12-h cold exposure on sleep regulation and cortical temperature in the rat. *Physiol. Behav.*, 54: 885–894.

Gottesman, C. (1992). Detection of seven sleep-waking stages in the rat. *Neurosci. Biobehav. Rev.*, 16: 31–38.

Gottesman, C. (1996). The transition from slow-wave sleep to paradoxical sleep: evolving facts and concepts of the neurophysiological processes underlying the intermediate stage of sleep. *Neurosci. Biobehav. Rev.*, 20: 367–387.

Greenspan, R.J., Tononi, G., Cirelli, C., and Shaw, J.P. (2001). Sleep and the fruit fly. *Trends Neurosci.*, 24: 142–145.

Gross, R.A. and Ferrendelli, J.A. (1980). Mechanisms of cyclic AMP regulation in cerebral anoxia and their relationship to glycogenolysis. *J. Neurochem.*, 34: 1309–1318.

Hartse, K.M. (1994). Sleep in insects and nonmammalian vertebrates. In: Kryger, M.H., Roth, T., and Dement, W.C. (Eds.). *Principles and Practice of Sleep Medicine*. Philadelphia: W.B. Saunders, pp. 95–104.

Horne, J.A. (2000). REM sleep by default? *Neurosci. Biobehav. Rev.*, 24: 777–797.

Jacobs, B.L. and Azmitia, E.C. (1992). Structure and function of the brain serotonin system. *Physiol. Rev.*, 72: 165–229.

Jouvet, M., Michel, F., and Courjon, J. (1959). Sur un stade de activité électrique cérébrale rapide au cours du sommeil physiologique. *C. R. Soc. Biol.*, 153: 101–103.

Kobayashi, T., Tsuji, Y., and Endo, S. (1985). Sleep cycles as a basic unit of sleep. In: Schulz, H. and Lavie, P. (Eds.). *Ultradian Rhythms in Physiology and Behavior. Exp. Brain Res.*, Berlin: Springer-Verlag, pp. 260–269.

Kripke, D.F., Reite, M.L., Pegram, L.M., Stephens, L.M., and Lewis, O.F. (1968). Nocturnal sleep in rhesus monkeys. *Electroencephalogr. Clin. Neurophysiol.*, 24: 582–586.

Landolt, H.-P. and Posthuma de Boer, L. (2001). Effect of chronic phenelzine treatment on REM sleep: report of three patients. *Neuropsychopharmacology*, 25: S63–S67.

Mandile, P., Vescia, S., Montagnese, P., Romano, F., and Giuditta, A. (1996). Characterization of transition sleep episodes in baseline EEG recordings of adult rats. *Physiol. Behav.*, 60: 1435–1439.

McGinty, D. and Szymusiak, R. (2001). Brain structures and mechanisms involved in the generation of NREM sleep: focus on the preoptic hypothalamus. *Sleep Med. Rev.*, 5: 323–342.

Merica, H. and Gaillard, J.M. (1991). A study of the interrupted REM episode. *Physiol. Behav.*, 50: 1153–1159.

Moore-Ede, M.C. (1986). Physiology of the circadian timing system: predictive versus reactive homeostasis. *Am. J. Physiol.*, 250: 735–752.

Moruzzi, G. (1969). Sleep and instinctive behavior. *Arch. Ital. Biol.*, 108: 175–216.

Mrosovsky, N. (1990). *Rheostasis. The Physiology of Change*. New York: Oxford University Press.

Myers, R.D. (1980). Hypothalamic control of thermoregulation. In: Morgane, P.J. and Panksepp, J. (Eds.). *Handbook of the Hypothalamus.* New York: Marcel Dekker, pp. 83–210.

Parmeggiani, P.L. (1968). Telencephalo-diencephalic aspects of sleep mechanisms. *Brain Res.,* 7: 350–359.

Parmeggiani, P.L. (1973). The physiological role of sleep. In: Koella, W.P. and Levin, P. (Eds.). *Sleep. Physiology, Biochemistry, Psychology, Pharmacology, Clinical Implications.* Basel: Karger, pp. 210–213.

Parmeggiani, P.L. (1977). Interaction between sleep and thermoregulation. *Waking Sleeping,* 1: 123–132.

Parmeggiani, P.L. (1980a). Behavioral phenomenology of sleep (somatic and vegetative). *Experientia,* 36: 6–11.

Parmeggiani, P.L. (1980b). Temperature regulation during sleep: a study in homeostasis. In: Orem, J. and Barnes, C.D. (Eds.). *Physiology in Sleep.* New York: Academic Press, pp. 97–143.

Parmeggiani, P.L. (1982). Regulation of physiological functions during sleep in mammals. *Experientia,* 38: 1405–1408.

Parmeggiani, P.L. (2003). Thermoregulation and sleep. *Front. Biosci.,* 8: 557–567.

Parmeggiani, P.L. and Rabini, C. (1967). Shivering and panting during sleep. *Brain Res.,* 6: 789–791.

Parmeggiani, P.L., Cianci, T., Calasso, M., Zamboni, G., and Perez, E. (1980). Quantitative analysis of short term deprivation and recovery of desynchronized sleep in cats. *Electroencephalogr. Clin. Neurophysiol.,* 50: 293–302.

Perez, E., Zamboni, G., and Parmeggiani, P.L. (1982). cAMP concentration in the rat's preoptic region and cerebral cortex during sleep deprivation and recovery induced by ambient temperature. *Exp. Brain Res.,* 47: 114–118.

Perez, E., Zamboni, G., Amici, R., Fadiga, L., and Parmeggiani, P.L. (1991). Ultradian and circadian changes in the cAMP concentration in the preoptic region of the rat. *Brain Res.,* 551: 132–135.

Perez, E., Zamboni, G., Amici, R., Jones, C.A., and Parmeggiani, P.L. (1995). cAMP accumulation in hypothalamus, cerebral cortex, pineal gland and brown fat across the wake-sleep cycle of the rat exposed to different ambient temperatures. *Brain Res.,* 684: 56–60.

Perkins, M.N., Rothwell, N.J., Stock, M.J., and Stone, T.W. (1981). Activation of brown adipose tissue thermogenesis by the ventromedial hypothalamus. *Nature,* 289: 401–402.

Rechtschaffen, A. and Bergmann, B.M. (2002). Sleep deprivation in the rat: an update of the 1989 paper. *Sleep,* 25: 18–24.

Rechtschaffen, A., Bergmann, B.M., Everson, C.A., Kushida, C.A., and Gilliland, M.A. (1989). Sleep deprivation in the rat: X. Integration and discussion of the findings. *Sleep,* 12: 68–87.

Roussel, B., Turrillot, P., and Kitahama, K. (1984). Effect of ambient temperature on the sleep-waking cycle in two strains of mice. *Brain Res.,* 294: 67–73.

Rusak, B. and Zucker, I. (1979). Neural regulation of circadian rhythms. *Physiol. Rev.,* 59: 449–526.

Sakaguchi, S., Glotzbach, S.F., and Heller, H.C. (1979). Influence of hypothalamic and ambient temperatures on sleep in kangaroo rats. *Am. J. Physiol.*, 237: 80–88.

Salin-Pascual, R., Gerashchenko, D., Greco, M.A., Blanco-Centurion, C., and Shiromani, P.-J. (2001). Hypothalamic regulation of sleep. *Neuropsychopharmacology*, 25: S21–S27.

Saper, C.B., Chou, T.C., and Scammell, T.E. (2001). The sleep switch: hypothalamic control of sleep and wakefulness. *Trends Neurosci.*, 24: 726–731.

Schulkin, J. (2003). Rethinking homeostasis. In: *Allostatic Regulation in Physiology and Pathophysiology*. Cambridge: The MIT Press.

Sichieri, R. and Schmidek, W.R. (1984). Influence of ambient temperature on the sleep-wakefulness cycle in the golden hamster. *Physiol. Behav.*, 33: 871–877.

Siegel, G.J., Agranoff, B.W., Albers, R.W., and Molinoff, P.B. (2000). *Basic Neurochemistry*. New York: Raven.

Silva, A.J., Kogan, J.H., Frankland, P.W., and Kida, S. (1998). CREB and memory. *Annu. Rev. Neurosci.*, 21: 127–148.

Tobler, I. (2000). Phylogeny of sleep regulation. In: Kryger, M.H., Roth, T., and Dement, W.C. (Eds.). *Principles and Practice of Sleep Medicine*. Philadelphia: W.B. Saunders, pp. 72–81.

Trachsel, L., Tobler, I., and Borbély, A.A. (1988). Electroencephalogram analysis of non-rapid eye movement sleep in rats. *Am. J. Physiol.*, 24: 27–37.

Ursin, R. (1970). Sleep stage relation within the sleep cycles in the cat. *Brain Res.*, 11: 91–97.

Vivaldi, E.A., Ocampo, A., Wyeneken, U., Roncagliolo, M., and Zapata, A.M. (1994). Short-term homeostasis of active sleep and the architecture of sleep in the rat. *J. Neurophysiol.*, 72: 1745–1755.

Walaas, S.L. and Greengard, P. (1991). Protein phosphorylation and neural function. *Pharmacol. Rev.*, 43: 299–349.

Woods, A.J. and Stock, M.J. (1996). Inhibition of brown fat activity during hypothalamic stimulation in the rat. *Am. J. Physiol.*, 266: R328–R337.

Wyatt, R.J., Fram, D.H., Kupfer, D.J., and Snyder, F. (1971). Total prolonged drug-induced REM sleep suppression in anxious-depressed patients. *Arch. Gen. Psychiatry*, 24: 145–155.

Zamboni, G., Perez, E., and Parmeggiani, P.L. (1982). Cyclic AMP concentration in the rat's preoptic region. *Experientia*, 38: 1188–1189.

Zamboni, G., Perez, E., Amici, R., and Parmeggiani, P.L. (1990). The short-term effects of dl-propranolol on the wake-sleep cycle of the rat are related to selective changes in preoptic cyclic AMP concentration. *Exp. Brain Res.*, 81: 107–112.

Zamboni, G., Jones, C.A., Amici, R., Perez, E., and Parmeggiani, P.L. (1996). The capacity to accumulate cyclic AMP in the preoptic-anterior hypothalamic area of the rat is affected by the exposition to low ambient temperature and the subsequent recovery. *Exp. Brain Res.*, 109: 164–168.

Zamboni, G., Perez, E., Amici, R., Jones, C.A., and Parmeggiani, P.L. (1999). Control of REM sleep: an aspect of the regulation of physiological homeostasis. *Arch. Ital. Biol.*, 137: 249–262.

Zamboni, G., Amici, R., Perez, E., Jones, C.A., and Parmeggiani, P.L. (2001). Pattern of REM sleep occurrence in continuous darkness following the exposure to low ambient temperature in the rat. *Behav. Brain Res.*, 122: 25–32.

Zamboni, G., Amici, R., Baracchi, F., Capitani, P., Cerri, M., Jones, C.A., Luppi, M., Perez, E., and Parmeggiani, P.L. (2003). Changes in the antidiuretic response to osmotic stimulation during REM sleep. *Sleep*, 26(abstracts suppl.): A63.

Zamboni, G., Jones, C.A., Domeniconi, R., Amici, R., Perez, E., Luppi, M., Cerri, M., and Parmeggiani, P.L. (2004). Specific changes in cerebral second messenger accumulation underline REM sleep inhibition induced by the exposure to low ambient temperature. *Brain Res.*, 1022: 62–70.

Zepelin, H. (2000). Mammalian sleep. In: Kryger, M.H., Roth, T., and Dement, W.C. (Eds.). *Principles and Practice of Sleep Medicine*. Philadelphia: W.B. Saunders, pp. 82–92.

Chapter 9

THE POWER OF BEHAVIORAL ANALYSIS IN UNDERSTANDING SLEEP MECHANISMS

Adrian R. Morrison[1]

The focus of this chapter is the important role behavioral observation has played in advancing understanding of sleep mechanisms and, for that matter, some disorders of sleep. Behavioral studies have been a major player and, I argue, will continue to be even as we move into the realms of genetic and molecular studies. A few examples supporting this assertion will be provided later.

Although sleep is organized in the brain, we sometimes forget that external and internal environmental influences play an important role in sleep's occurrence as they do various behaviors during wakefulness. Indeed, this book was designed to remind us of this fact. For example, hunger will drive an alert individual to seek food, and other than optimal temperatures can impede the onset of sleep. The latter fact was well demonstrated many years ago by Parmeggiani and colleagues, who revealed that environmental temperature was a major factor in controlling rapid-eye-movement (REM) sleep in cats (Parmeggiani, 1980), work that they have extended to rats (Amici *et al.*, 1994, 1998). A cold environment will reduce REM to its obligate level. Thus, it is well to remember that sleep does not occur in isolation, governed only by the interactions of certain neuronal groups within the brain, for these neuronal groups are, of course, modulated by stimuli

---

[1] armsleep@vet.upenn.edu

coming from within and without the body. Knowledge of an animal's physiology is most certainly critical for the understanding of sleep mechanisms.

To cite another example, by reasoning from the physiological state of an animal during sleep, we helped direct attention fixated on the caudal brainstem as the all-important region in which to study REM mechanisms to more rostral structures in the forebrain (Morrison and Reiner, 1985). During REM, a cat is in a nonhomeostatic, or at least a very reduced homeostatic, condition (Parmeggiani, 1980). The same can be said for cats decerebrated at the midbrain–pontine junction. Such cats exhibit periods of REM-like behavior, indicating that the peripheral elements of REM, such as atonia and REMs as well as a reduced homeostatic condition, can be organized in the pons and medulla (Jouvet, 1962; Villablanca, 1966).

Yet, this does not say that REM is initiated *de novo* in the pons in normal animals. Noting that REM can be stimulated to occur in decerebrates by various abnormal stimuli, such as the passing of a stomach tube or pinching an ear (Jouvet, 1964), we (Morrison and Reiner, 1985) reasoned that the caudal brainstem neurons responsible for generating the peripheral features of REM were in an unusual sensitized state. Thus, the early important work with decerebrate cats had fooled sleep researchers into neglecting more rostral brain structures, particularly in the hypothalamus, in the study of REM mechanisms. Obviously, critical changes had to be occurring prior to REM onset in the rostral brain, that is, some time in non-REM (NREM), in order to permit entrance into such a vulnerable state. Our reasoning stimulated a number of studies that demonstrated an important role for the hypothalamus in regulating the onset of REM in intact animals (Baghdoyan *et al.*, 1993; Sakai *et al.*, 1990; Marini *et al.*, 1990; Portas *et al.*, 1997).

We chose to examine another forebrain structure that connects heavily with autonomic and sleep-related structures in the caudal brainstem as well as the hypothalamus and basal forebrain, the amygdala (Morrison *et al.*, 2000). The amygdala serves as an interface between an environment replete with novel and/or threatening stimuli and an individual's reaction systems: it adds emotional flavor to experiences (Davis, 1992; LeDoux, 1992a,b). Clearly, activity in the amygdala should at the very least modulate sleep. Some of our results will be discussed later in the chapter.

Continuing Contributions of Behavioral Studies

Historically, behavioral observation was indispensable to the advancement of sleep research. What better example is there than the tedious observation of the eyes of sleeping infants that led to the recognition of REM (Aserinsky and Kleitman, 1953). Hess and then his student, Parmeggiani, used behavioral observations while electrically stimulating the brain to map out structures, such as the hypothalamus, hippocampus, and the caudate nucleus, which contributed to the full behavior of sleep (Parmeggiani *et al.*, 1985). As noted above, these and other studies of the forebrain were over shadowed by the strong emphasis on exploring the caudal brainstem in search of the controlling mechanisms of REM.

Much research on sleep has moved from cats to rats and now, increasingly, mice. The use of the last will increase as a search for relevant genes employ knockout mice with unknown behavioral phenotypes. And so, it will be important to know as much as possible about the behavior of these "new" animals if one is to interpret experiments accurately.

Also, differences in size or anatomy will dictate changes in approach to the study of sleep in these tiny animals. Mice are much smaller than cats and even rats so that the common use of a recording cable plugged into the head cap presents a problem, at least when amount or character of sleep following various manipulations is the issue. For example, (Tang and Sanford, 2002) have demonstrated that mice sleep more as recording cable weight is increased. If one uses telemetry or even a lighter cable, sleep decreases.

Observation of the behavior of mice will still be important as "new" mice are created as "knockouts" (Kas and Van Rhee, 2004). One need only think of the recent contribution of simple behavioral observation to the recognition of the role of the peptide orexin (hypocretin) in the pathophysiology of narcolepsy. Knockout mice being studied for determining the role of orexin in feeding behavior were fortunately videotaped during their night-time active period (Chemelli *et al.*, 1999). The mice were videotaped because the workers noticed that the mice were not eating at night. The videos revealed that the mice collapsed periodically during their active period at night. Although the initial thought was that the mice were having seizures, further analysis led to the realization that the behavior observed was characteristic of narcolepsy. This finding depended upon the experience of one who had spent many hours watching mice sleep (C. Sinton, personal communication). Electrographic recording then substantiated these behavioral observations. Now we know that the brains of narcoleptics exhibit a great loss of orexin-containing neurons (Peyron *et al.*, 2000; Thannickal *et al.*, 2000). Thus, behavioral observation played a key role in advancing our understanding of an important sleep disorder.

Behavioral observations were very important for the demonstration of sleep in yet smaller animals, fruit flies (*Drosophila melanogaster*). These animals present exciting possibilities for sleep research after already having provided important insights into the molecular mechanisms of circadian rhythms (Hendricks, 2003). Without benefit of the electrographic recordings standard in studies of vertebrate sleep, two groups simultaneously demonstrated through behavioral observations and manipulations, supplemented subsequently by other approaches, that flies sleep (Hendricks *et al.*, 2000; Shaw *et al.*, 2000). These groups have shown that flies exhibit all the features of sleep one can measure externally: "(1) consolidated circadian periods of immobility, (2) a species-specific posture and/or resting place, (3) an increased arousal threshold (although the state can be reversed by intense stimulation), and (4) a homeostatic regulatory system" (Hendricks, 2003). Furthermore, flies and mammals share genes that are upregulated after deprivation (Shaw *et al.*, 2000).

Contributions of REM without Atonia

Relatively small pontine lesions eliminate the normal atonia of skeletal muscles and release complex behaviors, such as walking and attack, during otherwise normal episodes of REM (Jouvet and Delorme, 1965; Villablanca, 1966; Henley and Morrison, 1974; Sastre and Jouvet, 1979; Hendricks *et al.*, 1982). We demonstrated that behaviors seen depended on the location of the lesions, indicating that more than removal of inhibition of spinal motor neurons was involved (Hendricks *et al.*, 1982). Observing the lesioned animals while they were awake revealed that they had a significant increase in exploratory behavior and did not demonstrate increased extensor tone, which strengthened our proposal that multiple systems were involved in the phenomenon.

The behavioral descriptions of this phenomenon created in cats were instrumental in the recognition of another sleep disorder, REM sleep behavior disorder (Schenck *et al.*, 1986). Knowing that cats could engage in complex behaviors during otherwise normal REM led the clinicians to recognize that some of their patients, who appeared to be epileptics, were, in fact, acting out their dreams during REM.

The REM without atonia phenomenon also contributed in a unique way to the demonstration of a dramatic decrease in homeostatic control of thermoregulation during REM. Although one could easily see the absence of panting during warming in REM (Parmeggiani, 1980), atonia prevented behavioral confirmation in the form of shivering, we took advantage of REM without atonia. Cats placed at 15°C kept a tightly curled posture, exhibited piloerection, and shivered violently during NREM. When they entered REM without atonia they left their protective posture, immediately stopped shivering and lost the piloerection (Hendricks *et al.*, 1977; Hendricks, 1982). These behavioral observations reinforced Parmeggiani's claim that responses to cold are also suppressed in cats during REM.

Yet another area of neuroscience benefited from behavioral observations in study of REM without atonia: the field of aggression. Our laboratory recognized that behaviors emerging during an episode of REM without atonia were not seen in all cats and were characteristic of particular cats' episodes (Henley and Morrison, 1974). Further work revealed that lesions extending more rostrally than other pontine lesions into the midbrain tegmentum resulted in expression of attack behavior that was predatory in nature, that is, the cats appeared to pounce on imaginary prey with no signs of affective display (Hendricks *et al.*, 1982). Their ears were pointed forward, and piloerection was not present: the piloerection and flattened ears of an angry, fearful cat characteristic of affective defense behavior were not observed. A later study revealed that of 28 cats with REM without atonia only eight exhibited predatory attack while awake (Morrison, 1986). Interestingly, six of these eight cats were aggressive toward other cats with which they had been either neutral or friendly, demonstrating the usual affective signs of "rage." They had to be restrained from full attack to prevent harm to the other cats.

We sought to determine what systems had been damaged, which resulted in these interesting behaviors. One of these is the amygdalofugal pathway to the caudal brainstem arising in the central nucleus (Hopkins and Holstege, 1978; Krettek and Price, 1978). We found that unilateral lesions of the central nucleus induced the same predatory-like attack during REM without atonia when combined with pontine lesions in areas that normally did not release attack behavior (Zagrodska *et al.*, 1998). Amygdalar lesions resulted in strong affective responses to con-specifics and sometimes to the experimenters when the cats were awake; but as previously determined nonmouse killers, the cats exhibited no increase in predation. Yet, during REM without atonia they demonstrated nonaffective, predatory attack behavior. Thus, two forms of agonistic behavior occurred simply by a change in behavioral state. The results suggested to Zagrodska *et al.* (1998) that depression of peripheral sympathetic activity and hypothalamic control during REM and REM without atonia could account for the lack of affective behavior during episodes of REM without atonia. "Cats can simply not mobilize the resources necessary for such behavior." This observation would seem to have important implications for research on neural systems involved in modulation of aggressive behavior. It suggests that the brain must receive information that there is an output to the visceral organs either from central feedback within the brain (an efferent copy) or via afferents from the periphery (Loewy, 1990). The latter might not happen in REM without atonia because of reduced sympathetic activity (Parmeggiani and Morrison, 1990) and possibly other forebrain controls (Morrison and Reiner, 1985) that characterize REM sleep. Thanks to the unique properties of REM without atonia, the necessarily labile nature of agonistic expression required for survival (Shaikh *et al.*, 1984) is revealed in a striking, if artificial way (Zagrodska *et al.*, 1998).

Solving the Mystery of PGO Waves

Having established that behavioral observation continues to play a role in sleep research — even specifically created knockout mice are not mere test tubes but are complex organisms with a rich behavioral repertoire — I will continue by describing the key role careful observations played in clarifying the nature of the one-time mysterious ponto-geniculo-occipital (PGO) spike or wave. Then I will turn to a discussion of how this insight led us to understand the linkage between wake-like neuronal activity during REM and skeletal muscle atonia and then to more recent results we have obtained in our studies of the amygdala.

PGO waves are macropotentials that appear spontaneously in the transition period just before the onset of REM and then throughout the subsequent episode. During REM one sees both isolated PGO waves and bursts, the latter clearly associated with REMs. Early interest in the use of REM as an avenue for the collection and study of dreams directed attention of sleep researchers toward brain regions associated with visual functions. As a result, PGO waves were very early recorded in the lateral geniculate body of cats (Mikiten *et al.*, 1961) although work by Bizzi and Brooks (1963) later demonstrated that they were driven from the pons and that those waves also recorded in the cerebral cortex did not depend upon the lateral geniculate body for their transmission. Then, Morrison and Pompeiano (1966) showed that the bursts of waves depended upon the occurrence of REMs when the REMs were eliminated by means of bilateral lesions of the vestibular nuclei, only the single waves of the transition periods and following episodes of REM appeared. Thus, the single wave seemed closer to being a fundamental unit of REM.

Careful observation of the behavior of sleeping cats, on the face of it an exercise with little prospect for interesting results, opened the door to understanding the operational significance of the PGO wave. Inspired by the insights that the ethologist, Nikko Tinbergen (1971), derived by careful observations of herring gulls, I decided, somewhat quixotically, simply to observe cats as they slept. The collapse of muscle tone as the cats entered REM was easily observed as were the already well-known twitches of vibrissae and digits and the REMs. But it then became evident that in the transition period between NREM and REM fasciculations of the forearm muscles were occurring before the collapse of tone and entrance into full REM and that they appeared within the same time frame as the transition period. What, if any, was their significance?

Fortunately, we were studying the effects of unilateral cerebellar cortical lesions in the forelimb area of the anterior lobe for another purpose, and these animals were available for study during sleep as well (Morrison and Bowker, 1975). In these cats the fasciculations turned into brief jerks of the forelimb ipsilateral to the lesion, disappearing as REM atonia ensued; and they showed a definite relationship to what we saw during neurological assessments when the cats were awake. The vestibular placing reflex, which is obtained by suddenly dropping a cat a few centimeters, results in a slight fanning of the digits. If the area of the cortex facilitating forelimb extensor motor neurons is damaged (the vermis), one observes an extensor thrust. On the other hand, if the area facilitating flexor motor neurons (the paravermis) is damaged instead, a dramatic, seemingly paradoxical, flexion occurs.

The diagram in Figure 1 illustrates schematically why these behaviors occurred. The Pürkinje cell output of the cerebellar cortex is inhibitory to deeper structures, including the deep cerebellar nuclei, which receive collateral inputs from various systems in addition to the reticular formation. With damage to the midline vermis or the more lateral paravermis one removes the Purkinje cell modulation, creating the possibility of exaggerated extensor or flexor movements, respectively (Chambers and Sprague, 1955). In the case of the vestibular placing reflex, external influences induce unmodulated activity in the deep cerebellar nuclei. But why do spontaneous flexor or extensor movements occur in the transition to REM following cerebellar lesions? Fortunately, we were recording PGO waves in the lateral geniculate body and observed that they appeared in a one-to-one relationship with the forelimb jerks (Figure 2). Apparently, the bursts of reticular formation activity heralding REM onset were the source of the excitations of the affected deep cerebellar nucleus.

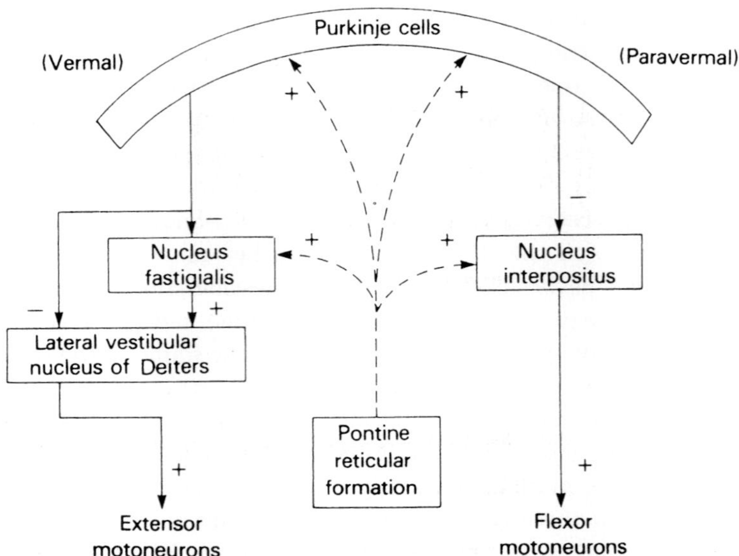

Figure 1. Schematic representation of neuronal circuitry involved in ponto-geniculo-occipital (PGO)-associated limb jerks. Removal of the cerebellar Purkinje cells in either the vermal or paravermal zones results in abolition of their inhibitory influence upon the deep cerebellar (and Deiter's) nuclei. Subsequent excitation by pontine reticular neurons (as during PGO spikes) exerts its effect upon these unregulated nuclei, thereby resulting in the limb jerks seen at the transition to REM. Reprinted from Figure 4 of Reiner and Morrison (1980).

By chance, we observed that sounds induced both jerks and PGO waves (Bowker and Morrison, 1976; Morrison and Bowker, 1975). The source of the first sound inducing both a jerk and a PGO wave was a collection of keys dropped on the floor. We then turned to a more controlled sound source, a tone generator. Surprisingly, it took a while for us to realize that cerebellar damage was not necessary: tones (90 dB) presented to normal cats elicited PGO waves, not only in NREM but also among the spontaneous waves of REM. This observation initiated a series of studies, which ultimately convinced us that the PGO waves are a sign of alerting, activity fundamental to the operation of the orienting reflex (Sanford *et al.*, 1993). Indeed, cats exhibiting REM without atonia that are capable of complex behaviors during that state without awakening demonstrated the same degree of orienting during REM without atonia as they did while awake (Morrison *et al.*, 1995). A yet-to-be-discovered process prevents the

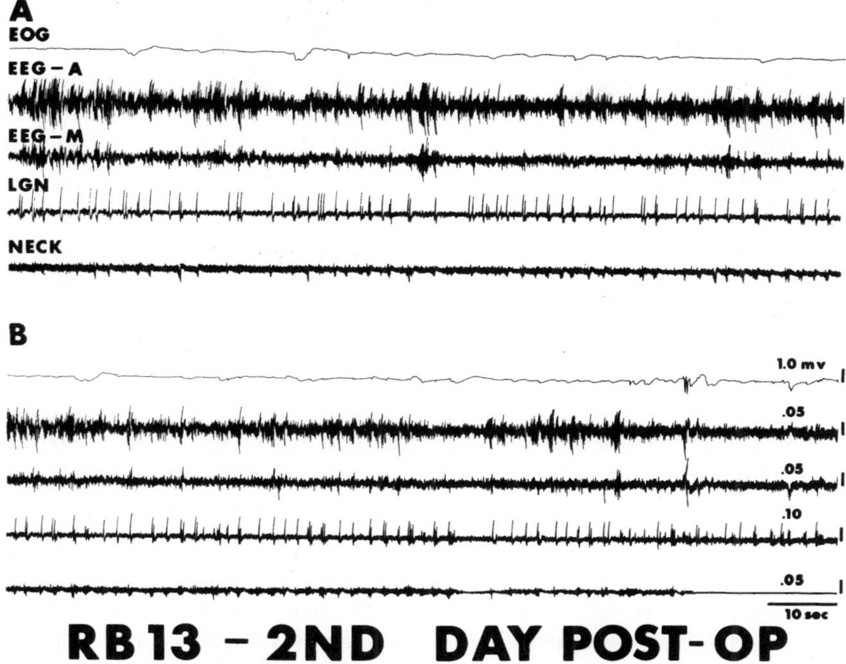

Figure 2. A continuous record, showing the transition to REM, in a cat with a large cerebellar lesion. The frequency of the jerks can be seen as artefacts in the neck muscle EMG tracing. They were accompanied by extensor thrusts of the right forelimb primarily. The prolonged transition period was sometimes observed in the first few postoperative days. Abbreviations: EEG-A and EEG-M, electroencephalograms recorded from the anterior suprasylvian and precruciate gyri: EOG, electro-oculograms; LGN, lateral geniculate nucleus; Neck, electromyogram from dorsal cervical muscles. Reprinted from Figure 4 of Morrison and Bowker (1975).

animals from awakening. Clearly, this would not depend on the usual atonia present in normal cats.

Returning to the discovery of the recognition of what PGO waves represent, we can add that behavioral observation helped us to understand that PGO waves in cats were not phenomena associated with visual function *per se* but were an expression of the very primitive function of alerting an animal to possible danger, heightening sensitivity in various systems. Indeed, the presence of PGO waves in the albino rat was in question in the mid-1970s. Reiner and I reasoned that if PGO waves were an expression of more general reticular activation and not a normal visual system, then cerebellar lesions should release jerks as they did in cats (Reiner and Morrison, 1980). This is what occurred — with one disconcerting feature: only four or five forelimb jerks appeared prior to REM. Ironically, another group had chanced on recording pontine waves with electrodes placed in the region of the locus coeruleus (LC), and recorded very few of them in the transition period, a number consistent with the extensor jerks in our study. Both results were reported at the same meeting (Farber *et al.*, 1976; Reiner and Morrison, 1976). Later work revealed that these waves recorded in the pons could also be elicited by sounds in albino rats (Kaufman and Morrison, 1981). PGO waves, then, are an expression of a fundamental property of REM: heightened activity of the reticular formation, which for unknown reasons is insufficient to awaken an animal until the episode has run its course.

One can reason that REM is an extreme expression of the orienting reflex. Ordinarily this reflex consists of a hesitation of movement followed by directed attention toward the stimulus. We can then view the collapse of antigravity tone as an extreme expression of the cessation of movement that is a part of orienting during wakefulness. Simply paying attention to one's own behavior can be instructive. For example, while walking across a street, one can experience a slight hesitation in the stance phase should a vehicle unexpectedly enter one's peripheral vision. These experiences first led me to the idea that general alerting of the nervous system was inextricably linked with suppression of movement, from slight to the point of collapse. The latter occurs in narcoleptics but is also possible in those not afflicted. It was just such an event that led me to the idea that REM is a variation on the theme of alerting (or, crudely, reticular activation) inducing suppression of movement to the extreme: atonia of antigravity muscles. While in a 100-yard freestyle swimming race in college, I saw my lead vanish as I was paralyzed in the water for a second or so. The excitement engendered a cataplectic attack. Then, thinking of that event years later after another experience crossing the street as a pedestrian, I had a "Eureka!" experience that had solved the problem of the atonia of REM: atonia in REM is an extreme expression of the orienting mechanism. The cataplectic attack associated with narcolepsy is an abnormal variant.

A Role for the Amygdala

The amygdala enters the picture at this point because it is the key interface between novel, interesting and/or dangerous signals from the external environment and the organism. A large body of literature supports the contention that the ability to attach emotional significance to sensory events and to influence resulting behavior resides in the amygdala (Davis, 1992; LeDoux, 1992a,b). Sensory information other than olfactory enters the amygdala through its lateral nucleus, an integral component of fear conditioning circuitry (LeDoux *et al.*, 1990). In addition to the amygdala's role in investing sensory events with *emotional* significance, more recent work implicates the amygdala in the regulation of attention, vigilance, and arousal state (Sanford *et al.*, 1995; Calvo *et al.*, 1996; Silvestri and Kapp, 1998; Holland and Gallagher, 1999). By influencing basal forebrain cholinergic systems, the major output nucleus of the amygdala, the central nucleus, contributes significantly to attentional function in conditioning (Holland and Gallagher, 1999).

Davis and Whalen (2001) have recently emphasized this new direction in thinking. They have reviewed the recent evidence from neuroimaging studies in humans that both positively and negatively valenced stimuli can affect the amygdala: they suggest that it may be particularly responsive to uncertain stimulus contingencies and to the presentation of biologically important stimuli (which often tend to produce strongly aversive emotional states). "More than functioning primarily for the production of strong emotional states, the amygdala would be poised to modulate the moment-to-moment vigilance level of the organism" (Davis and Whalen, 2001). Continuing this line of reasoning, Davis and Whalen propose that the amygdalar activation that has been seen in neuroimaging studies of human mood and anxiety disorders may reflect excessive vigilance rather than fear *per se.*

The amygdala originally captured our laboratory's attention regarding its possible role in the modulation of sleep and wakefulness because the central nucleus projects to the cholinergic basal forebrain (Zaborsky *et al.*, 1984), which is linked to the cortical activation of both W and REM and, indeed, enhancement of the states themselves (Cape *et al.*, 2000). The central nucleus also projects heavily to pontine neurons implicated in sleep control (Hopkins and Holstege, 1978; Krettek and Price, 1978; Moga and Gray, 1985). These neurons, in turn, project to various amygdalar nuclei (Bernard *et al.*, 1993; Saper and Loewy, 1980). The cholinergic basal forebrain projects densely to both central and basal nuclei (Heckers and Mesulam, 1994). Sleep- and wakefulness-related neurons have been reported in the lateral nucleus in rats (Bordi *et al.*, 1993). Permanent lesions of cells in this nucleus in rats (unpublished observations) as well as large amygdalar cell loss in the monkey (Benca *et al.*, 2000) significantly increased sleep. The serotonergic dorsal raphe (DR) nucleus modulates sleep partly through its efferent projections to the basolateral complex of the amygdala, which includes the lateral and basal nuclei and also projects, to a lesser degree, to the central nucleus (Fallon and Ciofi, 1992; Gao et al., 2002).

Thus, the amygdala may be a key structure in deciding whether alerting stimuli are important enough to arouse an animal into full wakefulness. Considering its anatomy in greater detail, the amygdala is well connected anatomically to mediate aspects of attention and, therefore sleep, dependent on reception of significant stimuli (Amaral et al., 1992; Price et al., 1987). The lateral nucleus projects medially to key nuclei (Pitkanen et al., 1995) that, in turn, project with it to the hippocampus (Pikkarainen et al., 1999), providing routes for the establishment of memories of emotion-provoking sensory stimuli and for the modulation of major sleep-organizing regions, not only via the aforementioned central nucleus, but, also, the hypothalamus, in particular the ventrolateral preoptic area (VLPO), directly via its medial nucleus (Csaki et al., 2000) and indirectly via other hypothalamic nuclei (Chou et al., 2002). The basolateral complex, consisting of the lateral and the basal nucleus, is interconnected with neocortical association areas of frontal and temporal regions (Pitkanen et al., 1995). These cortical structures, in turn, project directly and indirectly to the central nucleus, which also receives afferent fibers from the brainstem, primarily the pontine parabrachial area (Bernard et al., 1993). From the latter nucleus visceral information reaches the central nucleus.

Thus, an integration of exogenous, cognitive and visceral information can occur in the amygdala. The central nucleus, integrating information from many extrinsic sources (Jolkkonen and Pitkänen, 1998), projects to the hypothalamus and the dorsal pontine region that, we suggest, organizes orienting reactions (Morrison, 1979) and serves as the site of initiation of PGO waves (Datta et al., 1998).

Given that PGO waves may be considered as signs of alerting (but not necessarily arousal), one might expect that the amygdala would influence the neurons responsible for these waves. Indeed, bilateral electrical stimulation of the central nucleus in rats significantly increased the amplitudes of the spontaneous pontine waves occurring during REM. Waves recorded during wakefulness and NREM were not significantly affected (Figure 3) (DeBoer et al., 1998). Furthermore, electrical stimulation of the central nucleus significantly increased the amplitudes of sound-elicited PGO waves when the stimulation was delivered at the same time or no more than 100 ms

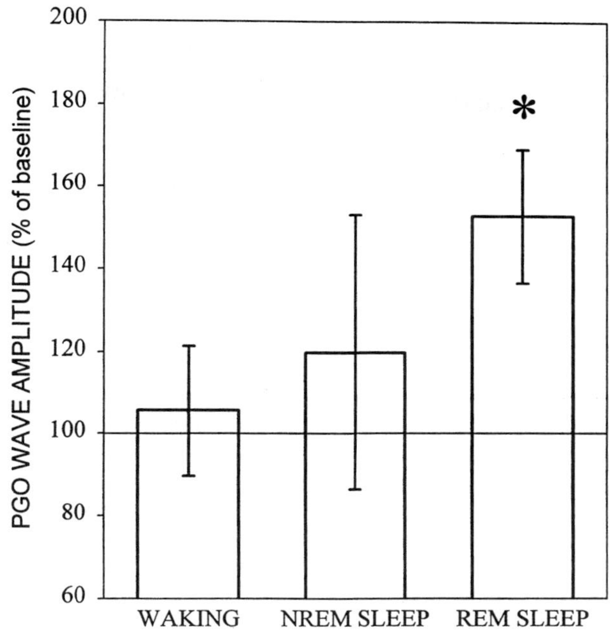

Figure 3. Effect of electrical stimulation in Ace during waking, NREM and REM on PGO wave amplitude. Data are expressed as percentage of control (means with standard errors). Significant differences from control are indicated by a star ($p < 0.05$, $n = 5$). Reprinted from Figure 3 of DeBoer *et al.* (1998).

prior to the sound (Figure 4). (DeBoer *et al.*, 1999). This pattern followed that of fear-potentiated startle (Rosen and Davis, 1988).

Because the amygdala is critical to the establishment of fear-conditioning, which can emphasize role the amygdala plays in sleep mechanisms, we have studied rats in two fear-conditioning paradigms (cued and contextual). In both studies the rats demonstrated a significant reduction in the amount of REM but not in total amount of sleep when tested the following day (Jha *et al.*, 2004; Pawlyk *et al.*, 2004). Sanford *et al.* (2003a,b) have described similar results with mice. For the cued condition, tones were paired with mild foot shocks. In the case of contextual conditioning, different groups of rats were shocked or not shocked in an "unsafe" chamber, and then sleep was recorded in that chamber 24 h later or in a "safe" chamber that had different lighting and bedding with rats always being handled by a different, "safe" person. That REM, and not NREM, was significantly reduced by fear

 A. R. Morrison

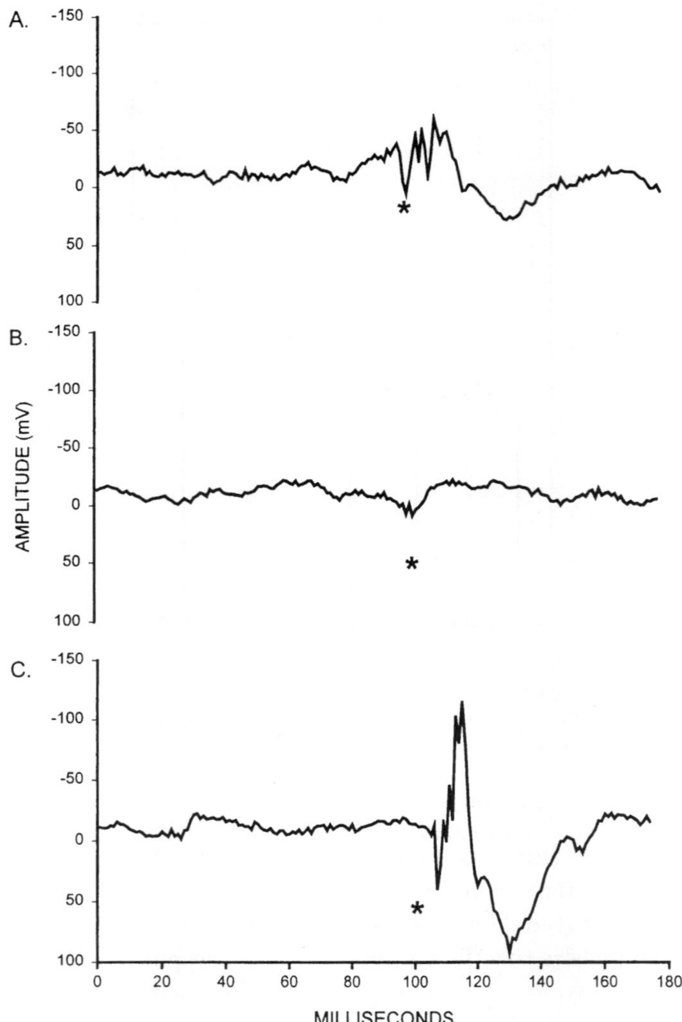

Figure 4. Representative responses from one rat demonstrating an elicited PGO wave in response to presentation of an auditory stimulus alone (A), no response when Ace was electrically stimulated without being paired with an auditory stimulus (B), and a relatively higher amplitude elicited PGO wave when the auditory stimulus was preceded 1.0 ms by electrical stimulation of Ace (C). Stars indicate the onset of the auditory stimulus (A, C) or of electrical stimulation of Ace (B). Reprinted from Figure 3 of DeBoer *et al.*, (1999).

conditioning suggests a special relationship between REM mechanisms and the external environment.

Thus, these new findings reinforce our major claim, that REM and alert wakefulness are each variations on the same theme: different expressions of a highly active brain (Morrison, 1983). Only through careful behavioral observations was this conclusion possible.

Acknowledgments

I wish to honor the memory of my professors, Drs James M. Sprague and William W. Chambers, who taught me the value of careful behavioral observations and whose seminal work on the cerebellum inspired some of the studies discussed in this chapter. I also thank my assistant of many years, Graziella L. Mann, and my various student colleagues, many cited among the references, who contributed so much to my laboratory. I owe special thanks to my colleague for more than 20 years, Richard J. Ross, MD, PhD. The laboratory's work has been generously supported by the National Institutes of Health, most recently by MH42903.

References

Amaral, D.G., Price, J.L., Pitkänen, A., and Carmichael, S.T. (1992). Anatomical organization of the primate amygdaloid complex. In: Aggleton, J.P. (Ed.). *The Amygdala: Neurobiological Aspects of Emotion, Memory, and Mental Dysfunction.* New York: Wiley-Liss, pp. 1–66.

Amici, R., Zamboni, G., Perez, E., Jones, C.A., Toni, I., and Culin, F. (1994). Pattern of desynchronized sleep during deprivation and recovery induced in the rat by changes in ambient temperature. *J. Sleep Res.*, 3: 250–256.

Amici, R., Zamboni, G., Perez, E., Jones, C.A., and Parmeggiani, P.L. (1998). The influence of a heavy thermal load on REM sleep in the rat. *Brain Res.*, 781: 252–258.

Aserinsky, E. and Kleitman, N. (1953). Periodic respiratory movements in conjunction with eye movements during sleep. *Science*, 150: 763–766.

Baghdoyan, H.A., Spotts, J.L., and Snyder, S.G. (1993). Simultaneous pontine and basal forebrain microinjections of carbachol suppress REM sleep. *J. Neurosci.*, 13: 229–242.

Benca, R.M., Obermeyer, W.H., Shelton, S.E., Droster, J., and Kalin, N.H. (2000). Effects of amygdala lesions on sleep in rhesus monkeys. *Brain Res.*, 879: 130–138.

Bernard, J.F., Alden, M., and Besson, J.M. (1993). The organization of the efferent projections from the pontine parabrachial area to the amygdaloid complex: a phaseolus vulgaris leucoagglutinin (PHA-L) study in rat. *J. Comp. Neurol.*, 329: 201–229.

Bizzi, E. and Brooks, D.C. (1963). Functional connections between pontine reticular formation and lateral geniculate nucleus during deep sleep. *Arch. Ital. Biol.*, 101: 666–680.

Bordi, F., LeDoux, J.E., Clugnet, M.C., and Pavlides, C. (1993). Single-unit activity in the lateral nucleus of the amygdala and overlying areas of the striatum in freely behaving rats: rates, discharge patterns, and responses to acoustic stimuli. *Behav. Neurosci.*, 107: 757–769.

Bowker, R.M. and Morrison, A.R. (1976). The startle reflex and PGO spikes. *Brain Res.*, 102: 185–190.

Calvo, J.M., Simón-Arceo, K., and Fernández-Mas, R. (1996). Prolonged enhancement of REM sleep produced by carbachol microinjection into the amygdala. *NeuroReport*, 7: 577–580.

Cape, E.G., Manns, I.D., Alonso, A., Beaudet, A., and Jones, B.E. (2000). Neurotensin-induced bursing of cholinergic basal forebrain neurons promotes cortical activity together with waking and paradoxical sleep. *J. Neurosci.*, 20: 8452–8461.

Chambers, W.W. and Sprague, J.M. (1955). Functional localization in the cerebellum. II. Somatotopic organization in cortex and nuclei. *Arch. Neurol. Psychiatry*, 4: 653–680.

Chemelli, R.M., Willie, J.T., Sinton, C.M., Elmquist, J.K., Scammell, T., Lee, C., Richardson, J.A., Williams, S.C., Xiong, Y., Kisanuki, Y., Fitch, T.E., Nakazato, M., Hammer, R.E., Saper, C.B., and Yanagisawa, M. (1999). Narcolepsy in orexin knockout mice: molecular genetics of sleep regulation. *Cell*, 98: 437–451.

Chou, T.C., Bjorkum, A.A., Gaus, S.E., Lu, J., Scammell, T.E., and Saper, C.B. (2002). Afferents to the ventrolateral preoptic nucleus. *J. Neurosci.*, 22: 977–990.

Csaki, A., Kocsis, K., Halasz, B., and Kiss, J. (2000). Localization of glutamatergic/aspartatergic neurons projecting to the hypothalamic paraventricular nucleus studied by retrograde transport of [3H]D-aspartate autoradiography. *Neuroscience*, 101: 637–655.

Datta, S., Siwek, D.F., Patterson, E.H., and Cipolloni, P.B. (1998). Localization of pontine PGO wave generation sites and their anatomical projections in the rat. *Synapse*, 30: 409–423.

Davis, M. (1992). The role of the amygdala in fear and anxiety. *Annu. Rev. Neurosci.*, 15: 353–375.

Davis, M. and Whalen, P.J. (2001). The amygdala: vigilance and emotion. *Mol. Psychiatry*, 6: 13–34.

DeBoer, T., Sanford, L.D., Ross, R.J., and Morrison, A.R. (1998). Effects of electrical stimulation in the amygdala on ponto-geniculo-occipital waves in rats. *Brain Res.*, 793: 305–310.

DeBoer, T., Ross, R.J., Morrison, A.R., and Sanford, L.D. (1999). Electrical stimulation of the amygdala increases the amplitude of elicited ponto-geniculo-occipital waves. *Physiol. Behav.*, 66: 119–124.

Fallon, J.H. and Ciofi, P. (1992). Distribution of monoamines within the amygdala. In: Aggleton, J.P. (Ed.). *The Amygdala: Neurobiological Aspects of Emotion, Memory and Mental Dysfunction.* New York: Wiley-Liss, pp. 97–114.

Farber, J., Marks, G., Barwise, C., and Roffwarg, H. (1976). Pontine sharp waves during REM sleep in the albino rat. *Sleep Res.*, 5: 21.

Gao, J., Zhang, J.X., and Xu, T.L. (2002). Modulation of serotonergic projection from dorsal raphe nucleus to basolateral amygdala on sleep–waking cycle of rats. *Brain Res.*, 945: 60–70.

Heckers, S. and Mesulam, M.-M. (1994). Two types of cholinergic projections to the rat amygdala. *Neuroscience*, 60: 383–397.

Hendricks, J.C. (1982). Absence of shivering in the cat during paradoxical sleep without atonia. *Exp. Neurol.*, 75: 700–710.

Hendricks, J.C. (2003). Sleeping flies don't lie: the use of Drosophila melanogaster to study sleep and circadian rhythms. *J. Appl. Physiol.*, 94: 1660–1672.

Hendricks, J.C., Bowker, R.M., and Morrison, A.R. (1977). Functional characteristics of cats with pontine lesions during sleep and wakefulness and their usefulness for sleep research. In: Koella, W.P. and Levin, P. (Eds.). *Sleep 1976*, Basel: Karger, pp. 6–10.

Hendricks, J.C., Morrison, A.R., and Mann, G.L. (1982). Different behaviors during paradoxical sleep without atonia depend on pontine lesion site. *Brain Res.*, 239: 81–105.

Hendricks, J.C., Finn, S.M., Panckeri, K.A., Chavkin, J., Williams, J.A., Sehgal, A., and Pack, A.I. (2000). Rest in Drosophila is a sleep-like state. *Neuron*, 25: 129–138.

Henley, K. and Morrison, A.R. (1974). A re-evaluation of the effects of lesions of the pontine tegmentum and locus coeruleus on phenomena of paradoxical sleep in the cat. *Acta Neurobiol. Exp.*, 34: 215–232.

Holland, P.C. and Gallagher, M. (1999). Amygdala circuitry in attentional and representational processes. *Trends Cogn. Sci.*, 3: 65–73.

Hopkins, D.A. and Holstege, G. (1978). Amygdaloid projections to the mesencephalon, pons and medulla oblongata in the cat. *Exp. Brain Res.*, 32: 529–547.

Jha, S.K., Brennen, F.X., Pawlyk, A.C., Ross, R.J., and Morrison, A.R. (2005). REM sleep: a sensitive index of fear conditioning in rats. *Eur. J. Neurosci.*, 21: 1077–1080.

Jolkkonen, E. and Pitkänen, A. (1998). Intrinsic connections of the rat amygdaloid complex: projections originating in the central nucleus. *J. Comp. Neurol.*, 395: 53–72.

Jouvet, M. (1962). Recherches sur les structures nerveuses et les mécanismes résponsables des differentes phases du sommeil physiologique. *Arch. Ital. Biol.*, 100: 125–206.

Jouvet, M. (1964). Cataplexie et sommeil paradoxal réflexes chez le chat pontine. *C. R. Soc. Biol.*, 159: 383–387.

Jouvet, M. and Delorme, F. (1965). Locus coeruleus et sommeil paradoxal. *C. R. Soc. Biol.*, 159: 895–899.

Kas, J.H. and Van Rhee, J.M. (2004). Dissecting complex behaviours in the postgenomic era. *TINS*, 27: 366–369.

Kaufman, L.S. and Morrison, A.R. (1981). Spontaneous and elicited PGO spikes in rats. *Brain Res.*, 214: 61–72.

Krettek, J.E. and Price, J.L. (1978). Amygdaloid projections to subcortical structures within the basal forebrain and brainstem in the rat and cat. *J. Comp. Neurol.*, 178: 225–254.

LeDoux, J.E. (1992a). Brain mechanisms of emotion and emotional learning. *Curr. Opin. Neurobiol.*, 2: 191–197.

LeDoux, J.E. (1992b). Emotion and the amygdala. In: Aggleton, J.P. (Ed.). *The Amygdala: Neurobiological Aspects of Emotion, Memory and Mental Dysfunction.* New York: Wiley-Liss, Inc., 339–351.

LeDoux, J.E., Cicchetti, E.P., Xagoraris, A., and Romanski, L.M. (1990). The lateral amygdaloid nucleus: sensory interface of the amygdala in fear conditioning. *J. Neurosci.*, 10: 1062–1069.

Loewy, A.D. (1990). Central autonomic functions. Loewy, A.D. and Spyer, K.M. (Eds.). *Central Regulation of Autonomic Functions.* Oxford: Oxford University Press, pp. 88–103.

Marini, G., Gritti, I., and Mancia, M. (1990). The role of some thalamic nuclei in sleep mechanisms: evidence from chemical lesions in the cat. In: Mancia, M. and Marini, M. (Eds.). *The Diencephalon and Sleep.* New York: Raven Press, pp. 279–292.

Mikiten, T.H., Niebyl, P.H., and Hendley, C.D. (1961). EEG desynchronization during behavioral sleep associated with spike discharges from the thalamus of the cat. *Fed. Proc.*, 20: 327.

Moga, M.M. and Gray, T.S. (1985). Evidence for corticotropin-releasing factor, neurotensin, and somatostatin in the neural pathway from the central nucleus of the amygdala to the parabrachial nucleus. *J. Comp. Neurol.*, 241: 275–284.

Morrison, A.R. (1979). Brainstem regulation of behavior during sleep and wakefulness. In: Sprague, J.M. and Epstein, A.W. (Eds.). *Progress in Psychobiology and Physiological Psychology.* New York: Academic Press, pp. 91–131.

Morrison, A.R. (1983). Paradoxical sleep and alert wakefulness: variations on a theme. In: Chase, M.H. and Weitzman, E.D. (Eds.). *Sleep Disorders, Basic and Clinical Research.* New York: Spectrum, pp. 95–127.

Morrison, A.R. (1986). Behavioral capabilities of cats during different behavioral states. Oomura, Y. (Ed.). *Emotions: Neuronal and Chemical Control.* Tokyo: Japan Scientific Societies Press, pp. 241–254.

Morrison, A.R. and Bowker, R.M. (1975). The biological significance of PGO spikes in the sleeping cat. *Acta Neurobiol. Exp.*, 35: 821–840.

Morrison, A.R. and Pompeiano, O. (1966). Vestibular influences during sleep IV: functional relations between vestibular nuclei and lateral geniculate nucleus during desynchronized sleep. *Arch. Ital. Biol.*, 104: 425–458.

Morrison, A.R. and Reiner, P.B. (1985). A dissection of paradoxical sleep. In: McGinty, D.J., Drucker-Colin, R., Morrison, A., and Parmeggiani, P.L. (Eds.). *Brain Mechanisms of Sleep.* New York: Raven Press, pp. 97–110.

Morrison, A.R., Sanford, L.D., Ball, W.A., Mann, G.L., and Ross, R.J. (1995). Stimulus-elicited behavior in rapid eye movement sleep without atonia. *Behav. Neurosci.,* 109: 972–979.

Morrison, A.R., Sanford, L.D., and Ross, R.J. (2000). The amygdala: a critical modulator of sensory influence on sleep. *Biol. Signals Recept.,* 9: 283–296.

Parmeggiani, P.L. (1980). Temperature regulation during sleep: a study in homeostasis. In: Orem, J. and Barnes, C.D. (Eds.). *Physiology in Sleep.* New York: Academic Press, pp. 97–143.

Parmeggiani, P.L. and Morrison, A.R. (1990). Alterations in autonomic functions during sleep. Loewy, A.D. and Spyer, K.M. (Eds.). *Central Regulation of Autonomic Functions.* Oxford: Oxford University Press, pp. 367–386.

Parmeggiani, P.L., Morrison, A.R., Drucker-Colin, R., and McGinty, D.J. (1985). Brain mechanisms of sleep: an overview of methodological issues. In: McGinty, D.J., Drucker-Colin, R., Morrison, A.R., and Parmeggiani, P.L. (Eds.). *Brain Mechanisms of Sleep.* New York: Raven Press, pp. 1–34.

Pawlyk, A.C., Jha, S.K., Brennan, F.X., Morrison, A.R., and Ross, R.J. (2005). A rodent model of sleep disturbances in the anxiety disorders: the role of context following fear conditioning. *Biol. Psychiatry,* 57: 268–277.

Peyron, C., Faraco, J., Rogers, W., Ripley, B., Overeem, S., Charnay, Y., Nevsimalova, S., Aldrich, M., Reynolds, D., Albin, R., Li, R., Hungs, M., Pedrazzoli, M., Padigaru, M., Kucherlapati, M., Fan, J., Maki, R., Lammers, G.J., Bouras, C., Kucherlapati, R., Nishino, S., and Mignot, E. (2000). A mutation in a case of early onset narcolepsy and a generalized absence of hypocretin peptides in human narcoleptic brains. *Nat. Med.,* 6: 991–997.

Pikkarainen, M., Ronkko, S., Savander, V., Insausti, R., and Pitkanen, A. (1999). Projections from the lateral, basal, and accessory basal nuclei of the amygdala to the hippocampal formation in rat. *J. Comp. Neurol.,* 403: 229–260.

Pitkanen, A., Stefanacci, L., Farb, C.R., Go, G.G., LeDoux, J.E., and Amaral, D.G. (1995). Intrinsic connections of the rat amygdaloid complex: projections originating in the lateral nucleus. *J. Comp. Neurol.,* 356: 288–310.

Portas, C.M., Thakkar, M., Rainnie, D.G., Greene, R.W., and McCarley, R.W. (1997). Role of adenosine in behavioral state modulation: a microdialysis study in the freely moving cat. *Neuroscience,* 79: 225–235.

Price, J.L., Russchen, F.T., and Amaral, D.G. (1987). The limbic region. II: the amygdaloid complex. In: Bjorklund, A., Hokfelt, T., and Swanson, L.W. (Eds.). *Handbook of Chemical Neuroanatomy. Integrated Systems of the CAN.* New York: Elsevier, pp. 279–375.

Reiner, P.B. and Morrison, A.R. (1976). Phasic phenomena in the albino rat. *Sleep,* 5: 32.

Reiner, P.B. and Morrison, A.R. (1980). Pontine-geniculate-occipital spikes in the albino rat: Evidence for the presence of the pontine component as revealed by cerebellar lesions. *Exp. Neurol.,* 69: 61–73.

Rosen, J.B. and Davis, M. (1988). Temporal characteristics of enhancement of startle by stimulation of the amygdala. *Physiol. Behav.*, 44: 117–123.

Sakai, K., Mansari, M.E., Lin, J.S., Zhang, G., and Vanni-Mercier, G. (1990). The posterior hypothalamus in the regulation of wakefulness and paradoxical sleep. In: Mancia, M. and Marini, M. (Eds.). *The Diencephalon and Sleep.* New York: Raven Press, pp. 171–198.

Sanford, L.D., Morrison, A.R., Ball, W.A., Ross, R.J., and Mann, G.L. (1993). The amplitude of elicited PGO waves: a correlate of orienting. *Electroencephalogr. Clin. Neurophysiol.*, 86: 438–445.

Sanford, L.D., Tejani-Butt, S.M., Ross, R.J., and Morrison, A.R. (1995). Amygdaloid control of alerting and behavioral arousal in rats: involvement of serotonergic mechanisms. *Arch. Ital. Biol.*, 134: 81–99.

Sanford, L.D., Tang, X., Ross, R.J., and Morrison, A.R. (2003a). Influence of shock training and explicit fear-conditioned cues on sleep architecture in mice: strain comparison. *Behav. Gen.* 33: 43–58.

Sanford, L.D., Yang, L., and Tang, X. (2003b). Influence of contextual fear on sleep in mice: a strain comparison. *Sleep*, 26: 527–540.

Saper, C.B. and Loewy, A.D. (1980). Efferent connections of the parabrachial nucleus in the rat. *Brain Res.*, 197: 291–317.

Sastre, J.P. and Jouvet, M. (1979). Le comportment oneirique du chat. *Physiol. Beh.*, 22: 979–989.

Schenck, C.H., Bundlie, S.R., Ettinger, M.G., and Mahowald, M.W. (1986). Chronic behavioral disorders of human REM sleep: a new category of parasomnia. *Sleep*, 9: 293–308.

Shaikh, M.B., Brutus, M., Siegel, H.E., and Siegel, A. (1984). Differential control of aggression by the midbrain. *Exp. Neurol.*, 83: 436–442.

Shaw, P.J., Cirelli, C., Greenspan, R.J., and Tononi, G. (2000). Correlates of sleep and waking in Drosophila melanogaster. *Science*, 287: 1834–1837.

Silvestri, A.J. and Kapp, B.S. (1998). Amygdaloid modulation of mesopontine peribrachial neuronal activity: implications for arousal. *Behav. Neurosci.*, 112: 571–588.

Tang, X. and Sanford, L.D. (2002). Telemetric recording of sleep and home cage activity in mice. *Sleep*, 25: 691–699.

Thannickal, T.C., Moore, R.Y., Nienhuis, R., Ramanathan, L., Gulyani, S., Aldrich, M., Cornford, M., and Siegel, J.M. (2000). Reduced number of hypocretin neurons in human narcolepsy. *Neuron*, 27: 469–474.

Tinbergen, N. (1971). *The Herring Gull's World.* New York: Basic Books.

Villablanca, J. (1966). Behavioral and polygraphic study of "sleep" and "wakefulness" in chronic decerebrate cats. *Electroencephalogr. Clin. Neurophysiol.*, 21: 562–577.

Zaborsky, L., Leranth, C., and Heimer, C. (1984). Ultrastructural evidence of amygdalofugal axons terminating on cholinergic cells of the rostral forebrain. *Neurosci. Lett.*, 52: 219–225.

Zagrodzka, J., Hedberg, C.E., Mann, G.L., and Morrison, A.R. (1998). Contrasting expressions of aggressive behavior released by lesions of the central nucleus of the amygdala during wakefulness and rapid eye movement sleep without atonia. *Beh. Neurosci.*, 112: 589–602.

Chapter 10

ANIMAL SLEEP: PHYLOGENETIC CORRELATIONS

Susana Esteban, María C. Nicolau, Antoni Gamundi, Mourad Akaârir, and Rubén V. Rial[1]

The theory of evolution as it was explained by Charles Darwin is probably one of the greatest examples of human genius of all times. However, it involves a task of extraordinary difficulty because beings have to be studied that lived immense times ago — a task that will probably always remain incomplete. Irremediably, this present review will only be able to present a little of the data and some of the hypotheses about how sleep might have evolved — from the simplest alternation of activity and rest to the complex organisation of a mammal's sleep. The reader must bear in mind that it is very difficult to reach any sure conclusions on the basis of present knowledge and there will therefore be specialists who would not accept the scientific nature of many of the statements that will be presented. It is perhaps surprising, however, that the evolution of sleep is a topic that attracts the curiosity of sleep specialists. The reason for their interest lies in the hope that if the evolution of sleep can be successfully deciphered then an answer can probably be found to the big question: Why do we sleep?

---

[1]rvrial@uib.es

Sleep as Behaviour

To review the characteristics of sleep that are applicable to the entire animal kingdom, one needs first to reach a precise definition of sleep. We recognise by introspection sleep in ourselves and we usually have no difficulty in recognising it in other human beings and even in the mammals that man has domesticated. This indubitably means that there exist numerous coincidences between our own sleep and that of the animals with which we share some phylogenetic proximity.

But coincidences between our own sleep and that of animals get fuzzier as we observe more distant species: Do fish sleep? Flies? Paramecia? Some sort of definition is therefore needed to allow us to recognise the presence or absence of sleep throughout the animal kingdom. In 1913, Piéron defined sleep as a reversible state, with motor repose and elevated sensory thresholds. Added to these characteristics were specific postures, the existence of protected sleeping sites (Flanigan *et al.*, 1973) and circadian organisation. The final characteristic to be added was regulation: both "hunger" and "satiety" are general characteristics of sleep and have been demonstrated in many species (Tobler, 1984). In view of the multiplicity of the characteristics of sleep, Bruce-Durie (1981) proposed that an animal that has a certain minimum number of these characteristics should be considered to be a sleeper, while species with a lower number should be regarded as presenting states of rest–activity, but not true sleep.

However, the decision to include or exclude sleep in a species on the basis of a greater or lesser number of characteristics seems somewhat arbitrary. Instead, it would seem more promising to arrange the different characteristics according to how they are related to each other. Figure 1 shows, for example, the last level of poikilotherm sleep — motor inhibition, elevated sensory thresholds (sensory blocking), posture control, and sleeping place selection. Above this level (to the left in the figure) is that of reversibility, with the possibility of switching from sleep to wakefulness, and above that, the two forms of regulation — circadian, which is probably the oldest, and homeostatic, which is more modern. Benington (2000) observed that it was just this existence of regulation that should allow one to recognise the function of sleep: if a state is regulated, the organism must be attempting to reach a stationary level in some of the parameters defined by that state. In accordance with this idea, therefore, since by sleeping the animal either achieves motor and sensory rest or maintains the part of its territory that it uses as a sleeping place as a base-camp for its daily activity, its sleep regulating systems must be seeking to adjust the immobility, the

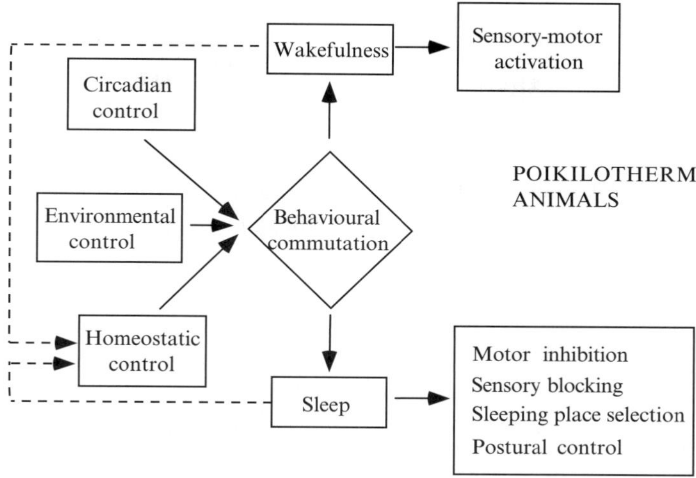

Figure 1. Model representing the characteristics that define sleep and its organisational hierarchy in poikilotherms. The dashed lines represent homeostatic feedback loops.

sensory information flow, and the establishment of a suitable base-camp to the characteristics of the species' ecological niche.

The elements of this model are of two types: (i) regulators and coordinators and (ii) a set of effectors. The former most likely exist in all animals that have true sleep, while the latter may be different and variable between species. An important detail of the model we have just outlined is that none of the effectors that come into action during sleep are exclusive to that state. On the contrary, motor rest, selection of a sleeping site (or of any other site), adoption of the typical sleeping posture, and even sensory blocking can occur during wakefulness. One must therefore conclude that the system that switches between sleep and wakefulness must have an additional function — the coordination of the full set of effectors in a unitary state. We shall see later, however, that this coordination does not occur in all animals and there occur types of behaviour that one could apparently qualify as sleep, but which are uncoordinated and in which these effectors are variable between episodes.

The Sleep of Mammals

The simple model of Figure 1 does not carry over to mammals, since in these animals there is not one sleep state, but two — REM and NREM. The differences between them are so marked that many researchers would say

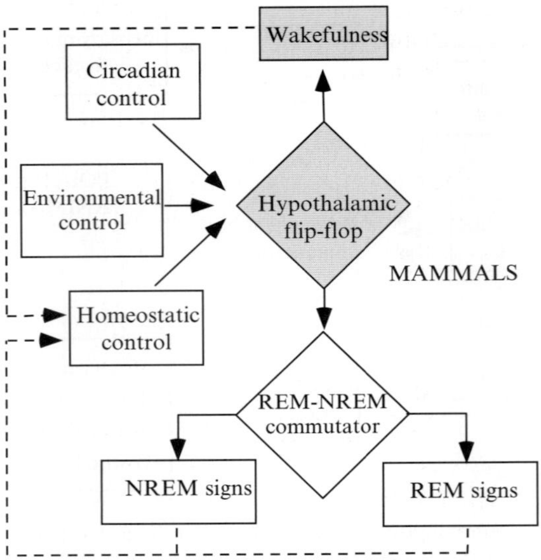

Figure 2. Model of sleep in mammals. As in Figure 1, the feedback loops are represented by dashed lines. There is little doubt that REM and NREM sleep have independent regulatory mechanisms, but these have been left out of the diagram for the sake of simplicity. The hypothalamic flip-flop and cortical arousal modules are shaded for reasons that will be explained in page 235.

that the situation is better described by considering that there exist not two, but three states of wakefulness, each with its own homeostatic and circadian regulatory mechanisms. This model, similar to that of Figure 1 but specific now to mammals, is represented in Figure 2. It is easy to see that mammalian sleep possesses all of the features shown in Figure 1 and that the difference between the two lies in the extra characteristics of the mammalian case. In particular, the new scheme shows two types of sleep — NREM and REM.

In conclusion, a definition applicable to the entire animal kingdom would be that sleep is a state of alternative behaviour to wakefulness and that it is regulated by homeostatic and circadian systems. Together, they control the transitions into and out of sleep and as an end result determine at certain moments a reduced motor activity, increased sensory thresholds, the choice of suitable sleeping places, and patterns of behaviour in which specific postures are favoured. The structures and mechanisms represented in Figure 1 only determine the alternation between activity and rest in simple animals, but in more complex animals they coordinate a greater number of features. Finally, in mammals, they determine the existence of not two, but three states — wakefulness, REM, and NREM — each defined by a complex constellation of physiological and behavioural signs. Furthermore, in these animals the coordination between the effectors is very effective and the occurrence of dissociated states is far less frequent than in the poikilotherms. One of the questions that the present review will attempt to answer is when, how, and why the poikilotherm model of sleep was modified to attain the characteristics of the mammalian sleep.

Evolution

Evolution is fundamentally determined by the production of variations in the descendants of individuals and the subsequent selection of the fittest. In accordance with evolution, it is possible to recognise the family relationships amongst not only the different species that are observable today, but also those that are extinct. These relationships are usually represented in the form of phylogenetic trees (Figure 3).

Knowledge of evolution has not only allowed trees such as these to be constructed, relating species and groups to each other, but it has also made it possible to make similar trees for any structure or function that is present in a group of living beings. For example, it has been possible to establish how the tetrapod limb appeared, beginning as a fin, continuing as a leg,

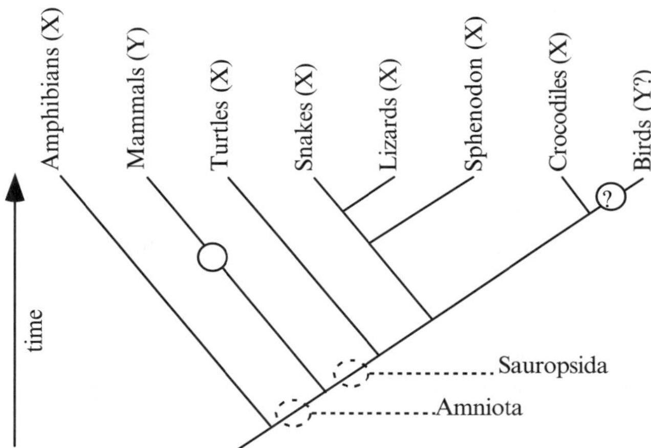

Figure 3. Tree showing the phylogenetic relationships between the main tetrapod groups. Explanation in the text.

and then even being converted into the wing of a bat or returning full circle to become the fin of a dolphin.

Various strategies are followed in order to reconstruct phylogenetic trees. The first is based on palaeontology — the study of the fossil record. It is a task that will never be completed because of the gaps that will always exist in this record. This is particularly regrettable with respect to the changes that the structure and function of the nervous system have undergone. The reason, of course, is the rarity of fossil remains of soft parts of the body and, even more so, the complete absence of fossilisation of behaviour. This means that it is impossible to know whether a certain extinct animal slept and, if it did, how it slept and what structures controlled its sleep.

The second strategy uses a comparative method based on making transversal observations in the nervous system of modern, phylogenetically related species. For instance, by comparing the sleep of modern reptiles and mammals one can infer what the sleep must have been like of the primitive reptile that, some 280 million years ago, was at the base of the bifurcation from which the two groups arose. The inferences obtained by this method should be treated with a degree of caution, however, because modern reptiles may be as different from that primitive ancestor as are modern mammals — there is no proof that the motor of evolution has come to a halt for some and continues to run for others.

The comparative method is still an important tool, and this drawback can perhaps be avoided. For example, if a characteristic exists in modern reptiles, fish, and amphibians, but is different in mammals, then the most parsimonious explanation would be that this characteristic should have existed in the entire series so that the change must have occurred at some moment of the transition from reptiles to mammals (open circle in Figure 3). Any other interpretation would require more changes and, hence, be less parsimonious. Naturally, this does not imply that another interpretation is not true, just that it is less likely.

A third strategy is based on the analysis of the differences in the development of the embryo of related species. These studies have undergone remarkable advances in the last decades and have received the name of "evolutionary developmental (Evo-Devo) Studies".

Whichever method is used, the construction of phylogenetic trees is founded on two fundamental classical concepts — analogy and homology. Two organs are said to be analogous when they fulfil the same mission, independently of any evolutionary relationship between them. Homology, however, refers only to the family relationships of phylogeny with no account taken of function. For example, the wings of birds and of insects are analogous but not homologous — they have the same function but there is no evolutionary relationship between the two. On the contrary, the wings of birds and the forelimbs of horses are homologous, and even though the former are used to walk and the latter to fly, they share a common ancestor. Often, an organ will be homologous and analogous at the same time, as are the limbs of all land mammals. But there are also occasions when the concepts are relative: the wings of birds and the wings of bats are homologous as forelimbs, but only analogous as wings, because there was no winged ancestor common to the two animals.

Phylogenetic trees can only take account of homologies and, with respect to the evolution of sleep, all of the interest lies in finding homologies between the features that define sleep and wakefulness in different animals. The following pages will describe the results of applying the comparative and the embryological methods to the study of the evolution of sleep. For obvious reasons, the palaeontological methods have a very limited application in the study of the phylogeny of sleep.

Comparative Phenomenology of Sleep

Do all vertebrates sleep?

The first step in a comparative analysis of sleep should be to determine whether sleep is a universally obligatory state for animals. Both popular observation and the specialist literature seem to agree that it is. Nonetheless, exceptions probably do exist — animals that either never sleep or go long sleepless periods without showing the sleep debt that most sleepers would show in the subsequent sleep. Table 1 presents some of the reported exceptions. These cases may have great importance. Science advances by inductive reasoning, obtaining general laws starting out from limited observations. Applied to sleep, there is no question but that many species have been found to sleep, and from there the generalisation is made: All species sleep. But this statement is exposed to the appearance of a single species that does not sleep, a finding that has in fact occurred and has been known for quite some time. Probably, in many species sleep is necessary for survival. But it also has to be recognised that in particular environments there exist animals that have developed the capacity for prolonged survival in the absence of sleep, and therefore that evolution has resources to offset the effects of prolonged insomnia, whatever those effects might be.

Table 1. Some animals in which prolonged insomnia and/or absence of rebound after sleep deprivation has been observed.

Group	Species	Reference
Chondrichthyes	*Galeorhinus galeus*	Compagno (1984)
	Galeorhinus canis	Weber (1961)
	Mustelus canis	Herald (1972)
	Notorhynchus maculatus	Lythgoe and Lythgoe (1991)
	Odontaspis taurus	Lythgoe and Lythgoe (1991)
Osteichthyes	*Typhlobagrus kroney*	Pavan (1946)
	Pimodella kronei	Pavan (1946)
	Anoptichthys jordani	Gertychowa (1970)
	Tunnus thynnus	Weber (1961)
	Sarda chiliensis	Costeau and Cousteau (1971)
	Scomber scombrus	Weber (1961)
	Osteoglossum bicirrhosum	Weber (1961)
	Acipenser sturio	Weber (1961)
	Acipenser rutheus	Weber (1961)
	Tilapia mossambica[a]	Shapiro and Hepburn (1976)
Amphibians	*Rana catesbiana*[b]	Hobson (1967)
	Proteus anguinus	Roth and Schlegel (1988)
Reptiles	*Caretta caretta*[b]	Susic (1972)
	Testudo denticulata[b]	Walker and Berger (1973)
	Alligator mississippiensis[c]	Van Twyver (1973)
Mammals	*Platanista indi*[d]	Pilleri (1979)
	Herbivores[e]	Ruckebush (1976)
Birds	Birds in flight or swimming	Amlaner and Ball (1994)
	King penguin[f]	Jouvet (1999)
	Pigeon[a]	Berger and Phillips (1994)

[a]Under continuous light.
[b]Activity–rest cycles were present but no changes in sensory threshold were found.
[c]Activity–rest cycles were absent under constant temperature.
[d]Sleep (?) while continuously swimming.
[e]No sleep during prolonged habituation to the recording procedures and no subsequent debt recovery.
[f]Clear sleep in isolated animals, but no sleep for several months in the colony.

There would seem to be little difficulty in accepting the capacity to survive without sleep in many fishes, amphibians, and even reptiles — animals with simple brains — but it is surprising that it also occurs in mammals, such as horses and dolphins. Studies on the sleep of a species are always carried out by providing the experimental animal with every facility to sleep under optimal conditions. In its natural habitat, however, there may arise circumstances in which the animal has to survive without sleep, exactly as has been observed in certain cases. Sleep has been studied in only a few hundred species of mammals, perhaps only 3% of the existing species. Even then, in-depth studies have only been performed on a very few species, maybe only three — the rat, the cat, and man — in which sleep seems to be obligatory. Given that in other species, a significant proportion of cases have been found to be either non-sleepers or atypical sleepers, the total number could well be very high.

The Sleep and Wakefulness of Poikilotherm Vertebrates

Behavioural sleep

Relative to mammals, very few poikilotherm vertebrates have as yet been studied. The published reports present a general lack of agreement about the polygraphic aspects of sleep, but a general agreement about the behavioural aspects. Motor repose, stereotyped posture, reversibility, and increased sensory thresholds have been recognised in most cases. Also, most poikilotherms are known to have specific resting places. Finally, physiological regulation has also been observed in the form of increased sleep after rest deprivation (Flanigan, 1973, 1974; Flanigan *et al.*, 1973, 1974; Tobler and Borbely, 1985). The evidence supporting regulation may not be decisive, however, for two reasons. Firstly, the procedures used to produce the sleep deprivation do not exclude the appearance of mere sensory and/or motor fatigue, so that the subsequent immobility may not really have been a recovery from a sleep debt. The reciprocal experiments would need to be done in which the production of sleep is increased in some form to look for a rebound of wakefulness, perhaps like that performed by Gamundí *et al.* (1998), who observed rest satiety after several days under constant light. Secondly, in some cases there is room for doubt as to whether what is really regulated in poikilotherms is sleep or simply periods of motor rest. The difference between the two phenomena is well known in mammals, but it could be a problem to distinguish them in simpler animals.

REM sleep (paradoxical sleep)

Several studies have reported eye movements and motor automatisms in sleeping foveate fish (Tauber *et al.*, 1969), but Peyreton and Dusan-Peyreton (1967) failed to find REM signs in the tench. In reptiles, various REM signs — eye movements, muscle twitches, and reduction in

EEG amplitude — have been reported by Tauber *et al.* (1966, 1968), Vasilescu (1970), Huntley *et al.* (1977), Romo *et al.* (1978), Karmanova (1982), Ayala-Guerrero (1985), Ayala-Guerrero *et al.* (1988), and Ayala-Guerrero and Huitron-Resendiz (1991), but, on the contrary, no REM was found by Herman *et al.* (1964), Karmanova and Churnosov (1972), Meglasson and Huggins (1979), or Peyreton and Dusan-Peyreton (1969). Moreover, Flanigan (1973, 1974) and Flanigan *et al.*, (1973, 1974) observed that many supposed eye movements recorded during behavioural rest in reptiles by means of electro-oculography were in reality artefacts — eye retractions and tongue, eyelid, or nictating membrane movements — which, when recorded, would be easily mistaken for true eye movements if they had not been directly observed. However, it is still possible that the transitory muscle activations typical of reptilian REM do not show up as eye movements. The oculo-motor system is, in phylogenetic terms, very old and has been well conserved over the course of evolution. There are, however, two motor variants used for visual stabilisation — non-mammals predominantly use compensatory head movements, while mammals mainly use the oculo-motor system which provides more degrees of freedom in the pursuit of moving images (Dieringer and Meie, 1994). Another REM sign — the hippocampal theta rhythm — has been observed in only one study (Servit and Strejcková, 1979), but it was not found after a careful search performed by Gaztelu *et al.* (1991).

In sum, there exist three possibilities: (i) the mammalian differentiation between REM and NREM could truly be absent in poikilotherms, (ii) the observed eye movements are real REM signs, or (iii) REM and NREM could exist in an unrecognised form. The main traits of REM sleep are well known in mammals, but even so there is a wide variation between species (Siegel, 1995). Although it is philosophically somewhat risky to require "essences" in a sleep stage (Blumberg and Lucas, 1996), it does seem reasonable to think that there must have existed an animal that was the first to show REM in evolution. It is also reasonable to assume that this animal would have shown only a "rudimentary" form of REM, so to speak. It would therefore be very useful to establish a minimal set of REM features. Siegel *et al.* (1998) proposed that REM be defined as a state of sleep in which there is a repetitive phasic activation of the reticulo-motor systems of the brain stem and that basic REM should only be recognised in the firing mode of reticular neurons. Work in this line (Eiland *et al.*, 2001) found that the firing mode of the reticular neurons in the turtle showed mixed characteristics between REM and NREM, indicative of a lack of differentiation between the two phases. Another way to recognise non-mammalian REM is to look for rhombencephalic descendant motor inhibition and rhombencephalic cholinergic control of motor automatisms (Nicolau *et al.*, 2000). Were these signs to be found in poikilotherms, their relationship to mammalian REM would be extremely suggestive. Some promising findings have been made in protochordates, where weak electrical stimulation of their hindbrain primordium causes long-lasting spinal inhibition, while de-cerebration increases motor activity and reactivity to environmental stimuli (Guthrie, 1977). Also, in fish and reptiles, injection of cholinergic agonists and antagonists produces changes in the rest state and influences the production of motor automatisms, both actions supposedly controlled by pontine structures (Karmanova, 1982). A significant number of cholinergic neurons have been found in the rhombencephalon of lizards and turtles (Medina *et al.*, 1993) and the presumed function of the cholinergic systems seems to be highly preserved in the transition from poikilotherms to mammals (Hoogland and Vermeulen-Vanderzee, 1990; Powers and Reiner, 1993).

NREM sleep

The search for NREM sleep in poikilotherms has not been successful. Several studies have looked for EEG delta activity, and while some authors describe its existence during sleep (Tauber *et al.*, 1968; Romo *et al.*, 1978; Warner and Huggins, 1978; Meglasson and Huggins, 1979) or wakefulness (Rial *et al.*, 1993; De Vera *et al.*, 1994), others cannot confirm its existence during sleep (Belekhova and Zagorulko, 1964; Herman *et al.*, 1964; Peyreton and Dusan-Peyreton, 1969; Vasilescu, 1970; Flanigan *et al.*, 1973, 1974; Hartse and Rechtschaffen, 1974, 1982; Ayala-Guerrero, 1985; Ayala-Guerrero *et al.*, 1988). The reptilian EEG power spectra is always dominated by low frequencies, although the amplitude seldom reaches the level required to be classed as delta EEG. These discrepancies can probably be explained if one takes some important characteristics of poikilotherm neurophysiology into account. One of these factors is body temperature. Many authors have observed that the absolute amplitude of the EEG is high when the body temperature is high and vice versa (Hunsaker and Lansing, 1962; Parson and Huggins, 1965a,b; Burr and Lange, 1973; Andry *et al.*, 1971; Huntley *et al.*, 1977; González *et al.*, 1978; De Vera *et al.*, 1994). Another factor that determines the amplitude of the EEG is the animal's state. Unlike the case for mammals, the EEG amplitude of poikilotherms decreases with decreasing alertness and is at a maximum during alert wakefulness (Enger, 1957; Bert and Godet, 1963; Belekhova and

Zagorulko, 1964; Herman *et al.*, 1964; De Juan and Segura, 1966; Segura and de Juan, 1966; Segura, 1966; Hobson *et al.*, 1968; Tauber *et al.*, 1968; Goodman and Weinberger, 1969; Lucas *et al.*, 1969; Peyreton and Dusan-Peyreton, 1969; Vasilescu, 1970; Flanigan, 1973, 1974; Flanigan *et al.*, 1973, 1974; Laming, 1980; Ayala-Guerrero, 1985; Huntley, 1987; Ayala-Guerrero *et al.*, 1988). Furthermore, the EEG amplitude increases along the phylogenetic line from fish to mammals (Bullock and Basar, 1988).

One may draw three principal conclusions from these results: (i) there exist slow frequencies in the poikilotherm EEG; (ii) the maximum amplitude of these EEG waves indubitably occurs in active and warm animals, i.e., not during sleep; and (iii) although reptilian slow waves might have amplitudes too low to be classified as delta EEG, their existence should be considered the mark of a general trend, which only reaches full expression in mammals.

Besides the slow waves, mammalian NREM also shows sleep spindles in the sigma (14 Hz) range. Two types of high-frequency spindles in the poikilotherm EEG have been reported. The first type is evoked in the olfactory bulb following the respiratory cycle and has been used simply as a sign to register the movements of breathing (De Vera and González, 1986). Other authors, however, have also described non-respiratory spindles. The two types can be recorded in animals that are awake and at different anatomical positions in the telencephalic cortex of the same animal (Gaztelu *et al.*, 1991) and the non-respiratory spindles can be produced either spontaneously or after sensory (optical and acoustical) stimulation (González and Rial, 1977). According to Servit *et al.* (1971) and Servit and Strejkova (1972), the non-respiratory spindles recorded in reptiles share a great many features with mammalian sleep spindles: both can be recorded simultaneously in the thalamus and in the cortex; both are under inhibitory GABA-ergic control; and both can transform into high voltage spikes and self-sustained spike and wave complexes, in all cases with a great similarity to paroxysmal epileptic events recorded in rats (Van Luijtelaar *et al.*, 1987; Nicolau *et al.*, 2000). Sleep spindles are considered to be signs of the blockade of information transfer between the thalamus and the cortex. Given that the reptilian spindles are observed only during wakefulness, and taking into account the low functional importance of the reptilian cortex in the wakefulness, the meaning of the reptilian spindles could well be different from that of the mammalian ones.

Another reported sign of NREM is the so-called high-voltage spike (HVS). According to some authors, HVS frequency increases during sleep

(Tauber *et al.*, 1966; Ayala Guerrero, 1985; Flanigan, 1973, 1974; Flanigan *et al.*, 1973, 1974). Hartse and Rechtschaffen (1974, 1982), proposed that reptilian HVS is equivalent to the limbic spike of NREM sleeping mammals and that it is the only sign of NREM in reptiles. However, its relationship with sleep seems to be dubious both in mammals (Buzsaki, 1986) and in reptiles in which several workers have observed the spikes irrespective of the state (Tauber *et al.*, 1968; Peyreton and Dusan-Peyreton, 1969; Van Twyver, 1973; Huntley *et al.*, 1977, 1978 (in amphibians); Warner and Huggins, 1978; Meglasson and Huggins, 1979; Huntley and Cohen, 1980; Eiland *et al.*, 2001).

As was noted above for REM, the absence of clear NREM signs also seems to be an unexpected result, because the poikilotherm brain possesses most of the brain centres and neurotransmitter systems (Wolters *et al.*, 1984, 1985) known to play a role in the control of this sleep phase. For instance, the reef wrasse shows a circadian rhythm in its search for a cave to sleep in and this behaviour is enhanced by the administration of serotonin (Lenke, 1998). Also, the zebrafish has a well-developed catecholaminergic system (Ma, 1994a,b) and in *Rana ridibunda* there is a state-dependent modification of serotonin synthesis (Kulikov *et al.*, 1994).

The Sleep and Wakefulness of Birds

Avian sleep seems to have the same phases as that of mammals — NREM and REM. A careful review of the published work, however, shows that this similarity may be misleading, for which reason in Figure 3 a question mark was put on the evolutionary path towards birds.

The aspect of NREM sleeping birds seems to be remarkably similar to that of light sleeping mammals (the guinea pig, for instance), because a high level of vigilance is always maintained and it is almost impossible to observe a sleeping bird without alerting it, and hence it is always necessary to use closed-circuit video monitoring (Klein *et al.*, 1963). The EEG shows in some brain locations, but not in all, high-voltage slow waves. However, the amplitude differences between wakefulness and NREM are lower than in mammals, to the point that Tradardi (1966) pointed out that in effect there exists no clear difference between the EEGs of awake and sleeping birds. This was confirmed by other workers who found high-voltage EEG waves, not only during sleep but also in awake animals (Rojas-Ramírez and Tauber, 1970; Van Twyver and Allison, 1972). However, other reports have affirmed that the EEG sign of sleep in birds consists of a discrete increase in amplitude (not so clear as in mammals) and a reduction in frequency (Walker *et al.*, 1983). In general, it has been found that the EEG activity of birds relies heavily on the state of the eyes — when they close there is an increase in the amplitude of the EEG (Campbell and Tobler, 1984) — and environmental light (Berger and Phillips, 1994) up to the point of a complete sleep suppression without rebound.

Most authors have also failed to record sleep spindles (Amlaner and Ball, 1994). In addition, the EMG shows no clear correlation with the sleeping state. For instance, Van Luijtelaar *et al.* (1987) scored NREM simply when the EMG was not higher than during wakefulness. The data relative to the changes in the slow-wave power during a sleep episode are also discordant. In the pigeon the power remained unchanged throughout the night and did not increase after sleep deprivation (Tobler and Borbely, 1988). On the contrary, in hens (Van Luijtelaar *et al.*, 1987) and in the European blackbird it was lower at the end of the night. However, in this latter species the arousal threshold increased in the contrary sense to the slow-wave power (Szymczak *et al.*, 1996), which is the opposite to what is known in mammals (Neckerman and Ursin, 1993).

Eye movements are the clearest sign of REM, although they may also be recorded (less frequently) during NREM (Amlaner and Ball, 1994). A reduction in EEG amplitude and an increase in frequency is also recognised. The EMG usually shows a decrease in tonic amplitude, but this is only visible in a low proportion of REM episodes (Susic and Kovacevic, 1973) and not in all species (Amlaner and Ball 1994). No theta rhythm has been described in birds (Van Twyver and Allison, 1972; Susic and Kovacevic, 1973).

Additional evidence has been sought with pharmacological experiments. An increase in REM has been found after the administration of acetylcholine agonists but the NREM was also affected (Voronov *et al.*, 1975; Karmanova, 1982). As also in mammals, in the parakeet, reserpine and parachlorophenylalanine cause insomnia (Vasconcelos-Dueñas and Ayala-Guerrero, 1983). Caffeine and adenosine increase and reduce, respectively, motor activity in the turtle dove (Esteban, unpublished results).

In view of these findings, the presence of the two sleep stages could be considered as dubious. Moreover, the reports of sleep in the platypus and the echidna (Siegel *et al.*, 1998, 1999) cast serious doubts on the value of the EEG in distinguishing between NREM and REM. In conclusion, one feels inclined to propose that there is at present no conclusive evidence for the existence of NREM in birds. Previous sections have described the predominance of the low-frequency end of the EEG power spectra in reptiles and a very similar pattern is observed in birds (Amlaner and Ball, 1994, Figure 7-5). We also saw that the amplitude of the reptile EEG depends on two fundamental factors — temperature and activation. Since birds are homeotherms, the temperature factor can be discarded, but the changes in amplitude of their EEG may still be the result of simple arousal changes.

Phylogenetic Aspects of Sleep in Mammals

Mammals are classified into Prototheria (with only three species, the duck-billed platypus and two echidnas), Metatheria (marsupials), and Eutheria (placental mammals). The mammals are relatively homogeneous with respect to sleep, since both the Metatheria and the Eutheria present the two states with similar characteristics. There are marked differences, however, in the Prototheria. The first studies on the echidna *Tachyglossus aculeatus* reported the existence of major amounts of NREM sleep, but a total absence of REM (Allison *et al.*, 1972). This was surprising because it suggested that NREM was older than REM despite the archaic aspect of REM. It hence seemed to be settled that NREM must have arisen in reptiles and, from them, was transmitted to birds and mammals, which in an independent, and surprisingly similar form, developed REM. This was the almost undisputed opinion until the end of the last century. But in 1997 the first studies were published on sleep in the platypus (*Ornithorhynchus anatinus*) (Siegel *et al.*, 1997, 1998, 1999). This species presented two very striking characteristics. Firstly, it has an unusually large proportion of REM — more than 60% of the total sleep time. This finding was subsequently repeated in the echidna (Siegel *et al.*, 1998). Secondly, while it was possible to define the REM unequivocally by behavioural criteria, the animal's EEG showed a surprising abundance of slow waves of great amplitude during a major fraction of the REM. On the contrary, at no time during REM were mixed frequencies and low amplitudes observed, i.e., like those of wakefulness, which, by the way, showed no major differences with those of other mammals.

The presence of large amounts of REM in a mammal with many reptilian characteristics had multiple consequences: (i) REM is probably older than NREM, (ii) REM ought to be found in reptiles, (iii) it is evident that the EEG has a very limited value as a sign of sleep in non-mammals, and (iv) reptiles can show REM that is not definable by the EEG.

The Evolution of Wakefulness

Very few reviews dealing with the evolution of sleep have approached the evolution of wakefulness and indeed its evolutionary continuity between different groups has always been taken for granted. Most studies have supposed that the wakefulness of mammals comes from that of reptiles which comes in turn from that of amphibians, and so on. There is no reason, however, for this to be taken as self-evident. One should ask oneself, for example, whether the centres responsible for wakefulness in a fish are the same as those in a reptile or in a mammal, just as we asked ourselves above whether the centres that control REM in mammals exist in reptiles. Given that the evolution of the brain of mammals has mostly occurred by the superposition of new structures that were practically nonexistent in the brains of their predecessors, it is quite possible that not only REM and NREM have changed, but also changes of similar importance have occurred with respect to wakefulness. Just because a shark, a crocodile, and a cat may be awake does not mean that the three are using homologous regions of the brain to control their wakefulness. In this sense, the presence of the cortex in mammals, a structure with very little precedence, is a crucial aspect.

An essential characteristic of mammalian wakefulness is the reduction in EEG voltage and synchronisation that appears after sensory stimulation and of course exists neither in poikilotherms nor in undeveloped mammals (Villablanca, 1965). The EEG arousal reaction of adult mammals is known to depend on two inputs to the cortex — one cholinergic coming from the basal telencephalon and the other serotonergic coming from the mid-brain raphe (Dringenberg and Vanderwolf, 1998). Cholinergic neurons are well developed in the basal telencephalon of reptiles (Medina *et al.*, 1993) and the same is true for the serotonergic raphe system (Kiehn *et al.*, 1992). It is evident from the different activation mode found in both poikilotherms and immature mammals that these systems have changed over the course of evolution and embryonary development. It has also long been known (Wikler, 1952) that cholinergic blocking can suppress the arousal reaction. However, the cortical dysfunction observed when the wakefulness EEG slows down runs parallel to impaired performance in cognitive ability (Dringenberg and Diavolitsis, 2002), thus emphasising the importance of an active cortex for the full wakefulness behaviour in adult animals. In sum, it seems clear that the homology between the wakefulness of animals with an undeveloped cortex and the cortical one of mammals is doubtful.

Ontogeny and Phylogeny

Karl von Baer — the father of modern embryology — observed that the early embryos of many animals were practically indistinguishable. This observation was considered to be a fundamental morphogenetic law. Haeckel extended von Baer's law to evolution with his famous law of recapitulation: "Ontogeny recapitulates phylogeny." Many evolutionary changes can be explained by this law, but there are also many others that do not seem to fit. The problem with Haeckel's law of recapitulation began to be resolved with W. Garstang's modification in 1922 stating that: "Changes in ontogeny create phylogeny." This revised formulation is in marked contrast with the erroneous, although still generalised, opinion that evolution is based on transformations in the form of adult individuals. On the contrary, it is now beginning to be accepted that in order to understand evolution, it is necessary to recognise, describe, and analyse all of a species' embryological stages in order to compare them with the corresponding stages of related species. Today, modern techniques of molecular genetics allow one to experiment with genes acting during development and how these changes (micro-evolution) may determine major changes in the final form (macro-evolution). Evidently, Von Baer's observational morphogenetic law fits well into modern understanding since it is reasonable to expect that early changes in an animal's development can have great transcendence and that in many cases their outcome will be lethal, so that such changes cannot be very frequent. On the contrary, the outcomes of changes at a later stage of development are more likely to be viable, which is why they are more abundant.

The methods of Evo-Devo biology are currently being applied to the study of the evolution of the vertebrate nervous system (Nieuwenhuis, 2002), the divergence of the reptilian and mammalian brain (Aboitiz *et al.*, 2002), and the evolution of the mammalian cortex (Montagnini and Treves, 2003). It is now well established that the development of the multi-layered mammalian isocortex from the reptilian brain design obeys the phylogenetic law fairly well.

A basic concept in Evo-Devo studies is that of heterochrony. This holds that differences in the development of phylogenetically related animals are due to different rates of embryonic development. Sometimes development is slowed down and the adult shows embryonic traits — a phenomenon known as paedomorphosis or neoteny. These cases evidently do not fulfil Haeckel's law. On the contrary, at other times development is accelerated, after which

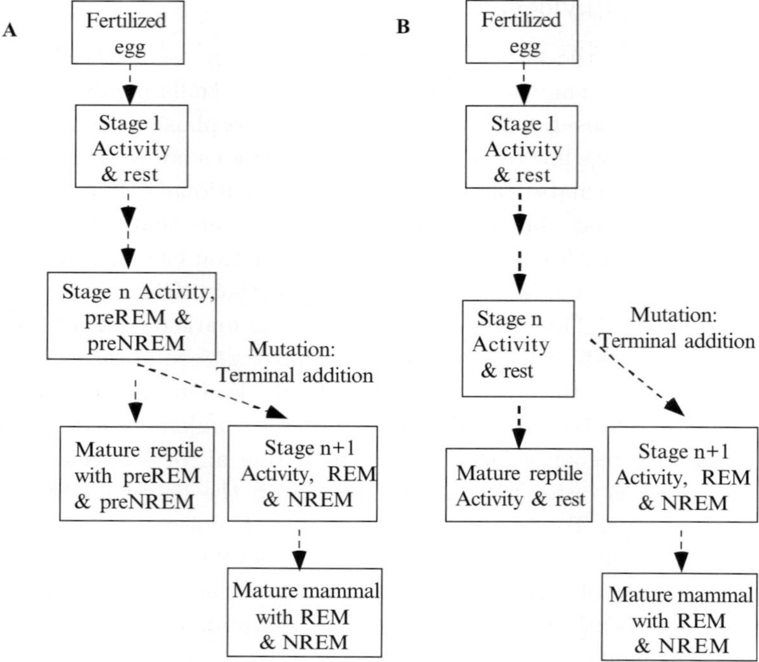

Figure 4. The two types of mammalian sleep were the result of a terminal addition which could have occurred in either of two ways. See the explanation in the text.

new traits appear in the adult organism — this is called peramorphosis or terminal addition and does satisfy the law of recapitulation.

Some results of applying the concept of heterochrony to the evolution of sleep are represented in Figure 4. The first option (panel A) assumes that primitive reptiles had both sleep states in an incomplete form and in this case the heterochrony would have consisted of an acceleration of the final stages of development with which the two states were perfected as a terminal addition. But if this is how things indeed occurred, then some of the signs indicative of the two sleep states should be recognisable in modern reptiles. The second option (panel B) assumes that the heterochrony occurred before the separation of the two states. In this case, the terminal addition of REM and NREM would have been completely new and without precedent in the reptiles. Given that the search for REM and NREM signs in reptiles has led to no clear results, this second option may well be correct. It is not, however, a parsimonious solution, as Figure 5 shows. If both

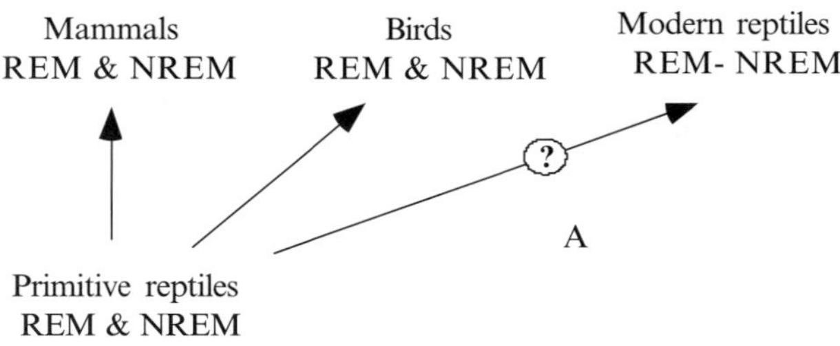

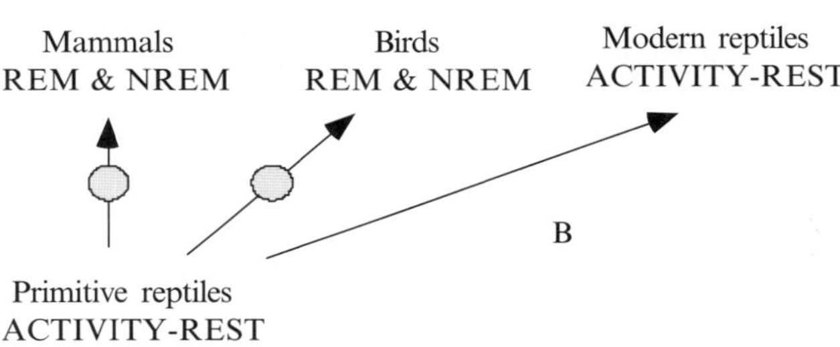

Figure 5. Alternative trees representing the phylogenetic relationships between modern reptiles, birds, and mammals. (Explanation in text.)

phases existed in the primitive reptiles (panel A), only a single mutation (circle with a question mark) would be required to explain their loss in modern reptiles (are they really absent?). Nevertheless, given the heterogeneity of these animals (recall Figure 3), it seems difficult to accept that the loss occurred in the entire group. On the contrary, if the two phases did not exist in the primitive reptiles (panel B), two mutations would have been required for them to arise independently in mammals and in birds. In sum, the more parsimonious hypothesis requires both states to exist in modern reptiles and hence the interest in continuing with these studies.

From what we have seen up to this point, it is difficult to draw any firm conclusion from the phylogenetic trees shown in Figure 5. To try to resolve the problem, we shall consider the embryology of sleep in mammals.

With the first studies on mammalian sleep, it was immediately accepted that REM sleep is the dominant state in immature mammals. However, the signs that are indicators of sleep in young animals do not exactly coincide with those of adults of the same species. For this reason, instead of the terms REM and NREM, one prefers to use active sleep (AS) and quiet sleep (QS) and it is usually accepted that there is a continuum between the two respective types of sleep in the adult and in the immature animal. As was observed above, this process would be a paradigmatic example of heterochrony by terminal addition. Nonetheless, Frank and Heller (2003) consider that the difference between AS and QS is not real; instead, the two states constitute a single undifferentiated state from which develops first NREM and then, a little later, REM. Seen in this way, the process can also be explained as a terminal addition, although in this case it would be double. The following paragraphs will briefly review the state of knowledge concerning these questions.

The Ontogeny of Sleep

Since the intra-uterine development of mammals makes it difficult to study them in stages prior to birth, it is not easy either to study the comparative embryology of sleep. Nevertheless, there have been some observations made on premature humans and on the newborn of altricial species, as well as some direct *in utero* observations.

Premature infants

Parmelee and Stern (1972) made the first observations on premature infants and their results have been confirmed by Dreyfus-Brisac and Monod (1975) and Lamblin *et al.* (1999). Before 28 weeks of gestational age, the infant shows periods of activity and rest in an undifferentiated state that simultaneously presents characteristics of QS and AS. "The infant is active all the time but does not seem to be awake ... Does he really sleep? What is sleep at this age?" (Dreyfus-Brisac and Monod, 1975). The EEG shows bursts of very slow waves — between 0.3 and 1 Hz — lasting from 3 to 20 s between which are sandwiched short, moderate-voltage, 8- to 14-Hz bursts. The pattern is discontinuous, alternating with periods of silence of 2–3 min.

The clear differentiation between wakefulness, AS, and QS begins to emerge between 32 and 35 weeks. At this age, the EEG presents a pattern of slow waves with an occasional superposition of 16-Hz waves — a pattern interrupted by periods of silence. There are also, however, periods of irregular activity including eye movements and slow waves with ripples in the EEG. A permanent slow-wave EEG is observed throughout wakefulness. From 35 weeks onwards, the wakefulness, AS, and QS states can be correlated with specific EEG patterns similar to those of the full-term neonate (Niedermeyer, 1993).

Full-term neonates

Wakefulness

During wakefulness, the neonate EEG shows low-amplitude (15–60 μV) delta and theta waves with some alpha components. This EEG is very similar to that observed during AS, particularly when the latter is recorded following a cycle of QS. In the full-term infant, 29% of the time is spent in wakefulness and 71% total in sleep. Two-thirds of this sleep is AS and one-third QS. Although electrophysiological differentiation between the two states is usually difficult because the EOG has a very low amplitude, visual observation allows them to be distinguished easily (Niedermeyer, 1993). The slow waves of wakefulness increase in amplitude up to 3 years, at which age they merge with the alpha rhythm precursor. This first appears at 3–4 months as a basic 4 to 6-Hz occipital rhythm, but does not reach the typical frequency of 10–11 Hz until 6 years of age (Niedermeyer, 1993). The most usual arousal response in infants of 3–17 weeks involves spinal and respiratory reflexes; cortical arousal, when present, is always manifest as an increase in high-frequency EEG components (McNamara *et al.*, 1998) with no change in the delta range amplitude.

Active sleep

In the first few weeks, it is most common for the normal neonate to fall asleep directly into AS, like cataleptic adults. Similarly, an AS phase always precedes awakening. When the baby is in AS, it shows: (i) a large amount of phasic motor activity with affective components such as smiling, grimacing, and crying; (ii) clusters of rapid eye movements, most commonly lateral; (iii) irregular respiration, often with brief periods of central-type apnea; (iv) a fall in muscle tone; and (v) changes in cardiac rate and skin resistance and penile erections. There are two main EEG patterns: (i) a fairly continuous, more or less rhythmic activity, occurring at the onset of sleep with a dominant frequency in the delta and theta ranges and small amounts of higher frequencies and EEG amplitudes varying between 40 and 100 μV and (ii) an EEG pattern occurring after a cycle of QS that consists of a lower-voltage (20–50 μV) mixture of theta and delta activity with some faster ripples (Lombroso, 1993; Niedermeyer, 1993). The loss of synchronisation, typical of the adult REM, with mixed frequencies and low amplitude, begins to be visible at 6 years, but complete maturity is not reached until adolescence (Harper *et al.*, 1981; Sterman *et al.*, 1982). Theta rhythm is rare before 3 years of age and again does not reach full development until adolescence (Niedermeyer, 1993).

Quiet sleep

In this sleep stage, a healthy infant (i) lies quietly with only occasional movements which may resemble startles, (ii) produces rare single eye movements, (iii) breathes regularly, and (iv) has a continuous level of tonic muscle activity. There are also two EEG patterns. The first is properly known by the term *tracé alternant*. It shows slow waves (1–4 Hz, 50–200 µV) with random faster transients. This pattern appears roughly every 4–5 s and lasts for 2–4 s. Between bursts, the EEG is of low voltage (20–40 µV) in the theta range. The second QS pattern shows a continuous slow-wave EEG (0.5–4 Hz, 50–200 µV). The continuous slow-wave EEG steadily increases to predominate by 3–4 weeks after birth (Lombroso, 1993; Niedermeyer, 1993).

Sleep spindles are observed from 7 weeks onwards (Metcalf, 1970), but do not acquire their typical form until 3–5 years of age. Instead, at earlier ages they often show a sharp negative component while the positive component is rounded (comb spindles), an element that has also been observed in reptiles (Nicolau *et al.*, 2000). The K-complexes are not observed until 5 months, when they are fairly large and blunt, showing an increasingly large and sharp component after 5–6 years.

Sleep in Young Mammals

Some reviews have compared the sleep characteristics of newborn mammals (Zepelin and Rechtschaffen, 1974; Allison and Chichetti, 1976; Meddis, 1983; Zepelin, 1994). In general, they describe major variations that depend on three factors: (i) the altricial–precocial dimension, (ii) the safety of the sleeping place, and (iii) the prey–predator status. These three factors are closely related, however, since prey are usually precocial and sleep in the open, while predators are usually altricial and have well-protected nests (Eisemberg, 1981).

The sleep of immature animals has been studied especially in depth in the cat and the rat (Jouvet-Mounier *et al.*, 1970; McGinty *et al.*, 1977). These species are born even less mature than humans, so that a major part of their embryonic development occurs after birth. The results, however, are similar to those described above for the human infant. In all cases, low frequencies dominate the EEG independently of the state of sleep or wakefulness.

The changes in the indicator signs of sleep and wakefulness are probably due to the processes of maturation of the brain, fundamentally to myelinisation (Paus *et al.*, 2001) and to reorganisation of the thalamo-cortical neurons (Warren and Jones, 1997). It is well established that the phylogenetically most modern regions of the brain are the last to mature, so that it is natural that the embryo shows none of the cortical signs of sleep and wakefulness of the adult.

Altricial (immature born) animals spend more time in sleep and show a very high proportion of REM. In the rat, myoclonic twitching of the limbs is the first sign of this phase. There are at least two mechanisms that generate muscular contractions in the rat embryo (Blumberg and Lucas, 2002). One is located in the spinal cord and produces movements that occur at random and the other is more rostral — perhaps in the medulla — and produces movements quickly and in an as yet undetermined pattern. Nonetheless, it is illustrative how the intact, sleeping animal presents coherent behaviour, with its limbs in synchrony. After birth, however, they are only observed during AS (Narayanan *et al.*, 1971).

According to Blumberg and Lucas (1996), the myoclonic twitching is probably involved in regulating the neuron apoptosis that occurs during development, to differentiate the different types of muscle fibres and finally to enable the formation of topographical maps, a factor which has received recent confirmation (Grillner, 2004). Of course, it is possible that the adult REM and the neonate AS are qualitatively different, so that the aforementioned functions may only be applicable to neonate sleep. But if only the EEG is taken into account to distinguish the phases of sleep, one would then also have to assume that neonate slow-wave wakefulness is different from adult wakefulness, an aspect that we shall return to later. The hypotheses distinguishing neonate sleep and that of adults are not parsimonious because they multiply the number of states. By itself, however, this is not reason enough to reject them. Instead, one must study the development and function of every component of sleep and wakefulness. Each component appears independently and for its own reasons, but when it acts in concert with the rest it generates complexity. This is the systems dynamics approach, according to which no causal priority should be assigned to any of a system's components. In sum, one should avoid favouring any given component — the EEG, eye movements, or the lack of muscle tone — as being essential to a phase of sleep and then assigning to it a causal priority to affirm or deny the existence of a determined state. There can be no essences in sleep states and no indicator is either the cause or the effect of the others. Each matures at its own rate and all are eventually integrated into the REM or NREM of the adult.

One aspect that has attracted the attention of many researchers is the magnitude of the total time of sleep, especially of REM, in immature animals. According to the most generally accepted ideas, it is an indicator of the need for REM in the development and differentiation of the nervous system. But it is also possible that immaturity itself constrains the animal to show only the simplest forms of behaviour. Sleep as behaviour is clearly much simpler than wakefulness, so that in order to produce sleep, less quantity of brain would be required than is necessary to produce the variety of behaviours that come into play during wakefulness. The immaturity of the nervous system could therefore be correlated more with the inability to maintain a continuous and complete wakefulness than with a true need for sleep. Most authors, however, have only considered relatively complex hypotheses, without taking into account the simplest one.

Unlike altricial animals, precocial animals have sensory and motor systems that are fully developed immediately after birth. There have been post-natal and *in utero* studies in some of these species. In sheep, cortical differentiation begins at 110 gestational days (term is at approximately 147 days) and is shown by the superposition of a large-amplitude, 3–10 Hz, activity on another of low voltage (Clewlow *et al.*, 1983). Between 130 and 133 gestational days, the EEG of the two sleep stages is well consolidated, with desynchronisation and mixed frequencies in the REM and slow waves in the NREM, i.e., the full set of adult mammalian sleep traits.

Summary

1. Behaviourally, sleep is flexible, with characteristics that vary between different animals, from the total absence of sleep in some species to the typical mammalian sleep with its two phases and complex regulatory mechanisms. The variability of sleep is probably driven by the characteristics of the ecological niche occupied by each animal, with no definite phylogenetic correlations.
2. Most vertebrates show signs of behavioural sleep and traits have been added by evolution, from mere changes in motor activity (probably the only sleep sign found in small-brained animals) to the complex traits recognised in mammals.

3. Fish, amphibians, reptiles, and young mammals present similar EEG features that are clearly different from those of adult mammals. This supports the idea that there were no fundamental changes in the evolution of sleep–wakefulness from fish to modern reptiles.

4. It seems safe to summarise the basic features of the poikilotherm EEG: (i) the amplitude depends on the body temperature; (ii) irrespective of the behavioural state, the EEG always shows a dominance of low frequencies; (iii) the maximum amplitude is observed during active wakefulness; and (iv) sensory activation always causes an increase in amplitude and synchronisation. Points ii–iv are also characteristic of immature mammals.

5. In poikilotherms, only two states are clearly recognised — rest and wakefulness — but the transition between them cannot be defined as it is in mammals and there is a continuous variation between the deepest sleep state and the most active wakefulness. This suggests that, unlike in mammals, either the switch between wakefulness and sleep does not exist or it is fairly undeveloped and does not coordinate the production of discrete states.

6. The EEG of non-mammalian animals has only limited usefulness as an indicator of sleep. Low frequencies dominate the spectrum in all states and only in mature mammals is there the EEG difference between REM and NREM or the reduction in voltage following behavioural activation.

7. There has been a general acceptance that the sleep of birds has the same phases as that of mammals. The data supporting this equivalence must, however, be called into question because of the similarity in the phenomenology of reptilian and avian sleep. Avian wakefulness has a slow-wave EEG similar to that of the supposed NREM, with the result that the polygraphic difference between the two states can be as fuzzy as between reptilian sleep and wakefulness. The same may be said about the distinction between REM and NREM. Avian sleep is heavily dependent on the state of the eyes, so that internal regulatory mechanisms may have less importance than in mammals.

8. The EEG of the first stages of mammalian ontogeny always shows dominance of the low-frequency end of the spectrum, with features that are similar to those that exist in mature reptiles, whereas the typical characteristics of wakefulness, NREM, and REM are only observed when the mammal has reached maturity. The two stages are thus most probably the result of a terminal addition.

9. The homology between the different types of vertebrate wakefulness has seldom been called into question. However, given that the vertebrate brain has evolved by the superposition of structures that did not exist in the previous stages, it is probable that there is really no such homology and that the cortical wakefulness of mammals is an acquisition that is only analogous with the wakefulness of other vertebrates.

Final Conclusions

Reptiles

The results summarised in the previous section allow us to present a tree of the phylogeny of sleep which is different from what has been accepted until now (Figure 6). Poikilotherms only have activity and rest and the EEG of the two states is similar with major differences only in amplitude. Some of the characteristics of REM probably exist during the rest of these animals, even though they are not observable in all the species. Poikilotherm rest may show REM with extensive dominance of tonic traits and a reduced amount of phasic signs, the latter observable in some species only [see "REM Sleep (Paradoxical Sleep)"]. This pre-REM rest phase is probably under cholinergic rhombencephalic control. These animals' wakefulness is coordinated by sensory and motor regions distributed throughout the nervous system. Of these regions, the telencephalon is of minor importance (Belekhova, 1979; Aboitiz *et al.*, 2002).

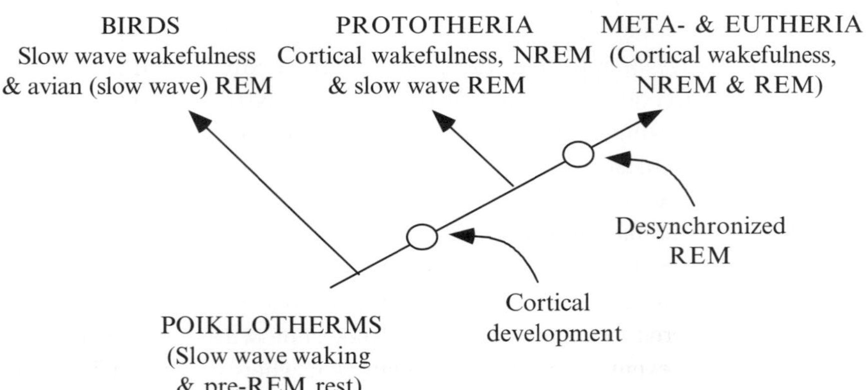

Figure 6. The most probable phylogenetic tree in accordance with the characteristics of vertebrate sleep. See explanation in the text.

Birds

It is possible that the characteristics of reptiles were conserved without major changes in birds (Figure 6) and it is doubtful that NREM exists in these animals. For this reason, in Figure 3 the evolution of the two states was labelled with a question mark. As we have seen, the existence of a delta-type EEG is in no way a definitive factor, especially considering that it is not only manifested during sleep, but is also present during wakefulness. It also has to be admitted that, apart from the EEG, there are very few objective data indicative of the existence of NREM in birds. On the contrary, it is possible that what has been thought to be NREM is really REM with a slow-wave EEG, as is the situation observed in the platypus. If platypus and echidna REM data had been known 30 years ago, the reality of avian NREM would not have been accepted without there having been many additional studies called for. But if it is indeed the case that birds really lack NREM, the general evolution of the states of sleep and wakefulness becomes beautifully simple. On the contrary, if NREM exists in birds, one has to assume that birds have also developed a telencephalic wakefulness that would be analogous, but not homologous (because, instead of depending on the cortex, it would depend on the striatal complex), to that of mammals (Nicolau *et al.*, 2000).

Avian wakefulness might also be similar to that of reptiles since both maintain sensory–motor control distributed throughout the length of the brain. It is possible of course that the development of their striatal complex gives them the capacity for multisensorial-motor associations, which are able to determine more complex behaviour than that of their ancestors (Divac and Ober, 1979); in electrophysiological terms this can be manifested as the already mentioned small changes in the telencephalic EEG.

Mammals

In this group, the most important change has been not the acquisition of two types of sleep, but that of a new wakefulness without precedent in the poikilotherm ancestors. This new state was the consequence of the development of the multi-layered isocortex. The development of olfaction is believed to have been a key event in early mammalian evolution (Jerison, 1973, 1990; Kemp, 1982). It has been postulated (Aboitiz *et al.*, 2002) that the lateral, mediodorsal, and hippocampal cortices of primitive mammals were put to use to make relatively elaborate, largely olfactory-based representations of space in which specific odours labelled particular objects, places, and routes, leading to an increasing importance of the development of multi-sensorial maps of space. In later stages, the visual and auditory representations, already present in the dorsal reptilian cortex, were developed in columnar form, establishing retinotopic and sound localisation areas. Most probably, these changes were caused by the adoption of a nocturnal lifestyle, quite different from that of reptiles whose activity is entirely dependent on external heat sources, i.e., it is diurnal. However, switching from diurnal to nocturnal activity was only possible after the development of endothermic metabolism. Thus, homeothermy and olfaction were the key events in the separation between mammals and reptiles and these changes were the consequence of a lifestyle change, from diurnal to nocturnal.

It has always been thought that the changes described in the above paragraph were the determinants of the division of sleep into two phases. It seems more probable, however, that they involved reorganisation of wakefulness, since (i) the telencephalic cortex was the anatomical structure that underwent the most important modifications of the entire nervous system and (ii) changes in the structure of the cortex determined profound alterations in the control of the activities typical of wakefulness (Rial *et al.*, 1993; De Vera *et al.*, 1994; Nicolau *et al.*, 2000). Added to the changes in the structure of the cortex were very effective mechanisms to determine entry into and exit from sleep, something that is absent in poikilotherms. As we have seen, there are no discrete states in poikilotherms. According to McGinty and Szimusiak (2001), entering and leaving sleep in mammals is controlled from the basal telencephalon and the hypothalamus where there are sleep-triggering and arousal-triggering executive neurons connected by mutually inhibitory interactions. They thus act as a bistable switch — a flip-flop, as shown in Figure 2 — reducing the existence of intermediate states. This explains one of the problems in the appearance of the two types of sleep. All animals have executive regions, but only mammals have well-coordinated on–off switches. The sleep and wakefulness executive neurons are warmth-sensitive, further evidence that they might have arisen in coincidence with thermoregulation (Parmeggiani and Morrison, 1990; McGinty *et al.*, 2001). Another essential change was the development of the cholinergic and serotoninergic systems that are responsible for the cortical arousal. It is notable that the cholinergic neurons responsible for REM cortical activation are also located in the basal telencephalon (Dringenberg and Vanderwolf, 1998). Most probably, cortical arousal appeared in two phases (shown in Figure 6), neither of which are present in immature mammals.

The first change must have occurred before the branching of monotremes and produced the cortical arousal during waking. The second change was responsible for the cortical arousal typical of REM. Although the EEG voltage reduction seen in waking and in REM sleep is presently thought to be produced by a single mechanism (Siegel *et al.*, 1999), it has been shown that, in phylogeny, the two have developed at different rates. The platypus has the wakefulness EEG voltage reduction, but it is not well developed during REM (Siegel *et al.*, 1999). However, no ontogenic difference between the two has been reported.

These relationships can be described by comparing Figures 1 and 2. The general opinion has always been that the difference between poikilotherm and mammalian sleep is that the undifferentiated sleep of the former split into the two phases — REM and NREM. The present review has argued, however, that the change consisted in mammals' acquisition of the hypothalamic flip-flop module and cortical arousal (represented in Figure 2 with shading). With this, the switch between activity and rest of the poikilotherms was the same as the mammalian switch between NREM and REM, respectively.

As a result of these acquisitions, the first reptile-like mammals may have found themselves faced with two different types of wakefulness — the old reptilian type, based on the activity of distributed sensory–motor centres, and the new type, fundamentally dependent on cortical activity. This situation is likely to have been unsustainable and the forced solution was involution of the coordinating centres of reptilian wakefulness. That this involution occurred in morphological terms is well known and indeed its paradigm is the involution of the tectal visual system against the development of the visual cortex. But there is no doubt that similar changes occurred in the other sensory systems and in the motor systems. In functional terms, the reptilian sensory–motor system responsible for wakefulness was left blind, deaf and paralysed, which is perhaps a good definition of mammalian NREM.

Further Consequences

The scheme shown in Figure 6 has some notable advantages. One is that it reduces to a minimum the number of evolutionary stages in the development of sleep from the first vertebrates to the most modern ones — mammals and birds. Moreover, while one might consider this advantage to be purely philosophical, all the states of wakefulness are now correlated with perfectly well-established changes in both the general physiology (thermoregulation) and the structure of the nervous system (isocortex development).

Another advantage of this proposed evolutionary path is that no alternative hypotheses really exist. Indeed, there are data that are not entirely coherent with the picture, but it is possible that many of the older reports are not very precise, while it seems difficult to deny the validity of the data summarised in "The Sleep and Wakefulness of Birds" paragraph (page 219). For some decades there were two counterposed possibilities with respect to the evolution of sleep — one that REM was the primitive sleep and the other that NREM was. For a short while, it was also supposed that there was a simultaneous evolution of the two states from an intermediate undifferentiated state, but the discovery of REM in the monotremes left no room for doubt about REM's antiquity. Meanwhile, none of the afore-mentioned possibilities took the evolution of wakefulness into account, which is perhaps one of the principal contributions of the scheme proposed in the present review. With the ideas that have been put forward, we have painted a coherent and unitary picture of the evolution of the wake–sleep continuum in the vertebrates. The result is a rather heterodox proposal, but there comes to mind Sherlock Holmes's advice to Dr Watson in *The Sign of Four*: "When you have eliminated the impossible, that which remains, *however improbable*, must be the truth."

To conclude, the proposed pathway for the evolution of wakefulness and sleep also provides an easy answer to the most important question in sleep research: Why do we sleep? The surprisingly simple answer is that our far too complex sleep is a mere consequence of having acquired a cortical wakefulness. In essence, the complex mammalian sleep has turned out to be a mere by-product of the evolution of wakefulness, serving no other purpose than to continue providing the simple rest and activity present in all animals, i.e., to divide time into cyclic periods of rest and activity, as Aschoff proposed just 40 years ago. In 1971, Rechtschaffen stated that "if sleep does not serve an absolute vital function, then it is the biggest mistake the evolutionary process ever made." However, there is no support for the expectation that a biological process should perform in a simple way. There are many examples of extreme complexity used to attain a simple function. There is the puzzle of mammalian foetal circulation in which, except for the short umbilical veins, pure oxygenated blood is never found and the placenta is in parallel, not in series, with the main organs and tissues — a fools' design from an engineer's viewpoint. The same can be said for the inverted vertebrate retina, or for the middle ear bone chain which resulted from the transformation of the fish jaw's articulation. The structure and function of the nervous system has evolved as an immensely complex patchwork in which cellular aggregations have been developed, discarded, and reused time and again for many different, and even opposing, functions and this may also be the case for the evolution of sleep and wakefulness.

Acknowledgments

This work has been in part supported by a grant of the Spanish Government DGCYT BFI2002-04583-C02-02.

References

Aboitiz, F., Montiel, J., Morales, D., and Concha, M. (2002). Evolutionary divergence of the reptilian and the mammalian brains: consideration on connectivity and development. *Brain Res. Rev.*, 39: 141–153.

Allison, T. and Chichetti, D.V. (1976). Sleep in mammals: ecological and constitutional correlates. *Science*, 194: 732–734.

Allison, T., Van Twyver, H., and Goff, W.R. (1972). Electrophysiological studies of the echidna, *Tachyglossus aculeatus*. I. Waking and sleep. *Arch. Ital. Biol.*, 110: 145–184.

Amlaner, C.J. and Ball, N.J. (1994). Avian sleep. In: Kryger, M.H., Roth, T., and Dement, W.C. (Eds.). *Principles and Practice of Sleep Medicine.* Philadelphia: W.B. Saunders, pp. 81–94.

Andry, M.L., Luttges, M.W., and Gamow, I. (1971). Temperature effects on spontaneous and evoked neural activity in the garter snake. *Exp. Neurol.*, 31: 32–44.

Aschoff, J. (1964). Survival value of diurnal rhythms. *Symp. Zool. Soc. Lond.*, 13: 79–98.

Ayala-Guerrero, F. (1985). Sleep in a chelonian reptile (*Kinosteron* sp). *Sleep Res.*, 14: 83.

Ayala-Guerrero, F. and Huitron-Resendiz, S. (1991). Sleep patterns in the lizard *Ctenosaura pectinata*. *Physiol. Behav.*, 49: 1305–1307.

Ayala-Guerrero, F., Calderon, A., and Perez, M. (1988). Sleep patterns in a chelonian reptile (*Gopherus flavomarginatus*). *Physiol. Behav.*, 44: 333–337.

Belekhova, M.G. (1979). Neurophysiology of the forebrain. In: Gans, C., Northcut, R.G., and Ulinski, P.S. (Eds.). *Biology of The Reptilia.* London: Academic Press, pp. 287–359.

Belekova, M.G. and Zagorul'ko, T.M. (1964). Correlations between background electrical activity, after-discharge and EEG activation response to photic stimulation in tortoise brain (*Emys lutaria*). *Zh. Vyssh. Nerv. Deyat. im. I.P. Pavlova*, 14: 1028–1032.

 S. Esteban et al.

Benington, J.H. (2000). Sleep homeostasis and the function of sleep. *Sleep*, 23: 959–966.

Berger, R.J. and Phillips, N.H. (1994). Constant light suppresses sleep and circadian rhythms in pigeons without consequent sleep rebound in darkness. *Am. J. Physiol.*, 267: R945–R952.

Bert, J. and Godet, R. (1963). Réaction d'eveil télencéphalique d'un Dipneuste. C.R. Societé de Biologie de l'ouest Africain, Séance July 12, pp. 1787–1790.

Blumberg, M.S. and Lucas, D.E. (1996). A developmental and component analysis of active sleep. *Dev. Psychobiol.*, 29: 1–22.

Blumberg, M.S. and Lucas, D.E. (2002). Dual mechanisms of twitching during sleep in neonatal rats. *Behav. Neurosci.*, 108: 1196–1202.

Bruce Durie, D.J. (1981). Sleep in animals. In: Wheatley, D. (Ed.). *Psychopharmacology of Sleep*. New York: Raven Press, pp. 1–18.

Bullock, T.H. and Basar, E. (1988). Comparison of ongoing compound field potentials in the brain of invertebrates and vertebrates. *Brain Res. Rev.*, 13: 57–75.

Burr, W. and Lange, H. (1973). Spontaneous brain activity in some species of amphibians and a reptile. *Electroencephalogr. Clin. Neurophysiol.*, 34: 735.

Buzsáki, G. (1986). Hippocampal sharp waves: their origin and significance. *Brain Res.*, 398: 242–252.

Campbell, S.S. and Tobler, I. (1984). Animal sleep: a review of sleep duration across phylogeny. *Neurosci. Biobehav. Rev.*, 8: 269–300.

Clewlow, F., Dawes, G.S., Johnston, B.M., and Walker, D.W. (1983). Changes in breathing, electrocortical and muscle activity in unanaestethized fetal lambs with age. *J. Physiol.*, 341: 463–476.

Compagno, L.J.V. (1984). FAO species catalogue. Vol. 4. Sharks of the world. An annotated and illustrated catalogue of shark species known to date. Hexanchiformes to Lamniformes. *FAO Fish. Synop.*, 125: 1–249.

Costeau, J.I. and Cousteau, P. (1971). The Shark, Splendid Savage of The Deep. New York: Doubleday and Co.

De Juan, A.O.R. and Segura, E.T. (1966). Proyección telencefálica de estímulos sensoriales en batracios. *Acta Physiol. Latinoam.*, 16: 40.

De Vera, L. and González, J. (1986). Effect of body temperature on the ventilatory responses in the lizard *Gallotia gallotti*. *Respir. Physiol.*, 65: 29–37.

De Vera, L., González, J., and Rial, R.V. (1994). Reptilian waking EEG: slow waves, spindles and evoked potentials. *Electroencephalogr. Clin. Neurophysiol.*, 90: 298–303.

Dieringer, N. and Meie, R.K. (1994). Strategies for simultaneous image stabilization and gaze orientation in different vertebrates. In: Delgado-García, J.M., Godaux, E., and Vidal, P.P. (Eds.). *Information Processing Underlying Gaze Control*. Oxford: Pergamon, pp. 429–437.

Divac, I. and Ober, G. (1979). The Neostriatum. New York: Pergamon Press.

Dreyfus-Brisac, C. and Monod, N. (1975). Electroencephalogran of full term newborns and premature infants. In: Reymons, A. (Ed.). *Handbook of Electroencephalography and Clinical Neurophysiology*. Amsterdam: Elsevier, pp. 6–23.

Dringenberg, H.C. and Diavolitsis, P. (2002). Electroencephalographic activation by fluoxetine in rats: role of 5-HT1A receptors and enhancement of concurrent acetylcholinesterase inhibitor treatment. *Neuropharmacology*, 42: 154–161.

Dringenberg, H.C. and Vanderwolf, C.H. (1998). Involvement of direct and indirect pathways in electrocorticographic activation. *Neurosci. Biobehav. Rev.*, 22: 243–257.

Eiland, M.M., Lyamin, O.I., and Siegel, J.M. (2001). State related discharge of neurons in the brainstem of freely moving box turtles *Terrapene carolina major*. *Arch. Ital. Biol.*, 139: 23–36.

Eisemberg, J.F. (1981). *The Mammalian Radiations: An Analysis of Trends in Evolution, Adaptation, and Behavior.* Chicago: The University of Chicago Press.

Enger, P.S. (1957). The electroencephalogram of codfish (*Gadus callarias*). *Acta Physiol. Scand.*, 39: 55–72.

Flanigan, W.F. (1973). Sleep and wakefulness in iguanid lizards, *Ctenosaura pectinata* and *Iguana iguana*. *Brain Behav. Evol.*, 8: 401–436.

Flanigan, W.F. (1974). Sleep and wakefulness in Chelonian reptiles II. the red-footed tortoise, *Gechelone carbonaria*. *Arch. Ital. Biol.*, 112: 253–277.

Flanigan, W.F., Wilcox, R.H., and Rechtschaffen, A. (1973). The EEG and behavioral continuum of the crocodilian *Caiman sclerops*. *Electroencephalogr. Clin. Neurophysiol.*, 34: 521–538.

Flanigan, W.F., Knight, C.P., Hartse, K.M., and Rechtschaffen, A. (1974). Sleep and wakefulness in chelonian reptiles I. the box turtle, *Terrapene carolina*. *Arch. Ital. Biol.*, 112: 227–252.

Frank, M.G. and Heller, C. (2003). The ontogeny of mammalian sleep: a reappraisal of alternative hypotheses. *J. Sleep Res.*, 12: 25–34.

Gamundí, A., Roca, C., Bernácer, R., Nicolau, M.C., and Rial, R.V. (1998). Behavioural sleep and environmental factors in reptiles (*Gallotia galloti*) *J. Physiol.*, 509: 88P.

Garstang, W. (1922). The theory of recapitulation: A critical re-statement of the biogenetic law. *Zool. J. Linnean Soc. Lond.*, 35: 81–101.

Gaztelu, J.M., García-Austt, E., and Bullock, T. (1991). Electrocorticograms of hippocampal and dorsal cortex of two reptiles: comparison with possible mammalian homologs. *Brain Behav. Evol.*, 37: 144–160.

Gertychowa, R. (1970). Studies on the ethology and space orientation of the blind cave fish *Anoptichthys jordani*. *Folia Biol.*, 18: 9–69.

González, J. and Rial, R.V. (1977). Electrofisiología de la corteza telencefálica de reptiles (*Lacerta galloti*): EEG y potenciales evocados. *Rev. Esp. Fisiol.*, 33: 239-248.

González, J., Vera, L.M., García-Cruz, C.M., and Rial, R.V. (1978). Efectos de la temperatura en el electroencefalograma y los potenciales evocados de los reptiles (*Lacerta galloti*). Rev. Esp. Fisiol., 34: 153–158.

Goodman, D.A. and Weinberger, N.M. (1969). An electroencephalographic study of *Necturus maculosus* (mudpuppy). *Physiol. Zool.*, 42: 398–410.

Grillner, S. (2004). Muscle twitches during sleep shape the precise modules of the withdrawal reflex. *Trends Neurosci.*, 27: 169–171.

Guthrie, D.M. (1977). The Physiology and structure of the nervous system of Amphioxus (*Branchiostoma lanceolatum Pallas*). In: Barrington, E.J.W., and Jeffries, R.P.S. (Eds.). *Protochordates Symposium of Zoological Society of London.* London: Academic Press, pp. 43–80.

Harper, R.M., Leake, B., Miyahara, L., Hoppenbrouwers, T., Sterman, M.B., and Hodgman, J. (1981). Development of ultradian periodicity and coalescence at 1 cycle per hour in electroencephalographic activity. *Exp. Neurol.*, 73: 127–143.

Hartse, K.M. and Rechtschaffen, A. (1974). Effect of atropine sulfate on the sleep related EEG spike activity of the tortoise (*Geochelone carbonaria.*). *Brain Behav. Evol.*, 9: 81–94.

Hartse, K.M. and Rechtschaffen, A. (1982). The effect of amphetamine, nembutal, alpha-methyl thyrosine and parachlorophenylalanine on sleep related spike activity of the tortoise, (*Geochelone carbonaria*) and on the cat ventral hippocampus spike. *Brain Behav. Evol.*, 21: 199–222.

Herald, E.S. (1972). Fishes of North America. New York: Doubleday and Co.

Hermann, H., Jouvet, M., and Klein, M.M. (1964). Analyse polygraphyque du sommeil de la tortue. *C. R. Acad. Sci. Paris*, 258: 2175–2178.

Hobson, J.A. (1967). Electrographic correlates of behavior in the frog with special reference to sleep. *Electroencephalogr. Clin. Neurophysiol.*, 22: 113–121.

Hobson, J.A., Goin, O.B., and Goin, C.J. (1968). Electrographic correlates of behavior in tree frogs. *Nature*, 220: 386–387.

Hoogland, P.V. and Vermeulen-Vanderzee, E. (1990). Distribution of choline acetyltransferase immunoreactivity in the telencephalon of the lizard *Gekko gecko. Brain Behav. Evol.*, 36: 378–390.

Hunsaker, D. and Lansing, R.W. (1962). Electroencephalographic studies in reptiles. *J. Exp. Zool.*, 49: 21–32.

Huntley, A.C. (1987). Electrophysiological and behavioral correlates of sleep in the desert iguana, *Dipsosaurus dorsalis hallowell. Comp. Biochem. Physiol.*, 86A: 325–330.

Huntley, A.C. and Cohen, H.B. (1980). Further comments on "sleep" in the desert iguana *Dipsosaurus dorsalis. Sleep Res.*, 9: 111.

Huntley, A.C., Friedman, J.K., and Cohen, H.B. (1977). Sleep in an Iguanid lizard (*Dipsosaurus dorsalis*). *Sleep Res.*, 6: 104.

Huntley, A.C., Donnelly, M., and Cohen, H.B. (1978). Sleep in the western toad (*Bufo boreas*). *Sleep Res.*, 7: 141.

Jerison, H.J. (1973). Evolution of brain and intelligence. New York: Academic Press.

Jerison, H.J. (1990). Fossil evidence on the evolution of the neocortex. In: Jones, E.G., and Peters, G. (Eds.). *Cereb. Cortex.* Plenun New York, pp. 285–309.

Jouvet, M. (1999). *The Paradox of Sleep. The Story of Dreaming.* Cambridge, MA: MIT Press.

Jouvet-Mounier, D., Astic, L., and Lacote, D. (1970). Ontogenesis of the sates of sleep in the rat, cat and guinea pig during the first postnatal month. *Dev. Psychobiol.*, 2: 216–239.

Karmanova, I.G. (1982). *Evolution of Sleep: Stages of the Formation of the Wakefulness-Sleep Cycle in Vertebrates.* Basel: Karger.

Karmanova, I.G. and Churnosov, E.V. (1972). Electrophysiological studies on natural sleep and wakefulness in turtles and hens. *Neurosci. Behav. Physiol.*, 6: 83–90.

Kemp, T.S. (1982). *Mammal-Like Reptiles and the Origin of Mammals.* London: Academic Press.

Kiehn, O., Rostrup, R., and Moller, M. (1992). Monoaminergic systems in the brainstem and spinal chord of the turtle *Pseudemys scripta* elegans as revealed by antibodies against serotonin and tyrosine hydroxilase. *J. Comp. Neurol.*, 325: 527–547.

Klein, M., Michel, F., and Jouvet, M. (1963). Etude polygraphique du sommeil chez les oiseaux. *C.R. Soc. Biol. (Paris)*, Séance, December 16, pp. 99–103.

Kulikov, A.V., Karmanova, I.G., Kozlachkova, E.Y., Voronova, I.P., and Popova, N.K. (1994). The brain tryptophan hydroxilase activity in the sleep like state in the frog. *Pharmacol. Biochem. Behav.*, 49: 277–279.

Lamblin, M.D., André, M., Challamel, M.J., Cursi-Dascalova, L., d'Allest, A.M., Giovanni, E., Moussalli-Salefrenque, F., Navelet, Y., Plouin, P., Radvany-Bouvet, M.F., Samson-Dollfus, D., and Cecchierini-Blineau, M.F. (1999). Electroencephalography of the premature and term newborn. Maturational aspects and glossary. *Neurophysiol. Clin.*, 29: 123–219.

Laming, P.R. (1980). Electroencephalographic studies on arousal in the goldfish (*Carassius auratus*). *J. Comp. Physiol. Psychol.*, 94: 238–254.

Lenke, R. (1998). Hormonal control of sleep-appetitive behaviour and diurnal rhythms in the cleaner wrasee *Labroides dimidiatus* (labridae, teleostei) *Behav. Brain Res.*, 27: 73–85.

Lombroso, C.T. (1993). Neonatal EEG poligraphy in normal and abnormal newborns. In: Niedermeyer, E., and Lopes Da Silva, F. (Eds.). *Electroencephalography.* Baltimore, MD: Williams and Wilkins, pp. 803–877.

Lucas, E., Sterman, M.B., and McGinty, D.J. (1969). The salamander EEG: a model of primitive sleep and wakefulness. *Psychophysiology*, 6: 230.

Lythgoe, J. and Lythgoe, G. (1991). Fishes of the Sea. Cambridge MA: MIT Press.

Ma, P.M. (1994a). Catecholaminergic systems in the zebrafish. I. Number, morphology and histochemical characteristics of neurons in the locus coeruleus. *J. Comp. Neurol.*, 344: 242–255.

Ma, P.M. (1994b). Catecholaminergic systems in the zebrafish. II. Projection pathways and pattern of termination in the locus coeruleus. *J. Comp. Neurol.*, 344: 256–269.

McGinty, D.J. and Szymusiak, R. (2001). Brain structures and mechanisms involved in the generation of NREM sleep: focus on the preoptic hypothalamus. *Sleep Med. Rev.*, 5: 323–342.

McGinty, D.J., Stevenson, M., Hoppenbrouwers, T., Harper, R.M., Sterman, M.B., and Hodgman, J. (1977). Polygraphic studies of kitten development: sleep state patterns. *Dev. Psychobiol.*, 10: 455–469.

McGinty, D.J., Alam, M.N., Szymusiak, R., Nakao, M., and Yamamoto, M. (2001). Hypothalamic sleep-promoting mechanisms. *Arch. Ital. Biol.*, 139: 63–75.

McNamara, F., Wulbrand, H., and Thach, B.T. (1998). Characteristics of the infant arousal response. *J. Appl. Physiol.*, 85: 2314–2321.

Meddis, R. (1983). The evolution of Sleep. In: Mayes, A. (Ed.). *Sleep Mechanisms in Humans and Animals: An Evolutionary Perspective.* London: Van Nostrand Reinhold. pp. 57–106.

Medina, L., Smeets, W.J.A.J., Hooglsand, P.V., and Puelles, L. (1993). Distribution of choline acetyltranferase inmunoreactivity in the brain of the lizard *Gallotia galloti. J. Comp. Neurol.*, 331: 261–285.

Meglasson, M.D. and Huggins, S.E. (1979). Sleep in a crocodilian (*Caiman sclerops*). *Comp. Biochem. Physiol.*, 63: 561–567.

Metcalf, D.R. (1970). EEG sleep spindle ontogenesis. *Neuropadiatrie*, 1: 428–33.

Montagnini, A. and Treves, A. (2003). The evolution of mammalian cortex, from lamination to arealization. *Brain Res. Bull.*, 60: 387–393.

Narayanan, C.H., Fox, M.V., and Hamburger, V. (1971). Prenatal development of spontaneous and evoked activity in the rat (*Rattus norwegicus*). *Behaviour*, 40: 100–134.

Neckerman, D. and Ursin, R. (1993). Sleep stages and EEG power spectrum in relation to acoustical stimuls arousal threshold in the rat. *Sleep*, 1: 6–82.

Nicolau, M.C., Akaârir, M., Gamundí, A., González, J., and Rial, R.V. (2000). Why we sleep: the evolutionary pathway to the mammalian sleep. *Prog. Neurobiol.*, 62: 379–406.

Niedermeyer, E. (1993). Maturation of the EEG: development of waking and sleep patterns. In: Niedermeyer, E. and Lopes Da Silva, F. (Eds.). *Electroencephalography.* Baltimore, MD: Williams and Wilkins, pp. 167–192.

Nieuwenhuys, R. (2002). Deuterostome brains: synopsis and commentary. *Brain Res. Bull.*, 57: 257–270.

Parmeggiani, P.L. and Morrison, A.R. (1990). Alterations in autonomic functions during sleep. In: Loewy, A.D. and Spyer, K.M. (Eds.). *Central Regulation of Autonomic Functions.* New York: Oxford University Press, pp. 367–386.

Parmelee, A.H. and Stern, E. (1972). Development of states in infants. In: Clemente, C.D., Purpura, D.P., and Mayer, F.E. (Eds.). *Sleep and Maturing Nervous System.* New York: Academic Press, pp. 200–228.

Parsons, L. and Huggins, S.E. (1965a). A study of spontaneous electrical activity in the brain of *Caiman sclerops. Proc. Soc. Exp. Biol. Med.*, 119: 397–400.

Parsons, L. and Huggins, S.E. (1965b). Effects of temperature on electroencephalogram of the Caiman. *Proc. Soc. Exp. Biol. Med.*, 120: 422–426.

Paus, T., Collins, D.L., Evans, A.C., Leonard, G., Pike, B., and Zijdenbos, A. (2001). Maturation of the white matter in the human brain: a review of magnetic resonance studies. *Brain Res. Bull.*, 54: 255–266.

Pavan, C. (1946). Observations and cave experiments on the cave fish *Pimodella kronei* and its relatives. *Am. Nat.*, 80: 346–361.

Peyreton, J. and Dusan-Peyreton, D. (1967). Etude polygraphique du cicle vieille-sommeil d'un teleosteén (*Tinca tinca*). *C. R. Soc. Biol. (Paris)*, 161: 2533.

Peyreton, J. and Dusan-Peyreton, D. (1969). Etude poligraphique du cycle vieille sommeil chez trois genres de reptiles. *C. R. Soc. Biol. (Paris)*, 163: 181–186.

Pieron, H. (1913). *Le probleme physiologique du sommeil.* Paris: Masson.

Pilleri, G. (1979). The Indus dolphin, platanista indi. *Endeavour*, 3: 48–56.

Powers, A.S. and Reiner, A. (1993). The distribution of cholinergic neurons in the central nervous system of turtles. *Brain Behav. Evol.*, 41: 326–345.

Rechtschaffen, A. (1971). The control of sleep. In: Hunt, W.A. (Ed.). *Human Behaviour and Its Control.* Cambridge, MA: Schenkman, pp. 75–92.

Rial, R.V., Nicolau. M.C., López-García, J.A., and Almirall, H. (1993). On the evolution of waking and sleeping. *Comp. Physiol. Biochem.*, 104: 189–193.

Rojas-Ramírez, J. and Tauber, E. (1970). Paradoxical sleep in two species of avian predator Falconiformes. *Science*, 167: 1754–1755.

Romo, R., Cepeda, C., and Velasco, M. (1978). Behavioral and electrophysiological patterns of wakefulness-sleep states in the lizard. *Phrinosoma regali. Bol. Estud. Med. Méx.*, 30: 13–18.

Roth, A. and Schlegel, P. (1988). Behavioral evidence and supporting electrophysiological observations for electroreception in the blind cave salamander *Proteus anguinus. Brain Behav. Evol.*, 32: 277–280.

Ruckebush, Y. (1976). Environment and sleep patterns in domestic animals. In: Koella, W.P. (Ed.). *Sleep.* Basel: Karger, pp. 159–163.

Segura, E.T. (1966). Estudios electroencefalográficos en anfibios. *Acta Physiol. Latinoamer.*, 16 (suppl.): 277–282.

Segura, E.T. and de Juan, A. (1966). Electroencephalographic studies in Toads. *Electroencephalogr. Clin. Neurophysiol.*, 21: 373–380.

Servit, Z. and Strejkova, A. (1972). Thalamocortical relations and the genesis of epileptic electrographic phenomena in the forebrain of the turtle. *Exp. Neurol.*, 35: 50–60.

Servit, Z. and Strejcková, A. (1979). Theta (RSA) activity in the brain of the turtle. *Physiol. Bohemoslov.*, 28: 17–24.

Servit, Z., Strejkova, A., and Volanschi, D. (1971). Epileptic focus in the forebrain of the turtle (*Testudo graeca*). Triggering of focal discharges with different sensory stimuli. *Physiol. Bohemoslov.*, 20: 221–228.

Shapiro, C.M. and Hepburn, H.R. (1976). Sleep in a schooling fish *Tilapia mossambica. Physiol. Behav.*, 16: 613–615.

Siegel, J.M. (1995). Phylogeny and the function of REM sleep. *Behav. Brain Res.*, 69: 29–34.

Siegel, J.M., Manger, P.R., Nienhuis, R., Fahringer, H.M., and Pettigrew, J.D. (1997). The platypus has REM sleep. *Sleep Res.*, 26: 177.

Siegel, J.M., Manger, P.R., Nienhuis, R., Fahringer, H.M., and Pettigrew, J.D. (1998). Monotremes and the evolution of rapid eye movement sleep. *Philos. Trans. R. Soc. Lond.*, 353: 1147–1157.

Siegel, J.M., Manger, P.R., Nienhuis, R., Fahringer, H.M., Shalita, T., and Pettigrew, J.D. (1999). Sleep in the platypus. *Neuroscience*, 91: 391–400.

Sterman, M.B., McGinty, D.J., Harper, R.M., Hoppenbrouwers, T., and Hodgman, J.E. (1982). Developmental comparison of sleep EEG power spectral patterns in infants at low and high risk for sudden death. *Electroencephalogr. Clin. Neurophysiol.*, 53: 166–181.

Susic, V. (1972). Electrographic and behavioral correlations of the rest-activity cycle in the sea turtle *Caretta caretta* L. (Chelonia). *J. Exp. Mar. Biol. Ecol.*, 10: 81–87.

Susic, V.T. and Kovacevic, R.M. (1973). Sleep patterns in the owl (*Strix aluco*) *Physiol. Behav.*, 11: 313–317.

Szymczak, J.T., Kaiser, W., Helb, H.W., and Beszczynska, B. (1996). A study of sleep in the European blackbird. *Physiol. Behav.*, 60: 1115–1120.

Tauber, E.S., Roffwarg, H.P., and Weitzman, E.D. (1966). Eye movements and electroencephalographic activity during sleep in diurnal lizards. *Nature*, 212: 1612–1613.

Tauber, E.S., Rojas-Ramirez, J., and Hernández-Peón, R. (1968). Electrophysiological and behavioral correlates of wakefulness and sleep in the lizard, *Ctenosaura pectinata*. *Electroencephalogr. Clin. Neurophysiol.*, 24: 424–433.

Tauber, E.S., Weitzman, E.D., and Korey, S.R. (1969). Eye movements during behavioral inactivity in certain bermuda reef fish. *Commun. Behav. Biol.*, 3: 131–135.

Tobler, I. (1984). Evolution of the sleep processes: a phylogenetic approach. *Exp. Brain Res.*, 8: 207–226.

Tobler, I. and Borbely, A.A. (1985). Effect of rest deprivation on motor activity of fish. *J. Comp. Physiol.*, 157: 817–822.

Tobler, I. and Borbely, A.A. (1988). Sleep and EEG spectra in the pigeon (*Columba livia*) under baseline conditions and after sleep deprivation. *J. Comp. Physiol.*, 163: 769–738.

Tradardi, V. (1966). Sleep in the pigeon. *Arch. Ital. Biol.*, 104: 516–521.

Van Luijtelaar, E.L.J.M., Van der Grinten, C.P.M., Blokuis, H.J., and Coenen, A.M.L. (1987). Sleep in the domestic hen (*Gallus domesticus*). *Physiol. Behav.*, 41: 409–414.

Van Twyver, H. and Allison, T. (1972). A polygraphic and behavioral study of sleep in the pigeon (*Columba livia*). *Exp. Neurol.*, 35: 138–153.

Van Twyver, H. (1973). Poligraphic studies of the American alligator. *Sleep Res.*, 2: 87.

Vasconcelos-Dueñas, I. and Ayala-Guerrero, F. (1983). Effects of PCPA on sleep in parakeets (*Aratinga canicularis*). *Proc. West Pharmacol. Soc.*, 26: 365–368.

Vasilescu, E. (1970). Sleep and wakefulness in the tortoise (*Emys orbicularis*). *Rev. Roum. Biol. Zool.*, 15: 177–179.

persons surely undergo changes in their central auditory neuronal networks organisation — cortical plasticity — which, in turn, would affect many other brain cell assemblies/networks. After an intra-cochlear implant, the hearing recovery would produce networks re-organisation, which in turn, could provoke the sleep architecture to shift to different sleep stage percentages (Velluti *et al.*, 2003).

Analysing human auditory responses

During sleep, a normal reaction to any supra-threshold sensory stimulation drives back to a wakeful condition. Human auditory responses recorded from the vertex have been reported by several investigators. In all subjects, the major changes observed in the auditory evoked response, when changing from the awake state to the four stages of SWS sleep consisted on a steady increase in peak to peak amplitude while during PS the amplitude was lower and approximated that of the awake state (Vanzulli *et al.*, 1961; Williams *et al.*, 1963; Weitzman and Kremen, 1965; Ornitz *et al.*, 1967). The early evoked auditory responses, reflecting the activation of the cortical level, exhibited an amplitude decrement in Stage II (Mendel and Goldstein, 1971), while they remained unmodified in a report by Erwin and Buchwald (1986). Using different stimulus rates, an attenuation of the early cortical response was obtained with fast stimulation frequency (Campbell, 1992), while a triphasic Pa wave response with a stimulus rate of 3–5 Hz was reported during sleep (Deiber *et al.*, 1989).

Experimental data gathered by using the far-field-potential recording technique in humans showed no sleep effects on the brainstem auditory evoked potentials (Amadeo and Shagass, 1973; Picton *et al.*, 1974; Osterhammel *et al.*, 1985; Bastuji *et al.*, 1988; Bastuji and García-Larrea, 1999). In addition, the constancy of the response was maintained whether sound stimuli were of high or low intensity (Campbell and Bartoli, 1986).

The brainstem auditory evoked potential — a human far-field recorded activity — is a technical coarse image that cannot reveal the effects of sleep. However, the significant unitary firing shifts produced during sleep in the brainstem auditory nuclei, described in guinea pigs, are surely present although not reflected by the human far-field technique (Velluti *et al.*, 1989; Velluti and Pedemonte, 2002, Chapter 22).

In addition, another phenomenon also aims at sleep actions on the auditory receptor itself, namely the transiently evoked oto-acoustic emission (sound emitted by the cochlea reflecting the outer hair cell motility controlled by the auditory efferent system). It has been reported in humans as being modified in general during sleep although independently of the sleep phase (Froehlich *et al.*, 1993).

The far-field technique data on the sleep effects on middle latency auditory evoked potentials — perhaps arising from the reticular formation, thalamus, and primary cortex — are much less consistent. While early studies indicated that these components were either not affected or only slightly affected by sleep, more recent reports showed marked changes, most notably on the later evoked potential components (Osterhammel *et al.*, 1985; Erwin and Buchwald, 1986; Ujszászi and Halász, 1986; Campbell, 1992). The late components of the evoked potential, also called the slow potentials or late auditory evoked responses, are most altered during sleep. As reported in the Chapter 23 by Bastuji and García-Larrea, a high amplitude complex waveform dominates in Stages II and III–IV which are the result of summed K-complexes evoked by sensory stimuli.

Semantic information is possible in Stage II and PS (Bastuji *et al.*, 2002), whereas the presence of P3 seems to be essential to stimulus encoding, despite the fact that the question if W and sleep P3 could be considered equivalent, remains to be studied (Bastuji and García-Larrea, Chapter 23).

The mismatch negativity was reported in SWS (Campbell, 1992) and during PS (Atienza and Cantero, 1997). Moreover, this negativity has recently also been reported in "quiet sleep" of newborns and linked to learning (Cheour *et al.*, 2002).

Conclusions and Final Proposal

Sleep and sensory input in general

The analysis of sensory functions during sleep–wake cycle leads to the conclusion that normal sleep depends in many ways on the sensory input. It is suggested that the sleep and waking control networks are modulated by several inputs, and therefore a proportion of "passive" effects must be associated with active functions for entering into and maintaining normal sleep. Among the many possible inputs, the sensory is a relevant one. Thus, the total amount of sleep increases under some experimental conditions: (a) continuous somatosensory stimulation induces EEG synchronisation and sleep; (b) total darkness increases sleep although only during a few days; (c) total silence, after bilateral cochlear destruction, increases the amount of sleep and episode frequency; (d) sleep stages percentages are different when deaf humans are compared with themselves after recovery of hearing with an intracochlear implant (Velluti *et al.*, 2003).

Furthermore, partial increments in the frequency of specific sleep stages are observed: (a) when rats are stimulated with sounds during any sleep stage; (b) during stimulation with bright light, which produces SWS increases in humans; (c) during electrical stimulation of the olfactory bulb, which produces SWS increases in cats (for a review, see Velluti, 1997).

On the other hand, the sensory influence on sleep are, e.g., the abolition or decrement of a sleep sign or stage produced by: (a) continuous light stimulation in rats that decreases PS for ~20 days; (b) bilateral lesions of some vestibular nuclei that abolishes rapid eye movements during PS for up to 36 days; (c) a long exposure to cold that produces decrement of PS leading to PS deprivation; (d) olfactory bulbectomy that decreases PS frequency episodes and its total amount for up to 15 days (for a review, see Velluti, 1997).

The lack of sensory inputs as well as their enhancement can produce sleep/waking imbalances, augmenting or diminishing their proportions. Thus, the changes induced in the waking and sleep networks lead to the cited imbalances not simply for passive sleep production but introducing sensory sleep-active influences.

1. Sleep and sound are closely related. Environmental noise as well as regular, monotonous, auditory stimuli, e.g., mother lullaby, are influences impeding or facilitating sleep.
2. The CNS and auditory system bioelectrical field activity — evoked potentials — shown from the early electrophysiological studies, vary in close correlation with W epochs and specially during sleep stages. The mismatch negativity is also related to memory in sleep and possible in newborn auditory learning.
3. The auditory system neuronal firing exhibits a variety of changes in all of its nuclei and primary cortical *loci* linked to the sleep–wakefulness cycle in many ways: i.e., increasing or decreasing their firing on passing to sleep, firing as during W, changing the discharge pattern, exhibiting theta rhythm phase-locking, while no auditory neurone stopped firing on passing to sleep. Edeline *et al.* (2001) also reported changes in the receptive field of cortical auditory neurones. Therefore, it can be concluded that when asleep many auditory units are sleep-active, probably associated with diverse sleep relevant cell assemblies. Moreover, when

functionally shifting into a different neuronal network/cell assembly, a unit may contribute to the sleep process just by increasing, decreasing, or showing no firing shift, according to the new role in the new cell association.

4. A magnetoencephalographic (MEG) approach described amplitude changes and anatomical place shifts of the sound evoked dipole in the human primary auditory cortex (Figure 4) on passing from W to sleep Stage II (Kakigi *et al.*, 2003). The dipole anatomical position shift obtained with MEG implicated a change to a new neuronal group already indirectly supported by unitary studies. The evoked activity during sleep — its dipole — appears in a different cortical region from that during W, thus suggesting a new cell assembly/neuronal network participation.

5. The functional magnetic resonance imaging (fMRI), when combined with EEG recording, showed that the auditory stimuli produce bilateral activation in the human auditory cortex (Figure 4) and other areas, both during W and sleep (all Stage II and SWS were collapsed into one because of technical reasons) (Portas *et al.*, 2000).

The data exhibited by fMRI strongly support the notion that the sleeping brain is able to process information, and detect meaningful events, as it can be observed in the unitary response in guinea pigs when a complex stimulus (the animal call) is played normally or in reverse (Figure 4; Chapter 22).

Some sleep researchers are, unconsciously, looking for a "sleep centre" that does not exist. A CNS centre may be real and useful for controlling functions such as the cardiovascular, the respiratory, etc., while, on the other hand, sleep is not a function but a complete different CNS state. This means different brains for the diverse W conditions, for sleep Stages I, II and SWS, and for PS with or without phasic components. Hence, sleep means a whole change of networks/cell assemblies, a new cooperative interaction among them, considering that a single network may sub-serve several different functions.

Getting (1989), postulated that "... If these network, synaptic, and cellular mechanisms are under modulatory control, then an anatomical network may be configured into any one of several *modes* ... The term *modes* is intended to imply a manner in which a network processes information or generates an output pattern..." (Figure 3). When afferent or modulating inputs alter the properties of the basic constituents of a set of networks, a transition among modes may occur, e.g., in our case passing from W to

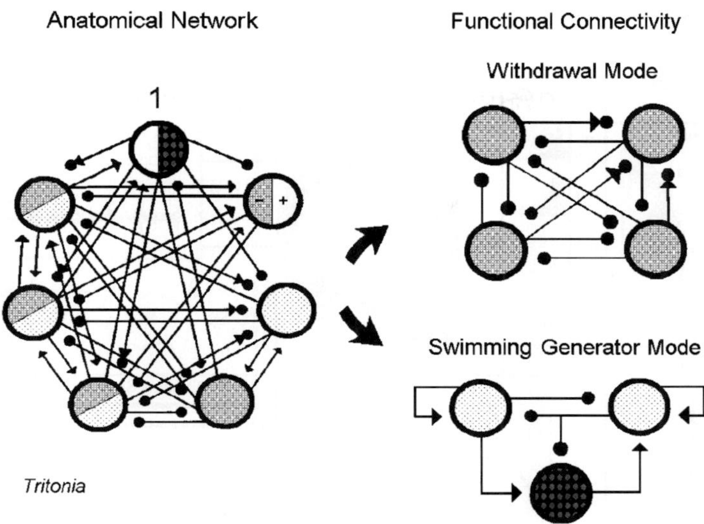

Figure 3. Neuronal network of the *Tritonia* anatomical monosynaptic connectivity — excitatory and inhibitory — and the two possibilities for functional–behavioural networks acting as: (a) withdrawal mode and (b) swimming generator mode. The neurone 1 (top, left) activation–deactivation is the first action to produce the functional and, therefore anatomical organisation shift, changing the animal behaviour (Modified from Getting, 1989).

sleep. A neurone as a basic constituent of a network or cell assembly may fire an action potential or not, or may increase or decrease firing while still belonging to the same network although participating in a new particular function. Thus, increasing firing does not necessarily mean that a cell is sub-serving to sleep or waking, because in the sleep case, for instance, the recorded neurone may belong to a network in which it, although engaged in sleep, should play a decreasing firing *mode.*

Further, the imbalance introduced by cell 1 in the *Tritonia* (Figure 3) may be provoked, in a complex brain, by a summation of factors that provokes, after some signal — perhaps decreasing light intensity — a group of neuronal networks/cell assemblies to progressively begin to condition the system. Partially supporting this assumption is the observation that when a human or an animal is entering into sleep, the many variables recorded never occur in synchrony, but appear with seconds of differences between them, e.g., EEG slow activity, electromyogram decrement, eye movements, hippocampal theta rhythm frequency and amplitude, heart rate shifts, arterial pressure changes, breathing rhythm alterations, and so on.

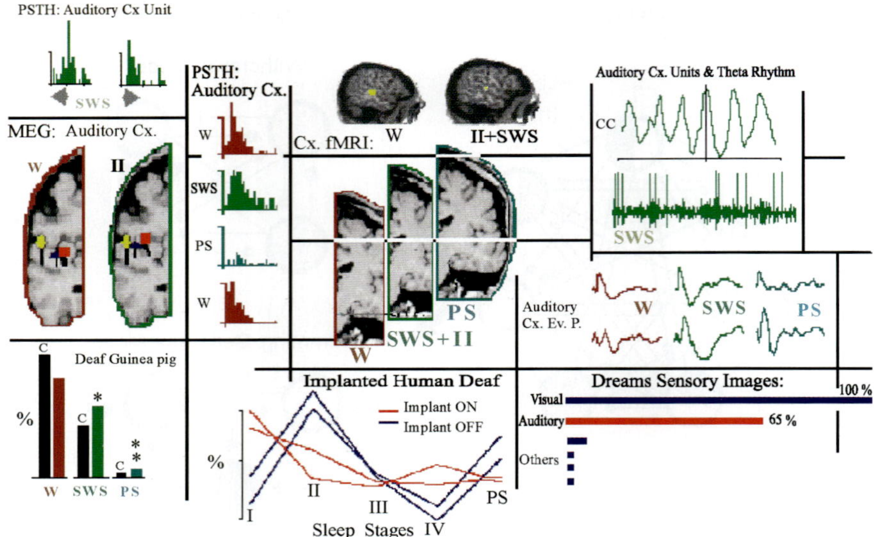

Figure 4. Diverse technical approaches supporting the postulated notion of the importance and possible active participation of the auditory input on sleep processes. Three human half brain tomographic cuts (centre) represent the three main functional possibilities: wakefulness (W), slow-wave sleep (SWS), and paradoxical sleep (PS). Post-stimulus time histogram (PSTH) changes of a cortical auditory neurone firing shift when stimulated with natural sound played directly or backwards (Pérez-Perera *et al.*, 2001). PSTH of a cortical unit on passing from wakefulness (W) to slow-wave sleep (SWS) and paradoxical sleep (PS) exhibits firing and pattern shifts (Peña *et al.*, 1999). Human auditory cortical imaging (fMRI) demonstrate activity during sleep (modified from Portas *et al.*, 2000). The cortical auditory neurones can be phase-locked to hippocampal theta rhythm (Pedemonte *et al.*, 2001). Rat auditory cortical evoked potentials through the sleep–wake cycle show amplitude changes (Hall and Borbély, 1970). The dream auditory "images" are present in 65% of dream recalls (Hoffman and McCarley, 1981). Human and guinea pig deafness influence sleep. The human recorded with the intra-cochlear implant off and on shows different sleep stages percentages while the guinea pig exhibited (bars) an increase in sleep time with decreasing wakefulness (Pedemonte *et al.*, 1996b; Velluti *et al.*, 2003). The human magnetoencephalography (MEG) shows a place shift of the dipole evoked by three sound stimulating frequencies on passing to sleep Stage II, demonstrating a change of neuronal network/cell assembly (modified from Kakigi *et al.*, 2003).

A special point is the environmental reduction of sensory information, as occurs during the night, allowing the auditory system neurones to become engaged, as I am postulating, in active sleep-related processes. Thus, the sensory input is not only a passive but also an active contributor to the whole brain change on passing from W to sleep, although maintaining the environment monitoring.

The many technical approaches (Figure 4) reviewed support the notion of the sensory information, in general, and the auditory incoming information, in particular, as exerting influences on sleep through a dynamic neuronal participation in different sleep-related cell assemblies. We have previously postulated that the auditory neurones firing in sleep at the same rate and pattern as during W are those neurones that monitor the environment. These cells increase their percentages at the auditory primary cortical level (Figure 2). At the brainstem, on the other hand, the auditory *loci* firing percentages are approximately divided by thirds, perhaps participating more closely in sleep-promoting regions. The units that increase or decrease their firing are postulated to be sleep-related neurones, at cortical as well as at brainstem levels.

Acknowledgments

I am grateful to Prof. J.M. Monti for reading the manuscript and his valuable suggestions and also to the Program for Basic Science Development (Uruguay) for partial support.

References

Amadeo, M. and Shagass, C. (1973). Brief latency click-evoked potentials during waking and sleep in man. *Psychophysiology*, 10: 244–250.

Atienza, M. and Cantero, J.L. (1997). The mismatch negativity component reveals the sensory memory during REM sleep in humans. *Neurosci. Lett.*, 237: 21–24.

Bastuji, H. and García-Larrea, L. (1999). Evoked potentials as a tool for the investigation of human sleep. *Sleep Med. Rev.*, 3: 23–45.

Bastuji, H., García-Larrea, L., Bertrand, O., and Mauguière, F. (1988). BAEP latency changes during nocturnal sep are not correlated with sep stages but with body temperature variations. *Electroencephalogr. Clin. Neurophysiol.*, 70: 9–15.

Bastuji, H., Perrin, F., and García-Larrea, L. (2002). Semantic analysis of auditory input during sep: studies with event related potentials. *Int. J. Psychophysiol.*, 46: 243–255.

Bremer, F. (1935). Cerveau "isole" et physiologie du sommeil. *C. R. Soc. Biol.*, 118: 1235–1241.

Campbell, K. (1992). Evoked potentials measures of information processing during natural sleep. In: Broughton, R. and Ogilvie, R. (Eds.). *Sleep, Arousal and Performance*. Boston: Birkhauser, pp. 88–116.

Campbell, K. and Bartoli, E. (1986). Human auditory evoked potentials during natural sleep. *Electroencephalogr. Clin. Neurophysiol.*, 65: 142–149.

Cardinali, D.P. and Pevet, P. (1998). Basic aspects of melatonin action. *Sleep Med. Rev.*, 2: 175–190.

Cirelli, C. and Tononi, G. (2000). On the functional significance of *c-fos* induction during sleep–wake cycle. *Sleep*, 23: 453–469.

Croome, D.J. (1977). Noise and sleep. In: *Noise, Building and People*. London: Pergamon Press, pp. 101–109.

Cheour, M., Martynova, O., Naatanen, R., Erkkola, R., Sillanpaa, M., Kero, P., Raz, A., Kaipio, M.-L., Hiltunen, J., Aaltonen, O., Savela, J., and Hamalainen, H. (2002). Speech sounds learned by sleeping newborns. *Nature*, 415: 599–600.

Clemente, C.D. and Sterman, M.B. (1963). Cortical synchronization and sleep patterns in acute restrained and chronic behaving cats induced by basal forebrain stimulation. *Electroencephalogr. Clin. Neurophysiol.*, 24: 172–187.

Dana, B.B. (1916). Morbid somnolence and its relation to the endocrine glands. *N. Y. J. Med. Rec.*, 89: 1–5.

Deiber, M.P., Ibañez, V., Bastuji, H., Fischer, C., and Mauguière, F. (1989). Changes of middle latency auditory evoked potentials during natural sleep in humans. *Neurology*, 39: 806–813.

Dikshit, B.B. (1934). Action of acetylcholine on the "sleep centre". *J. Physiol.*, 83: 42.

Edeline, J.M., Dutrieux, G., Manunta, G., and Hennevin, E. (2001). Diversity of receptive field changes in auditory cortex during natural sleep. *Eur. J. Neurosci.* 14: 1865–1880.

Froehlich, P., Collet, L., Valaxt, J.L., and Morgon, A. (1993). Sleep and active cochlear micromechanical properties in human subjects. *Hear. Res.*, 66: 1–7.

Erwin, R. and Buchwald, J. (1986). Midlatency auditory evoked responses: Differential effects of sleep in the human. *Electroencephalogr. Clin. Neurophysiol.*, 65: 383–392.

George, R., Haslett, W.L., and Jenden, D.J. (1964). A cholinergic mechanism in the brainstem reticular formation: induction of paradoxical sleep. *Int. J. Neuropharmacol.*, 3: 541–552.

Getting, P.A. (1989). Emerging principles governing the operation of neural networks. *Annu. Rev. Neurosci.*, 12: 185–204.

Hall, R.D. and Borbély, A.A. (1970). Acoustically evoked potentials in the rat during sleep and waking. *Exp. Brain Res.*, 11: 93–110.

Hernández-Peón, R., Chávez Ibarra, G., Morgane, J.P., and Timo Iaria, C. (1963). Limbic cholinergic pathways involved in sep and emotional behavior. *Exp. Neurol.*, 8: 93–111.

Hess, W.R. (1944). Das schlafsyndrom als folge dienzephaler reizung. *Helv. Physiol. Pharamcol. Acta*, 2: 305–344.

Hoffman, E.A. and McCarley, R.W. (1981). REM sleep dreams and the activation-synthesis hypothesis. *Am. J. Psychiatry*, L38: 904–912.

Huttenlocher, P.R. (1960). Effects of the state of arousal on click responses in the mesencephalic reticular formation. *Electroencephalogr. Clin. Neurophysiol.*, 12: 819–827.

Jouvet, M. (1961). Telencephalic and rombencephalic sleep in the cat. In: Wostenholme, G.E.W. and O'Connor, C.M. (Eds.). *The Nature of Sleep.* London: Churchill.

Jouvet, M. (1962). Recherches sur les structures nerveuses et les mecanismes responsables de differentes phases du sommeil physiologique. *Arch. Ital. Biol.*, 100: 125–206.

Kakigi, R., Naka, D., Okusa, T., Wang, X., Inui, K., Qiu, Y., Diep Tran, T., Miki, K., Tamura, Y., Nguyen, T.B., Watanabe, S., and Hoshiyama, M. (2003). Sensory perception during sleep in humans: a magnetoencephalograhic study. *Sleep Med.*, 4: 493–507.

Maquet, P. (2000). Functional neuroimaging of normal human sleep by positron emission tomography. *J. Sleep Res.*, 9: 207–231.

McGinty, D. and Szymusiak, R. (2003). Hypothalamic regulation of sleep and arousal. *Front. Biosci.*, 8: 1074–1083.

Mendel, M.I. and Goldstein, R. (1971). Early components of the averaged electroencephalographic response to constant level clicks during all night sleep. *J. Speech Hear. Res.*, 14: 829–840.

Morales-Cobas, G., Ferreira, M.I., and Velluti, R.A. (1995). Sleep and waking firing of inferior colliculus neurons in response to low frequency sound stimulation. *J. Sleep Res.*, 4: 242–251.

Moruzzi, G. (1963). Active processes in the brainstem during sleep. *Harvey Lecture Series, 58.* New York: Academic Press, pp. 233–297.

Moruzzi, G. and Magoun, H. (1949). Brain stem reticular formation and activation of the EEG. *Electroencephalogr. Clin. Neurophysiol.*, 1: 455–473.

Muzet, A. and Naitoh, P. (1977). Sommeil et bruit. *Confront. Psychiatr.*, 15: 215–235.

Ornitz, E.M., Panman, L.M., and Walter, R.D. (1967). The variability of the auditory averaged evoked responses during sleep and dreaming in children and adults. *Electroencephalogr. Clin. Neurophysiol.*, 22: 514–524.

Osterhammel, P., Shallop, J., and Terkildsen, K. (1985). The effects of sleep on the auditory brainstem response (ABR) and the middle latency response (MLR). *Scand. Audiol.*, 14: 47–50.

Parmeggiani, P.L., Lenzi, P., Azzaroni, A., and D'Alessandro, R. (1982). Hippocampal influence on unit responses elicited in the cat's auditory cortex by acoustic stimulation. *Exp. Neurol.*, 78: 259–274.

Pearson, K.S., Berber, D.S., Tabachnick, B.G., and Fidell, S. (1995). Predicting noise-induced sleep disturbances. *J. Acoust. Soc. Am.*, 97: 331–338.

Pedemonte, M. and Velluti, R.A. (2005). Sleep hippocampal theta rhythm and sensory processing. In: Lader, M., Cardinali, D.P., and Perumal, P. (Eds.). *Sleep and Sleep Disorders: A Neuropsychopharmacological Approach.* Georgetown, TX: Landes Biosciencies, pp. 8–12.

Pedemonte, M., Peña, J.L., Morales-Cobas, G., and Velluti, R.A. (1994). Effects of sleep on the responses of single cells in the lateral superior olive. *Arch. Ital. Biol.*, 132: 165–178.

Pedemonte, M., Peña, J.L., and Velluti, R.A. (1996a). Firing of inferior colliculus auditory neurons is phase-locked to the hippocampus theta rhythm during paradoxical sleep and waking. *Exp. Brain Res.*, 112: 41–46.

Pedemonte, M., Peña, J.L., Torterolo, P., and Velluti, R.A. (1996b). Auditory deprivation modifies sleep in guinea pig. *Neurosci. Lett.*, 223: 1–4.

Pedemonte, M., Pérez-Perera, L., Peña, J.L., and Velluti, R.A. (2001). Auditory processing during sleep: correlation of cortical unitary activity with hippocampus theta rhythm. *Sleep Res. Online*, 4: 52–57.

Peña, J.L., Pedemonte, M., Ribeiro, M.F., and Velluti, R. (1992). Single unit activity in the guinea pig cochlear nucleus during sleep and wakefulness. *Arch. Ital. Biol.*, 130: 179–189.

Peña, J.L., Pérez-Perera, L., Bouvier, M., and Velluti, R.A. (1999). Sleep and wakefulness modulation of the neuronal firing in the auditory cortex of the guinea pig. *Brain Res.*, 816: 463–470.

Pérez-Perera, L., Bentancor, C., Pedemonte, M., and Velluti, R.A. (2001). Auditory cortex unitary activity correlated to sleep-wakefulness and theta rhythm in response to natural sounds. *Acta de Fisiologia*, 7: 187.

Picton, T.W., Hillyard, S.A., Krausz, H.I., and Galambos, R. (1974). Human auditory evoked potentials. I. Evaluation of components. *Electroencephalogr. Clin. Neurophysiol.*, 36: 179–190.

Portas, C.M., Krakow, K., Allen, P., Josephs, O., Armony, J.L., and Frith, C.D. (2000). Auditory processing across the sleep–wake cycle: simultaneous EEG and fMRI monitoring in humans. *Neuron*, 28: 991–999.

Reiter, R.J. and Tan, D.X. (2003). What constitutes a physiological concentration of melatonin? *J. Pineal Res.*, 34: 79–80.

Sakurai, Y. (1999). How do cell assemblies encode information in the brain? *Neurosci. Biobehav. Rev.*, 23: 785–796.

Soca, F. (1900). Sur un cas de sommeil prolongé pendant sept mois par un tumeur de l'hypophyse. *Nouv. Iconogr. Salpêtrière*, 2: 101–115.

Terzano, M.G., Parrino, L., Fioriti, G., Orofiamma, B., and Depoortere, H. (1990). Modifications of sleep structure by increasing levels of acoustic perturbation in normal subjects. *Electroencephalogr. Clin. Neurophysiol.*, 76: 29–38.

Ujszászi, J. and Halász, P. (1986). Late component variants of single auditory evoked responses during NREM sleep stage 2 in man. *Electroencephalogr. Clin. Neurophysiol.*, 64: 260–268.

Vallet, M. (1982). La perturbation du sommeil par le bruit. *Soz. Praventivmed.*, 27: 124–131.

Vanzulli, A., Bogacz, J., and García-Austt, E. (1961). Evoked responses in man. III. Auditory response. *Acta Neurol. Latinoam.*, 7: 303–308.

Velluti, R.A. (1997). Interactions between sleep and sensory physiology. A review. *J. Sleep Res.*, 6: 61–77.

Velluti, R. and Hernández-Peón, R. (1963). Atropine blockade within a cholinergic hypnogenic circuit. *Exp. Neurol.*, 8: 20–29.

Velluti, R.A. and Pedemonte, M. (2002). *In vivo* approach to the cellular mechanisms for sensory processing in sleep and wakefulness. *Cell. Mol. Neurobiol.*, 22: 501–515.

Velluti, R.A., Pedemonte, M., and García-Austt, E. (1989). Correlative changes of auditory nerve and microphonic potentials throughout sleep. *Hear. Res.* 39: 203–208.

Velluti, R.A., Pedemonte, M., and Peña, J.L. (2000). Reciprocal actions between sensory signals and sleep. *Biol. Signals Recept.*, 9: 297–308.

Velluti, R.A., Pedemonte, M., Suárez, H., Inderkum, A., Rodríguez-Servetti, Z., and Rodríguez-Alvez, A. (2003). Human sleep architecture shifts due to auditory sensory input. *Sleep. Suppl.*, 26: 19.

Vinogradova, O.S. (2001). Hippocampus as comparator: role of the two input and two output systems of the hippocampus in selection and registration of information. *Hippocampus*, 11: 578–598.

Vital-Durand, F. and Michel, F. (1971). Effets de la desafferentation periphérique sur le cicle veille-sommeil chez le chat. *Arch. Ital. Biol.*, 109: 166–186.

Von Economo, C. (1930). Sleep as a problem of localization. *J. Nerv. Ment. Dis.*, 7: 249–259.

Weitzman, E.D. and Kremen, H. (1965). Auditory evoked responses during different stages of sleep in man. *Electroencephalogr. Clin. Neurophysiol.*, 18: 65–70.

Williams, H.L., Tepas, D.I., and Morloch, H.C. (1963). Evoked responses to clicks and electroencephalographic stages of sleep in man. *Science*, 138: 685–686.

Zubek, J.P. (1969). Physiological and biochemical effects. In: Zubek, J.P. (Ed.). *Sensory Deprivation: Fifteen Years of Research.* New York: Appleton-Century-Crofts, pp. 255–288.

Chapter 12

THE PROBLEM OF CAUSAL DETERMINATION OF SLEEP BEHAVIOUR

Pier Luigi Parmeggiani[1]

Well aware of the fact that sleep is a global behaviour of the organism, W.R. Hess, a pioneer in sleep research, felt it necessary to point out how he had approached the experimental study of sleep: "I have indeed for years been occupied with obtaining as many data as possible by experiments involving electrical stimulation and circumscribed lesions of specific brainstem areas. Surely such observations are indispensable in support of any comprehensive interpretation... it is essential that the data are interrelated and woven into a theoretical fabric. In this process of general theoretical integration I have repeatedly gained new insight particularly in respect to the organisation of the diencephalon. Coordination of the findings is also necessary, if the true significance of the data is to be ascertained; this is especially true in biology... scepticism toward a synthetizing approach to biology means neither more nor less than giving up hope ever to understand the integration of life functions — the alpha and omega of the unity of the individual organism... It is an illusion to suppose that simple facts have themselves the power to constitute a theory. It is only the inference based upon them that will advance our viewpoints" (Hess, 1965, p. 4). In this regard, we may wonder whether his approach has lost its utility at

---

[1]pier.parmeggiani@unibo.it

the present time characterised by an intense and fruitful analytical study of sleep behaviour. On this basis, the aim of the chapter is to examine general criteria by which a lawful determination of the physiologic events of a behavioural state is identified.

Theoretical Considerations

The observable behavioural continuum results from the combined activity of somatic and autonomic physiological effectors under the integrative control of the central nervous system. For practical purposes, this continuum may be divided into four behavioural states, namely active wakefulness (AW), quiet wakefulness (QW), non-rapid eye movement sleep (NREM sleep), and rapid eye movement sleep (REM sleep). A behavioural state entails a temporal dimension of functional stability that is experimentally measured by means of stimulus–response relationships in several physiological domains (cf. Parmeggiani, 2000). Such relationships reveal the nature of the general regulation paradigm actually underlying the process of moulding the multifarious activity of somatic and autonomic effectors to a global behaviour. This is a complex physiological pattern that results from the co-ordination of local auto-regulation, spinal reflex regulation, and brainstem and brain regulation.

At the level of single effector mechanisms, a fragmented intensive determination operates whereas at high integration levels determination is more extensive as it concomitantly affects several effector mechanisms, which taken together underlie the occurrence of the somatic and autonomic global pattern of the behavioural state. A sign of such integration is the presence, in some instances, of the same somatic and/or autonomic activity in different behaviours.

The term "determination" has been used instead of "causation" because the principle of *causation* (unsymmetrical constant and unique determination of the effect by the efficient cause) is only one, albeit very important principle in Science, among several categories of determination that are useful to describe lawful relationships among variables (cf. Bunge, 1979). "Scientific explanation has traditionally been regarded as causal explanation; the explanation of a fact was not usually deemed to be scientific unless its proximate and ultimate causes were assigned" (Bunge, 1979, p. 282). However, "Simple causation involves an artificial isolation or singling out of both factors and trends of evolution; it may reflect the central streamline but not the whole process. Isolation is a simplifying hypothesis rather than a fact. It is indispensable and even approximately valid in many cases; nevertheless, it is never rigorously true" and "Causal chains are valid along limited stretches; their validity is sooner or later ruined by branching, convergence, or discontinuity. Continuity is essential to causality, but no more essential to the world than discontinuity, with which it is intimately connected" (Bunge, 1979, pp. 146, 147). There are many other categories of lawful determination having scientific relevance in addition to causal determination (productive causation). According to Bunge (1979, pp. 17–19), they are: *quantitative self-determination* (determination of the consequent by the antecedent in the continuous unfolding of states that differ from one another in quantitative respects only), *interactive determination* (determination of the consequent by mutual action), *mechanical determination* (determination of the consequent by the antecedent with the addition of efficient causes and mutual actions), *statistical determination* (determination of the end result by the joint action of independent entities), and *structural determination* (determination of the parts by the whole).

An analytical approach to sleep physiology is necessary at any level of complexity to dissect the elementary molecular and cellular mechanisms of single physiological functions underlying the global phenomenology of behavioural states. However, it is often conceptually misleading to attach the rigid causal relationships of productive causation, fitting elementary processes, to integrative processes that generate the behavioural states of the living organism. According to Medawar (1996, pp. 126, 127), "If an explanation or interpretation of a phenomenon or state of affairs is to be fully satisfying and actable on, it must have a special, not merely a general relevance to the problem under investigation."

Molecular and cellular processes described by causal determination and constrained in small temporal and spatial dimensions characterise the *proximate determination* of elementary somatic and autonomic physiological phenomena. As already mentioned, it is epistemologically unjustified to proceed further to a direct conceptual identification of such elementary events with integrative processes underlying a behavioural state. This is a sort of "causal" reductionism, which not only lacks a physiological basis but also results in a misconception of the meaning of the word "sleep." This word ought to be used as a linguistic expression and not as a real entity like a single and well-defined biological object or an organ carrying out a specific physiological function. Considering sleep behaviour, no single physiological function should be privileged by overlooking many others. In fact, sleep, if identified correctly as a global behaviour, is the result of a multivariate system of functions whose properties are determined by many variables. This is the level of a complex *intermediate determination*, which by weaving together proximate cause–effect relationships occurring in the neuronal network of the central nervous system controls both the somatic and autonomic activities of the whole organism. No matter how productive causation underlies this functional complexity, the several categories of determination mentioned before are also necessary to explain the lawful determination of all the phenomena characterising a behavioural state. This is particularly true because such categories of intermediate determination adequately explain the characteristic flexibility, plasticity, and variability of a behavioural state yielding multifarious exogenous and endogenous influences. Moreover, the combination of graded and all or no bioelectrical and biochemical activity of neurones, the micro-compartmentalisation of neuronal and glia cell aggregates, and the complexity of neural and humoral interconnections between neurones underlie a good deal of functional indetermination that cannot be easily explained in behavioural terms by rigid causation.

Besides the level of intermediate determination, it is not clear whether a *remote determination* of sleep exists in terms of activity of a highly specific and segregated neuronal network. A role for such remote determination is of easy specification particularly because it would increase the constraints on intermediate determination to better control in its turn also proximate determination at molecular and cellular levels of sleep behaviour. In fact, although the concept of remote determination may be appealing to explain in a rather simplistic way the specific global integration of physiological functions in a behavioural state, a still open question is whether it corresponds to a physiological reality or is simply a revival of the old concept of "sleep centre". The main reason for this uncertainty is that the experimental demonstration of the physiological existence of this kind of remote determination is at most indirect or even purely inductive, since it is based on phenomena belonging to the same domain of the experimental validation of intermediate determination.

In conclusion, sleep appears to be a behavioural state resulting from dynamic interactions of different physiological functions in response to several endogenous (feeding, fatigue, temperature, instinctive drives) and exogenous (light–dark, temperature, food, season, social drives) cues. From the viewpoint of its determination, the mechanism appears so complex as to justify a theoretical distinction between *proximate, intermediate,* and *remote* aspects of determination of sleep behaviour. This gradual approach to sleep behaviour avoids extending the category of rigid causal determination beyond the molecular and cellular levels and forcing experimental results to fit a reductionistic theory in spite of the fact that many elementary physiological events characterising sleep behaviour are not specific to sleep alone. In other words, sleep, like wakefulness, is a function of other interactive functions and not the unique result of the compelling influence of a segregated and highly specific neuronal network of the central nervous system.

Practical Considerations

A few simple examples of application of the criteria discussed above to functional levels of increasing integrative complexity in the central nervous system will be considered next according to the categories of proximate, intermediate, and remote determination of the physiological phenomena of sleep behaviour. In this context, intermediate and remote determination underlie the expression of the behavioural phenotype and the behavioural genotype of sleep, respectively.

Proximate versus intermediate determination

The disappearance of shivering during REM sleep (Parmeggiani and Rabini, 1967) in terms of proximate determination may be considered a direct result of the tonic inhibition of spinal motorneurones underlying the postural muscle atonia during REM sleep. However, the disappearance of shivering during REM sleep without atonia (Hendricks *et al.*, 1977; Hendricks, 1982) shows that a change in the activity of the high integration levels underlying thermoregulation is specifically involved in this suppression. It has also been shown that the disappearance during REM sleep of thermoregulatory responses to direct thermal stimulation of the preoptic–hypothalamic area, like panting (Parmeggiani *et al.*, 1973), metabolic heat production (Glotzbach and Heller, 1976), and vasomotion (Parmeggiani *et al.*, 1977), is consistent with this conclusion. Thus, a reductionistic approach based on proximate determination alone is not satisfactory and intermediate determination is required involving brainstem and preoptic–hypothalamic integrative levels.

The ultradian sleep cycle (a single sequence of NREM sleep and REM sleep episodes) shows variability in duration and architecture depending on exogenous and endogenous factors beyond the boundaries of proximate determination. In particular, it is possible to define with adequate accuracy the end of the cycle with REM sleep by means of only a central (electroencephalogram) bioelectrical variable and a peripheral (electromyogram) bioelectrical variable. However, the beginning of the ultradian sleep cycle is much less distinctly appreciated in such variables. The extension of intermediate determination by adding the information obtained from thermal variables (e.g., hypothalamic and ear pinna temperatures) to that of bioelectrical variables marks a more reliable starting point of an undisturbed ultradian sleep cycle (Azzaroni and Parmeggiani, 1995). This predictive efficacy results from the fact that not every change in the bioelectrical variables of NREM sleep is indicative of co-ordinated changes in autonomic variables, the consistent and basic physiological features characterising the occurrence of a complete ultradian sleep cycle. In conclusion, the proximate determination of few biological variables does not yield correct information on the state of the system. This state is the result of the combination of many variables due to intermediate determination.

Intermediate versus remote determination

The effect of warming the preoptic–hypothalamic area (Von Euler and Söderberg, 1958; Roberts and Robinson, 1969; Roberts *et al.*, 1969; Sakaguchi *et al.*, 1979) shows that somatic and autonomic responses characterising heat loss behaviour are associated with electroencephalographic synchronisation and somatic and autonomic sleep behaviour. In this respect, the question may be whether the result supports the existence in this area of either a mechanism of remote determination or a mechanism of intermediate determination of NREM sleep. According to the concept of remote determination, the changes in the electroencephalogram are the primary event of NREM sleep and even the sign of productive causation of heat loss. Conversely, the concept of intermediate determination suggests the existence of an integrative mechanism underlying with no specific priority both electroencephalographic synchronisation and heat loss as common features of NREM sleep behaviour. In this case, a restraint in accepting the concept of remote determination of sleep is suggested by the fact that cooling of the same region induces the somatic, autonomic, and electroencephalographic changes characterising heat conservation and waking behaviour (Sakaguchi *et al.*, 1979). Moreover, other studies have shown that the differences in the spontaneous activity of cold- and warm-responsive neurones across QW, NREM sleep, and REM sleep are consistent with a direct involvement of such neurones also in sleep regulation (Alam *et al.*, 1997; McGinty *et al.*, 2001; Szymusiak *et al.*, 2001). On this basis, it is likely that different mechanisms would control behavioural state-related excitability and specific responsiveness in thermoresponsive neurones, which probably underlie several functions at the high integration level of the preoptic–hypothalamic structures (Parmeggiani *et al.*, 1987). Hence, it is reasonable to conclude that preoptic–hypothalamic mechanisms underlie the intermediate determination of the behavioural integration of both bioelectrical and temperature regulation in response to such thermal challenges.

In contrast, a sleep-specific neuronal network of remote determination ought to be anatomically and functionally distinct from and hierarchically superposed on the complex neuronal network effecting the systemic executive integration (intermediate determination) of brain bioelectrical activity and somatic and autonomic physiological functions. The artificial dissection of such a specific neuronal network of remote determination of sleep runs the risk of overlooking the conspicuous integrative overlap of the neuronal organisation of different basic physiological controls in the preoptic–hypothalamic area. Overlooking intermediate determination in favour of remote determination may suggest a new version of the old simplistic concept of "sleep centre."

Another example supporting the previous considerations is the falsification of the reductionistic causation of sleep based on its identification with the bioelectrical activity of the brain. Sleep defined only by such activity is virtually stripped of its characteristic somatic and autonomic physiologic phenomena and reduced to a mere term with linguistic value but scientifical inconsistency. The word sleep acquires a scientific objectivity if characterised by an adequate number of physiological variables, that is by the phenomenology controlled by intermediate determination. The "bioelectrical" reductionism of identifying the synchronisation of the electroencephalogram with sleep itself failed to define sleep properly. In 1953, the existence of a new feature of sleep behaviour showing a desynchronised electroencephalogram had to be seriously entertained (Aserinsky and Kleitman, 1953). Certainly, this awareness raises the problem of establishing an operational definition of sleep behaviour that is at the same time parsimonious for practical reasons and apt to avoid misleading reductionism. In the past, several sleep theories were derived directly from a single physiological effect of proximate or intermediate determination with the ensuing neglect of the global nature of sleep regulation in favour of a subordinated regulation (Parmeggiani, 1995). A conceptual danger ought to be pointed out, namely that of equating a global behavioural event, such as sleep, with the few phenomena on which its technical definition is necessarily based in providing a common scientific language. In conclusion, the analysis of sleep phenomena shows that the physiological and theoretical aspects of the process we call sleep can only be logically organised by taking into account several different criteria. It is, therefore, impossible to choose just one of these as being truly paradigmatic (Parmeggiani, 1980).

Remote determination

Concerning the remote determination of sleep behaviour, the question is to verify whether the concept is supportable by a mechanistic reality. A testable working hypothesis, however, ought to be conceived independently of the domain of intermediate determination. To this end, several criteria are necessary for a general and rational classification of the behavioural phenomena characterising the ultradian wake–sleep cycle (Table 1).

In particular, a functional model of hierarchical permutations (Table 2) can be surmised from the mechanistic viewpoint on the basis of the

Table 1. Classification criteria of the behavioural states of the ultradian wake–sleep cycle.

Criteria	QW	NREMS	REMS
Bioelectrical	Desynchronised	Synchronised	Desynchronised
Ethological	Appetitive (somatic)	Appetitive (autonomic)	Consummatory (somatic + autonomic)
Hierarchical	Prosencephalic	Diencephalic	Rhombencephalic
Operational	Closed loop	Closed loop	Open loop
Teleological	Homeostatic	Homeostatic	Poikilostatic

QW, quiet wakefulness; NREMS, non-rapid eye movement sleep; REMS, rapid eye movement sleep (from Parmeggiani, 1980).

Table 2. Permutations in functional hierarchical arrays.

Rank	MHA	FHA		
		QW	NREMS	REMS
I	T	T	D	R
II	D	D	R	T
III	R	R	T	D

MHA, morphological hierarchical array; FHA, functional hierarchical array; QW, quiet wakefulness; NREMS, non-rapid eye movement sleep; REMS, rapid eye movement sleep; D, diencephalon; R, rhombencephalon; T, telencephalon (from Parmeggiani, 1982).

morphological and functional organisation of the central nervous system as brought about by phylogenetic and ontogenetic processes (Parmeggiani, 1982). In particular, the states of the behavioural continuum are considered the functional landmarks of the discontinuous development of the mammalian encephalon characterised by the superimposition of increasingly complex integrative levels of physiological regulation. In mammals, the evolution of the ultradian wake–sleep cycle, from QW to NREM sleep to REM sleep, would reflect a stepwise functional regression of hierarchical dominance from telencephalon (QW) to diencephalon (NREM sleep) to rhombencephalon (REM sleep). The hierarchical array of the morphological organisation is, of course, invariant, whereas the hierarchical array of functional dominance is behavioural state-dependent as a result of permutations occurring in the functional relationships among phylogenetically different structures of the encephalon during the ultradian wake–sleep cycle (cf. Parmeggiani, 1982, 1994). Mechanisms that could underlie such hierarchical permutations are indeterminate at present, but the model may be useful as a single conceptual frame encompassing both functional changes during ontogenesis and physiological differences between mammalian species. At all events, such considerations point to the possibility of a genetic determination of sleep behaviour. After Claparède (1905), the work of ethologists in particular has shown many instinctive aspects of sleep behaviour (Holzapfel, 1940; Tinbergen, 1951; Hediger, 1959, 1969). From the viewpoint of remote determination, it is interesting to discuss briefly whether considering sleep an instinct supports a lawful organisation of the behavioural continuum.

The operative model of instinctive activity points out the basic importance of the consummatory act. The identification of such an act would allow sleep behaviour to be construed as an instinct (cf. Table 1). Unfortunately, sleep reveals no clear-cut physiological features of the occurrence of a consummatory act. This is a basic difference between sleep and classical instinctive patterns characterised by clearly manifested consummatory acts. However, if the consummatory act of sleep is a process effected within the nervous system as an introverted event, it may not show a behavioural pattern of somatic and autonomic interactions with the environment. To support this possibility, however, two fundamental properties of the consummatory act ought to be demonstrated in sleep behaviour. Firstly, that it is a prepotent process and, secondly, that it is defined not only in qualitative but also in quantitative terms. According to these criteria, the consistent expression of an endogenous need of the central nervous system was considered to be the occurrence of REM sleep (Parmeggiani, 1973) for the following reasons: (i) the process is physiologically prepotent because thermoregulation, a basic function in mammals, is suspended (Parmeggiani and Rabini, 1967) and (ii) the process is necessary on a quantitative temporal basis as shown by the effects of its temperature-dependent deprivation and recovery (Parmeggiani and Rabini, 1970; Parmeggiani *et al.*, 1980). Thus, REM sleep appears to be the best candidate for the role of consummatory act. On the other hand, the precise homeostatic regulation of physiological activity characterising NREM sleep appears consistent with an autonomic appetitive state controlling the occurrence of a consummatory act basically altering homeostatic regulation in mammals (Parmeggiani, 1980). The physiological study of the instinctive aspects of sleep behaviour (Parmeggiani, 1968; Moruzzi, 1969) points to a remote determination arising from genetic factors (Valatx *et al.*, 1972; Valatx and Bugat, 1974) lately under careful and promising scrutiny (Huber *et al.*, 2003).

Conclusion

The conclusion of this chapter is that many criteria are needed for a lawful determination of the processes underlying sleep behaviour. Much research still lies ahead to comply with the operative logic underlying the integrative complexity of the behavioural continuum.

References

Alam, M.N., McGinty, D., and Szymusiak, R. (1997). Thermosensitive neurons of the diagonal band in rats: relation to wakefulness and non-rapid eye movement sleep. *Brain Res.*, 752: 81–89.

Aserinsky, E. and Kleitman, N. (1953). Regularly occurring periods of eye motility and concomitant phenomena during sleep. *Science*, 118: 273–274.

Azzaroni, A. and Parmeggiani P. L. (1995). Synchronized sleep duration is related to tonic vasoconstriction of thermoregulatory heat exchangers. *J. Sleep Res.*, 4: 41–47.

Bunge, M. (1979). *Causality and Modern Science*. New York: Dover Publications.

Claparède, E. (1905). Esquisse d'une théorie biologique du sommeil. *Arch. Psychol.*, 4: 246–349.

Glotzbach, S.F. and Heller, H.C. (1976) Central nervous regulation of body temperature during sleep. *Science*, 194: 537–539.

Hediger, H. (1959). Wie Tiere schlafen. *Med. Klin.*, 20: 938–946.

Hediger, H. (1969). Comparative observations on sleep. *Proc. R. Soc. Med.*, 62: 153–156.

Hendricks, J.C. (1982). Absence of shivering in the cat during paradoxical sleep without atonia. *Exp. Neurol.*, 75: 700–710.

Hendricks, J.C., Bowker, R.M., and Morrison, A.R. (1977). Functional characteristics of cats with pontine lesions during sleep and wakefulness and their usefulness for sleep research. In: Koella, W. P. and Levin, P. (Eds.). *Sleep 1976*. Karger, Basel, pp. 6–10.

Hess, W.R. (1965). Sleep as a phenomenon of the integral organism. In: Akert, K., Bally, C., and Schadé, J.P. (Eds.). *Progress in Brain Research. Sleep Mechanisms*. Amsterdam: Elsevier, pp. 3–8.

Holzapfel, M. (1940). Triebbedingte Ruhezustände als Ziel von Appetenzhandlungen. *Naturwissenschaften*, 28: 273–280.

Huber, R., Hill, S.L., Holladay, C. Biesiadecki, M. Tononi, G., and Cirelli, C. (2004). Sleep homeostasis in *Drosophila melanogaster. Sleep*, 27: 628–639.

McGinty, D., Alam, M.N., Szymusiak, R., Nakao, M., and Yamamoto M. (2001). Hypothalamic sleep-promoting mechanisms: coupling to thermoregulation. *Arch. Ital. Biol.*, 139: 63–65.

Medawar, P. (1996). Further comments on psychoanalysis. In: Medawar, P.(Ed.). *The Strange Case of the Spotted Mice*. Oxford: Oxford University Press, pp. 120–131.

Moruzzi, G. (1969). Sleep and instinctive behavior. *Arch. Ital. Biol.*, 107: 175–216.

Parmeggiani, P.L. and Rabini, C. (1967). Shivering and panting during sleep. *Brain Res.*, 6: 789–791.

Parmeggiani, P.L. (1968). Telencephalo-diencephalic aspects of sleep mechanisms. *Brain Res.*, 7: 350–359.

Parmeggiani, P.L. (1973). The physiological role of sleep. In: Levin, P. and Koella, W.P. (Eds.). *Sleep*. Basel: Karger, pp. 210–216.

Parmeggiani, P.L. (1980). Behavioral phenomenology of sleep (somatic and vegetative). *Experientia*, 36: 6–11.

Parmeggiani, P.L. (1982). Regulation of physiological functions during sleep in mammals. *Experientia*, 38: 1405–1408.

Parmeggiani, P.L. (1994). The autonomic nervous system in sleep. In: Kryger, M.H., Roth, T., and Dement W.C.(Eds.). *Principles and Practice of Sleep Medicine*. Philadelphia: Saunders pp. 194–203.

Parmeggiani, P.L. (1995). A retrospective assessment of sleep research in the western world during the late 19th and early 20th centuries. In: Shiyi, L. and Inoué, S. (Eds.). *Sleep: Ancient and Modern*. Shangai: The Shanghai Scientific and Technological Literature Publishing House, pp. 89–99.

Parmeggiani, P.L. (2000). Physiological regulation in sleep. In: Kryger, M.H., Roth, T., and Dement, W.C. (Eds.). *Principles and Practice of Sleep Medicine*. Philadelphia: Saunders, pp. 169–178.

Parmeggiani, P.L. and Rabini, C. (1970). Sleep and environmental temperature. *Arch. Ital. Biol.*, 108: 369–387.

Parmeggiani, P.L., Franzini, C., Lenzi, P., and Zamboni, G. (1973). Threshold of respiratory responses to preoptic heating during sleep in freely moving cats. *Brain Res.*, 52: 189–201.

Parmeggiani, P.L., Zamboni, G., Cianci, T., and Calasso, M. (1977). Absence of thermoregulatory vasomotor responses during fast wave sleep in cats. *Electroenceph. Clin. Neurophysiol.*, 42: 372–380.

Parmeggiani, P.L., Cianci, T., Calasso, M., Zamboni, G., and Perez, E. (1980). Quantitative analysis of short term deprivation and recovery of desynchronized sleep in cats. *Electroenceph. Clin. Neurophysiol.*, 50: 293–302.

Parmeggiani, P.L., Cevolani, D., Azzaroni, A., and Ferrari, G. (1987). Thermosensitivity of anterior hypothalamic–preoptic neurons during the waking–sleeping cycle: a study in brain functional states. *Brain Res.*, 415: 79–89.

Roberts, W.W. and Robinson, T.C.L. (1969). Relaxation and sleep induced by warming of the preoptic region and anterior hypothalamus in cats. *Exp. Neurol.*, 25: 282–294.

Roberts, W.W., Bergquist, E.H., and Robinson, T.C.L. (1969). Thermoregulatory grooming and sleep-like relaxation induced by local warming of preoptic area and anterior hypothalamus in opossum. *J. Comp. Physiol. Psychol.*, 67: 182–188.

Sakaguchi, S., Glotzbach, S.F., and Heller, H.C. (1979). Influence of hypothalamic and ambient temperatures on sleep in kangaroo rats. *Am. J. Physiol.*, 294: R80–R88.

Szymusiak, R., Steiniger, T., Alam, M.N., and McGinty, D. (2001). Preoptic area sleep-regulating mechanisms. *Arch. Ital. Biol.* 139: 77–92.

Tinbergen, N. (1951). *The Study of Instinct.* Oxford: Oxford University Press.

Valatx, J.L. and Bugat, R. (1974). Facteurs génétique dans le déterminisme du cycle veille-sommeil chez le souris. *Brain Res.*, 69: 315–330.

Valatx, J.L., Bugat, R., and Jouvet, M. (1972). Genetic studies of sleep in mice. *Nature*, 238: 226–227.

Von Euler, C. and Söderberg, U. (1958). The influence of hypothalamic thermoceptive structures on the electroencephalogram and gamma motor activity. *Electroenceph. Clin. Neurophysiol.*, 42: 112–129.

II. PHYSIOLOGIC FUNCTIONS
IN SLEEP

Chapter 13

CONTROL OF MUSCLE TONE ACROSS THE SLEEP–WAKE CYCLE

Jerome M. Siegel[1]

During normal sleep, muscle tone in the skeletal muscles diminishes from prior waking levels. In non-rapid eye movement (REM) sleep residual muscle tone is normally present. In REM sleep muscle tone is generally abolished, with the exception of tone in the diaphragm and extraocular muscles. Abnormalities in the regulation of tone across the sleep–wake cycle lead to a number of pathologies that can have enormous effects on health and safety. I will first describe the major pathologies of muscle tone control over the sleep–wake cycle and then review what we know about the underlying physiology that is disrupted in these disorders.

Non-REM Sleep Pathologies

Sleep walking consists of recurrent episodes in which the subject arouses from non-REM sleep, typically during the first third of the night, and shows complex behavioral automatisms that include leaving the bed and walking for some distance. Although it was originally thought to represent the acting out of a dream, Gastaut and Broughton (1965) and Jacobson *et al.* (1965) independently confirmed that sleep walking occurs in non-REM sleep and is not normally associated with any dream-like mentation

---

[1] jsiegel@ucla.edu

or mentation regarding the executed movements. The link to deep non-REM sleep (stages 3–4) fits with the greater incidence in children, who have more deep slow-wave sleep than do adults. However, the disorder persists in adults with an incidence of 1% compared to the 15–30% incidence in children. Injuries are common and can be severe (Broughton, 2000).

Night terrors, arousals marked by screams, and associated motor activity can be linked to sleep walking or can occur independently and are always initiated in non-REM sleep. A number of drug treatments, including tricyclic benzodiazepines and carbamazepine, have been used to treat sleep walking and night terrors, but this treatment is not successful in many patients (Broughton, 2000).

The restless legs syndrome (RLS) is characterized by an irresistible desire to move the legs, usually associated with paresthesias/dysesthesias and motor restlessness. It is present in 5–10% of the adult population (Odin *et al.*, 2002). Most patients with RLS have periodic movements during non-REM sleep, a contraction of limb muscles especially prevalent in the tibialis anterior and that occurs every 10–30 s. Periodic limb movements (PLMs) are most numerous in the first half of the night. Although the vast majority of patients with RLS experience PLMs (PLMs in sleep), PLMs frequently occur independently of RLS. The RLS/PLMs syndrome produces profound insomnia (Hening, 2002; Parker and Rye, 2002; Trenkwalder, 2003). The etiology of the condition remains uncertain, but recent discoveries implicate dysfunction in areas of the nervous system from the spinal cord to the basal ganglia. Some current work has supported the hypothesis that the condition results from a deficiency of dopaminergic function based on abnormalities of iron transport and storage. Dopamine agonists are the most reliable treatment for severe cases, although other recent studies have used a number of other medications, including opioids and anticonvulsants (Hening, 2002). Dopamine agonists appear to act at the motoneuronal or adjacent spinal levels rather than in forebrain regions, since the phenomenon can be demonstrated in and reversed by dopamine agonists applied to the isolated spinal cord (Hening, 2002; Odin *et al.*, 2002). However, treatments are still unsatisfactory for most cases. A recent report found that RLS was associated with increased levels of hypocretin, making it the only neurological syndrome known to be associated with increased hypocretin and one of only a few syndromes associated with hypocretin abnormalities; narcolepsy, Guillain–Barre syndrome, and myotonic dystrophy being among the others (Ripley *et al.*, 2001; Allen *et al.*, 2002; Martínez-Rodríguez *et al.*, 2003). Our finding that hypocretin release is linked to motor activity (Wu *et al.*, 2002) suggests that this release and the release of other transmitters controlled by interactions with hypocretin (John *et al.*, 2003) may contribute to motor restlessness in waking as well as PLMs.

Nocturnal bruxism is a grinding or clenching of the teeth during sleep that differs from daytime parafunctional jaw muscle activity (Lavigne and Manzini, 2003). Not only does bruxism produce attrition of tooth height by as much as 50% and loss of buccal tooth surface, it also frequently produces painful chronic temporal mandibular joint dysfunction (Lobbezoo and Lavigne, 1997), headaches, tooth sensitivity, and disturbed sleep. Incidence in adults ranges from 3 to 13%, with higher levels in children. Sixty to 80% of sleep bruxism episodes occur during non-REM sleep stages 1 and 2 (Lavigne and Manzini, 2003). The incidence of sleep bruxism is higher in RLS patients (Lavigne and Montplaisir, 1994). Like RLS, sleep bruxism is sometimes improved by L-dopa treatment. The preponderance of evidence indicates that L-dopa acts by increasing dopamine availability at the motoneuronal level as it appears to do in RLS, i.e., the effect does not appear to be mediated by the basal ganglia or other forebrain regions (Lobbezoo *et al.*, 1997).

Sleep apnea affects more than 18 million Americans. Sleep apnea more than doubles the risk of heart failure, and 37% of patients with heart failure have obstructive sleep apnea (Javaheri *et al.*, 1998; Sin *et al.*, 1999; Shahar *et al.*, 2001; Bradley and Floras, 2003). Untreated sleep apnea is also linked to memory problems, weight gain, impotence, headaches, and motor vehicle crashes (Bedard *et al.*, 1993; Guilleminault, 1994; Naegele *et al.*, 1998; Salorio *et al.*, 2002).

Evidence for brain damage in obstructive sleep apnea

Sleep apnea patients whose respiratory problems are satisfactorily treated with continuous positive airway pressure (CPAP) or by other means show persistent cognitive deficits, including impairment of short-term memory, sleepiness, and problems with language comprehension and expression (Bedard *et al.*, 1993; Naegele *et al.*, 1998; Beebe and Gozal, 2002). A recent MRI study by Harper's group demonstrated that obstructive sleep apnea patients have diminished regional gray matter volume in frontal, parietal, cingulate and hippocampal cortex, and in the cerebellum (Macey *et al.*, 2002). Two startling observations were a unilateral loss of gray matter in cortical brain sites associated with control of the oral airway in the expression of speech (Broca's area), and that there are deficient functional responses in areas responsible for integration of sensory information for speech (Wernicke's area); those unexpected findings were coupled with the observation that nearly 40% of the obstructive sleep apnea subjects studied had a history of stuttering or speech impediment since childhood (vs. 8% of controls). Adults with persistent developmental stuttering show damage to speech-related brain regions, including Wernicke's area (Foundas *et al.*, 2001). The unilateral nature of the gray matter loss in well-perfused structures related to motor regulation of the upper airway suggests that this damage may be a cause rather than a consequence of obstructive sleep apnea. Harper's group found that obstructive sleep apnea is also associated with damage to CA1 regions of the hippocampus. Hippocampal structures are known to show significant changes in activity change prior to sigh-apnea sequences in animals (Poe *et al.*, 1996) and, on stimulation, will elicit marked changes in respiration, including apnea in a variety of species (Anand and Dua, 1956; Duffin and Hockman, 1972; Ruit and Neafsey, 1988). Damage was also consistently seen in vermal regions of the cerebellum, especially the deep cerebellar nuclei, most prominently in the fastigial nucleus. These regions have an important role in muscle tone control (Asanome *et al.*, 1998; Davis, 2000; Lazorthes *et al.*, 2002), and are regulated by monoaminergic inputs (Guglielmino and Strata, 1971; Doba and Reis, 1972; Moises and Woodward, 1980). Bilateral damage in other regions unrelated to respiratory control suggests that the chronic intermittent hypoxia resulting from sleep apnea may over time cause further degenerative changes in the brain. These degenerative changes may well exacerbate any initial neurological deficits, thereby contributing to further airway collapse.

The hypothesis that obstructive sleep apnea might cause brain damage has been tested in rats. Gozal *et al.* (2001) Subjected rats to chronic intermittent hypoxia for 12 h/day for up to 14 days. The level of chronic intermittent hypoxia used was adjusted to produce a reduction in arterial oxygenation comparable to that seen in human obstructive sleep apnea. Intermittent hypoxia resulted in increased levels of apoptosis in the CA1 region of the hippocampus and in neocortex, but not in the CA3 hippocampal region, after 1–2 days. A marked reduction in the number of cortical and CA-1 cells bearing N-methyl-D-aspartate (NMDA) glutamate receptor binding sites was seen. In a prior study, rats exposed to hypobaric hypoxia showed a >35% reduction in NMDA binding sites in cortex and hippocampus (Pichiule *et al.*, 1996). These results suggest that a glutamate-mediated excitotoxic process, killing cells with NMDA receptors, might be involved in mediating the effects of chronic intermittent hypoxia.

The implications of the findings of gray matter loss and altered neural processing of breathing and autonomic challenges in obstructive sleep apnea are profound. The findings suggest that brain damage underlies the cognitive deficits found in obstructive sleep apnea of both children and adults, the altered sensory processing found in obstructive sleep apnea, and produces the abnormal atonia and sequencing of muscle activation found in the syndrome.

Overview of pathological conditions

Multiple modes of failure of the sleep motor control system in non-REM sleep are consistent with the complexity of the system. The disorders discussed above may involve different patterns of neurotransmitter disturbance at the motoneuronal level, possibly resulting from different patterns of change in the activity of higher neural structures.

REM Sleep Pathologies

Regulation of muscle tone in REM sleep

Most studies of muscle tone regulation across the sleep–wake cycle have emphasized the determinants of REM sleep atonia. Here, we briefly summarize the major findings. Figure 1 presents an outline of some of the major systems we have studied.

Evidence for glycinergic involvement in the atonia of REM sleep

Chase's group was the first to document hyperpolarization of motoneurons during REM sleep (Nakamura *et al.*, 1978). Their studies have indicated a major involvement of glycine in the suppression of tone in skeletal muscles during REM sleep. They found that REM was accompanied by a bombardment of trigeminal and lumbar motoneurons with inhibitory postsynaptic potentials (IPSPs) (Chase and Morales, 1982). The glycine antagonist strychnine reversed these phasic potentials (Soja *et al.*, 1987), whereas the gamma aminobutyric acid (GABA) antagonists picrotoxin and bicuculine did not (Chandler *et al.*, 1980a,b; Chase *et al.*, 1980, 1989). Membrane hyperpolarization, combined with the attenuation of IPSPs by strychnine, led to the hypothesis that glycine release was primarily responsible for the hyperpolarization of trigeminal and lumbar motoneurons during REM sleep (Chase and Morales, 1990). Glycine not only inhibits motoneurons directly, but also facilitates the response of NMDA glutamate receptors on motoneurons (Berger and Isaacson, 1999). Phasic reversible IPSPs were not

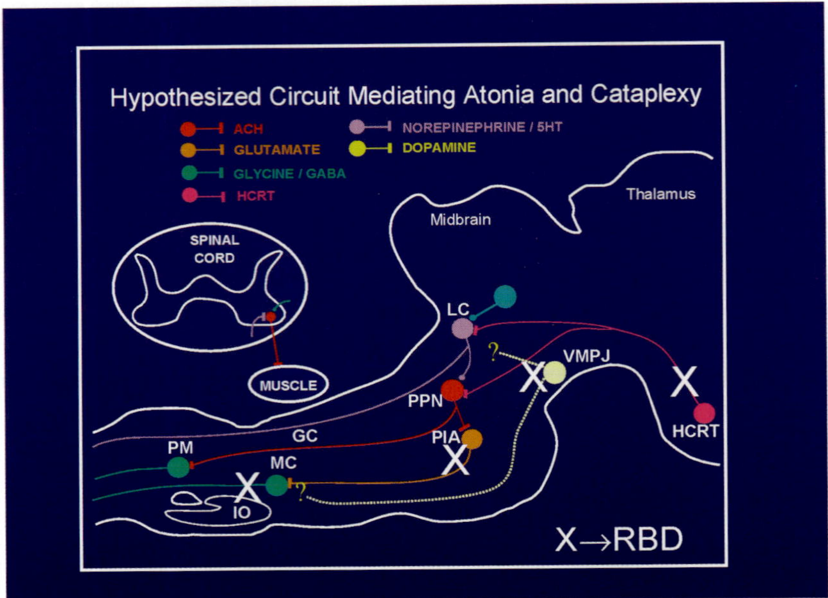

Figure 1. Some of the major pathways implicated in muscle tone control across the sleep–wake cycle. The systems are drawn on a sagittal section of the brainstem of the cat. See text for a description of the experimental evidence for the relationships illustrated. Xs illustrate points at which lesions are hypothesized to disrupt the mechanisms producing atonia, resulting in REM sleep without atonia. VMPJ, ventral mesopontine junction (Lai and Siegel, 2003); PPN, pedunculopontine nucleus; lc, locus coeruleus; GC, nucleus gigantocellularis; MC, nucleus magnocellularis; PM, nucleus magnocellularis.

seen in these studies in non-REM sleep, suggesting that either glycine is not released in non-REM sleep or that it is released tonically, in contrast to the phasic glycine release of REM sleep.

After making these observations in the intact animal, Chase *et al.*, developed an acute model of REM sleep atonia. Atonia was achieved by iontophoresing carbachol into the pons of the decerebrate cat (Morales *et al.*, 1987). This acute preparation allows a more rapid analysis of the REM atonia mechanism. The studies of Morales *et al.* indicated that glycine has a role in the IPSPs seen in the decerebrate animal, as it does in REM sleep in the intact cat.

Chase's group has focused on the phasic inhibitory potentials occurring during REM sleep. However, the "main event" from a sleep apnea viewpoint may be the tonic muscle tone changes in non-REM and REM sleep, rather than the phasic potentials during REM sleep that last only milliseconds. The work by Chase's group does not exclude the central participation of other transmitters in the overall regulation of muscle tone in REM sleep. It also says little about non-REM sleep muscle tone control.

Morrison *et al.* (2002) delivered transmitter agonists to the hypoglossal nucleus to determine whether muscle tone could be suppressed in urethane anesthetized animals. They found that glycine produced a suppression of muscle tone, supporting the idea that it could be responsible for the suppression of tone in REM sleep.

The role of GABA in motoneuron inhibition during sleep

GABA is thought to be the most common inhibitory neurotransmitter in the brain, being active at 20–40% of brain synapses (Bloom and Iverson, 1971). However, its possible role in the reduction of tone in non-REM sleep and in REM sleep has received little attention. In their work on lumbar motoneurons in REM sleep models, Chase *et al.* (1989) found that iontophoresis of the GABA antagonists picrotoxin and bicuculine did not prevent motoneuron IPSPs in REM sleep. However, they did note that the GABA antagonists substantially reduced the IPSP durations. In other work, Okabe *et al.* (1994) found inhibitory effects of GABA on hypoglossal motoneurons recorded from anesthetized rats. In the urethane anesthetized rat, Liu *et al.* (2003) and Morrison *et al.* (2003) found that GABA suppressed muscle tone in the hypoglossal nucleus. They further found that GABA antagonism was ineffective in blocking atonia during REM sleep but did increase genioglossus muscle tone in non-REM sleep. They did not examine GABA release in either non-REM or REM sleep. GABA and glycine may be released by the same axon terminals but may also be released independently (O'Brien and Berger, 1999).

In our *in vivo* microdialysis studies of the locus coeruleus (Nitz and Siegel, 1997a), raphe (Nitz and Siegel, 1997b), and posterior hypothalamus (Nitz and Siegel, 1996), we have shown that it is possible to measure GABA release across the sleep cycle. Moreover, we have found that there is a selective GABAergic inhibition of noradrenergic and serotonergic cell groups during REM sleep. This inhibition is likely to be responsible for the cessation of discharge in these cells during REM sleep. This cessation of serotonin neuron discharge, likely caused by GABA action on the raphe magnus, pallidus, and obscurus, results in disfacilitation of at least one motoneuron group (the hypoglossal nucleus) during REM sleep, as outlined below. However, this indirect effect of GABA does not rule out a direct effect of collaterals of these same cells, or of other GABAergic interneurons or projection neurons, on motoneurons. It has been reported that both GABA and glutamate release in the thalamus are increased in non-REM sleep (Kekesi *et al.*, 1997). It remains to be determined if a similar pattern of release is seen in motoneuron pools.

Evidence for serotonin involvement in the atonia of REM sleep

Kubin *et al.* (1993) used a version of the decerebrate carbachol model to study hypoglossal motor activity. They focused on the hypoglossal nucleus because of studies that showed that tongue hypotonia was one of the major causes of obstructive sleep apnea (Sauerland and Harper, 1976). Kubin *et al.* (1994) found that serotonin release in the hypoglossal nucleus was decreased during carbachol-triggered REM sleep. During carbachol atonia, injection of serotonergic agonists into the hypoglossal nucleus reduced the carbachol-induced suppression of tone (Kubin *et al.*, 1996). While serotonin manipulations had a potent effect on hypoglossal tone, injection of glycine antagonists during periods of carbachol triggered REM sleep did not block atonia (Kubin *et al.*, 1993). Kubin *et al.* concluded that the atonia mechanism in hypoglossal motoneurons was fundamentally different from that which had been seen by Chase and Morales in trigeminal and lumbar motoneurons. They concluded that serotonergic disfacilitation was the major factor responsible for REM sleep atonia in the hypoglossal nucleus, whereas glycinergic hyperpolarization was responsible for atonia in trigeminal and lumbar motoneurons.

Does the neurochemistry of REM sleep atonia in hypoglossal, trigeminal, and lumbar motor systems differ? The evidence listed above suggests that two distinct atonia mechanisms are operating in lumbar and trigeminal vs. hypoglossal motoneurons in REM sleep: amino acid-mediated active inhibition in lumbar motoneurons and serotonin-mediated disfacilitation in hypoglossal motoneurons. However, closer examination of the results suggests that atonia generation in these regions need not differ. Chase and Morales used iontophoresis to come to the conclusion that glycinergic mechanisms were involved. They reported that iontophoresis of strychnine reduced, but did not eliminate, the hyperpolarization seen in skeletal motoneurons (Soja *et al.*, 1987, 1991). Kubin *et al.* (1992) used microinjection of agonists and antagonists to substantiate the involvement of serotonin. Kubin *et al.* reported that, whereas much of the reduction in hypoglossal discharge could be countered by serotonin microinjection, some of the carbachol-induced reduction in tone remained. They concluded that the study "demonstrates that other, non-serotonergic mechanisms also contribute to the carbachol-induced suppression" (Kubin *et al.*, 1996). It may well be that hypoglossal motoneurons are subjected to phasic glycinergic IPSPs as are trigeminal motoneurons. Indeed, Yamuy *et al.* (1999) subsequently showed that hypoglossal motoneurons, like masseter and ventral horn motoneurons, receive glycinergic IPSPs during REM sleep. Conversely, the trigeminal and lumbar motoneurons receive an extensive serotonergic innervation (White *et al.*, 1996). Hyperpolarization in the trigeminal as well as hypoglossal motoneurons during REM sleep could be partially due to disfacilitation by serotonin (or norepinephrine or glutamate — see below), as well as glycinergic inhibition.

The serotonergic disfacilitation and glycinergic inhibition hypotheses are not mutually exclusive. *In vitro* studies by Umemiya and Berger (1995) indicate that glycinergic inhibition is enhanced in the absence of serotonin. Therefore, *in vivo*, serotonergic withdrawal and increased glycine release in REM sleep may act synergistically to hyperpolarize the motoneuron. Application of serotonin may eliminate most of the hyperpolarization of REM sleep, and blockade of glycine may also eliminate most of the hyperpolarization. It is also quite possible that a blockade of norepinephrine or other transmitters would also prevent most of the hyperpolarization; i.e., one should not expect these effects to sum up to 100%.

Supporting a role for serotonergic mechanisms in the atonia of the limb muscles is the preservation of the activity of serotonergic neurons during REM sleep without atonia. This is in contrast to their reduction of activity in non-REM sleep and cessation of activity during normal REM sleep (Trulson *et al.*, 1981). This suggests that some of the "inhibition" of skeletal motor activity occurring during normal REM sleep may in fact be disfacilitation. Lesions that produce REM sleep without atonia return serotonergic activity and perhaps motor facilitation to REM sleep. These mechanisms and interactions may also have a role in non-REM sleep motor dysfunction.

Role of norepinephrine in motoneuron facilitation

In acute studies, noradrenergic neurons in the locus coeruleus have been shown to depolarize motoneurons and increase muscle tone (Parkis *et al.*, 1995; Fung and Barnes, 1987; Lai *et al.*, 1989). Unilateral lesions of the locus coeruleus produce an ipsilateral reduction of muscle tone (D'Ascanio *et al.*, 1988). Noradrenergic cells of the locus coeruleus and of the more ventral and caudally located A5–A7 noradrenergic cell groups have projections to the brainstem, spinal motor, and cerebellar areas. One-third of locus coeruleus and a majority of non-locus coeruleus noradrenergic cells have spinal projections (Nygren and Olson, 1977; Satoh *et al.*, 1977; Reddy *et al.*, 1989; Jones, 1991), with terminals on spinal and brainstem motoneurons (Lyons *et al.*, 1989; Jones, 1991). Locus coeruleus neurons in humans become active in response to inspiratory loading, which simulates obstructive apnea (Gozal *et al.*, 1995).

Work has shown that locus coeruleus cells may not act through norepinephrine release alone. Eighty-six percent of the locus coeruleus neurons that project to spinal cord motoneuronal regions have glutamate as a co-transmitter (Liu *et al.*, 1995). Thus, motor facilitation resulting from locus coeruleus activation may involve a synergistic interaction between norepinephrine and glutamate. The extent to which such an interaction occurs can best be determined by measurement of the release of both transmitters.

Sleep-related activity of serotonergic and noradrenergic neurons

Studies of aminergic cells in behaving animals began with the work of McGinty and colleagues (McGinty and Sakai, 1973; McGinty and Harper, 1976). They found that serotonergic cells discharged regularly in waking, decreased discharge in non-REM sleep, and ceased discharge in REM sleep. Subsequent work showed that noradrenergic cells had a similar pattern of waking activity and cessation of discharge in REM sleep (McGinty and Sakai, 1973; Hobson *et al.*, 1975). Whereas there is overwhelming evidence that most noradrenergic and serotonergic neurons cease discharge during REM sleep, other evidence suggests that a subset of caudal serotonergic neurons in the nucleus raphe magnus may not cease discharge in REM sleep (Cespuglio *et al.*, 1981; Sakai *et al.*, 1983). It is certainly possible that some portion of noradrenergic neurons, particularly those in medullary regions adjacent to the hypoglossal motoneurons (A5–A7), do not show the REM sleep-off pattern that characterizes the pontine locus coeruleus population, although recordings from this region suggest that at least some of these cells may show the REM sleep-off pattern (Eguchi and Satoh, 1980).

Monoamine neurotransmitter release has been shown to be regulated not only by action potentials in the cell soma (Jacobs, 1991; Rueter and

Jacobs, 1996), but also by presynaptic control of release (Di Chiara *et al.*, 1996; Marshall *et al.*, 1997). This presynaptic regulation can attenuate or even reverse the release patterns that might be expected based on action potential activity of the afferent cells. For example, it has been shown that despite the midline locations of serotonergic neurons and their bilateral projections, strong interhemispheric asymmetries in release are present and are readily altered by eye closure and behavioral variables (Baxter *et al.*, 2001).

Role of glutamate in motoneuron facilitation during sleep

Current evidence indicates that the primary cell populations contributing to respiratory rhythmicity are glutamatergic, as are some cells projecting from respiratory centers to motoneurons (Bonham, 1995). Thus, the respiratory drive to the phrenic motoneurons, as well as that to the accessory respiratory musculature, such as the masseter muscle, may be due to glutamatergic input. It is likely that changes in glutamate release contribute to the reduction in tone in non-REM sleep in respiratory and non-respiratory motoneurons.

In studies of unrestrained animals, we have reported that the population of reticular and reticulospinal pontine and medullary cells as a whole reaches its lowest discharge level in non-REM sleep. They reach their highest discharge levels, exceeding mean waking values, in REM sleep (Siegel, 1979; Siegel and Tomaszewski, 1983; Siegel *et al.*, 1983). Much of this cell population is glutamatergic and sends axons both to other reticular and reticulospinal neurons, and to cranial and ventral horn motoneurons (Lai and Siegel, 1991; Lai *et al.*, 1993, 1999). Thus, the cessation or reduction of activity in glutamatergic neurons of the pontine and medial medullary reticular formation during non-REM sleep may contribute to the non-REM sleep related hypotonia that figures so prominently in sleep apnea, and the dysfunction of these cells may cause disorders of excessive motor activity in non-REM sleep.

Increased discharge of glutamatergic cells in REM sleep, to the extent that it changes levels of glutamate release onto respiratory motor systems, may ordinarily compensate for the loss of noradrenergic and serotonergic facilitation (and the likely co-release of glutamate from aminergic neurons) in this state. Silent respiratory-related reticular interneurons are converted into neurons with clear respiratory rhythmicity by iontophoresis of increased levels of glutamate (Foutz *et al.*, 1987). Glutamate delivery was particularly effective in non-REM sleep (Foutz *et al.*, 1987), a time when we would expect glutamate release to be minimal. In contrast, delivery of glutamate during REM sleep, a time when presumptive glutamatergic neurons are already active, produced little change in their respiratory rhythmicity. The level of glutamate release may be a key determinant of upper airway motoneuron activity and may contribute to non-REM sleep parasomnias, yet the pattern of release and the effects of glutamate agonists and antagonists at the motoneuronal level in both respiratory and non-respiratory related motoneurons is unknown.

Studies of transmitter release in decerebrate animals

Amino acids

We have used the acute decerebrate preparation to conduct the first studies of the release of amino acids and monoamines in the REM sleep-like atonic state that can be elicited by pontine stimulation.

We hypothesized that cessation of brainstem monoaminergic systems and an activation of brainstem inhibitory systems are both involved in pontine inhibitory area (PIA) stimulation-induced muscle atonia. Kodama *et al.* (2003) demonstrated an increase in inhibitory amino acid release in motor nuclei during electrical and chemical PIA stimulation in the decerebrate cat using *in vivo* microdialysis and high-performance liquid chromatography analysis techniques. Microinjection of acetylcholine into the PIA elicited muscle atonia and simultaneously produced a significant increase in both glycine and GABA release in the hypoglossal nucleus and in the lumbar ventral horn. Glycine release increased by 74% in the hypoglossal nucleus and by 50% in the spinal cord. GABA release increased by 31% in the hypoglossal nucleus and by 64% in the ventral horn during atonia induced by cholinergic stimulation of the PIA. Glutamate release in the motor nuclei was not significantly altered during atonia induced by electrical or acetylcholine stimulation of the PIA. We suggest that both glycine and GABA play important roles in the regulation of upper airway and postural muscle tone in REM sleep. A combination of decreased monoamine and increased inhibitory amino acid release in motoneuron pools causes PIA-induced atonia and may be involved in atonia linked to REM sleep (see below).

Monoamines

Lai *et al.* (2001) wanted to examine further the neurotransmitter environment of motoneurons during REM sleep. In this study, we addressed the issue of whether monoamine release was greater in hypoglossal than in ventral horn motoneurons in atonic states induced by pontine stimulation, using microdialysis in the decerebrate animal. Electrical stimulation and cholinergic agonist injection into the mesopontine reticular formation produced a suppression of tone in the postural and respiratory muscles and simultaneously caused a significant reduction of norepinephrine and serotonin release that was of similar magnitude in both the hypoglossal nucleus and the spinal cord. Norepinephrine and serotonin release in these motoneuron pools was unchanged when the stimulation was applied to brainstem areas that did not generate bilateral suppression of muscle tone. No change in dopamine release in the motoneuron pools was seen during mesopontine stimulation-induced atonia. We hypothesize that the reduction of monoamine release that we observe exerts a disfacilitatory effect on both ventral horn and hypoglossal motoneurons, and that this disfacilitatory mechanism contributes to the muscle atonia elicited in the decerebrate animal and in the intact animal during REM sleep. A combination of decreased norepinephrine and serotonin and increased glycine and GABA release is linked to pontine-triggered atonia. These changes in release occur to equal extents in the ventral horn and the hypoglossal nucleus.

The reduced release of serotonin and norepinephrine and simultaneous increase in release of glycine and GABA in the REM sleep-like state induced by pontine stimulation raises the issue of how these monoamine and amino acid changes are coupled. Mileykovskiy *et al.* (2000) determined the response of locus coeruleus cells to brainstem stimulation that suppressed muscled tone. Activation of the PIA or the medullary inhibitory area (gigantocellular reticular nucleus) (Gi) suppresses muscle tone in decerebrate animals (Lai and Siegel, 1988). Both PIA and Gi stimulation produced inhibition of locus coeruleus discharge. We conclude that activation of pontine and medullary inhibitory regions produces a coordinated reduction in the activity of LC units (and of cells in the midbrain locomotor region, which also facilitates muscle tone). This relation is particularly striking in the case of PIA stimulation, since stimulating electrodes that were effective in suppressing muscle tone reduced locus coeruleus activity, even though in many cases these stimulation electrodes were within a millimeter or two of the locus coeruleus, and therefore might be expected to excite these cells.

This study demonstrates a surprising inhibitory connection between pontine inhibitory regions, which work by triggering the release of inhibitory amino acids onto motoneurons, and the locus coeruleus, whose neurons release norepinephrine, which facilitates activity in motoneurons. Disturbance of the inhibitory coupling between these two systems may be a factor in motor disorders of REM sleep, but their role in non-REM sleep is unknown.

In a study of the physiology of the descending inhibitory system, we determined the conduction velocity of the descending inhibitory projections (Kohyama *et al.*, 1998a). In further work we showed that there is an ascending projection from the medullary inhibitory region to the region of the locus coeruleus (as suggested above). When we blocked this ascending pathway with lidocaine, sites in the medulla that had been inhibitory produced a net excitation. This work demonstrated the importance of the ascending pathway to locus coeruleus for motor inhibition (Kohyama *et al.*, 1998b).

Summary

The suppression of muscle tone during sleep involves a complex interplay of disfacilitatory and inhibitory processes. Although the normal mechanisms regulating this suppression in REM sleep are becoming understood, the factors regulating tone in non-REM sleep are less well known. The disruptions responsible for sleep motor pathologies are poorly understood.

Acknowledgement

This work was supported by the Medical Research Service of the US Department of Veterans Affairs, and USPHS grants NS14610, MH64109, and HL41370.

References

Allen, R.P., Mignot, E., Ripley, B., Nishino, S., and Earley, C.J. (2002). Increased CSF hypocretin-1 (orexin-A) in restless legs syndrome. *Neurology*, 59: 639–641.

Anand, B.K. and Dua, S. (1956). Circulatory and respiratory changes induced by electrical stimulation of limbic system (visceral brain). *J. Neurophysiol.*, 19: 393–400.

Asanome, M., Matsuyama, K., and Mori, S. (1998). Augmentation of postural muscle tone induced by the stimulation of the descending fibers in the midline area of the cerebellar white matter in the acute decerebrate cat. *Neurosci. Res.*, 30: 257–269.

Baxter, L.R.J., Clark, E.C., Ackermann, R.F., Lacan, G., and Melega, W.P. (2001). Brain mediation of anolis social dominance displays. ii. Differential forebrain serotonin turnover, and effects of specific 5-ht receptor agonists. *Brain Behav. Evol.*, 57: 184–201.

Bedard, M.A., Montplaisir, J., Malo, J., Richer, F., and Rouleau, I. (1993). Persistent neuropsychological deficits and vigilance impairment in sleep apnea syndrome after treatment with continuous positive airways pressure (CPAP). *J. Clin. Exp. Neuropsychol.*, 15: 330–341.

Beebe, D.W. and Gozal, D. (2002). Obstructive sleep apnea and the prefrontal cortex: towards a comprehensive model linking nocturnal upper airway obstruction to daytime cognitive and behavioral deficits. *J. Sleep Res.*, 11: 1–16.

Berger, A.J. and Isaacson, J.S. (1999). Modulation of motoneuron N-methyl-D-aspartate receptors by the inhibitory neurotransmitter glycine. *J. Physiol. Paris*, 93: 23–27.

Bloom, F. and Iverson, L. (1971). Localizing 3H-GABA in nerve terminals of rat cerebral cortex by electron microscopic autoradiography. *Nature*, 229: 628–630.

Bonham, A.C. (1995). Neurotransmitters in the CNS control of breathing. *Resp. Physiol.*, 101: 219–230.

Bradley, T.D. and Floras, J.S. (2003). Sleep apnea and heart failure: part II: central sleep apnea. *Circulation*, 107: 1822.

Broughton, R.J. (2000). NREM parasomnias. In: Kryger, M.H., Roth, T., and Dement, W.C. (Eds.). *Principles and Practice of Sleep Medicine*. Philadelphia: W.B. Saunders, pp. 693–706.

Cespuglio, R., Faradji, H., Gomez, M.E., and Jouvet, M. (1981). Single unit recordings in the nuclei raphe dorsalis and magnus during the sleep–waking cycle of semi-chronic prepared cats. *Neurosci. Lett.*, 24: 133–138.

Chandler, S.H., Chase, M.H., and Nakamura, Y. (1980a). Intracellular analysis of synaptic mechanisms controlling trigeminal motoneuron activity during sleep and wakefulness. *J. Neurophysiol.*, 44: 359–371.

Chandler, S.H., Nakamura, Y., and Chase, M.H. (1980b). Intracellular analysis of synaptic potentials induced in trigeminal jaw-closer motoneurons by pontomesencephalic reticular stimulation during sleep and wakefulness. *J. Neurophysiol.*, 44: 372–382.

Chase, M.H. and Morales, F.R. (1982). Phasic changes in motoneuron membrane potential during REM periods of active sleep. *Neurosci. Lett.*, 34: 177–182.

Chase, M.H. and Morales, F.R. (1990). The atonia and myoclonia of active (REM) sleep. *Annu. Rev. Psychol.*, 41: 557–584.

Chase, M.H., Chandler, S.H., and Nakamura, Y. (1980). Intracellular determination of membrane potential of trigeminal motoneurons during sleep and wakefulness. *J. Neurophysiol.*, 44: 349–358.

Chase, M.H., Soja, P.J., and Morales, F.R. (1989). Evidence that glycine mediates the postsynaptic potentials that inhibit lumbar motoneurons during the atonia of active sleep. *J. Neurosci.*, 9: 743–751.

D'Ascanio, P., Pompeiano, O., and Stampacchia, G. (1988). Noradrenergic and cholinergic mechanisms responsible for the gain regulation of vesibulospinal reflexes. In: *Progress in Brain Research*. Amsterdam: Elsevier Science, pp. 361–373.

Davis, R. (2000). Cerebellar stimulation for cerebral palsy spasticity, function, and seizures. *Arch. Med. Res.*, 31: 290–299.

Di Chiara, G., Tanda, G., and Carboni, E. (1996). Estimation of *in-vivo* neurotransmitter release by brain microdialysis: the issue of validity. *Behav. Pharmacol.*, 7: 640–657.

Doba, N. and Reis, D.J. (1972). Cerebellum: role in reflex cardiovascular adjustment to posture. *Brain Res.*, 39: 495–500.

Duffin, J. and Hockman, C.H. (1972). Limbic forebrain and midbrain modulation and phase-switching of expiratory neurons. *Brain Res.*, 39: 235–239.

Eguchi, K. and Satoh, T. (1980). Characterization of the neurons in the region of solitary tract nucleus during sleep. *Physiol. Behav.*, 24: 99–102.

Foundas, A.L., Bollich, A.M., Corey, D.M., Hurley, M., and Heilman, K.M. (2001). Anomalous anatomy of speech-language areas in adults with persistent developmental stuttering. *Neurology*, 57: 207–215.

Foutz, A.S., Boudinot, E., Morin-Surun, M.P., Champagnat, J., Gonsalves, S.F., and Denavit-Saubie, M. (1987). Excitability of 'silent' respiratory neurons during sleep–waking states: an iontophoretic study in undrugged chronic cats. *Brain Res.*, 404: 10–20.

Fung, S.J. and Barnes, C.D. (1987). Membrane excitability changes in hindlimb motoneurons induced by stimulation of the locus coeruleus in cats. *Brain Res.*, 402: 230–242.

Gastaut, H. and Broughton, R.J. (1965). A clinical and polygraphic study of episodic phenomena during sleep. *Biol. Psychiatry*, 7: 197–221.

Gozal, D., Omidvar, O., Kirlew, K.A., Hathout, G.M., Hamilton, R., Lufkin, R.B., and Harper, R.M. (1995). Identification of human brain regions underlying responses to resistive inspiratory loading with functional magnetic resonance imaging. *Proc. Natl. Acad. Sci.*, 92: 6607–6611.

Gozal, D., Daniel, J.M., and Dohanich, G.P. (2001). Behavioral and anatomical correlates of chronic episodic hypoxia during sleep in the rat. *J. Neurosci.*, 21: 2442–2450.

Guglielmino, S. and Strata, P. (1971). Cerebellum and atonia of the desynchronized phase of sleep. *Arch. Ital. Biol.*, 109: 210–217.

Guilleminault, C. (1994). Clinical features and evaluation of obstructive sleep apnea. In: *Principles and Practice of Sleep Medicine*. Philadelphia: W.B. Saunders Co, pp. 667–677.

Hening, W.A. (2002). Restless legs syndrome: a sensorimotor disorder of sleep/wake motor regulation. *Curr. Neurol. Neurosci. Rep.*, 2: 186–196.

Hobson, J.A., McCarley, R.W., and Wyzinski, P.W. (1975). Sleep cycle oscillation: reciprocal discharge by two brainstem neuronal groups. *Science*, 189: 55–58.

Jacobs, B.L. (1991). Serotonin and behavior: emphasis on motor control. *J. Clin. Psychiatry*, 52 (Suppl): 17–23.

Jacobson, A., Kales, A., Lehmann, D., and Zweizig, J.R. (1965). Somnambulism: all night electroencephalographic studies. *Science*, 148: 975–977.

Javaheri, S., Parker, T.J., Liming, J.D., Corbett, W.S., Nishiyama, H., Wexler, L., and Roselle, G.A. (1998). Sleep apnea in 81 ambulatory male patients with stable heart failure. Types and their prevalences, consequences, and presentations. *Circulation*, 97: 2154–2159.

John, J., Wu, M.-F., Kodama, T., and Siegel, J.M. (2003). Intravenously administered hypocretin-1 alters brain amino acid release: an *in vivo* microdialysis study in rats. *J. Physiol., (Lond.)*, 548(2): 557–562.

Jones, B.E. (1991). Noradrenergic locus coeruleus neurons: their distant connections and their relationship to neighboring (including cholinergic and GABAergic) neurons of the central gray and reticular formation. *Prog. Brain Res.*, 88: 15–30.

Kekesi, K.A., Dobolyi, A., Salfay, O., Nyitrai, G., and Juhasz, G. (1997). Slow wave sleep is accompanied by release of certain amino acids in the thalamus of cats. *Neuroreport*, 8: 1183–1186.

Kodama, T., Lai, Y.Y., and Siegel, J.M. (2003). Changes in inhibitory amino acid release linked to pontine-induced atonia: an *in vivo* microdialysis study. *J. Neurosci.*, 23: 1548–1554.

Kohyama, J., Lai, Y.Y., and Siegel, J.M. (1998a). Inactivation of the pons blocks medullary-induced muscle tone suppression in the decerebrate cat. *Sleep*, 21: 695–699.

Kohyama, J., Lai, Y.Y., and Siegel, J.M. (1998b). Reticulospinal systems mediate atonia with short and long latencies. *J. Neurophysiol.*, 80: 1839–1851.

Kubin, L., Tojima, H., Davies, R.O., and Pack, A.I. (1992). Serotonergic excitatory drive to hypoglossal motoneurons in the decerebrate cat. *Neurosci. Lett.*, 139: 243–248.

Kubin, L., Kimura, H., Tojima, H., Davies, R.O., and Pack, A.I. (1993). Suppression of hypoglossal motoneurons during the carbachol-induced atonia of REM sleep is not caused by fast synaptic inhibition. *Brain Res.*, 611: 300–312.

Kubin, L., Reignier, C., Tojima, H., Taguchi, O., Pack, A.I., and Davies, R.O. (1994). Changes in serotonin level in the hypoglossal nucleus region during carbachol-induced atonia. *Brain Res.*, 645: 291–302.

Kubin, L., Tojima, H., Reignier, C., Pack, A.I., and Davies, R.O. (1996). Interaction of serotonergic excitatory drive to hypoglossal motoneurons with carbachol-induced, REM sleep-like atonia. *Sleep*, 19: 187–195.

Lai, Y.Y. and Siegel, J.M. (1988). Medullary regions mediating atonia. *J. Neurosci.*, 8: 4790–4796.

Lai, Y.Y. and Siegel, J.M. (1991). Ponto-medullary glutamate receptors mediating locomotion and muscle tone suppression. *J. Neurosci.*, 11: 2931–2937.

Lai, Y.Y. and Siegel, J.M. (2003). Physiological and anatomical link between Parkinson-like disease and REM sleep behavior disorder. *Mol. Neurobiol.*, 27: 137–152.

Lai, Y.Y., Strahlendorf, H.K., Fung, S.J., and Barnes, C.D. (1989). The actions of two monoamines on spinal motoneurons from stimulation of the locus coeruleus in the cat. *Brain Res.*, 484: 268–272.

Lai, Y.Y., Clements, J., and Siegel, J. (1993). Glutamatergic and cholinergic projections to the pontine inhibitory area identified with horseradish peroxidase retrograde transport and immunohistochemistry. *J. Comp. Neurol.*, 336: 321–330.

Lai, Y.Y., Clements, J.R., Wu, X.Y., Shalita, T., Wu, J.P., Kuo, J.S., and Siegel, J.M. (1999). Brainstem projections to the ventromedial medulla in cat: retrograde transport horseradish peroxidase and immunohistochemical studies. *J. Comp. Neurol.*, 408: 419–436.

Lai, Y.Y., Kodama, T., and Siegel, J.M. (2001). Changes in monoamine release in the ventral horn and hypoglossal nucleus linked to pontine inhibition of muscle tone: an *in vivo* microdialysis study. *J. Neurosci.*, 21: 7384–7391.

Lavigne, G.J. and Manzini, C. (2003). Bruxism. In: Kryger, M., Roth, T., and Dement, W.C. (Eds.). *Principles and Practice of Sleep Medicine.* Philadelphia: W.B. Saunders, pp. 773–785.

Lavigne, G.J. and Montplaisir, J.Y. (1994). Restless legs syndrome and sleep bruxism: prevalence and association among Canadians. *Sleep*, 17: 739–743.

Lazorthes, Y., Sol, J.C., Sallerin, B., and Verdie, J.C. (2002). The surgical management of spasticity. *Eur. J. Neurol.*, 9 (Suppl 1): 35–41.

Liu, R.H., Fung, S.J., Reddy, V.K., and Barnes, C.D. (1995). Localization of glutamatergic neurons in the dorsolateral pontine tegmentum projecting to the spinal cord of the cat with a proposed role of glutamate on lumbar motoneuron activity. *Neuroscience*, 64: 193–208.

Liu, X., Sood, S., Liu, H., Nolan, P., Morrison, J.L., and Horner, R.L. (2003). Suppression of genioglossus muscle tone and activity during reflex hypercapnic stimulation by GABA(A) mechanisms at the hypoglossal motor nucleus *in vivo. Neuroscience*, 116: 249–259.

Lobbezoo, F. and Lavigne, G.J. (1997). Do bruxism and temporomandibular disorders have a cause-and-effect relationship? *J. Orofac. Pain*, 11: 15–23.

Lobbezoo, F., Lavigne, G.J., Tanguay, R., and Montplaisir, J.Y. (1997). The effect of catecholamine precursor L-dopa on sleep bruxism: a controlled clinical trial. *Mov. Disord.*, 12: 73–78.

Lyons, W.E., Fritschy, J.M., and Grzanna, R. (1989). The noradrenergic neurotoxin DSP-4 eliminates the coeruleospinal projection but spares projections of the A5 and A7 groups to the ventral horn of the rat spinal cord. *J. Neurosci.*, 9: 1481–1489.

Macey, P.M., Henderson, L.A., Macey, K.E., Alger, J.R., Frysinger, R.C., Woo, M.A., Harper, R.K., Yan-Go, F.L., and Harper, R.M. (2002). Brain morphology associated with obstructive sleep apnea. *Am. J. Respir. Crit. Care Med.*, 166: 1382–1387.

Marshall, D.L., Redfern, P.H., and Wonnacott, S. (1997). Presynaptic nicotinic modulation of dopamine release in the three ascending pathways studied by *in vivo* microdialysis: comparison of naive and chronic nicotine-treated rats. *J. Neurochem.*, 68: 1511–1519.

Martínez-Rodríguez, Lin, L., Iranzo, A., Genid, D., Marti, M.J., Santamaría, J., and Mignot, E. (2003). Decreased hypocretin-1 (orexin-A) levels in the cerebrospinal fluid of patients with myotonic dystrophy and excessive daytime sleepiness. *Sleep*, 26: 287–290.

McGinty, D.J. and Harper, R.M. (1976). Dorsal raphe neurons: depression of firing during sleep in cats. *Brain Res.*, 101: 569–575.

McGinty, D. and Sakai, K. (1973). Unit activity in the dorsal pontine reticular formation in the cat. *Sleep Res.*, 2: 33.

Mileykovskiy, B.Y., Kiyashchenko, L.I., Kodama, T., Lai., Y.Y., and Siegel, J.M. (2000). Activation of pontine and medullary motor inhibitory regions reduces discharge in neurons located in the locus coeruleus and the anatomical equivalent of the midbrain locomotor region. *J. Neurosci.*, 20: 8551–8558.

Moises, H.C. and Woodward, D.J. (1980). Potentiation of GABA inhibitory action in cerebellum by locus coeruleus stimulation. *Brain Res.*, 182: 327–344.

Morales, F.R., Engelhardt, J.K., Soja, P.J., and Pereda, A.E. (1987). Motoneuron properties during motor inhibition produced by microinjection of carbachol into the pontine reticular formation of the decerebrate cat. *J. Neurophysiol.*, 57: 1118–1129.

Morrison, J.L., Sood, S., Liu, X., Liu, H., Park, E., Nolan, P., and Horner, R.L. (2002). Glycine at hypoglossal motor nucleus: genioglossus activity, $CO(2)$ responses, and the additive effects of GABA. *J. Appl. Physiol.*, 93: 1786–1796.

Morrison, J.L., Sood, S., Liu, H., Park, E., Nolan, P., and Horner, R.L. (2003). GABA receptor antagonism at the hypoglossal motor nucleus increases genioglossus muscle activity in NREM but not REM sleep. *J. Physiol.*, 548: 569–583.

Naegele, B., Pepin, J.L., Levy, P., Bonnet, C., Pellat, J., and Feuerstein, C. (1998). Cognitive executive dysfunction in patients with obstructive sleep apnea syndrome (OSAS) after CPAP treatment. *Sleep*, 21: 392–397.

Nakamura, Y., Goldberg, L.J., Chandler, S.H., and Chase, M.H. (1978). Intracellular analysis of trigeminal motoneuron activity during sleep in the cat. *Science*, 199: 204–207.

Nitz, D. and Siegel. J.M. (1996). GABA release in the posterior hypothalamus of the cat as a function of sleep/wake state. *Am. J. Physiol.*, 40: 1707–1712.

Nitz, D. and Siegel, J.M. (1997a). GABA release in the cat locus coeruleus as a function of the sleep/wake state. *Neuroscience*, 78: 795–801.

Nitz, D. and Siegel, J.M. (1997b). GABA release in the dorsal raphe nucleus: role in the control of REM sleep. *Am. J. Physiol.*, 273: R451–R455.

Nygren, L. and Olson, L. (1977). A new major projection from locus coeruleus: the main source of noradrenergic nerve terminals in the ventral and dorsal columns of the spinal cord. *Brain Res.*, 132: 95–93.

O'Brien, J.A. and Berger, A.J. (1999). Cotransmission of GABA and glycine to brain-stem motoneurons. *J. Neurophysiol.*, 82: 1638–1641.

Odin, P., Mrowka, M., and Shing, M. (2002). Restless legs syndrome. *Eur. J. Neuro.*, Suppl 3: 59–67.

Okabe, S., Woch, G., and Kubin, L. (1994). Role of GABAb receptors in the control of hypoglossal motoneurons *in vivo. Neuroreport*, 5: 2573–2576.

Parker, K.P. and Rye, D.B. (2002). Restless legs syndrome and periodic limb movement disorder. *Nurs. Clin. North. Am.*, 337: 655–673.

Parkis, M.A., Bayliss, D.A., and Berger, A.J. (1995). Actions of norepinephrine on rat hypoglossal motoneurons. *J. Neurophysiol.*, 74: 1911–1919.

Pichiule, P., Chavez, J.C., Boero, J., and Arregui, A. (1996). Chronic hypoxia induces modification of the *N*-methyl-D-aspartate receptor in rat brain. *Neurosci. Lett.*, 218: 83–86.

Poe, G.R., Kristensen, M.P., Rector, D.M., and Harper, R.M. Hippocampal activity during transient respiratory events in the freely behaving cat. *Neuroscience*, 72: 39–48, 1996.

Reddy, V.K., Fung, S.J., Zhuo, H., and Barnes, C.D. (1989). Spinally projecting noradrenergic neurons of the dorsolateral pontine tegmentum: a combined immunocytochemical and retrograde labeling study. *Brain Res.*, 491: 144–149.

Ripley, B., Overeem, S., Fujiki, N., Nevsimalova, S., Uchino, M., Yesavage, J., Di Monte, D., Dohi, K., Melberg, A., Lammers, G.J., Nishida, Y., Roelandse, F.W., Hungs, M., Mignot, E., and Nishino, S. (2001). CSF hypocretin/orexin levels in narcolepsy and other neurological conditions. *Neurology*, 57: 2253–2258.

Rueter, L.E. and Jacobs, B.L. (1996). A microdialysis examination of serotonin release in the rat forebrain induced by behavioral/environmental manipulations. *Brain Res.*, 739: 57–69.

Ruit, K.G. and Neafsey, E.J. (1988). Cardiovascular and respiratory responses to electrical and chemical stimulation of the hippocampus in anesthetized and awake rats. *Brain Res.*, 457(2): 310–321.

Sakai, K., Mercier, G.V., and Jouvet, M. (1983). Evidence for the presence of PS-off neurons in the ventromedial medulla oblongata of freely moving cats. *Exp. Brain Res.*, 49: 311–314.

Salorio, C.F., White, D.A., Piccirillo, J., Duntley, S.P., and Uhles, M.L. (2002). Learning, memory, and executive control in individuals with obstructive sleep apnea syndrome. *J. Clin. Exp. Neuropsychol.*, 24: 93–100.

Satoh, K., Tohyama, M., Yamamoto, K., Sakumotot, T., and Shimizu, N. (1977). Noradrenaline innervation of the spinal cord studied by the horseradish peroxidase method combined with monoamine oxidase staining. *Exp. Brain Res.*, 30: 175–186.

Sauerland, E.K. and Harper, R.M. (1976). The human tongue during sleep: electromyographic activity of the genioglossus muscle. *Exp. Neurol.*, 51: 160–170.

Shahar, E., Whitney, C., Redline, S., Lee, E., Newman, A., Javier, N., O'Connor, G., Boland, L., Schwartz, J., and Samet, J. (2001). Sleep-disordered breathing and cardiovascular disease cross-sectional results of the sleep heart health study. *Am. J. Respir. Crit. Care Med.*, 163: 19.

Siegel, J.M. (1979). Behavioral relations of medullary reticular formation cells. *Exp. Neurol.*, 65: 691–698.

Siegel, J.M. and Tomaszewski, K.S. (1983). Behavioral organization of reticular formation: Studies in the unrestrained cat. I. Cells related to axial, limb, eye, and other movements. *J. Neurophysiol.*, 50: 696–716.

Siegel, J.M., Tomaszewski, K.S., and Wheeler, R.L. (1983). Behavioral organization of reticular formation: Studies in the unrestrained cat: II. Cells related to facial movements. *J. Neurophysiol.*, 50: 717–723.

Sin, D.D., Fitzgerald, F., Parker, J.D., Newton, G., Floras, J.S., and Bradley, T.D. (1999). Risk factors for central and obstructive sleep apnea in 450 men and women with congestive heart failure. *Am. J. Respir. Crit. Care Med.*, 160: 1101.

Soja, P.J., Morales, F.R., Baranyi, A., and Chase, M.H. (1987). Effect of inhibitory amino acid antagonists on IPSPs induced in lumbar motoneurons upon stimulation of the nucleus reticularis gigantocellularis during active sleep. *Brain Res.*, 423: 353–358.

Soja, P.J., López-Rodríguez, F., Morales, F.R., and Chase, M. (1991). The postsynaptic inhibitory control of lumbar motoneurons during the atonia of active sleep: effect of strychnine on motoneuron properties. *J. Neurosci.*, 11: 2804–2811.

Trenkwalder, C. (2003). Restless legs syndrome and periodic limb movements. *Adv. Neurol.*, 89: 145–151.

Trulson, M.E., Jacobs, B.L., and Morrison, A.R. (1981). Raphe unit activity during REM sleep in normal cats and in pontine lesioned cats displaying REM sleep without atonia. *Brain Res.*, 226: 75–91.

Umemiya, M. and Berger, A.J. (1995). Presynaptic inhibition by serotonin of glycinergic inhibitory synaptic currents in the rat brain stem. *J. Neurophysiol.*, 73: 1192–1201.

White, S.R., Fung, S.J., Jackson, D.A., and Imel, K.M. (1996). Serotonin, norepinephrine and associated neuropeptides: effects on somatic motoneuron excitability. *Prog. Brain Res.*, 107: 183–199.

Wu, M.F., John, J., Maidment, N., Lam, H.A., and Siegel, J.M. (2002). Hypocretin release in normal and narcoleptic dogs after food and sleep deprivation, eating, and movement. *Am. J. Physiol. Regul. Integr. Comp. Physiol.*, 283: 1079–1086.

Yamuy, J., Fung, S.J., Xi, M., Morales, F.R., and Chase, M.H. (1999). Hypoglossal motoneurons are postsynaptically inhibited during carbachol-induced rapid eye movement sleep. *Neuroscience*, 94: 11–15.

Chapter 14

NEURAL CONTROL OF BREATHING IN SLEEP

John M. Orem[1]

This chapter deals with the mechanisms by which the state of consciousness affects the respiratory system. The central idea is that state effects are the result of variations in tonic inputs to the respiratory system.

Neural Control of Respiration in Nonrapid Eye Movement (NREM) Sleep

In humans, there are four stages of NREM sleep. For consideration of the respiratory system, Krieger (2000) divided NREM sleep into unsteady (stages I and II) NREM sleep and steady (stages III and IV) NREM sleep. In unsteady NREM sleep, 40–80% of normal subjects have regular oscillations in the amplitude of breathing. The wavelength of the periodicity varies between 30 and 120 s. Although amplitude waxes and wanes, the frequency of breathing is generally constant. This pattern of breathing occurs during light NREM sleep and is associated with alternating patterns of arousal and sleep in the electroencephalogram. Large amplitude breaths are associated with arousal, and smaller amplitude breaths, or apnea, occur during sleep. Interpretations of this phenomenon generally rely on the importance of a wakefulness stimulus for the respiratory system that at sleep onset is lost, causing a reduction in breathing, and that upon arousal is regained,

---

[1]john.orem@ttuhsc.edu

303

and causes hyperventilation. Other evidences of the wakefulness stimulus are the reduced slope of the ventilatory response to CO_2 in NREM sleep (Douglas, 2000) and the post-hyperventilation apnea that occurs in NREM sleep but not wakefulness (Fink, 1961).

In steady NREM sleep, breathing is highly regular and minute ventilation decreases (Krieger, 2000). The decreased ventilation is not just the result of a decreased metabolic rate, because end tidal CO_2 is increased. Therefore, the hypoventilation is apparently the result of the loss of the wakefulness stimulus or inhibitory effects of (unknown) sleep processes. Krieger favors the latter interpretation because ventilation decreases progressively from light to deep NREM sleep and because the loss of wakefulness apparently occurs as a discrete event. However, the wakefulness stimulus may be an arousal stimulus related to the level of central nervous system (CNS) excitation that varies continuously in intensity from aroused wakefulness to deep sleep.

Studies in animals report results like those in steady NREM sleep in humans. In cat and dog, the frequency of breathing is lower and more regular in NREM sleep than in wakefulness (Orem et al., 1977; Phillipson, 1978). Peak instantaneous airflow rate and the peak negative pressure developed against a narrowed airway decrease whereas upper airway resistance increases. Tidal volume increases as the result of an increased duration of inspiration, but minute ventilation decreases and end-tidal CO_2 concentrations increase. These findings can be explained also by the loss of a wakefulness or arousal stimulus.

Studies of single respiratory neurons indicate that the arousal stimulus is tonic. There is a decrease in medullary respiratory neuronal activity in NREM sleep (Orem et al., 1974, 1985; Puizillout and Ternaux, 1974; Foutz et al., 1987). Neurons in both the ventral and dorsal respiratory groups are affected, but the effect depends on the amount of nonrespiratory (tonic) activity in the activity of a respiratory cell. Respiratory cells whose activity depends primarily on tonic inputs and only weakly on respiratory-modulated inputs are affected more by sleep than respiratory cells whose activity depends primarily on rhythmic, respiratory-related inputs (Figures 1 and 2). Among the former cells are some upper airway motor neurons (Orem et al., 1985). In contrast, neurons whose activity is primarily determined by rhythmic, respiratory inputs do not show dramatic changes in activity in NREM sleep compared to relaxed wakefulness. The persistence of respiratory activity but the loss of tonic activity in NREM sleep is shown also by experiments in which glutamate is applied to respiratory cells

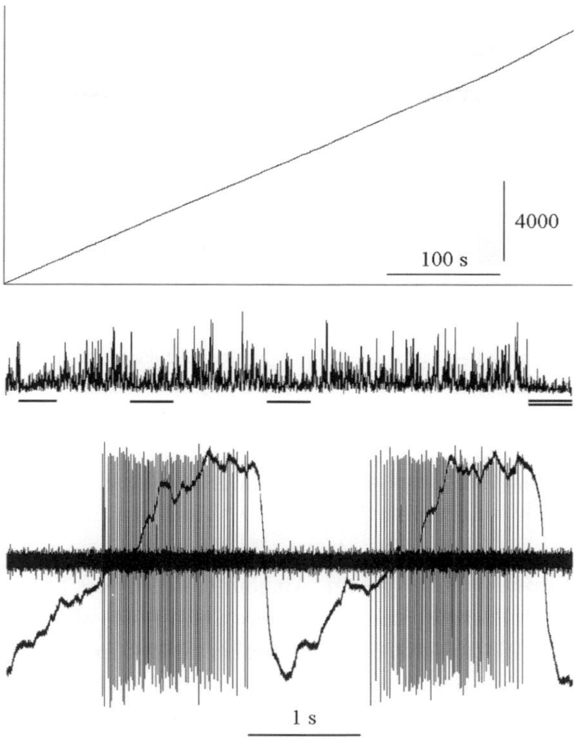

Figure 1. Activity of an expiratory–inspiratory neuron from wakefulness to the onset of REM sleep. (Top) Cumulative action potential counts as a function of time. The tracing below this plot shows the half-wave rectified electroencephalogram. Periods of arousal are underscored. REM sleep onset is denoted by double underscoring. (Bottom) The activity of the cell superimposed on airflow. Inspiratory airflows are signified by upward deflections of the airflow tracing. Note that the activity of this cell is invariant (the slope of the cumulative count curve is constant) throughout the alternating periods of wakefulness and NREM sleep but increases at the onset of REM sleep. A straight line through the cumulative count curve shows the invariance of the activity in wakefulness/NREM sleep. In REM sleep, the slope of the curve increases and the curve departs from the straight line. (From Orem *et al.*, 2002.)

that are silent during sleep. The cells become rhythmically active following application of the excitatory neurotransmitter (Foutz *et al.*, 1987). This indicates that respiratory-modulated inputs to the cells are still present in sleep but are subthreshold because of a loss of tonic excitatory inputs.

In conclusion, respiratory activity in NREM sleep is reduced because of the loss of arousal-dependent stimuli (the wakefulness stimulus) that

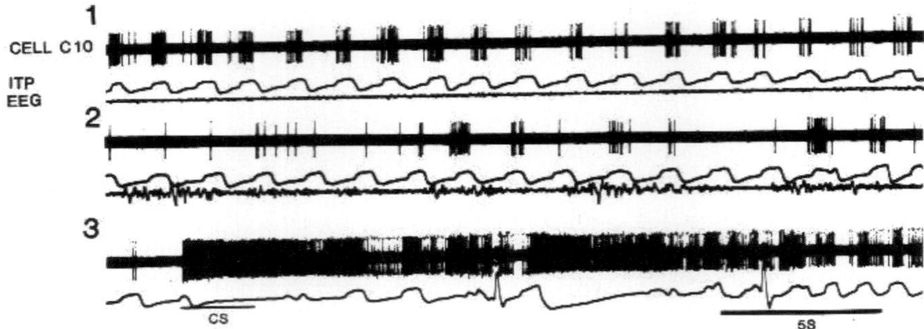

Figure 2. A medullary inspiratory cell that was sleep sensitive. (1) Spontaneous activity of the cell during wakefulness; *top trace*, action potentials of the cell; *middle trace*, intratracheal pressure, negative pressures indicated by upward deflections; *lower trace*, electroencephalogram. (2) Spontaneous activity of the cell during drowsiness or NREM sleep. Note that the respiratory activity of the cell decreased in drowsiness/NREM sleep. (3) Intense activation of the cell during and after behavioral inhibition of inspiration elicited by a conditioning stimulus (CS). (From Orem, 1989.)

provide tonic inputs to the system. Although all sources of tonic inputs are not known, the following will be addressed here: (1) the brainstem reticular formation; (2) the collection of higher structures that exert behavioral control on the respiratory system; (3) aminergic brainstem nuclei; and (4) hypothalamic orexin-containing neurons. All excite the respiratory system and may individually or collectively constitute an arousal stimulus for breathing that is lost in sleep. Central neurons sensitive to pH/CO_2 also excite breathing but their identity and the effects of sleep on their activity are not known.

Reticular formation

Stimulation of the reticular formation excites the respiratory system. Midbrain reticular stimulation causes a reduction in the duration of expiration and an increased rate of rise and amplitude of phrenic nerve activity (Hugelin and Cohen, 1963). Reticular stimulation causes also an increase in laryngeal abductor activity, converting it from patterns characteristic of NREM sleep to those of wakefulness, and, like wakefulness, reticular stimulation preferentially facilitates the activity of the muscles of the upper airway rather than the muscles of the diaphragm (Orem and Lydic, 1978). These results imply that, during the transition from wakefulness to NREM sleep, the muscles of the upper airway may lose their tonic excitatory inputs to a greater extent than the diaphragm. This could lead to occlusive collapse of the airway during sleep.

The differential effects of reticular stimulation on upper airway and diaphragmatic activity explain also results showing that upper airway motor neurons are more sensitive than those of phrenic motor neurons to the depressive effects of ethanol, diazepam, pentobarbital, halothane, hypocapnia, chemical stimuli, and thermal depression of neuronal activity near the ventral medullary surface (Bonora *et al.*, 1984, 1985; St. John and Bledsoe, 1985; St. John, 1986; St. John *et al.*, 1986). Also, the systems controlling the upper airway muscles are more sensitive than those of the diaphragm to the excitatory effects of protriptyline, strychnine, cyanide, and doxapram.

The preferential effect of arousal on upper airway muscles compared to the diaphragm is seen also in responses to occlusions of the airway applied during sleep (Orem *et al.*, 1980; Brouillette and Thach, 1979a,b; Mezzanotte *et al.*, 1992; Wheatley *et al.*, 1993). The progressive response of the genioglossus muscle to occlusion, as well as the response to hypoxia and hypercapnia, is quantitatively greater than the diaphragmatic response (Brouillette and Thach, 1979a,b). In addition, dilations of the airways to negative pressure during sleep are weak compared to those in wakefulness.

Behavioral control

Behavioral control of breathing may be reflexive, as occurs in sneezing, coughing, vomiting, and eructation, or voluntary, as during speaking, breath holding, and playing a wind instrument. These behavioral acts require the integration of nonrespiratory inputs into circuits of the respiratory oscillator, and generally occur only in wakefulness. For example, mechanical and chemical stimulation of the larynx (Sullivan *et al.*, 1979a) and bronchopulmonary stimulation (Sullivan *et al.*, 1979b) cause coughing in wakefulness but not in sleep (Anderson *et al.*, 1996). It is not known why these responses can occur in wakefulness but not sleep, but it may be that the readiness of behavioral control in wakefulness constitutes a stimulus for the respiratory system that is lost in sleep. This may be relevant to obstructive sleep apnea if what is lost in sleep is a wakefulness-dependent behavioral compensation for a high upper airway resistance.

The list of structures that can contribute to behavioral control of brainstem and spinal respiratory neurons includes structures from all levels of the neuraxis. The controls exerted by some telencephalic structures, for

example, the amygdala and the central gray, may occur in relation to
emotional and volitional acts (Reis and McHugh, 1968; Eldridge *et al.*,
1981; Plum and Leigh, 1981). Little is known about the neurophysiology
of behavioral control. Respiratory cells involved in this control may be less
active in sleep. Studies in cats show that behavioral inhibition of inspiration
does not depend on cells within the central pattern generator that inhibit
inspiration during spontaneous breathing but rather on a class of cells that
is excited primarily by tonic sources and that is affected greatly by sleep
(Figure 2). Furthermore, in patients with obstructive sleep apnea, dilation
of the upper airways to a degree sufficient to overcome obstruction may
be a behavioral compensatory response that depends on wakefulness and is
lost in sleep (Mezzanotte *et al.*, 1992).

Aminergic systems

The activities of serotonin (5-hydroxytryptamine [5-HT])- and
norepinephrine-containing neurons of the brainstem decrease during sleep
(Heym *et al.*, 1982; Trulson and Trulson, 1982). These cells have extensive
axonal projections to respiratory regions. Both central respiratory neurons
and respiratory motor neurons have receptors for 5-HT and norepinephrine.
5-HT has excitatory effects on motor neurons, including those innervating
the upper airway and respiratory pump muscles (Kubin *et al.*, 1992a). Similar to 5-HT, norepinephrine is predominantly excitatory to motor neurons,
but its effect on medullary respiratory neurons is inhibitory (Champagnat
et al., 1979; Funk *et al.*, 1994). The magnitude of the excitatory effect of
5-HT on different groups of upper airway motor neurons varies (Fenik *et al.*,
1997), and the same might be the case for norepinephrine. These differences
could account for differences in the magnitude of the suppressant effect of
sleep on different upper airway muscles.

Hypothalamic orexinergic neurons

The hypothalamus controls the respiratory system to maintain homeostasis during thermoregulation, in response to changes in metabolism, and
during motor activation. A group of hypothalamic neurons containing excitatory peptides, orexins (also known as hypocretins), have been described
in the perifornical region of the posterior hypothalamus. These cells have
widespread axonal projections that target wakefulness-related neuronal
groups (serotonergic, noradrenergic, histaminergic, and cholinergic), as well
as motor neurons and sympathetic preganglionic neurons (Peyron *et al.*,

1998). The activity of orexin neurons and orexin release are maximal during wakefulness, especially in relation to motor activation (Estabrooke *et al.*, 2001; Yoshida *et al.*, 2001; Kiyashchenko *et al.*, 2002; Torterolo *et al.*, 2003). Thus, orexins have the potential to enhance respiratory output in wakefulness by their direct actions on motor neurons and indirectly by stimulating the activity of brainstem aminergic neurons.

Conclusion

Breathing is reduced and can fail in NREM sleep. Dilation of the extrathoracic airway may be insufficient and/or respiratory efforts can stop altogether. The loss of tonic inputs that constitute an arousal or waking stimulus to the respiratory system may be the cause of the reduction and, in sleep apnea, failure of breathing in NREM sleep. The possible sources of tonic inputs include structures throughout the CNS. However, evidence of tonic excitatory roles is particularly strong for the collections of structures in the brain stem that are essential for wakefulness (reticular formation from the rostral pons to the posterior hypothalamus) and that have state-dependent activity (aminergic neurons of the raphe nuclei and locus coeruleus).

Neural Control of Breathing in Rapid Eye Movement (REM) Sleep

Breathing is in some ways excited and in other ways inhibited in REM sleep. Excitation is evident from the rapid and irregular rate and from, in cat at least, lower end tidal CO_2 levels signifying hyperventilation (Orem *et al.*, 1977, 2000; Phillipson, 1978). The irregular breathing pattern of REM sleep is evidently the result of internal processes, because it does not depend on variations in chemoreceptor (Gauzzi and Freis, 1969), vagal (Dawes *et al.*, 1972; Remmers *et al.*, 1976; Foutz *et al.*, 1979), or thoracic (Netick and Foutz, 1980) afferent activity. These processes may also blunt ventilatory responses to chemical stimuli and other respiratory reflexes, such as the responses to occlusions (Phillipson, 1978; Orem *et al.*, 1980). Inhibitory processes are in part the result of the atonia of the state. In cats (Parmeggiani and Sabattini, 1972) and adolescent humans (Tabachnik *et al.*, 1981), but not in rats (Megirian *et al.*, 1987), atonia of the intercostal muscles reduces or eliminates costal breathing in REM sleep. Many upper airway respiratory muscles are also atonic or hypotonic (Orem and Lydic, 1978). Postinspiratory diaphragmatic activity in cat also decreases in REM sleep (Lovering *et al.*, 2003), but in general the diaphragm is spared the atonia. Obstructive episodes are the longest, and blood oxygen desaturations most severe, during REM sleep in patients with obstructive sleep apnea. Similarly, oxygen desaturations are generally most severe during REM sleep in patients with lung disease.

Here we consider the internal excitatory and inhibitory processes that affect the respiratory system in REM sleep.

Increased respiratory neuronal activity in REM sleep: Endogenous excitatory drive

Central respiratory neurons, like most cells throughout the nervous system, are more active in REM sleep than in NREM sleep (Figure 3). Medullary respiratory neurons activated in REM sleep include augmenting and late inspiratory cells (Orem, 1994) and some augmenting expiratory cells, which are active even during the very short expirations that occur during periods of irregular and rapid breathing (Orem, 1998) (Figure 4).

Excitation of respiratory cells in REM sleep is the result of endogenous drive(s). Excitation occurs even when mechanical and chemical variables (e.g., airway resistance, chest wall compliance, CO_2 tensions) are removed or held constant by mechanical ventilation (Figures 5 and 6) (Orem, *et al.*, 2000). Thus, the excitatory drive is not reflexive and must have an internal source, and possibly an internal source that is specific to REM sleep — an idea supported by positive relations between the activity of some respiratory neurons and phasic REM sleep activity (Orem, 1980) and between the rate of breathing in REM sleep and the activity of REM sleep-specific neurons (Netick *et al.*, 1977). The anatomical sources of the endogenous excitatory drive are unknown. It has been proposed that the drive may cause the first respiratory movements *in utero* (Ioffe *et al.*, 1993) and the rapid, irregular breathing characteristic of REM sleep (Orem *et al.*, 2000).

Endogenous drive may be the result of activation of behavioral mechanisms during dreams. Evidence of this comes from reported relations between the pattern of breathing and the content of the dream. Just as eye movements have been related to a dream involving visual scanning, the pattern of breathing is sometimes appropriate to physical activity in the dream. One study found that the probability of a dream report and the vividness, emotional content, and amount of physical activity in the dream were higher when breathing rates were high and variable. They found also that specific respiratory content was twice as likely when the subject

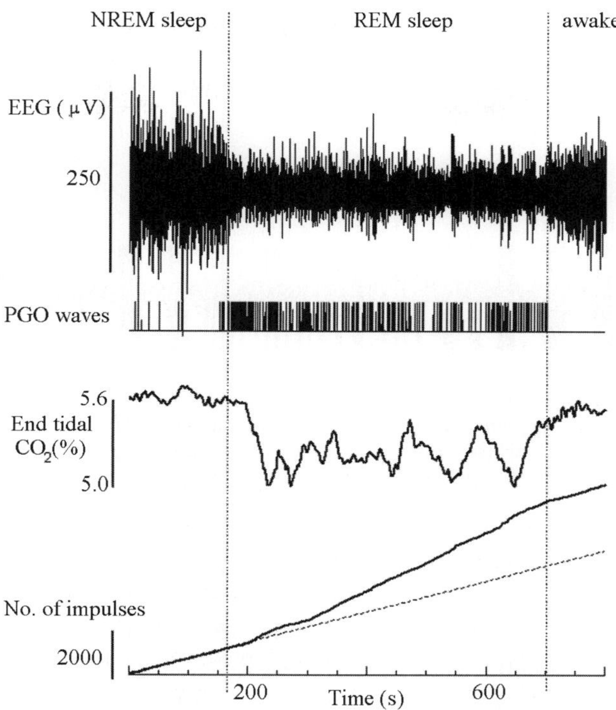

Figure 3. End-tidal CO$_2$ percentage and activity of a respiratory neuron during spontaneous breathing in NREM and REM sleep and wakefulness. Neuronal activity is shown as cumulative impulses from the beginning of the record. The dashed line is 8 impulses per second. In REM sleep the mean discharge rate increased to 14 impulses per second. The neuron was an augmenting inspiratory cell with an η^2 value of 0.9. (From Orem *et al.*, 2000.)

was awakened following apnea as compared to following other respiratory patterns (Hobson *et al.*, 1965). Other studies found that highly variable rates of breathing were associated with reports of the sleeper having little active participation in the dream and of little physical aggression in it, but large-amplitude breaths were associated with the sleeper having intense active participation in the dream, and variability in amplitude was associated with dreams containing a high degree of physical aggression (Baust and Engel, 1971). These results support the idea that breathing patterns may parallel the content of the dream. Other literature is less convincing. Hauri and Van de Castle (1973) examined heart rate, the galvanic skin response, and breathing in relation to dream emotionality, physical activity in the

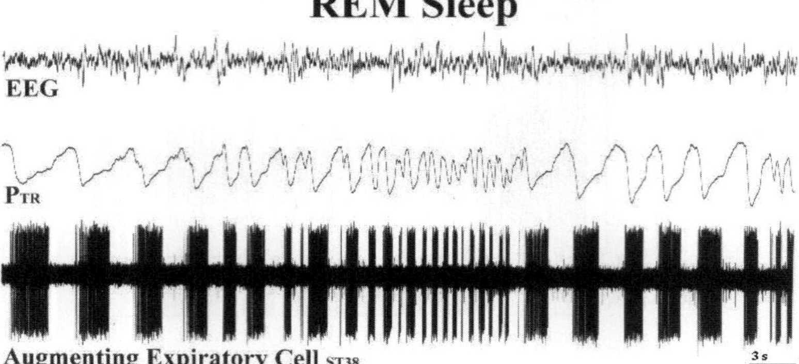

Figure 4. Activity of an augmenting expiratory cell in REM sleep. EEG, electroencephalogram; P_{TR}; tracheal pressure. The entire episode shown here is 27 s in length. The rapid breathing in the middle of the tracings has a frequency of approximately 180 breaths per minute. (From Orem, 1998.)

dream and dream intensity. Respiration rate was related to emotionality and to dream intensity, but there was no significant relation between physical activity in the dream and the rate of breathing. Furthermore, mentation (dreaming) indistinguishable from that in REM sleep occurs also in NREM sleep (Pace-Schott *et al.*, 2003). If endogenous drive is the result of behavioral activation, then it should appear in NREM sleep as well as in REM sleep.

The existence of a REM sleep dependent endogenous excitatory drive to the respiratory system is not in doubt, but it is uncertain whether this drive is the result of behavioral or other processes. Correlations between dreams and breathing patterns have been found in some but not in other studies, and correlations between REM sleep events, such as pontogeniculo-occipital waves, and respiratory activity are statistically weak (Dunin-Barkowski and Orem, 1998; Orem *et al.*, 2000). It may be then that endogenous drive has many sources and many causes. The endogenous drive may be clinically important. At times it can be so intense that it causes hypoventilation as a result of respiratory fibrillation (Figure 4). Respiratory rates can exceed $200\,\mathrm{min}^{-1}$, and tidal volumes are so small that only dead space is ventilated.

The atonia of REM sleep

Atonia of intercostal muscles occurs in REM sleep in cats (Parmeggiani and Sabattini, 1972) and adolescent humans (Tabachnik *et al.*, 1981), but not in

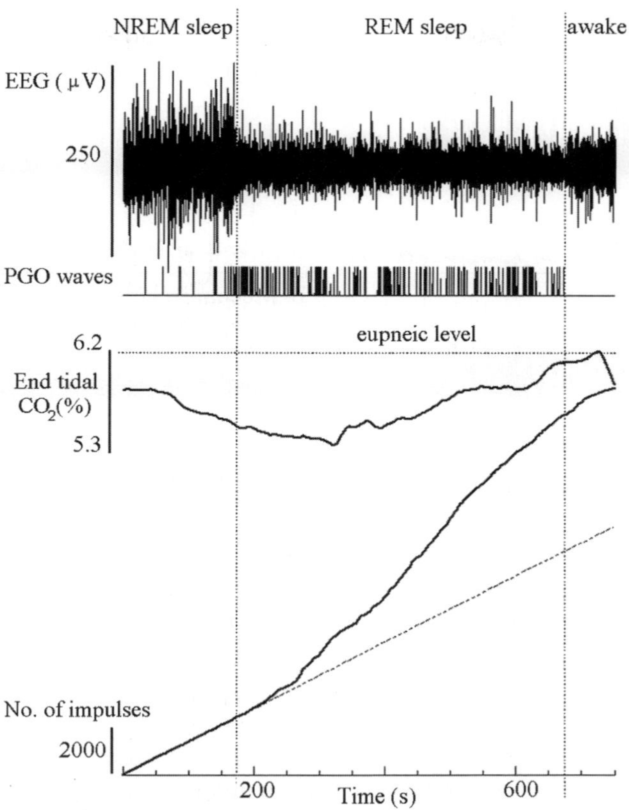

Figure 5. Excitation in REM sleep of a respiratory neuron during mechanical ventilation. The dashed line is NREM sleep discharge rate of 16.7 impulses per second. The cell is an expiratory–inspiratory phase spanning cell with an η^2 value of 0.9. (From Orem *et al.*, 2000.)

rats (Megirian *et al.*, 1987). Other accessory respiratory muscles such as the scalene and sternocleidomastoid muscles are also atonic in REM sleep (e.g., Johnson and Remmers, 1984), but the diaphragm is largely spared. Presumably this atonia, like that affecting other spinal motor neurons (Glenn *et al.*, 1978), is the result of active inhibition mediated by glycine (see Pompeiano, 1967, for an early review proposing that atonia is the result of active inhibition) and involves pathways from the dorsolateral pons into the medullary reticular formation and spinal cord. Lesions of the pontine region of locus coeruleus and subcoeruleus produce a syndrome of REM sleep without atonia (Sastre and Jouvet, 1979). Stimulation of medullary

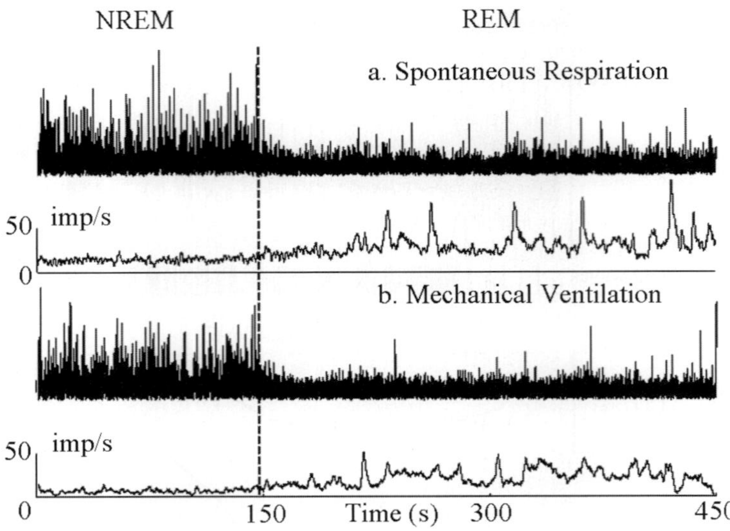

Figure 6. Half-wave rectified electroencephalograms and instantaneous discharge rate of an inspiratory neuron in NREM and REM sleep during spontaneous respiration (a) and during mechanical ventilation (b). The figure shows that in REM sleep this neuron is driven by endogenous tonic inputs that account for much of the activity of the neuron during spontaneous breathing. (From Orem *et al.*, 2002.)

reticular formation produces nonreciprocal inhibition of spinal motor neurons (Jankowska *et al.*, 1968), and the activity of single medullary neurons is correlated with the atonia of REM sleep (Sakai *et al.*, 1979).

Accessory respiratory muscles may become active, apparently overcoming the atonia, in REM sleep in subjects with diaphragm paralysis. Dogs subjected to bilateral phrenicotomies developed, over a period of months, activity in muscles that were atonic prior to and immediately following the phrenicotomies (Issa and Bitner, 1992). Similarly, there is a recent report on patients with bilateral diaphragm paralysis but with accessory respiratory muscle activity in REM sleep. These results suggest a reorganization of the neural elements that control breathing in that state (Bennett *et al.*, 2004).

Atonia of hypoglossal motor neurons in a carbachol-induced state, which may be a model of REM sleep (see George *et al.*, 1964; Vanni-Mercier *et al.*, 1989; Vertes *et al.*, 1993), is caused, not by active inhibition, but rather primarily by disfacilitation as the result of loss of aminergic excitation (Kubin *et al.*, 1994, 1996). In the carbachol state, pharyngeal motor neurons are profoundly suppressed whereas phrenic and laryngeal motor neurons are relatively unaffected (Fenik *et al.*, 1998), and the activity of medullary inspiratory neurons is minimally suppressed, or even increased (Kubin *et al.*, 1992b, Woch *et al.*, 2000). However, the respiratory rate is reduced and regular in the carbachol model, whereas it is greatly accelerated and irregular during natural REM sleep.

In chronically instrumented, behaving animals, recordings from upper airway muscles innervated by hypoglossal motor neurons support the idea that atonia is caused by disfacilitation. For example, antagonism of serotonergic excitatory effects during wakefulness reduced the activity of geniohyoid and sternohyoid muscles in the English bulldog, which is a natural model of obstructive sleep apnea (Veasey *et al.*, 1996), and perfusion of the hypoglossal nucleus with 5-HT attenuated the suppression of genioglossal muscle activity during sleep in rats (Jelev *et al.*, 2001). The applicability of these findings to the behavior of other upper airway motor neurons during natural REM sleep remains to be determined, as do the implications for treatment of obstructive sleep apnea. To date, clinical trials to test the salutory effects of aminergic excitation with, for example, serotonin reuptake inhibitors, have yielded weak or negative results, perhaps because they have not targeted the appropriate combinations of aminergic receptors. The main receptors mediating the excitatory effects of 5-HT and norepinephrine in upper airway motor neurons have now been identified as type 5-HT_{2A} and alpha_{1B} adrenergic, respectively (Okabe *et al.*, 1997; Volgin *et al.*, 2001). Interestingly, in one study in the English bulldog, the results of a systemic treatment that had a partial preference toward 5-HT_2 receptors were more promising than in other trials (Veasey *et al.*, 1999). Nevertheless, the prospects for pharmacotherapy for obstructive sleep apnea are complicated by the fact that the same excitatory aminergic receptors that mediate wakefulness-related excitatory effects in upper airway motor neurons are also present in many other brain regions and subserve many other functions, including sleep. Thus, targeting selected combinations of receptors may be insufficient and a successful therapeutic intervention may require new methods of selective drug delivery to the desired sites of their action.

Neural control of breathing in REM sleep and the patient with lung disease

Patients with lung disease commonly hypoventilate more in REM sleep than in other states. The many explanations of this phenomenon are based on much of what is known of the physiology of breathing in REM sleep.

Koo *et al.* (1975) proposed that patients with chronic obstructive pulmonary disease (COPD) retain secretions in REM sleep because of slowed mucociliary clearance and suppressed coughing. This, they argued, caused an increase in alveoli that were perfused but not ventilated — thereby decreasing oxygen saturation of the blood. They proposed also that the desaturation was aggravated by an increase in metabolic rate in REM sleep, which had been reported by Brebbia and Altshuler (1965).

Wynne *et al.* (1979) concluded that desaturation in REM sleep in patients with COPD was the result of atonia of intercostal muscles. They noted that patients with COPD have shorter, flatter, and less effective diaphragms and that therefore they rely more on intercostal muscles for ventilation. In REM sleep, however, the intercostal muscles are atonic, and the patient with COPD must ventilate with only an inadequate diaphragm. Johnson and Remmers (1984) extended this idea and showed that the scalene and sternocleidomastoid muscles, which are recruited in patients with COPD, are atonic also in REM sleep.

Early findings of impaired ventilatory responses in REM sleep (Phillipson, 1978) were applied to the interpretation of the REM-related desaturation: Douglas *et al.* (1979) found that blue bloaters but not pink puffers desaturated in REM sleep, and they attributed the difference to the presence or absence of a ventilatory response to CO_2 in REM sleep. Fleetham *et al.* (1980) concurred showing an inverse relation between the degree of desaturation in REM sleep and the waking ventilatory response to CO_2. They proposed also that intercostal atonia would lower lung volumes and increase airway resistance, which would contribute to hypoventilation.

George *et al.* (1987) found that patients with COPD desaturated most during periods of eye movements in REM sleep. Millman *et al.* (1988) noted that ventilation was reduced during eye movements in REM sleep in healthy young adults because of an increased rate and decreased depth of breathing. Finally, we propose here that the associations observed by Millman and George and their colleagues are caused by the endogeneous excitatory drive that occurs in REM sleep and that can cause respiratory fibrillation. Douglas (1994), before us, concluded that hypoventilation in REM sleep by patients with lung disease was caused by a disorganization of the output of the central pattern generator.

Conclusion

Both excitatory and inhibitory tonic processes affect the respiratory system in REM sleep. The rapid and irregular breathing of the state can be explained by tonic endogenous excitatory drive(s) of unknown origin(s). In contrast, tonic inhibitory or disfacilitatory processes cause changes in lung mechanics, obstructive events, and oxygen desaturations of patients with lung disease. The tonic inhibition or disfacilitation is evidently subject to modifications, as occur in subjects with diaphragm paralysis.

Acknowledgments

This work was made possible by grants HL21257, HL62589, NS46062 from the National Heart, Lung, and Blood Institute of the National Institutes of Health.

References

Anderson, C.A., Dick, T.E., and Orem, J. (1996). Respiratory responses to tracheobronchial stimulation during sleep and wakefulness in the adult cat. *Sleep*, 19: 472–478.

Baust, W. and Engel, R. (1971). The correlation of heart and respiratory frequency in natural sleep of man and their relation to dream content. *Electroenceph. Clin. Neurophysiol.*, 30: 262–263.

Bennett, J.R., Dunroy, H.M.A., Corfield, D.R., Hart, N., Simonds, A.K., Pokey, M.I., and Morrell, M.J. (2004). Respiratory muscle activity during REM sleep in patients with diaphragm paralysis. *Neurology*, 62: 134–137.

Bonora, M., Shields, G.I., Knuth, S.L., Bartlett, D.J., and St. John, W.M. (1984). Selective depression by ethanol of upper airway respiratory motor activity in cats. *Am. Rev. Respir. Dis.*, 130: 156–161.

Bonora, M., St. John, W.M., and Bledsoe, T.A. (1985). Differential elevation by protriptyline and depression by diazepam of upper airway respiratory motor activity. *Am. Rev. Respir. Dis.*, 131: 41–45.

Brebbia, D.R. and Altshuler, K.Z. (1965). Oxygen consumption rate and electroencephalographic stage of sleep. *Science*, 150: 1621–1623.

Brouillette, R.T. and Thach, B.T. (1979a). A neuromuscular mechanism maintaining extrathoracic airway patency. *J. Appl. Physiol.*, 46: 772–779.

Brouillette, R.T. and Thach, B.T. (1979b). Effects of chemoreceptors and pulmonary mechanoreceptors on the respiratory activity of the genioglossus muscle. *Fed. Proc.*, 38: 1142.

Champagnat, J., Denavit-Saubié, M., Henry, J.L., and Leviel, V. (1979). Catecholaminergic depressant effects on bulbar respiratory mechanisms. *Brain Res.*, 160: 57–68.

Dawes, G.S., Fox, H.E., Leduc, B.M., Liggins, G.C., and Richards, R.T. (1972). Respiratory movements and rapid eye movement sleep in the foetal lamb. *J. Physiol. (Lond.)*, 220: 119–143.

Douglas, N.J. (1994). Chronic obstructive pulmonary disease. In: Kryger, M.H., Roth, T., and Dement, W.C. (Eds.). *Principles and Practice of Sleep Medicine*. New York: W.B. Saunders, pp. 965–975.

Douglas, N.J. (2000). Respiratory physiology: control of ventilation. In: Kryger, M.H., Roth, T., and Dement, W.C. (Eds.). *Principles and Practices of Sleep Medicine.* New York: W.B. Saunders, pp. 221–228.

Douglas, N.J., Calverley, P.W., Leggett, R.J., Brash, H.M., Flenley, D.C., and Brezinova, V. (1979). Transient hypoxaemia during sleep in chronic bronchitis and emphysema. *Lancet*, 1: 1–4.

Dunin-Barkowski, W.L. and Orem, J.M. (1998). Suppression of diaphragmatic activity during spontaneous ponto-geniculo-occipital waves in cat. *Sleep*, 21: 671–675.

Eldridge, F.L., Millhorn, D.E., and Waldrop, T.G. (1981). Exercise hyperpnea and locomotion: parallel activation from the hypothalamus. *Science*, 211: 844–846.

Estabrooke, I.V., McCarthy, M.T., Ko, E., Chou, T.C., Chemelli, R.M., Yanagisawa, M., Saper, C.B., and Scammell, T.E. (2001). Fos expression in orexin neurons varies with behavioral state. *J. Neurosci.*, 21: 1656–1662.

Fenik, V., Kubin, L., Okabe, S., Pack, A.I., and Davies, R.O. (1997). Differential sensitivity of laryngeal and pharyngeal motoneurons to iontophoretic application of serotonin. *Neuroscience*, 81: 873–885.

Fenik, V., Davies, R.O., Pack, A.I., and Kubin, L. (1998). Differential suppression of upper airway motor activity during carbachol-induced, REM sleep-like atonia. *Am. J. Physiol.*, 275: 1013–1024.

Fink, B.R. (1961). Influence of cerebral activity in wakefulness on regulation of breathing. *J. Appl. Physiol.*, 16: 15–20.

Fleetham, J.A., Mezon, B., West, P., Bradley, C.A., Anthonisen, N.R., and Kryger, M.H. (1980). Chemical control of ventilation and sleep arterial oxygen desaturation in patients with COPD. *Am. Rev. Respir. Dis.*, 122: 583–589.

Foutz, A.S., Netick, A., and Dement, W.C. (1979). Sleep state effects on breathing after spinal cord section and vagotomy in the cat. *Respir. Physiol.*, 37: 89–100.

Foutz, A.S., Boudinot, E., Morin-Surin, M.-P., Champagnat, J., Gonsalves, S.F., and Denavit-Saubie, M. (1987). Excitability of "silent" respiratory neurons during sleep–waking states: an iontophoretic study in undrugged chronic cats. *Brain Res.*, 171: 135–141.

Funk, G.D., Smith, J.C., and Feldman, J.L. (1994). Development of thyrotropin-releasing hormone and norepinephrine potentiation of inspiratory-related hypoglossal motoneuron discharge in neonatal and juvenile mice *in vitro. J. Neurophysiol.*, 72: 2538–2541.

Gauzzi, M. and Freis, E.D. (1969). Sino-aortic reflexes pH, pO_2, and pCO_2 in wakefulness and sleep. *Am. J. Physiol.*, 217: 1623–1627.

George, C.F., West, P., and Kryger, M.H. (1987). Oxygenation and breathing pattern during phasic and tonic REM in patients with chronic obstructive pulmonary disease. *Sleep*, 10: 234–243.

George, R., Haslett, W.L., and Jenden, D.J. (1964). A cholinergic mechanism in the brainstem reticular formation: induction of paradoxical sleep. *Int. J. Neuropharmacol.*, 3: 541–552.

Glenn, L.L., Foutz, A., and Dement, W.C. (1978). Membrane potential of spinal motoneurons during natural sleep in cats. *Sleep*, 1: 199–204.

Hauri, P. and Van de Castle, R.L. (1973). Psychophysiological parallels in dreams. *Psychosom. Med.*, 35: 297–308.

Heym, J., Steinfels, G.F., and Jacobs, B.L. (1982). Activity of serotonin-containing neurons in the nucleus raphe pallidus of freely moving cats. *Brain Res.*, 251: 259–276.

Hobson, J.A., Goldfrank, F., and Snyder, F. (1965). Respiration and mental activity in sleep. *J. Psychiatry Res.*, 3: 79–90.

Hugelin, A. and Cohen, M.I. (1963). The reticular activating system and respiratory regulation in the cat. *Ann. N. Y. Acad. Sci.*, 109: 586–603.

Issa, F.G. and Bitner, S. (1992). Restructuring of sleep and reversal of REM-induced supraspinal hypotonia of respiratory muscles following bilateral phrenicotomy. *Neurosci. Lett.*, 139: 231–233.

Ioffe, S., Jansen, A.H., and Chernick, V. (1993). Fetal respiratory neuronal activity during REM and NREM sleep. *J. Appl. Physiol.*, 75: 191–197.

Jankowska, E., Lund, S., Lundberg, A., and Pompeiano, O. (1968). Inhibitory effects evoked through ventral reticulospinal pathways. *Arch. Ital. Biol.*, 106: 124–140.

Jelev, A., Sood, S., Liu, H., Nolan, P., and Horner, R.L. (2001). Microdialysis perfusion of 5-HT into hypoglossal motor nucleus differentially modulates genioglossus activity across natural sleep–wake states in rats. *J. Physiol. (Lond.)*, 532: 467–481.

Johnson, M.W. and Remmers, J.E. (1984). Accessory muscle activity during sleep in chronic obstructive pulmonary disease. *J. Appl. Physiol.*, 57: 1011–1017.

Kiyashchenko, L.I., Mileykovskiy, B.Y., Maidment, N., Lam, H.A., Wu, M.F., John, J., Peever, J., and Siegel, J.M. (2002). Release of hypocretin (orexin) during waking and sleep states. *J. Neurosci.*, 22: 5282–5286.

Koo, K.W., Sax, D.S., and Snider, G.L. (1975). Arterial blood gases and pH during sleep in chronic obstructive pulmonary disease. *Am. J. Med.*, 58: 663–670.

Krieger, J. (2000). Respiratory physiology: breathing in normal subjects. In: Kryger, M.H., Roth, T., and Dement, W.C. (Eds.). *Principles and Practices of Sleep Medicine*. New York: W.B. Saunders, pp. 229–241.

Kubin, L., Kimura, H., Tojima, H., Pack, A.I., and Davies, R.O. (1992a). Behavior of VRG neurons during the atonia of REM sleep induced by pontine carbachol in decerebrate cats. *Brain Res.*, 592: 91–100.

Kubin, L., Tojima, H., Davies, R.O., and Pack, A.I. (1992b). Serotonergic excitatory drive to hypoglossal motoneurons in the decerebrate cat. *Neurosci. Lett.*, 139: 243–248.

Kubin, L., Kimura, H., Tojima, H., Pack, A.I., and Davies. R.O. (1994). Changes in serotonin level in the hypoglossal nucleus region during the carbachol-induced atonia. *Brain Res.*, 645: 291–302.

Kubin, L., Tojima, H., Reignier, C., Pack, A.I., and Davies, R.O. (1996). Interaction of serotonergic excitatory drive to hypoglossal motoneurons with carbachol-induced, REM sleep-like atonia. *Sleep*, 19: 187–195.

Lovering, A.T., Dunin-Barkowski, W.L., Vidruk, E.H., and Orem, J.M. (2003). Ventilatory response of the cat to hypoxia in sleep and wakefulness. *J. Appl. Physiol.*, 95: 545–554.

Megirian, D., Pollard, M.J., and Sherrey, J.H. (1987). The labile respiratory activity of ribcage muscles of the rat during sleep. *J. Physiol. (Lond.)*, 389: 99–110.

Mezzanotte, W.S., Tangel, D.J., and White, D.P. (1992). Waking genioglossal electromyogram in sleep apnea patients versus normal controls (a neuromuscular compensatory mechanism). *J. Clin. Invest.*, 89: 1571–1579.

Millman, R.P., Knight, H., Kline, L.R., Shore, E.T., Chung, D.C., and Pack, A.I. (1988). Changes in compartmental ventilation in association with eye movements during REM sleep. *J. Appl. Physiol.*, 65: 1196–1202.

Netick, A. and Foutz, A.S. (1980). Respiratory activity and sleep-wakefulness in the deafferented paralyzed cat. *Sleep*, 3: 1–12.

Netick, A., Orem, J., and Dement, W. (1977). Neuronal activity specific to REM sleep and its relationship to breathing. *Brain Res.*, 120: 197–207.

Okabe, S., Mackiewicz, M., and Kubin, L. (1997). Serotonin receptor mRNA expression in the hypoglossal motor nucleus. *Respir. Physiol.*, 110: 151–160.

Orem, J. (1980). Medullary respiratory neuron activity: relationship to tonic and phasic REM sleep. *J. Appl. Physiol.*, 48: 54–65.

Orem, J. (1989). Behavioral inspiratory inhibition: inactivated and activated respiratory cells. *J. Neurophysiol.*, 62: 1069–1078.

Orem, J. (1994). Central respiratory activity in rapid eye movement sleep: augmenting and late inspiratory cells. *Sleep*, 17: 665–673.

Orem, J. (1998). Augmenting expiratory neuronal activity in sleep and wakefulness and in relation to duration of expiration. *J. Appl. Physiol.*, 85: 1260–1266.

Orem, J. and Lydic, R. (1978). Upper airway function during sleep and wakefulness: experimental studies on normal and anesthetized cats. *Sleep*, 1: 49–68.

Orem, J., Montplaisir, J., and Dement, W. (1974). Changes in the activity of respiratory neurones during sleep. *Brain Res.*, 82: 309–315.

Orem, J., Netick, A., and Dement, W.C. (1977). Breathing during sleep and wakefulness in the cat. *Respir. Physiol.*, 30: 265–289.

Orem, J., Dick, T., and Norris, P. (1980). Laryngeal and diaphragmatic responses to airway occlusion in sleep and wakefulness. *Electroenceph. Clin. Neurophysiol.*, 50: 151–164.

Orem, J., Osorio, I., Brooks, E., and Dick, T. (1985). Activity of respiratory neurons during NREM sleep. *J. Neurophysiol.*, 54: 1144–1156.

Orem, J., Lovering, A.T., Dunin-Barkowski, W., and Vidruk, E.H. (2000). Endogenous excitatory drive to the respiratory system in rapid eye movement sleep in cats. *J. Physiol.*, 527: 365–376.

Orem, J., Lovering, A.T., Dunin-Barkowski, W., and Vidruk, E.H. (2002). Tonic activity in the respiratory system in wakefulness, NREM and REM sleep. *Sleep*, 25: 488–496.

Pace-Schott, E., Solms, M., Blagrove, M., and Harnad, S. (2003). *Sleep and Dreaming. Scientific Advances and Reconsiderations*. Cambridge: Cambridge University Press.

Parmeggiani, P.L. and Sabattini, L. (1972). Electromyographic aspects of postural, respiratory and thermoregulatory mechanisms in sleeping cats. *Electroenceph. Clin. Neurophysiol.*, 33: 1–13.

Peyron, C., Tighe, D.K., van den Pol, A.N., de Lecea, L., Heller, H.C., Sutcliffe, J.G., and Kilduff, T.S. (1998). Neurons containing hypocretin (orexin) project to multiple neuronal systems. *J. Neurosci.*, 18: 9996–10015.

Phillipson, E.A. (1978). Control of breathing during sleep. *Am. Rev. Respir. Dis.*, 118: 909–939.

Plum, F. and Leigh, R.J. (1981). Abnormalities of central mechanisms. In: Hornhein, T.F. (Ed.). *Regulation of Breathing*. New York, NY: Marcel Dekker, pp. 989–1067.

Pompeiano, O. (1967). The neurophysiological mechanisms of the postural and motor events during desynchronized sleep. *Proc. Assoc. Res. Nerve. Ment. Dis.*, 45: 351–423.

Puizillout, J.J. and Ternaux, J.P. (1974). Variations d'activités toniques, phasiques et respiratoires au niveau bulbaire pendant l'endormement de la préparation encéphale isolé. *Brain Res.*, 66: 67–83.

Reis, D.J. and McHugh, P.R. (1968). Hypoxia as a cause of bradycardia during amygdala stimulation in monkey. *J. Appl. Physiol.*, 214: 601–610.

Remmers, J.E., Bartlett, D. Jr., and Putnam, M.D. (1976). Changes in the respiratory cycle associated with sleep. *Respir. Physiol.*, 28: 227–238.

Sastre, J.P. and Jouvet, M. (1979). Le compretment onirique du chat. *Physiol. Behav.*, 22: 979–989.

Sakai, K., Kanamore, N., and Jouvet, M. (1979). Activite unitaires specifique due someil paradoxal dans lar formation reticulee bulbaire chez le chat non-restreint. *C.R. Acad. Sci. (Paris)*, 289: 557–561.

St. John, W.M. (1986). Influence of reticular mechanisms upon hypoglossal, trigeminal and phrenic activities. *Respir. Physiol.*, 66: 27–40.

St. John, W.M. and Bledsoe, T.A. (1985). Comparison of respiratory-related trigeminal, hypoglossal and phrenic activities. *Respir. Physiol.*, 62: 61–78.

St. John, W.M., Bartlett, D.J., Knuth, K.V., Knuth, S.L., and Daubenspeck, J.A. (1986). Differential depression of hypoglossal nerve activity by alcohol. Protection by pretreatment with medoxyprogesterone acetate. *Am. Rev. Respir. Dis.*, 133: 46–48.

Sullivan, C.E., Kozar, L.F., Murphy, E., and Phillipson, E.A. (1979a). Arousal, ventilatory, and airway responses to bronchopulmonary stimulation in sleeping dogs. *J. Appl. Physiol.*, 45: 681–689.

Sullivan, C.E., Zamel, N., Kozar, L.F., Murphy, E., and Phillipson, E.A. (1979b). Regulation of airway smooth muscle tone in sleeping dogs. *Am. Rev. Respir. Dis.*, 119: 87–99.

Tabachnik, E., Muller, N.L., Bryan, A.C., and Levison, H. (1981). Changes in ventilation and chest wall mechanics during sleep in normal adolescents. *J. Appl. Physiol.*, 51: 557–564.

Torterolo, P., Yamuy, J., Sampogna, S., Morales, F.R., and Chase, M.H. (2003). Hypocretinergic neurons are primarily involved in activation of the somato-motor system. *Sleep*, 26: 25–28.

Trulson, M.E. and Trulson, V.M. (1982). Activity of nucleus raphe pallidus neurons across the sleep-waking cycle in freely moving cats. *Brain Res.*, 237: 232–237.

Vanni-Mercier, G., Sakai, K., Lin, J.S., and Jouvet, M. (1989). Mapping of cholinoceptive brainstem structures responsible for the generation of para-doxical sleep in the cat. *Arch. Ital. Biol.*, 127: 133–164.

Veasey, S.C., Panckeri, K.A., Hoffman, E.A., Pack, A.I., and Hendricks, J.C. (1996). The effect of serotonin antagonists in an animal model of sleep-disordered breathing. *Am. J. Respir. Crit. Care Med.*, 153: 776–786.

Veasey, S.C., Fenik, P., Panckeri, K., Pack, A.I., and Hendricks, J.C. (1999). The effects of trazodone with L-trytophan on sleep-disordered breathing in the English bulldog. *Am. J. Respir. Crit. Care Med.*, 160: 1659–1667.

Vertes, R.P., Colom, L.V., and Fortin, W.J. (1993). Brainstem sites for the car-bachol elicitation of the hippocampal theta rhythm in the rat. *Exp. Brain Res.*, 96: 419–429.

Volgin, D.V., Mackiewicz, M., and Kubin, L. (2001). α_{1B} Receptors are the main postsynaptic mediators of adrenergic excitation in brainstem motoneurons, a single-cell RT-PCR study. *J. Chem. Neuroanat.*, 22: 157–166.

Wheatley, J.R., Mezzanotte, W.S., Tangel, D.J., and White, D.P. (1993). Influ-ence of sleep on genioglossus muscle activation by negative pressure in nor-mal men. *Am. Rev. Respir. Dis.*, 148: 597–605.

Woch, G., Ogawa, H., Davies, R.O., and Kubin, L. (2000). Behavior of hypoglossal inspiratory premotor neurons during the carbachol-induced, REM sleep-like suppression of upper airway motoneurons. *Exp. Brain Res.*, 130: 508–520.

Wynne, J.W., Block, A.J., Hemenway, J., Hunt, L.A., and Flick, M.R. (1979). Disordered breathing and oxygen desaturation during sleep in patients with chronic obstructive lung disease (COLD). *Am. J. Med.*, 66: 573–579.

Yoshida, Y., Fujiki, N., Nakajima, T., Ripley, B., Matsumura, H., Yoneda, H., Mignot, E., and Nishino, S. (2001). Fluctuation of extracellular hypocretin-1 (orexin A) levels in the rat in relation to the light-dark cycle and sleep-wake activities. *Eur. J. Neurosci.*, 14: 1075–1081.

Chapter 15

REFLEX CARDIOVASCULAR CONTROL IN SLEEP

Alessandro Silvani and Pierluigi Lenzi[1]

Ventilatory, cardiac, and vascular functions are regulated to respond to body metabolic needs in terms of nutrient supply and waste removal. Sleep limits the variability in local metabolic needs associated with behavioural engagement with the external environment. In addition, sleep entails dramatic changes in the activity of the central nervous system, potentially altering the neural integration of cardioventilatory control. On the other hand, cardioventilatory challenges influence the sleep process, which in turn, may further modify the regulatory capacity. Extreme challenges usually determine awakening, which increases the cardioventilatory regulatory efficacy. Arousal may thus be considered as an intermediate mechanism of the cardioventilatory regulation. The mean level and fluctuations around the mean of respiratory and cardiovascular variables depend on the wake–sleep state and are not of exclusive physiological interest. Rather, the features of cardioventilatory regulation during sleep (Verrier *et al.*, 1996) and of their transition to the regulatory pattern of morning awakening (George, 2000) may play a role in the pathophysiology of acute myocardial syndromes, stroke, and sudden death. Moreover, sleep may be of value as an autonomic stress test for the cardiovascular system (Verrier *et al.*, 1996) in that a pathological pattern of cardiovascular regulation may become evident

---

[1]plenzi@biocfarm.unibo.it

earlier during sleep than in wakefulness. Evidence supporting this hypothesis has been gained regarding myocardial infarction (Vanoli *et al.*, 1995), sudden infant death syndrome (Franco *et al.*, 1998), and neurological disorders (Ferini-Strambi *et al.*, 1995).

In spite of the relevance of cardioventilatory regulation during sleep for the basic and clinical science and of four decades of extensive research, it may be surprisingly difficult to draw a consistent picture of the topic. Indeed, the field is still open to experimental and theoretical work aimed at reconciling some inconsistencies between the reported results.

This chapter will mainly deal with evidence concerning reflex cardiovascular control during the wake–sleep cycle. Ventilatory regulation will also be considered as it is strictly linked to cardiovascular regulation. As a premise, the physiological and technical factors that may underlie some discrepancies between published results will be presented.

Cardiovascular Regulatory Mechanisms

Cardiovascular regulation is exerted at multiple hierarchical levels. At the lowest level, vascular resistance changes as a function of the local physical and chemical environment. As a result, blood flow is relatively independent of perfusion pressure (autoregulation), and is coupled to the local rate of energy utilisation (flow–metabolism coupling), such coupling also depending on partial pressures of oxygen and carbon dioxide (chemical regulation). The intermediate level of cardiac and vascular control is exerted by autonomic reflexes, which originate from peripheral tissues and from the cardiovascular system itself. The integrated reflex control of the cardiovascular and ventilatory functions allows an effective buffering of alterations in systemic arterial pressure, arterial blood gas concentration, and body temperature, and contributes to maintain the constancy of the internal environment (homeostasis). The highest level of cardiovascular control is exerted by the central nervous system, which imposes autonomic commands (Spyer, 1994) on cardiac, vascular, and ventilatory effectors. In general, central autonomic commands contribute to adapt cardiovascular regulation to changing behavioural needs, as in physical exercise or in defence reaction. In other instances, however, no adaptive function can be envisaged for autonomic commands, so that their cardiovascular effects may be considered as disturbances [as in phasic events during rapid eye movement (REM) sleep, see below].

The interactions between local, reflex, and central cardiovascular regulatory mechanisms are ubiquitary and complex, and many of the control mechanisms involved are intrinsically non-linear (Malpas, 2002; Ursino and Magosso, 2003). This may lead to divergent results at the level of the cardiovascular end-variables measured in similar experiments due to quantitative differences in controller or effector responses that shift the balance among interacting regulatory mechanisms. Such differences may occur not only between different species, but also between different animal strains (Campen *et al.*, 2002) or human ethnic groups (Crisostomo *et al.*, 1998). Although the basic features of cardiovascular control appear constant among species and groups, genetic differences may affect the balance among the controls involved and may explain some inconsistencies among experimental results.

Summing up, the neural control of the cardiovascular system is accomplished by the autonomic outflow to the heart (sympathetic + parasympathetic) and vessels (sympathetic). The autonomic outflow includes both the reflex contribution of peripheral factors, such as baro-, chemo-, thermoreceptors, pulmonary afferents, etc., and also central commands that change as a function of the behavioural state such as the wake–sleep states, the defence reaction, and emotional states. The summation of these influences on the autonomic cardiovascular outflow makes it difficult to evaluate the effect of a single factor, such as baro- or chemo-receptor activation and the gain of feedback loop regulations. In spite of these theoretical difficulties, the gain of homeostatic regulations has been tentatively measured in different behavioural states, with differences between measures depending on other uncontrolled peripheral or central influences, different techniques utilised, and different species studied.

Heterogeneity of the Wake–Sleep States

The wake–sleep cycle is segmented into the main behavioural states of wakefulness, REM sleep and non-REM sleep. Classification helps to understand sleep physiology, as it focuses on differences among states. However, the very concept of a state is hardly applicable to the continuum of sleep-related changes in physiological variables. Hence, by neglecting the heterogeneity within states, conventional classification allows but a step of approximation to the understanding of sleep physiology, and may be the basis of some inconsistencies in the literature on cardiovascular control during sleep.

Cardiovascular control during sleep is often compared with that during wakefulness, although wakefulness entails a wide repertoire of physiological responses. The heterogeneity of the waking state is generally reduced by requiring that waking be quiet. The definition of quiet wakefulness is rather loose, however, and does not exclude the confounding effects of drowsiness or the experimental setting. Although comparisons between sleep states appear more reliable than those versus wakefulness, sleep periods show a distinct within-state heterogeneity, too. Non-REM sleep, which is further divided into four stages in humans, shows an evolving microstructure that includes changes in electroencephalographic patterns [K-complexes, microarousals, and periods of cyclic alternating pattern (CAP)] as well as distinct changes in cardiovascular and ventilatory functions (Somers *et al.*, 1993; Quattrochi *et al.*, 2000; Iellamo *et al.*, 2004). On the other hand, REM sleep consists of tonic periods interspersed with periods of phasic neural, cardiovascular, and ventilatory changes (Gassel *et al.*, 1964; Mancia *et al.*, 1971; Parmeggiani, 1980; Sei and Morita, 1999; Silvani *et al.*, 2005). Phasic episodes may be underrepresented in some experimental work, as the interest for steady data may lead to discard periods characterised by irregularities in ventilation, heart rate, and arterial pressure. Finally, cardiovascular features of both non-REM sleep and REM sleep change during the night (Legramante *et al.*, 2003), possibly depending on both prior sleep time and circadian factors.

Technical Issues

The study of cardiovascular control in sleep is complicated by the need to analyse closed-loop preparations without disturbing the sleep state. The different measurement procedures and the different mathematical techniques for data analysis may further confound the interpretation of the experimental results.

Early studies on cardiovascular control in sleeping cats and rats were performed after a relatively short period of postoperative recovery, which was subsequently proved to deeply affect cardiovascular regulation during sleep (Sei and Morita, 1999). Furthermore, surgical denervation of sino-aortic afferents in experimental animals, which has been widely used as a tool to understand reflex cardiovascular control in sleep, does not allow to discriminate between baroceptive and chemoceptive cardiovascular effects. Similarly, the effects of temporary carotid occlusion, which has been applied to unload carotid baroreceptors during sleep, also reflect changes in the discharge of chemoreceptors and of aortic baroreceptors. Finally, a large number of studies have quantified the chronotropic baroreflex responses to a change in arterial pressure during sleep. In this regard, a confounding factor is represented by the choice of heart rate or of heart period as the dependent variable, because these two reciprocal quantities are related by a hyperbolic function. Moreover, while some studies induced arterial pressure changes by injection of vasoactive drugs or mechanical means, others relied on spontaneous fluctuations in arterial pressure to probe the baroreflex function in sleep. These latter studies utilised a variety of mathematical techniques for data analysis, ranging from linear regression and correlation to parametric modelling and spectral analysis. The estimates obtained with different techniques show some degree of similarity, but it must be emphasised that they also reflect different and complementary aspects of baroreflex control (Parati *et al.*, 2000). For example, the cardiac baroreflex response to wide changes in arterial pressure may differ from the response to moderate fluctuations of blood pressure around its physiological value. More confounding factors arise from subtle differences among the techniques of analysis, and will be addressed in the following section.

Baroreceptor Reflexes

Fluctuations in arterial blood pressure induce changes in the arterial wall tension, which are sensed by stretch receptors in arterial walls, particularly at the carotid sinus and along the aortic arch. Baroreceptors or stretch receptors are also present in vascular districts with low transmural pressure, as in the wall of the pulmonary veins and around cardiac atria, where they mainly sense changes in atrial filling, depending on central blood volume. The following discussion will only deal with arterial baroreceptors, because the role of cardiopulmonary baroreceptors in the reflex cardiovascular control during sleep has not been clarified. However, stimuli used to test the arterial baroreflex during sleep may also engage the cardiopulmonary baroreceptor reflex. In this regard, the lack of an effective cardiopulmonary baroreflex in newborn life (Merrill *et al.*, 1995) adds to the difficulty of extrapolating information on cardiovascular baroreflex control in sleep across developmental stages.

Afferent impulses from arterial baroreceptors reach the nucleus tractus solitarii in the medulla oblongata. These impulses modulate vagal and sympathetic efferent activity to the heart and vessels as well as ventilation, hormone release, and arousal. The autonomic effects of the baroreflex on the cardiovascular system depict a negative feedback control. A rise in arterial pressure slows down heart rhythm, reduces cardiac contractility, and dilates peripheral resistance and capacitance vessels (Sagawa, 1984). Besides cardiovascular effects, baroreceptor stimulation also inhibits pulmonary ventilation (Stella *et al.*, 2001), which in turn affects heart rhythm and arterial pressure (Kara *et al.*, 2003). The gain of the baroreceptor reflex is defined as the change in the controlled variable (arterial pressure or heart period) per unit change in the independent variable (pressure that causes stretch of baroreceptors). Measuring the baroreflex gain is simpler with regard to the control of heart period than for the control of arterial pressure, which is the end-variable of the reflex. The gain of the arterial pressure — heart period baroreflex loop may be measured by evaluating the change in heart period induced by a 1 mmHg change in arterial pressure. The latter may be directly evaluated in experimental settings with isolated carotid sinus by comparing the changes in sinus pressure with the resulting changes in central arterial pressure (Dworkin *et al.*, 2000). This and other similar techniques are invasive and laborious, not suitable for studying the baroreceptor–arterial pressure reflex during the wake–sleep cycle. Simpler indirect techniques have been envisaged, studying the changes in local sympathetic nerve activity and vascular resistance in response to changes in arterial pressure. However, these techniques too are difficult to apply during sleep and provide indexes that are only unsafe estimates of the baroreceptor–arterial pressure gain. In fact, while vascular sympathetic activation is generally aimed at regulating sistemic arterial pressure, there are instances in which the resistance of a given vascular bed changes in the opposite direction to that of total peripheral resistance. This occurs during the transition between wake–sleep states, when a re-patterning of vascular autonomic outflow occurs, as indicated by the wide changes observed in regional blood flow and vascular resistance (Lenzi *et al.*, 1987, 1989; Zoccoli *et al.*, 1992, 1994). In spite of the unavoidable theoretical and practical problems, some data on baroreceptor regulation of regional sympathetic activity will however be considered.

Baroreflex control of the vasculature

In non-REM sleep, the tonic level of muscle sympathetic nerve activity decreases in human subjects with respect to wakefulness despite a blood pressure decrease (Somers *et al.*, 1993). In addition, the tonic level of renal sympathetic nerve activity correlates positively with arterial pressure in rats across the behaviours of non-REM sleep and quiet and active wakefulness (Miki *et al.*, 2003). Combs *et al.* (1986) computed the gain of the baroreflex control of vascular resistance in sleeping baboons by means of bilateral carotid occlusion, which unloads carotid baroreceptors. Renal baroreflex vasoconstriction was reduced during (behaviourally determined) quiet sleep compared with quiet wakefulness, whereas both leg and terminal aortic baroreflex vasoconstriction, which refer to the perfusion of muscle, skin, and visceral tissues, were independent of the behavioural state (Combs *et al.*, 1986). These results indicate that baroreflex gain of local vascular control may be lower during non-REM sleep than in wakefulness, albeit with regional differences. Accordingly, the baroreflex gain of muscle sympathetic nerve activity was lower in non-REM sleep than in wakefulness in a study by Nakazato *et al.* (1998), who computed the relationship between spontaneous fluctuations in muscle sympathetic nerve activity and those in diastolic blood pressure in healthy human subjects. A decrease in baroreflex control of muscle sympathetic nerve activity during non-REM sleep may also explain why the burst properties of sympathetic nerve activity to the muscle and skin, which are independent during wakefulness, become synchronised with the deepening of non-REM sleep (Kodama *et al.*, 1998). Accordingly, a reduced differentiation between sympathetic activities to different tissues, which characterises non-REM sleep, may be observed after anaesthesia of the glossopharingeal and vagus nerves, which carry baroceptive (as well as chemoceptive and lung receptor) afferents (Fagius *et al.*, 1985). Moreover, sensory stimuli do not increase muscle sympathetic nerve activity during wakefulness, whereas they do so both in non-REM sleep, in association with K-complexes (Somers *et al.*, 1993), and after cervical spinal cord lesions (Stjernberg *et al.*, 1986), which interrupt baroreflex pathways.

For what concerns REM sleep, no difference with respect to wakefulness was found in the gain of baroreflex control of vascular nerve activity by Nakazato *et al.* (1998). It is, however, clear that the control pattern of peripheral vascular beds in REM sleep is profoundly shaped by central autonomic commands and by reflexes other than the baroreflex (Baccelli *et al.*, 1974; Parmeggiani, 1980). Regional blood flows are thus deeply modified by the wake–sleep state and ambient temperature (Lenzi *et al.*, 1987, 1989; Zoccoli *et al.*, 1992, 1994). In most reports, arterial pressure increases in REM sleep with respect to non-REM sleep, because of vasoconstriction in skeletal muscles (Mancia *et al.*, 1971; Miki *et al.*, 2004), which compensates for a modest vasodilatation in the mesenteric (Mancia *et al.*, 1971; Miki *et al.*, 2004) and renal beds (Mancia *et al.*, 1971; Yoshimoto *et al.*, 2004). The tonic increase in muscle vascular resistance is paralleled by an increase in muscle sympathetic nerve activity (Hornyak *et al.*, 1991; Somers *et al.*, 1993; Miki *et al.*, 2004). The latter was attributed to a reflex effect that originates bilaterally from the atonic muscles, because it was abolished in cat hindlimbs after their deafferentation (Baccelli *et al.*, 1974). In the renal vascular bed, the slight vasodilatation during REM sleep is accompanied by a substantial reduction in renal sympathetic nerve activity (Yoshimoto *et al.*, 2004). Renal sympathetic nerve activity during REM sleep is lower than that predicted by the tonic value of arterial pressure on the basis of the relationship that applies to the other states (Miki *et al.*, 2003). Moreover, the decrease in renal sympathetic nerve activity during REM sleep precedes the increase in arterial pressure, and hence is not simply a baroreflex response (Miki *et al.*, 2003). In midcollicular-decerebrate cats in a REM-sleep-like state, muscle sympathetic nerve activity increases and both renal and splanchnic sympathetic nerve activities decrease irrespective of sinoaortic denervation, vagotomy, and paralysis (Futuro-Neto and Coote, 1982). These results suggest that the changes in regional sympathetic activity during REM sleep may occur in the absence of baroreflex resetting and of reflexes elicited by muscle atonia, and may thus represent the result of central autonomic commands issued by brainstem structures. Similarly, central autonomic commands underlie the phasic hypertensive events (arterial pressure surges), which are superimposed upon the tonic level of arterial pressure in REM sleep. Arterial pressure surges have been observed in REM sleep in experimental animals (cat, Mancia *et al.*, 1971; rat, Sei and Morita, 1999; mouse, Campen *et al.*, 2002; lamb, Fewell, 1993; Silvani *et al.*, 2005), and in human subjects, and may exceed the maximum pressure values recorded during wakefulness (Coccagna *et al.*, 1971). During the pressure surges, peripheral vascular resistance increases (Fewell, 1993). The increase in resistance also occurs in the coronary vascular bed (Fewell, 1993), in spite of the greater cardiac metabolic demand during these hypertensive events. The concomitant increase in muscle vascular resistance (Mancia *et al.*, 1971) is abolished by sympathectomy but not by limb deafferentation, indicating that local reflexes are not necessary for its origin (Baccelli *et al.*, 1974). In cats after total transection of the brainstem core at the ponto-mesencephalic junction, phasic hypertensive events are still noted during REM sleep, although they lose their temporal relationship with muscle twitches (Kanamori *et al.*, 1995). Thus, the control by brain structures rostral to the pons is not needed to produce pressure surges in REM sleep, although it deeply affects both their frequency and their relationship with other phasic sleep phenomena. The baroreceptor reflex may also play a role in shaping blood pressure surges in REM sleep, as suggested by the finding that muscle sympathetic nerve activity increases before the surges, but abruptly ceases during their course (Somers *et al.*, 1993).

To summarise, baroreflex control of the vasculature is effective during sleep, although its gain may be reduced during non-REM sleep. In REM sleep, central autonomic commands play a substantial role in the tonic and phasic control of vascular resistance.

Baroreflex control of the heart

Baroreceptor stimulation elicits an increase in vagal activity and a withdrawal of sympathetic activity to the heart. The resultant decrease in heart rate and contractility reduces cardiac output and counteracts the increase in arterial pressure that originated the reflex response (Sagawa, 1984). Owing to the ease of obtaining heart rate recordings and to the development of reliable, yet non-invasive devices to measure arterial pressure in human subjects, a substantial number of studies have investigated baroreflex control of heart rate during sleep. Much of this experimental work focused on the relationship between spontaneous fluctuations in arterial pressure and those in heart rate, to exploit the opportunity of a totally non-invasive approach.

Although with some variation among species and experimental series (see, Silvani *et al.*, 2003; Iellamo *et al.*, 2004 for recent references), heart rate tends to decrease from wakefulness to non-REM sleep despite a slight reduction in arterial pressure, and remains lower than in wakefulness after the transition to REM sleep, when arterial pressure rises again. The tonic changes in heart rate during non-REM sleep may be ascribed either to baroreflex resetting or to the effects of central autonomic commands. The latter may be prominent, as heart rate still decreases substantially from wakefulness to non-REM sleep in rats after sinoaortic denervation (Sei *et al.*, 1999). Conversely, central autonomic commands cannot explain the tonic decrease in heart rate during REM sleep with respect to wakefulness, which is not observed after sinoaortic denervation (Horne *et al.*, 1991; Sei *et al.*, 1999).

The transduction of vagal activity at the sinoatrial node is fast enough to allow beat-to-beat control of heart rhythm (Berger *et al.*, 1989). Conversely, the sinoatrial node responds more slowly to sympathetic activity, acting as a low-pass filter with a corner frequency of 0.01–0.02 Hz coupled to a time delay of 1.7 s (Berger *et al.*, 1989). The vast majority of the results reported on short-term changes in heart rhythm reflect predominantly or solely the baroreflex control of parasympathetic vagal activity (Parati *et al.*, 2000). Early studies in human subjects evaluated the regression coefficient between heart period and arterial pressure after injection of a pressor drug, typically angiotensin. Pickering *et al.* (1968) reported that the gain of the cardiac baroreflex increased significantly during REM sleep and — in most subjects — also during non-REM sleep with respect to wakefulness. Interestingly, the increase in gain during REM sleep was the greatest during bursts of rapid eye movements (Pickering *et al.*, 1968), which may be associated with blood pressure surges (Somers *et al.*, 1993). These results were replicated by Smyth *et al.* (1969). However, another paper by the same group (Bristow *et al.*, 1969) still reported an increase in baroreflex gain in REM sleep with respect to wakefulness, but found evidence of baroreflex resetting rather than of changes in baroreflex gain in non-REM sleep. Accordingly, parallel shifts of the baroreceptor–cardiac reflex response function continuously occur during the night, and are associated with changes in the tonic levels of heart period and arterial pressure (Kasting *et al.*, 1987). Cardiac baroreflex gain was again found to be higher in stages 2 and 3 of non-REM sleep than in wakefulness in a later study (Conway *et al.*, 1983). Subsequent work on cardiac baroreflex gain in sleeping human subjects was mainly based on the analysis of spontaneous fluctuations in heart period and blood pressure. Parati *et al.* (1988) computed baroreflex gain by the so-called sequence method (Parati *et al.*, 2000), i.e., as the regression coefficient between spontaneous parallel changes in heart period and arterial pressure, but did not perform polygraphic recordings. Baroreflex gain increased substantially during the night in healthy human subjects (Parati *et al.*, 1988). These results reflect short-term cardiovascular control, because the length of most of the spontaneous sequences considered was three heart beats. A later study by Nakazato *et al.* (1998), which combined the sequence method with polygraphic discrimination of sleep states in healthy subjects, did not find any significant difference in cardiac baroreflex gain among wake–sleep states, either considering responses to pressure rises or to pressure falls. In recent reports, cardiac baroreflex gain in response to spontaneous decreases in pressure did not differ among wake–sleep states in human subjects, whereas baroreflex gain to pressure increases was higher in non-REM sleep than in wakefulness (Legramante *et al.*, 2003; Iellamo *et al.*, 2004). These findings raise the hypothesis that the cardiac baroreflex does not always work in the linear portion of the arterial pressure — heart period function in physiological conditions; in fact, if it did, results concerning the gain of baroreflex responses to pressure changes in either directions would be similar. The lack of changes in the cardiac baroreflex response to spontaneous decreases in pressure may blunt state-related differences when the sequence method is applied both to increasing and to decreasing spontaneous pressure changes. Baroreflex gain to increases in pressure was the highest during the last cycle of REM sleep in the night, but during the first cycle of REM sleep it did not differ from the gain in wakefulness and was even lower than the gain in the first cycle of non-REM sleep (Legramante *et al.*, 2003). The mechanisms that underlie differences in baroreflex gain during REM sleep in the course of the night are unclear, as baroreflex responsiveness in human subjects does not show substantial circadian variability (Kasting *et al.*, 1987). Differences in the distribution of phasic neural and cardiovascular events between REM sleep cycles might contribute to the results. Similarly, some inconsistencies concerning cardiac baroreflex gain in non-REM sleep may be ascribed to the heterogeneity of this state. Iellamo *et al.* (2004) showed that cardiac baroreflex gain to spontaneous increases in pressure progressively decreased from REM sleep to stage 2 non-REM sleep and further to stages 3 and 4 non-REM sleep, and reached its lowest value in wakefulness. Moreover, cyclic alternating pattern during non-REM sleep increased cardiac baroreflex gain to the values in REM sleep (Iellamo *et al.*, 2004).

On the basis of spontaneous fluctuations in blood pressure and heart period, baroreflex gain has also been computed in the frequency domain as the modulus of the transfer function between the two signals (α coefficient) in a given frequency range (Parati *et al.*, 2000). Van de Borne *et al.* (1994) computed the α coefficient in sleeping healthy subjects in the low-frequency range (0.07–0.14 Hz), which reflects cardiac baroreflex control at a longer term than that covered by the sequence method. Baroreflex gain was the highest during REM sleep, whereas in non-REM sleep it was not significantly different from that during wakefulness (Van de Borne *et al.*, 1994). These results were confirmed with a very similar technique by Monti *et al.* (2002). In this report, the α coefficient was also computed at frequencies around the breathing rate, and found to be higher during both non-REM sleep and REM sleep than during wakefulness (Monti *et al.*, 2002). However, the interpretation of the α coefficient in the high-frequency band requires caution, because central commands play a relevant role in shaping cardiovascular variability around the breathing rate (Parati *et al.*, 2000).

The results of studies performed on animal models do not substantially clarify the picture obtained in human subjects. In baboons, cardiac baroreflex responses either to carotid sinus occlusion (Combs *et al.*, 1986) or to cyclic constriction of the descending aorta at low frequencies (Stephenson *et al.*, 1981) are more marked during (behaviourally determined) sleep with respect to eating and exercise, with a predominant vagal contribution (Stephenson *et al.*, 1981). Thus, the increase in cardiac barore-flex gain that is frequently observed during sleep in human subjects also characterises sleep in a non-human primate. Similar results were reported by Vatner *et al.* (1971), who stimulated the carotid sinus nerve in conscious dogs, eliciting a baroreflex bradycardia that was enhanced in (behaviourally determined) sleep with respect to wakefulness. Conversely, cardiac barore-flex gain in response to the pressor effects of angiotensin was substantially lower in REM sleep than in quiet wakefulness in cats (Knuepfer *et al.*, 1986). A high variability in cardiac baroreflex gain was also reported during REM sleep in cats and could not be linked to any electrophysiological or behavioural parameter (Knuepfer *et al.*, 1986). In cats, Del Bo *et al.* (1985) found that the cardiac baroreflex response to either carotid sinus disten-sion or occlusion was unchanged during quiet sleep with respect to fight-ing and quiet wakefulness. However, some potentiation of the cardiac reflex response to baroreceptor unloading was inferred in non-REM sleep, in which baseline blood pressure was lower than in the other states (Del Bo *et al.*, 1985). During REM sleep, cardiac baroreflex gain was unchanged following carotid sinus distension but depressed following carotid occlusion (Del Bo *et al.*, 1985). These results do not agree with those of Rector *et al.* (2000), who concluded that in cats, especially during depressor challenges, the ven-tral medullary surface is released in REM sleep from neural influences that dampen baroreflexes. In other species, the available evidence does not point toward major changes in cardiac baroreflex gain during sleep. In newborn lambs, no change in gain was found among wake–sleep states following the constriction of an aortic cuff, which induced pressure increases (Horne *et al.*, 1991). It must be noted, however, that REM sleep episodes with frequent phasic events were excluded from the analysis in that study. In rats, cardiac baroreflex gain, as computed by the sequence method, did not show any significant relation to the wake–sleep state (Zoccoli *et al.*, 2001). In neuro-muscularly blocked rats, cardiac baroreflex gain in response to stimulation of the aortic depressor nerve increased with electroencephalographic activ-ity in the delta, but not in the theta frequency band (Dworkin and Dworkin, 2004). Although spectral power in the delta frequency band characterises non-REM sleep and power in the theta band is prominent during REM sleep in rats, the interpretation of these results in terms of wake–sleep states requires caution, because of the non-physiological condition of the model.

To summarise, the prevailing view in the literature both on human sub-jects and on animal models is that cardiac baroreflex gain increases dur-ing sleep, and particularly during REM sleep, with respect to wakefulness.

However, the finding is not constant either within or between species, suggesting that any difference in cardiac baroreflex gain among wake–sleep states is not substantial. Cardiac baroreflex gain during the night may be affected by sleep microstructure and by phasic cardiovascular events occurring during sleep, thus adding a confounding factor when one attempts to compare the results of different studies. Moreover, state-related differences in baroreflex gain to rises, but not to decreases in pressure suggest that shifts in the working point of the cardiac baroreflex may occur during the night. In particular, the working point may be near the upper saturating portion of the arterial pressure — heart period function during wakefulness, and may progressively shift downward and leftward along the linear portion of the curve during non-REM sleep and REM sleep. Targeted studies are needed to test this hypothesis.

Whereas the results concerning cardiac baroreflex gain during sleep need some clarification, it is clear that heart rhythm is deeply affected by non-baroreflex, central autonomic commands during sleep as well as during wakefulness. In cats, heart rate surges were reported in correspondence with the bursts of rapid eye movements in REM sleep, and were rarely accompanied by modest increases in arterial pressure (Gassel *et al.*, 1964). In dogs, during REM sleep, phasic surges and pauses in heart rate may not be preceded by blood pressure changes (Dickerson *et al.*, 1993), suggesting that autonomic control of the heart may be phasically independent from that of the circulation during this state. On the other hand, heart rate surges accompany surges in blood pressure during REM sleep (Sei and Morita, 1996; Silvani *et al.*, 2005), indicating that an integrated, non-baroreflex cardiovascular control may also prevail in this state. The effects of such a control on heart rate and arterial pressure are analogous to those that characterise the defence reaction (Spyer, 1994) or the onset of dynamic exercise (DiCarlo and Bishop, 2001) during wakefulness. In rats (Sei and Morita, 1996), heart rate tends to rise during the pressure surges in REM sleep, and increases significantly thereafter. In newborn lambs (Silvani *et al.*, 2005), heart rate starts to rise concomitantly with the increase in blood pressure, but decreases below control levels thereafter during the course of the pressure surge. Thus, in newborn lambs, baroreflex control of heart rate prevails late in the course of the pressure surges, when arterial pressure is still above control levels, arguing against a major role of baroreflex resetting (cf. DiCarlo and Bishop, 2001) in the generation of the blood pressure surges in REM sleep. The qualitative notion that central autonomic commands act on the heart and on blood vessels during REM sleep has been recently quantified by assessing the role played by central commands and by the baroreflex in the control of heart rhythm during sleep (Zoccoli *et al.*, 2001; Silvani *et al.*, 2003, 2005). In particular, parallel changes in heart period and blood pressure (e.g., a pattern of hypertension and cardiac slowing) indicate that heart rhythm control is mainly exerted by the baroreceptor reflex, whereas opposite changes in the two variables (e.g., a pattern of hypertension and tachycardia, like that observed during pressure surges in REM sleep) indicates that central autonomic commands prevail over the baroreflex in controlling heart rhythm (Zoccoli *et al.*, 2001). The linear regression and the linear correlation coefficients yield information on the sign and strength of the relationship between heart period and arterial pressure within a given time window, which may be suited to the length of the sleep episodes in the model studied. In adult rats, central autonomic commands on the heart and blood vessels prevail in REM sleep as a whole over the control exerted by the baroreceptor reflex (Zoccoli *et al.*, 2001; Silvani *et al.*, 2003). Their prevalence is linked to slow oscillations in heart period, which reflect its sympathetic modulation (Zoccoli *et al.*, 2001). These results cannot be attributed to sleep-related changes in cardiac baroreflex gain, which are negligible in this model (Zoccoli *et al.*, 2001). Following acoustic stimuli, primary pressure changes occur in all wake–sleep states, and elicit strong cardiac baroreflex responses (Silvani *et al.*, 2003). Accordingly, the prevalence of central autonomic commands in the control of heart rhythm during REM sleep almost disappears after cardiovascular regulation has been perturbed by acoustic stimulation during sleep, even though no clear-cut prevalence of baroreflex control emerges in this state (Silvani *et al.*, 2003). On the other hand, during non-REM sleep, heart rhythm is under prevalent baroreflex control both in control conditions and after acoustic stimulation (Zoccoli *et al.*, 2001; Silvani *et al.*, 2003). Thus, sleep-related changes in the prevalence of baroreflex control of heart rhythm persist despite cardiovascular perturbations. These sleep-related changes may be observed across species and developmental stages. In fact, baroreflex coupling between heart period and arterial pressure is stronger in non-REM sleep than in REM sleep also in newborn lambs (Silvani *et al.*, 2005), in which again no major changes in cardiac baroreflex gain occur across sleep states (Horne *et al.*, 1991). In newborn lambs, however, central autonomic commands do not prevail over the baroreceptor reflex in REM sleep as a whole (Silvani *et al.*, 2004), at variance with the results reported in rats in control conditions (Zoccoli *et al.*, 2001; Silvani *et al.*, 2003). To summarise, the role of the baroreceptor reflex in controlling heart rhythm is greater in non-REM sleep than in REM sleep. On the other hand, during REM sleep, the prevalence of central autonomic commands in the control of heart rhythm is inconstant, and mirrors the features of cardiovascular control during the phasic events in this state.

Theoretical issue

Taking into account the different central and peripheral influences to the heart and vessels (see Zoccoli *et al.*, 2001) it is possible to discuss the concept of "baroreflex resetting" frequently utilised to describe the presumable shift of the baroreflex set-point (see, for instance, Kasting *et al.*, 1987). Let us consider the following diagramatic scheme, corresponding to that proposed by Zoccoli and coworkers (Zoccoli *et al.*, 2001):

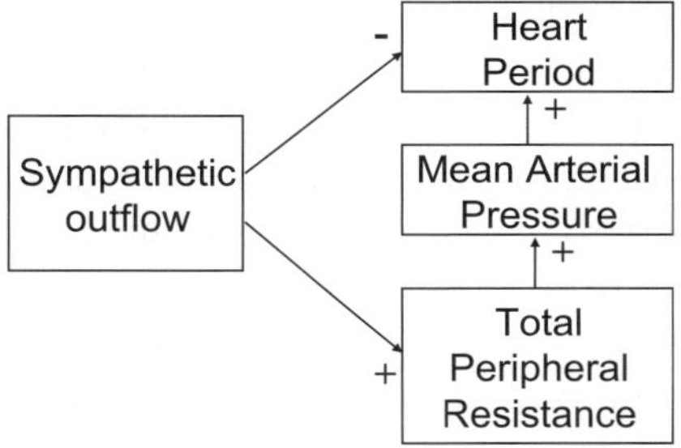

If a tonic increase occurs in the sympathetic outflow to the heart and vessels, an increase in total peripheral resistance and mean arterial pressure will occur, though dampened by the baroreceptor-arterial pressure reflex. The heart period will be influenced in opposite directions by the increase in sympathetic outflow to the heart and the increase in mean arterial pressure, respectively. The new mean value of the heart period may be higher or lower than the previous one, depending on the relative strength of central and baroreflex drives. In this new condition the fluctuations of mean arterial pressure will influence the heart period with a gain that, in the hypothesis of linearity, is unchanged. The transition to this new condition, characterised by the same baroreflex gain as before, but different central values for mean arterial pressure and heart period, is commonly referred to as "baroreflex resetting." Thus a putative "baroreflex resetting" may actually reflect a change in the tonic value of the autonomic output to the heart and vessels.

Chemoreceptor Reflexes

Chemoreceptor location

Peripheral and central chemoreceptors exert a profound effect on ventilation and cardiovascular regulation during wakefulness and especially during sleep. The peripheral arterial chemoreceptors, located in the carotid and aortic bodies (glomi) at the carotid bifurcation and near the arch of aorta, respectively, send chemoceptive information towards medullary centers including the nucleus tractus solitarii (for reviews, see Kara *et al.*, 2003; Timmers *et al.*, 2003). Because of their anatomic location, aortic bodies have been less extensively studied and their function appears to be similar, though less powerful, to that of the carotid bodies. Peripheral chemoreceptors respond to changes in O_2, CO_2, and H^+ concentration. Although peripheral chemoreceptors are primarily responsible for O_2 sensing, they are also important for CO_2 sensing (Timmers *et al.*, 2003). Central chemoreceptors are distributed in many regions from the brain stem to the thalamus (Haxhiu *et al.*, 2001; Nattie and Li, 2002; Neubauer and Sunderram, 2004) and mostly contribute to CO_2/H^+ sensing, even if O_2 sensing neurons are also present (Neubauer and Sunderram, 2004). Central chemoception appears to depend on the wake–sleep state (Li *et al.*, 1999; Nattie and Li, 2002). In spite of the extensive research done on this topic, the exact mechanisms involved in chemoreceptor activation remain unclear for both peripheral and central chemoreceptors.

Effects of chemoreceptor activation

Chemoreceptors had been initially studied for their manifest effects on ventilation, but it was soon evident that they also exert profound effects on cardiovascular control. Chemoreceptor activation induces hyperventilation, but also increases vagal outflow to the heart and sympathetic outflow to blood vessels, thus inducing bradycardia and hypertension. Hypertension, in turn, acts on the heart and vessels through the baroreceptor reflex, which tends to further lower heart rate and to dampen the increase in arterial pressure. Concomitantly, the increased ventilation exerts an opposite effect on the heart and vessels, stimulating heart rate and reducing peripheral resistance and arterial pressure (Kara *et al.*, 2003). The balance of the different contributions is obviously complex, since the different chemical stimuli (O_2, CO_2, and H^+ concentrations) activate with different thresholds peripheral and central chemoreceptors, which in turn may exert different ventilatory and cardiovascular effects, while the behavioural state also plays a role in this balance. A further complicating factor is the duration of chemoreceptor activation, since the different regulations adapt with different time constants and the tonic effects of chemoreceptor stimulation may be different from the phasic ones. In any case, ventilatory disturbances that lead to hypoxic and/or hypercapnic episodes also determine important cardiovascular effects, so that they are worth considering in the study of cardiovascular control. Depressed chemical drives facilitate the development of central apneas and hypoventilation, while strong drives may lead to periodic breathing and central apneas as well (De Backer, 1998). Acute exposure to hypobaric hypoxia at high altitude increases sympathetic activity and blood pressure, these effects outlasting the exposure period and remaining after return to the sea level (Hansen and Sander, 2003). The cardiovascular effects of hypoxaemia are larger if hypoxaemia is produced by apnea than if it is produced by breathing a hypoxic mixture (Kara *et al.*, 2003) because in the first instance there is not the dampening effect of ventilation. The effects of exposure to hypoxia are not limited to the cardioventilatory regulation, but also include the activation of mechanisms ranging from molecular to cell to system levels (Sarkar *et al.*, 2003). The sympathetic adjustments induced by mild hypoxia are initiated by activation of peripheral chemoreceptors, while more severe hypoxia activates the sympathetic outflow via direct effects on the brain stem (Guyenet, 2000). In patients whose carotid body had been resected because of a neoplasia, the normocapnic hypoxic responsiveness was completely abolished, while a residual responsiveness to hypoxaemia during simultaneous hypercapnia was present and could originate from the aortic bodies (Timmers *et al.*, 2003). The timing of hypoxic changes is also relevant: in rats, exposure to chronic intermittent hypoxia induces long term facilitation of carotid body sensory activity (Peng *et al.*, 2003) and increases arterial pressure well over the stimulation period (Hui *et al.*, 2003), whereas these effects are not evoked by sustained hypoxia. The increase in arterial pressure associated with intermittent hypoxia is blocked by carotid body denervation, sympathetic nerve ablation, renal sympathectomy, adrenal medullectomy and angiotensin II receptor blockade. Apparently, the adrenergic and renin–angiotensin system overactivity is required for the appearance of the hypertensive effects of intermittent hypoxia in rats, and similarly for the development of hypertension associated with obstructive sleep apneas in patients (Fletcher, 2001). As far as hypercapnic stimuli are concerned, the cardioventilatory response mostly relies on central chemoreceptors, but carotid chemoreceptor also contribute, since carotid denervation reduces this response by 30% (Timmers *et al.*, 2003).

Chemoreceptor activation and the wake–sleep states

Chemoreflex sensitivity is wake–sleep state dependent. The ventilatory responses to hypercapnia and hypoxia are generally reduced during sleep compared to wakefulness (Corfield *et al.*, 1999). Thus, in rats, CO_2 microdialysis in the retrotrapezoid nucleus increases breathing in wakefulness but not in sleep (Li *et al.*, 1999). Sleep deprivation *per se* does not decrease the hypercapnic ventilatory response in humans (Spengler and Shea, 2000). While during wakefulness ventilation also relies on other drives, during sleep it essentially depends on chemoreceptor activation. Subjects lacking chemoreceptor control breathe adequately during many waking behaviours, but seriously hypoventilate during non-REM sleep (Shea, 1997). Post-hyperventilation apneas occur during sleep but not during wakefulness in human subjects (Skatrud and Dempsey, 1983). Hypoxia causes periodic breathing during non-REM sleep, but not during wakefulness (Berssenbrugge *et al.*, 1983). Peripheral chemoreceptors play a fundamental role in ventilatory regulation during sleep and their role also changes with the wake–sleep state. Thus, periodic breathing during sleep is favoured by high peripheral chemoreflex sensitivity (Lahiri *et al.*, 1983). Peripheral chemoreceptor activity contributes to the amplification of changes in ventilation related to the wake–sleep state in human subjects (Dunai *et al.*, 1996). During non-REM sleep, post-hyperventilation apnea does not occur in chemoreceptor denervated dogs (Nakayama *et al.*, 2003). Peripheral chemoreceptor deactivation by hypocapnia-alkalosis decreases tidal volume during wakefulness and non-REM sleep and, if hypocapnia is severe enough, during REM sleep in dogs (Smith *et al.*, 1997). In goats, following carotid body denervation, ventrolateral medullary cooling caused prolonged apneas during non-REM sleep but only brief apneas in the awake state (Ohtake *et al.*, 1996). However, in lambs, alveolar hypoxia produced similar cardioventilatory responses during the different wake–sleep states (Fewell *et al.*, 1984).

Hypoxia affects sleep by inducing periodic breathing and central apneas, increasing arousals, reducing total sleep time and determining a shift toward lighter sleep stages, with marked decrements in slow-wave and REM sleep. The poor sleep quality may account for worsened daytime performance at high altitude (Mizuno *et al.*, 1993; Salvaggio *et al.*, 1998; Wickramasinghe and Anholm, 1999; Barash *et al.*, 2001; Weil, 2004) in human subjects. Sleep disturbances may be reduced by enrichment of room air with O_2 (Barash *et al.*, 2001). Peripheral chemoreceptors contribute to the disruption of REM sleep under hypoxic conditions (Ryan and Megirian, 1982).

Chemoreceptor activation may determine awakening, the mechanisms of arousal depending on chemical and/or mechanical stimuli. For example, mechanical stimuli are stronger with obstructive than with central apneas (for a review, see Berry and Gleeson, 1997). O_2 and CO_2 interact in producing awakening in human subjects: the time to awakening in response to airway occlusion is increased while breathing an hyperoxic mixture and decreased by a hypercapnic mixture (Berry and Light, 1992; Berry *et al.*, 1993). Carotid chemoreceptors and baroreceptors play a major role in producing awakening during hypoxic and/or hypercapnic stimulation. In fact, in carotid denervated cats exposed to rapid hypoxia, awakening occurred at arterial O_2 saturation lower than 50% (Neubauer *et al.*, 1981). Following carotid denervation, in lambs exposed to hypoxia or hypercapnia the awakening delay increased, being longer in REM sleep than in non-REM sleep and further increasing with repeated hypoxic stimulations. Most importantly, following carotid denervation, awakening failed to occur in the majority of cases of hypoxic and hypercapnic stimulation in lambs and dogs (Bowes *et al.*, 1981; Fewell *et al.*, 1989, 1990). On the contrary, following airway occlusion, awakening occurred almost always in lambs, but it took longer to occur (Fewell *et al.*, 1990).

Chronic intermittent hypoxia determines the persistent ventilatory, cardiovascular and metabolic effects that are normally associated wits continuous exposure to hypoxia. Though considered to provide beneficial effects in certain diseases, to improve exercise performances in athletes and to enhance the ventilatory response to acute hypoxia, chronic intermittent hypoxia causes detrimental effects such as arterial hypertension, neuropathological and cognitive deficits, enhanced susceptibility to oxydative injury, and possibly myocardial and cerebral infarction (for reviews, see Neubauer, 2001; Kara *et al.*, 2003). Sleep apneas (either obstructive or central) frequently occur in human subjects and cause these adverse effects, too. In sleep apnea patients, the peripheral chemoreflex response to hypoxia and hypercapnia is enhanced, while tonic activation of peripheral chemoreceptors contributes to the high levels of sympathetic activity and arterial pressure observed even during normoxic daytime wakefulness. The tonic increase in sympathetic activity possibly depends on adaptation processes occurring within the sympathoexcitatory region of the rostral ventrolateral medulla, where neurons are sensitive to direct effects of hypoxia. The long-term changes generated by exposure to chronic intermittent hypoxia, as well as those consequent to sustained hypobaric hypoxia at high altitude, may have an adaptive value and improve the ability to survive in the extreme conditions experienced. However, neurocognitive deficits may develop with sustained or chronic intermittent hypoxia (Neubauer, 2001). This suggests that hypoxic damage occurs in neural tissue, likely due to mitochondrial oxygen deficiency, leading to cell energy deficit, adverse metabolic changes and damage at a cellular level. Hypoxic functional impairment of neural tissue is also suggested by poor sleep quality and reduced work efficiency at high altitude, while air oxygen enrichment appears to improve sleep quality (Barash *et al.*, 2001). The hypothesis that oxygen mitochondrial deficiency is caused by the limitation of oxygen diffusion is worth considering (Lenzi *et al.*, 2000).

Some conclusions may now be drawn. Chemoreceptor activation in response to chemical drives stimulates adaptive changes in regulatory functions. Some responses appears to be beneficial for survival, for instance the increase in ventilation in hypoxic or hypercapnic conditions. Some responses may be adverse, e.g., the generation of reactive free radicals during hypoxia may lead to neuronal damage. Some other responses may be at the same time beneficial and adverse. For instance, the increase in arterial pressure evoked by the chemoreflex may help increase blood flow to critical tissues under acute hypoxic or hypercapnic conditions, but becomes dangerous for the heart and vessels when lasting for a long time. However, even this last point may be discussed. In fact, if extreme environmental conditions are long lasting, long-lasting adaptations, such as the increase in arterial pressure, are adequate to enhance survival, even at the price of worsening cognitive and circulatory long-term performance. The basic point is that extreme conditions are intrinsically dangerous for the organism and that the regulatory mechanisms may only do their best to help survival. The resulting quality of survival is possibly far less than optimal.

References

Baccelli, G., Albertini, R., Mancia, G., and Zanchetti, A. (1974). Central and reflex regulation of sympathetic vasoconstrictor activity to limb muscles during desynchronized sleep in the cat. *Circ. Res.*, 35: 625–635.

Barash, I., Beatty, C., Powell, F., Prisk, G., and West, J. (2001). Nocturnal oxygen enrichment of room air at 3800 meter altitude improves sleep architecture. *High Alt. Med. Biol.*, 2: 525–533.

Berger, R., Saul, J., and Cohen, R. (1989). Transfer function analysis of autonomic regulation I. Canine atrial rate response. *Am. J. Physiol.*, 256: H142–152.

Berry, R. and Gleeson, K. (1997). Respiratory arousal from sleep: mechanisms and significance. *Sleep*, 20: 654–675.

Berry, R. and Light, R. (1992). Effect of hyperoxia on the arousal response to airway occlusion during sleep in normal subjects. *Am. Rev. Respir. Dis.*, 146: 330–334.

Berry, R., Mahutte, C., and Light, R. (1993). Effect of hypercapnia on the arousal response to airway occlusion during sleep in normal subjects. *J. Appl. Physiol.*, 74: 2269–2275.

Berssenbrugge, A., Dempsey, J., Iber, C., Skatrud, J., and Wilson, P. (1983). Mechanisms of hypoxia-induced periodic breathing during sleep in humans. *J. Physiol.*, 343: 507–526.

Bowes, G., Townsend, E., Kozar, L., Bromley, S., and Phillipson, E. (1981). Effect of carotid body denervation on arousal response to hypoxia in sleeping dogs. *J. Appl. Physiol.*, 51: 40–45.

Bristow, J., Honour, A., Pickering, T., and Sleight, P. (1969). Cardiovascular and respiratory changes during sleep in normal and hypertensive subjects. *Cardiovasc. Res.*, 3: 476–485.

Campen, M.J., Tagaito, Y., Jenkins, T.P., Smith, P.L., Schwartz, A.R., and O'Donnel, C.P. (2002). Phenotypic differences in the hemodynamic response during REM sleep in six strains of inbred mice. *Physiol. Genomics*, 11: 227–234.

Coccagna, G., Mantovani, M., Brignani, F., Manzini, A., and Lugaresi, E. (1971). Arterial pressure changes during spontaneous sleep in man. *Electroencephalogr. Clin. Neurophysiol.*, 31: 277–281.

Combs, C., Smith, O., Astley, C., and Feigl, E. (1986). Differential effect of behavior on cardiac and vasomotor baroreflex responses. *Am. J. Physiol.*, 251: R126–136.

Conway, J., Boon, N., Vann Jones, J., and Sleight, P. (1983). Involvement of the baroreceptor reflexes in the changes in blood pressure with sleep and mental arousal. *Hypertension*, 5: 746–748.

Corfield, D., Roberts, C., Griffiths, M., and Adams, L. (1999). Sleep-related changes in the human 'neuromuscular' ventilatory response to hypoxia. *Respir. Physiol.*, 117: 109–120.

Crisostomo, I., Zayyad, A., Carley, D.W., Abubaker, J., Onal, E., Stepanski, E.J., Lopata, M., and Basner, R.C. (1998). Chemo- and baroresponses differ in African-Americans and Caucasians in sleep. *J. Appl. Physiol.*, 85: 1413–1420.

De Backer, W. (1998). Methods and clinical significance of studying chemical drives. *Respir. Physiol.*, 114: 75–81.

Del Bo, A., Baccelli, G., Cellina, G., Fea, F., Ferrari, A., and Zanchetti, A. (1985). Carotid sinus reflexes during postural changes, naturally elicited fighting behavior and phases of sleep in the cat. *Cardiovasc. Res.*, 19: 762–769.

DiCarlo, S.E. and Bishop, V. (2001). Central baroreflex resetting as a means of increasing and decreasing sympathetic outflow and arterial pressure. *Ann. N. Y. Acad. Sci.*, 940: 324–337.

Dickerson, L., Huang, A., Nearing, B., and Verrier, R. (1993). Primary coronary vasodilation associated with pauses in heart rhythm during sleep. *Am. J. Physiol.*, 264: 186–196.

Dunai, J., Wilkinson, M., and Trinder, J. (1996). Interaction of chemical and state effects on ventilation during sleep onset. *J. Appl. Physiol.*, 81: 2235–2243.

Dworkin, B.R. and Dworkin, S. (2004). Baroreflexes of the rat. III. Open-loop gain and electroencephalographic arousal. *Am. J. Physiol.*, 286: R597–605.

Dworkin, B.R., Dworkin, S., and Tang, X. (2000). Carotid and aortic baroreflexes of the rat: I. Open-loop steady-state properties and blood pressure variability. *Am. J. Physiol.*, 279: R1910–1921.

Fagius, J., Wallin, B.G., Sundlof, G., Nerhed, C., and Englesson, S. (1985). Sympathetic outflow in man after anaesthesia of the glossopharyngeal and vagus nerves. *Brain*, 108: 423–438.

Ferini-Strambi, L., Rovaris, M., Oldani, A., Martinelli, V., Filippi, M., Smirne, S., Zucconi, M., and Comi, G. (1995). Cardiac autonomic function during sleep and wakefulness in multiple sclerosis. *J. Neurol.*, 242: 639–643.

Fewell, J., Williams, B., and Hill, D. (1984). Sleep does not affect the cardiovascular response to alveolar hypoxia in lambs. *J. Dev. Physiol.*, 6: 401–405.

Fewell, J., Kondo, C., Dascalu, V., and Filyk, S. (1989). Influence of carotid denervation on the arousal and cardiopulmonary response to rapidly developing hypoxemia in lambs. *Pediatr. Res.*, 25: 473–477.

Fewell, J., Taylor, B., Kondo, C., Dascalu, V., and Filyk, S. (1990). Influence of carotid denervation on the arousal and cardiopulmonary responses to upper airway obstruction in lambs. *Pediatr. Res.*, 28: 374–378.

Fewell, J.E. (1993). Influence of sleep on systemic and coronary hemodynamics in lambs. *J. Dev. Physiol.*, 19: 71–76.

Fletcher, E. (2001). Physiological consequences of intermittent hypoxia: systemic blood pressure. *J. Appl. Physiol.*, 90: 1600–1605.

Franco, P., Szilwowski, H., Dramaix, M., and Kahn, A. (1998). Polisomnographic study of the autonomic nervous system in potential victims of sudden infant death syndrome. *Clin. Auton. Res.*, 8: 243–249.

Futuro-Neto, H.A., and Coote, J.H. (1982). Changes in sympathetic activity to heart and blood vessels during desynchronized sleep. *Brain Res.*, 252: 259–268.

Gassel, M.M., Ghelarducci, B., Marchiafava, P.L., and Pompeiano, O. (1964). Phasic changes in blood pressure and heart rate during the rapid eye movement episodes of desynchronized sleep in unrestrained cats. *Arch. Ital. Biol.*, 102: 530–544.

George, C.F.P. (2000). Hypertension, ischemic heart disease, and stroke. In: Kryger, M.H., Roth, T., and Dement W.C. (Eds.). *Principles and Practice of Sleep Medicine.* Philadelphia: W.B. Saunders Company, pp. 1030–1039.

Guyenet, P. (2000). Neural structures that mediate sympathoexcitation during hypoxia. *Respir. Physiol.*, 121: 147–162.

Hansen, J. and Sander, M. (2003). Sympathetic neural overactivity in healthy humans after prolonged exposure to hypobaric hypoxia. *J. Physiol.*, 546: 921–929.

Haxhiu, M., Tolentino-Silva, F., Pete, G., Kc, P., and Mack, S. (2001). Monoaminergic neurons, chemosensation and arousal. *Respir. Physiol.*, 129: 191–209.

Horne, R., De Preu, N., Berger, P., and Walker, A. (1991). Arousal responses to hypertension in lambs: effect of sinoaortic denervation. *Am. J. Physiol.*, 260: 1283–1289.

Hornyak, M., Cejnar, M., Elam, M., Matousek, M., and Wallin, G. (1991). Sympathetic muscle nerve activity during sleep in man. *Brain*, 114: 1281–1295.

Hui, A.S., Striet, J.B., Gudelsky, G., Sovkhova, G.K., Gozal, E., Beitner-Johnson, D., Guo, S.Z., Sachleben, L.R., Haycock, J.W., Gozal, D., and Czyzyk-Kazeska, M.F. (2003). Regulation of catecholamines by sustained and intermittent hypoxia in neuroendocrine cells and sympathetic neurons. *Hypertension*, 42: 1130–1136.

Iellamo, F., Placidi, F., Marciani, M.G., Romigi, A., Tombini, M., Aquilani, S., Massaro, M., Galante, A., and Legramante, J.M. (2004). Baroreflex buffering of sympathetic activation during sleep. Evidence from autonomic assessment of sleep macroarchitecture and microarchitecture. *Hypertension*, 43: 1–6.

Kanamori, N., Sakai, K., Sei, H., Bouvard, A., Salvert, D., Vanni-Mercier, G., and Jouvet, M. (1995). Effects of decerebration on blood pressure during paradoxical sleep in cats. *Brain Res. Bull.*, 37: 545–549.

Kara, T., Narkiewicz, K., and Somers, V. (2003). Chemoreflexes — physiology and clinical implications. *Acta Physiol. Scand.*, 177: 377–384.

Kasting, G., Eckberg, D., Fritsch, J., and Birkett, C. (1987). Continuous resetting of the human carotid baroreceptor-cardiac reflex. *Am. J. Physiol.*, 252: 732–736.

Knuepfer, M., Stumpf, H., and Stock, G. (1986). Baroreceptor sensitivity during desynchronized sleep. *Exp. Neurol.*, 92: 323–334.

Kodama, Y., Iwase, S., Mano, T., Cui, J., Kitazawa, H., Okada, H., Takeuchi, S., and Sobue, G. (1998). Attenuation of regional differentiation of sympathetic nerve activity during sleep in humans. *J. Auton. Nerv. Syst.*, 74: 126–133.

Lahiri, S., Maret, K., and Sherpa, M. (1983). Dependence of high altitude sleep apnea on ventilatory sensitivity to hypoxia. *Respir. Physiol.*, 52: 281–301.

Legramante, J.M., Marciani, M.G., Placidi, F., Aquilani, S., Romigi, A., Tombini, M., Massaro, M., Galante, A., and Iellamo, F. (2003). Sleep-related changes in baroreflex sensitivity and cardiovascular autonomic modulation. *J. Hypertens.*, 21: 1555–1561.

Lenzi, P., Cianci, T., Guidalotti, P.L., Leonardi, G.S., and Franzini, C. (1987). Brain circulation during sleep and its relation to extracerebral hemodynamics. *Brain Res.*, 415: 14–20.

Lenzi, P., Cianci, T., Leonardi, G.S., Martinelli, A., and Franzini, C. (1989). Muscle blood flow changes during sleep as a function of fibre type composition. *Exp. Brain Res.*, 74: 549–554.

Lenzi, P., Zoccoli, G., Walker, A.M., and Franzini, C. (2000). Cerebral circulation in REM sleep: is oxygen a main regulating factor? *Sleep Res. Online*, 3: 77–85.

Li, A., Randall, M., and Nattie, E. (1999). CO(2) microdialysis in retrotrapezoid nucleus of the rat increases breathing in wakefulness but not in sleep. *J. Appl. Physiol.*, 87: 910–919.

Malpas, S.C. (2002). Neural influences on cardiovascular variability: possibilities and pitfalls. *Am. J. Physiol.*, H282: 6–20.

Mancia, G., Baccelli, G., Adams, D.B., and Zanchetti, A. (1971). Vasomotor regulation during sleep in the cat. *Am. J. Physiol.*, 220: 1086–1093.

Merrill, D., McWeeny, O., Segar, J., and Robillard, J. (1995). Impairment of cardiopulmonary baroreflexes during the newborn period. *Am. J. Physiol.*, 268: 1343–1351.

Miki, K., Kato, M., and Kajii, S. (2003). Relationship between renal sympathetic nerve activity and arterial pressure during REM sleep in rats. *Am. J. Physiol.*, 284: 467–473.

Miki, K., Oda, M., Kamijyo, N., Kawahara, K., and Yoshimoto, M. (2004). Lumbar sympathetic nerve activity and hindquarter blood flow during REM sleep in rats. *J. Physiol.*, 557: 261–271.

Mizuno, K., Asano, K., and Okudaira, N. (1993). Sleep and respiration under acute hypobaric hypoxia. *Jpn. J. Physiol.*, 43: 161–175.

Monti, A., Medigue, C., Nedelcoux, H., and Escourrou, P. (2002). Autonomic control of the cardiovascular system during sleep in normal subjects. *Eur. J. Appl. Physiol.*, 87: 174–181.

Nakayama, H., Smith, C., Rodman, J., Skatrud, J., and Dempsey, J. (2003). Carotid body denervation eliminates apnea in response to transient hypocapnia. *J. Appl. Physiol.*, 94: 155–164.

Nakazato, T., Shikama, T., Toma, S., Nakajima, Y., and Masuda, Y. (1998). Nocturnal variation in human sympathetic baroreflex sensitivity. *J. Auton. Nerv. Syst.*, 70: 32–37.

Nattie, E. and Li, A. (2002). CO2 dialysis in nucleus tractus solitarius region of rat increases ventilation in sleep and wakefulness. *J. Appl. Physiol.*, 92: 2119–2130.

Neubauer, J. (2001). Physiological and pathophysiological responses to intermittent hypoxia. *J. Appl. Physiol.*, 90: 1593–1599.

Neubauer, J. and Sunderram, J. (2004). Oxygen-sensing neurons in the central nervous system. *J. Appl. Physiol.*, 96: 367–374.

Neubauer, J., Santiago, T., and Edelman, N. (1981). Hypoxic arousal in intact and carotid chemodenervated sleeping cats. *J. Appl. Physiol.*, 51: 1294–1299.

Ohtake, P., Forster, H., Pan, L., Lowry, T., Korducki, M., and Whaley, A. (1996). Effects of cooling the ventrolateral medulla on diaphragm activity during NREM sleep. *Respir. Physiol.*, 104: 127–135.

Parati, G., Di Rienzo, M., Bertinieri, G., Pomidossi, G., Casadei, R., Groppelli, A., Pedotti, A., Zanchetti, A., and Mancia, G. (1988). Evaluation of the baroreceptor-heart rate reflex by 24-hour intra-arterial blood pressure monitoring in humans. *Hypertension*, 12: 214–222.

Parati, G., Di Rienzo, M., and Mancia, G. (2000). How to measure baroreflex sensitivity: from the cardiovascular laboratory to daily life. *J. Hypertens.*, 18: 7–19.

Parmeggiani, P.L. (1980). Behavioral phenomenology of sleep (somatic and vegetative). *Experientia*, 36: 6–11.

Peng, Y., Overholt, J., Kline, D., Kumar, G., and Prabhakar, N. (2003). Induction of sensory long-term facilitation in the carotid body by intermittent hypoxia: implications for recurrent apneas. *Proc. Natl. Acad. Sci. USA*, 100: 10073–10078.

Pickering, G.W., Sleight, P., and Smyth, H.S. (1968). The reflex regulation of arterial pressure during sleep in man. *J. Physiol.*, 194: 46P–48P.

Quattrochi, J.J., Shapiro, J., Verrier, R.L., and Hobson, J.A. (2000). Transient cardiorespiratory events during NREM sleep: a feline model for human microarousals. *J. Sleep Res.*, 9: 185–191.

Rector, D.M., Richard, C.A., Staba, R.J., and Harper, R.M. (2000). Sleep states alter ventral medullary surface responses to blood pressure challenges. *Am. J. Physiol.*, 278: 1090–1098.

Ryan, A. and Megirian, D. (1982). Sleep–wake patterns of intact and carotid sinus nerve sectioned rats during hypoxia. *Sleep*, 5: 1–10.

Sagawa, K. (1984). Baroreflex control of systemic arterial pressure and vascular bed. In: Geiger, S.R. and Wiedeman, M.P. (Eds.). *Handbook of Physiology*. Bethesda, MD: Am. Physiol. Soc., pp. 453–496.

Salvaggio, A., Insalaco, G., Marrone, O., Romano, S., Braghiroli, A., Lanfranchi, P., Patruno, V., Donner, C., and Bonsignore, G. (1998). Effects of high-altitude periodic breathing on sleep and arterial oxyhaemoglobin saturation. *Eur. Respir. J.*, 12: 408–413.

Sarkar, S., Banerjee, P., and Selvamurthy, W. (2003). High altitude hypoxia: an intricate interplay of oxygen responsive macroevents and micromolecules. *Mol. Cell. Biochem.*, 253: 287–305.

Sei, H. and Morita, Y. (1996). Acceleration of EEG theta wave precedes the phasic surge of arterial pressure during REM sleep in the rat. *NeuroReport*, 7: 3059–3062.

Sei, H. and Morita, Y. (1999). Why does arterial blood pressure rise actively during REM sleep? *J. Med. Invest.*, 46: 11–17.

Sei, H., Morita, Y., Tsunooka, K., and Morita, H. (1999). Sino-aortic denervation augments the increase in blood pressure seen during paradoxical sleep in the rat. *J. Sleep Res.*, 8: 45–50.

Shea, S. (1997). Life without ventilatory chemosensitivity. *Respir. Physiol.*, 110: 199–210.

Silvani, A., Bojic, T., Cianci, T., Franzini, C., Lodi, C.A., Predieri, S., Zoccoli, G., and Lenzi, P. (2003). Effects of acoustic stimulation on cardiovascular regulation during sleep. *Sleep*, 2: 201–205.

Silvani, A., Asti, V., Bojic, T., Ferrari, V., Franzini, C., Grant, D.A., Lenzi, P., Walker, A.M., and Zoccoli, G. (2005). Sleep-dependent changes in the coupling between heart period and arterial pressure in newborn lambs. *Pediatr. Res.*, 57: 108–114.

Skatrud, J. and Dempsey, J. (1983). Interaction of sleep state and chemical stimuli in sustaining rhythmic ventilation. *J. Appl. Physiol.*, 55: 813–822.

Smith, C., Harms, C., Henderson, K., and Dempsey, J. (1997). Ventilatory effects of specific carotid body hypocapnia and hypoxia in awake dogs. *J. Appl. Physiol.*, 82: 791–798.

Smyth, H., Sleigth, P., and Pickering, G. (1969). Reflex regulation of arterial pressure during sleep in man. *Circ. Res.*, 24: 109–121.

Somers, V.K., Dyken, M.E., Mark, A.L., and Abboud, F.M. (1993). Sympathetic nerve activity during sleep in normal subjects. *N. Engl. J. Med.*, 328: 303–307.

Spengler, C. and Shea, S. (2000). Sleep deprivation *per se* does not decrease the hypercapnic ventilatory response in humans. *Am. J. Respir. Crit. Care Med.*, 166: 1005.

Spyer, K. (1994). Central nervous mechanisms contributing to cardiovascular control. *J. Physiol.*, 474: 1–19.

Stella, M., Knuth, S., and Bartlett, D. (2001). Respiratory response to baroreceptor stimulation and spontaneous contractions of the urinary bladder. *Respir. Physiol.*, 124: 169–178.

Stephenson, R., Smith, O., and Scher, A. (1981). Baroreceptor regulation of heart rate in baboons during different behavioral states. *Am. J. Physiol.*, 241: R277–285.

Stjernberg, L., Blumberg, H., and Wallin, B.G. (1986). Sympathetic activity in man after spinal cord injury. Outflow to muscle below the lesion. *Brain*, 109: 695–715.

Timmers, H., Wieling, W., Karemaker, J.M., and Lenders, J.W. (2003). Denervation of carotid baro- and chemoreceptors in humans. *J. Physiol.*, 553: 3–11.

Ursino, M. and Magosso, E. (2003). Role of short-term cardiovascular regulation in heart period variability: a modeling study. *Am. J. Physiol.*, 284: H1479–1493.

Van de Borne, P., Nguyen, H., Biston, P., Linkowski, P., and Degaute, J. (1994). Effects of wake and sleep stages on the 24-h autonomic control of blood pressure and heart rate in recumbent men. *Am. J. Physiol.*, 266: H548–554.

Vanoli, E., Adamson, P.B., Ba-Lin, M.B.H., Pinna, G.D., Lazzara, R., and Orr, W.C. (1995). Heart rate variability during specific sleep stages. A comparison of healthy subjects with patients after myocardial infarction. *Circulation*, 91: 1918–1922.

Vatner, S., Franklin, D., and Braunwald, E. (1971). Effects of anesthesia and sleep on circulatory response to carotid sinus nerve stimulation. *Am. J. Physiol.*, 220: 1249–1255.

Verrier, R.L., Muller, J.E., and Hobson, J.A. (1996). Sleep, dreams, and sudden death: the case for sleep as an autonomic stress test for the heart. *Cardiovasc. Res.*, 31: 181–211.

Weil, J. (2004). Sleep at high altitude. *High Alt. Med. Biol.*, 5: 180–189.

Wickramasinghe, H. and Anholm, J. (1999). Sleep and breathing at high altitude. *Sleep Breath.*, 3: 89–102.

Yoshimoto, M., Sakagami, T., Nagura, S., and Miki, K. (2004). Relationship between renal sympathetic nerve activity and renal blood flow during natural behavior in rats. *Am. J. Physiol.*, 286: R881–887.

Zoccoli, G., Cianci, T., Lenzi, P., and Franzini, C. (1992). Shivering during sleep: relationship between muscle blood flow and fiber type composition. *Experientia*, 48: 228–230.

Zoccoli, G., Bach, V., Cianci, T., Lenzi, P., and Franzini, C. (1994). Brain blood flow and extracerebral carotid circulation during sleep in rat. *Brain Res.*, 641: 46–50.

Zoccoli, G., Andreoli, E., Bojic, T., Cianci, T., Franzini, C., Predieri, S., and Lenzi, P. (2001). Central and baroreflex control of heart rate during the wake–sleep cycle in rat. *Sleep*, 24: 753–758.

REGULATION OF CEREBRAL CIRCULATION DURING SLEEP

Giovanna Zoccoli[1], Tijana Bojic, and Carlo Franzini

The regulation of physiological systems changes with state (wakefulness, non-rapid eye movement (NREM) sleep, and rapid eye movement (REM) sleep) (Parmeggiani, 1980a). This has been demonstrated in studies of thermoregulation (Parmeggiani, 1980b), respiration (Phillipson and Bowes, 1986), peripheral circulation (Franzini *et al.*, 1996), and cerebral circulation (Zoccoli *et al.*, 2002). The sleep process primarily involves the brain, and changes in cerebral activity are the primary events of sleep. Thus, brain circulation during sleep has been the focus of many studies, with the assumption that its understanding might shed light on the elusive issue of sleep function. The main conclusions are the following:

1. It is assumed that change in neuronal activity and oxygen consumption or anaerobic energy usage of the tissue proportionally induces changes in cerebral blood flow (CBF, flow–activity coupling).
2. Brain activity and CBF mostly decrease during NREM sleep with respect to wakefulness, and rise again markedly in REM sleep. Thus, flow–activity coupling exists also during sleep.
3. CBF fluctuations during the wake–sleep cycle result from changes in vascular resistance, but the mechanism is not known. They are independent

---

[1] giovanna.zoccoli@unibo.it

of systemic haemodynamic changes, particularly the redistribution of blood flow in other peripheral beds.

4. In central core structures (brain stem, mesencephalic tectum, thalamus, and basal forebrain), CBF increases during REM sleep while in NREM and anaesthesia CBF decreases. This speaks for central core structure functional unity both in sleep and anaesthesia, with a different pattern of activation between NREM sleep and REM sleep.

5. Changes of cortical CBF are more variable, with deactivation of hetero-modal frontoparietal association cortices as a common characteristic of both REM and NREM sleep.

6. The regulation of cerebral circulation during sleep reveals no specific, state-dependent features, flow–activity coupling being the prevailing mechanism, with O_2 as a candidate for the metabolic mediator in multiple mechanisms of flow–metabolism coupling.

CBF has been considered since many years as a marker of neuronal activity (Roy and Sherrington, 1890). During brain activation, a local increase in oxygen consumption is followed by a larger increase in blood flow: CBF changes describe changes in activity of local neuronal population. Recent data show that the increased energy expense produced by neuronal activity is mainly utilised for reversing the ion movements that generate postsynaptic currents and actions potentials (Attwell and Iadecola, 2002). In theory, extrinsic and intrinsic innervations to brain vessels can produce CBF changes uncoupled to changes in local activity. Even though recent data show that the activity of sympathetic nervous system exerts a tonic restrain on cerebral circulation during sleep (Loos *et al.*, 2005), there are no evidences that neurogenic CBF control might dissociate blood flow and activity in physiological conditions. Thus, CBF studies can be used to obtain information about levels of brain activity during behavioural conditions like sleep.

Flow–Activity Coupling: Data Obtained during the Wake–Sleep Cycle

Blood flow, O_2 consumption, and glucose uptake undergo directionally similar changes in the brain in different conditions of wakefulness (quiet wakefulness and active wakefulness: sensory stimulation, selective attention) and sleep (NREM and REM sleep) (cf. Lenzi *et al.*, 1999).

The available data on brain neuronal firing, metabolism, and blood flow during NREM and REM sleep are compatible with the hypothesis that mechanisms regulating flow–activity coupling are the same in sleep as in wakefulness. For instance, the changes in blood flow and substrate uptake (glucose, O_2) accompanying the transition from NREM to REM sleep closely match those occurring in wakefulness in the transition to higher activation levels (Lenzi *et al.*, 2000). Data obtained in sleep studies allow identifying some important features of the relationship between brain blood flow, metabolism, and glucose and oxygen uptake:

1. CBF increases more than O_2 uptake when brain metabolism increases in REM sleep. Data from Santiago *et al.* (1986) and Chao *et al.* (1989), showing a significant decrease in cerebral arteriovenous O_2 difference during REM sleep, have been confirmed by near-infrared spectroscopy (NIRS) studies. NIRS has been used to assess O_2 saturation and estimate CBF changes during sleep. In the transition from wakefulness to NREM sleep oxygenated haemoglobin is unchanged; in the transition from NREM to REM sleep oxygenated haemoglobin is increased in accordance with a CBF increase exceeding O_2 consumption increment (Onoe *et al.*, 1991).

2. In REM sleep, glucose uptake increases more than O_2 uptake, thus leading to anaerobic glucose metabolism and lactate production. In foetal lambs (Clapp *et al.*, 1980; Chao *et al.*, 1989), during low-voltage fast activity (REM sleep equivalent), both O_2 and glucose consumption increase, but cerebral glucose uptake exceeds O_2 uptake. The increased glucose/O_2 quotient indicates a modest but significant anaerobic component in brain metabolism, which is accompanied by an increase in the magnitude of the lactate arteriovenous difference (Chao *et al.*, 1989).

3. The relationship between glucose and O_2 cerebral uptake is modified by the occurrence of sleep. Comparison of pre-sleep and post-sleep brain glucose and O_2 metabolism (Boyle *et al.*, 1994) showed a greater decrease in glucose than in O_2 utilisation after sleep, suggesting the appearance of a relative decrease in anaerobic metabolism. Reduced metabolism, reduced flow (Droste *et al.*, 1993; Hajak *et al.*, 1994; Braun *et al.*, 1997), and reduced anaerobic glycolysis all agree with the "restorative" function of sleep (see below). Wu *et al.* (1991), however, found no differences in mean cerebral glucose utilisation during wakefulness before and after sleep deprivation. This discrepancy should be resolved, because it is central to the issue of a "recovery" function of sleep.

As far as the identification of the mediators between neuronal activity, metabolism, and blood flow is concerned, both glucose and O_2 are potential candidates, because CMR_{glu} and $CMRO_2$ increase during REM sleep. Studies on brain microcirculation during sleep indicate that no capillary recruitment accompanies the sleep–wake cycle: brain capillary surface area for exchanges of substances between blood and brain remains constant (Zoccoli et al., 1996). Even if recent data speak for invariability of blood–brain barrier permeability to glucose between quiet wakefulness and REM sleep (Silvani et al., 2005), the low extraction coefficient, and the high diffusion capacity of this substrate are inconsistent with the idea that glucose might couple flow and metabolism. Accordingly, the rate-limiting reaction for glucose catabolism is the rate of phosphorilation, and glucose transport does not represent the rate-limiting step in glycolysis.

Oxygen seems to be a better candidate. The current view is that O_2 utilisation is normally set by tissue metabolic activity and glucose oxidation is near maximal capacity at rest (*oxidative capacity limitation*); therefore, during brain activation, extra energy requirements are to be satisfied by non-oxidative glucose utilisation (Fox et al., 1988). The same hypothesis may be invoked to explain the excess glucose uptake in REM sleep: little reserve would be available in oxidative machinery for a further increase in glucose oxidation and extra energy requirements are met by non-oxidative metabolism and lactate production. However, this "metabolic" hypothesis cannot explain why when arterial PO_2 augments beyond $100\,mmHg$ up to $\sim 300\,torr$ brain tissue PO_2 increases, accompanied by a parallel decrease of tissue H^+ concentration and CBF (Shinozuka et al., 1989).

A different hypothesis was a proposed (Lenzi et al., 1999) that a limit may exist in the capacity of O_2 to pass from erythrocytes to mitochondria (*oxygen diffusion limitation*). Due to O_2 diffusion limitation, brain microregions lying at mid-distance between capillaries may become hypoxic. In these hypoxic micro-regions, when the metabolic rate rises during activation, or ambient PO_2 decreases, PO_2 can fall to values as low as zero. As a consequence, non-oxidative glucose metabolism develops, accounting for the increase in lactate and H^+ production. With arterial PO_2 increasing beyond $100\,mmHg$, O_2 diffusion would improve due to the increased blood–tissue PO_2 difference and both H^+ and lactate tissue concentration would decrease (Shinozuka et al., 1989).

Hypoxic micro-regions generated by the effect of oxygen diffusion limitation may be the site of origin of vasodilatatory commands helping keep blood flow adequate to metabolic needs.

The important effect of oxygen on CBF and metabolism during sleep is stressed by the effect of hypoxia on sleep, in particular REM sleep. Ambient hypoxia reduces "total sleep time" and the percentage of REM sleep in humans (Mizuno *et al.*, 1993), cats (Baker and McGinty, 1979), and rats (Pappenheimer, 1977), while an increased ambient PO_2 reduces sleep disturbances (West, 1995).

In conclusion, hypoxic micro-regions generated by O_2 diffusion limitation may supply signals for regulating CBF to levels adequate to activity and then to metabolic needs. Obviously, the feedback regulation based on O_2 utilisation by the tissue may coexist with other regulations, including not only feedback, but also anticipatory regulations, characterised by arteriolar vasodilatation directly controlled by neuronal activation. However, oxygen remains a primary candidate for coupling CBF and activity during REM sleep; in turn, oxygen deficiency, through intermediate steps (changes in anaerobic glucose metabolism and H^+concentration in brain tissue) activates potent vasodilatatory agents. As reported above, the available evidences indicate also that the haemodynamic responses to neuronal activity are not initiated by signals arising *directly* from the energy deficits of the tissue but rather are driven (a) locally, by fast glutamate-mediated signalling processes and (b) globally, by amine- and acetylcholine-mediated systems (Attwell and Iadecola, 2002).

Finally, another substance that could be important in coupling blood flow and neuronal activity during sleep is represented by nitric oxide (NO). In fact, the first study to probe the role of NO in CBF regulation during sleep by inhibiting NO synthase concluded that NO is the major determinant of CBF differences occurring across the sleep–wake states (Zoccoli *et al.*, 2001).

Regional Cerebral Blood Flow Changes during Sleep

Positron emission tomography (PET) and Doppler flowmetry studies have shed light on the spatial and temporal dimensions of CBF changes during sleep (Maquet, 2000; Zoccoli *et al.*, 2002).

Maquet *et al.* (1996) found an increased regional blood flow during REM sleep in pontine tegmentum, dorsal mesencephalon, thalamic nuclei, amygdala, anterior cingulate, and entorhinal cortex. They interpreted these focal activations as bearing on different aspects of REM sleep neuro- and psycho-physiology; the REM sleep brain activation pattern partly explains specific autonomic phenomenology of this state. This accounts for the partial overlap of brain structures' (brainstem, anterior cingulate, prefrontal cortex) activation in REM sleep and in states of autonomic cardiovascular arousal during wakefulness (Critchley *et al.*, 2000). PET studies point out to the centrencephalic (brainstem, thalamus, basal forebrain) origin of the state and its participation in reprocessing and long-term consolidation of recent, non-declarative, and emotional memory in humans (Maquet, 2001). Recent data (Peigneux *et al.*, 2003) define further the nature of the reprocessed memorised information. They claim that during REM sleep it is reinforced high-order information contained in probabilistic rules of defined visual stimuli and not its basic visuomotor component. Critical neuroanatomical structures, cuneus and striatum, are also activated in a quantitative manner with respect to information acquisition.

A companion study from the same group examined previously the "functional neuroanatomy of human slow wave sleep" (Maquet *et al.*, 1997). A significant negative correlation was found between the occurrence of NREM sleep and regional CBF in central core structures (pons, mesencephalon, and thalamus). These results were confirmed by other authors (Kajimura *et al.*, 1999; Kjaer *et al.*, 2002), and a further distinction was made between early deactivation (light sleep: pons and thalamus) and late deactivation (deep sleep: encompassing also midbrain and neocortex) with respect to wakefulness levels (Kajimura *et al.*, 1999).

In NREM sleep, a negative correlation has also been reported between sigma (spindle) and delta activities and regional flow in the brainstem reticular formation, cerebellum, and thalamus, whereas at the cortical level, both positive and negative correlations of CBF with delta activity were demonstrated (Hofle *et al.*, 1997). Principal component analysis also indicates decreased thalamic perfusion in NREM sleep (Andersson *et al.*, 1998). These studies extend to human beings the evidence of a reduced metabolic cost of synchronising modes of operation in the thalamo-cortical circuitry, which was first shown by measurements of brain glucose uptake in other species (Franzini, 1992). The central role of the thalamus in the genesis of cortical synchronous activity is well established (Steriade *et al.*, 1994) and is confirmed by studies on sleep pathology (e.g., fatal familial insomnia; Lugaresi *et al.*, 1986).

The brainstem-thalamo-cortical circuits responsible for the synchronisation-desynchronisation (S–D) pattern operate not only in sleep, but also in other functional conditions (e.g., anaesthesia). When different inhalational anaesthetic agents are utilised, a common pattern of reduced 18-fluorodeoxyglucose utilisation results in the same anatomical structures (midbrain reticular formation, thalamus, basal forebrain), suggesting that different anaesthetics must affect the same anatomical targets to exert their action (Alkire *et al.*, 2000). The hypothesis is further supported by a study with an anaesthetic of a different class (intravenous) reporting "an EEG pattern very similar to stage IV sleep" and "a significant covariation between the thalamic and midbrain blood flow changes, suggesting a close functional relationship between the two structures" (Fiset *et al.*, 1999). These structures therefore represent the "common final path" for the S–D pattern both in NREM sleep and in anaesthesia. Thus, sleep and anaesthesia seem to share neurophysiological and pharmacological mechanisms, both in humans and animals (Tung and Mendelson, 2004).

CBF changes in central core structures are similar in different studies (Maquet *et al.*, 1996, 1997; Braun *et al.*, 1997; Hofle *et al.*, 1997; Andersson *et al.*, 1998); a stereotyped circulatory and metabolic pattern links specific brain structures (brainstem, thalamus) into new functional units during the sleep cycle with respect to wakefulness. In contrast, greater variability across studies is apparent in cortical CBF data. Differences in cortical activation or deactivation often ascribed to differences in the species studied or methods used might well result from inter-individual or even intra-individual variability intrinsic to the single sleep cycle.

At a cortical level (Braun *et al.*, 1997), heteromodal frontoparietal association cortices were deactivated during both NREM and REM sleep. This deactivation "may be a defining characteristic of sleep itself that involves the highest integrative processes of the brain." Its uniformity across sleep states might relate, in very general terms, to the fact that important features of sleep mental activity are shared by both NREM and REM sleep (Bosinelli, 1995). On the other hand, deactivation of the primary sensory cortex has been reported in NREM sleep (visual and auditive: Czisch *et al.*, 2002) and in REM sleep (parietal: Maquet *et al.*, 1996, and visual: Braun *et al.*, 1998).

CBF is rapidly restored in the centrencephalic brainstem-thalamic regions during the process of awakening (Balkin *et al.*, 2002). Awakening from sleep entails rapid re-establishment of consciousness followed by the relatively slow re-establishment of alertness. Functional brain imaging investigation on sleep deprivation (Thomas *et al.*, 2000) suggests that maintenance of alertness varies primarily as a function of thalamus and prefrontal cortices' activation levels. The role of thalamus and prefrontal cortices, studied as a function of the hypothesised "sleep debt," is further investigated during re-establishment of alertness, i.e. awakening. On awakening, "sleep debt" is at minimal level, but similar psychomotor and cognitive deficits are observed, due to intrusion of sleep maintenance mechanisms into waking state ("sleep inertia": Tassi and Muzet, 2000). During transition from sleep to full alertness, Balkin *et al.* (2002) observed a 15-min time delay of anterior cortical activation with respect to most rapidly activated centrencephalic structures. Concomitant changes in patterns of regional interconnectivity across the awakening process are consistent with the notion that increasing alertness is an emergent product of orchestrated inter-regional activation pattern. It is suggested that functional uncoupling of reticular formation and prefrontal cortex and re-establishment of functional coherence in the prefrontal cortico-striatal thalamo-cortical circuit represents a dynamic neurophysiological correlate of the re-establishment of normal alertness (Balkin *et al.*, 2002).

In addition, Braun *et al.* (1997) reported significantly lower CBF values during post-sleep wakefulness than during pre-sleep wakefulness; the effect was more pronounced in cortical and limbic structures. The sleep process might thus reset the circulatory and metabolic activities of the brain to a lower level, in accordance with a "restorative" function of sleep (see later).

Spinal cord blood flow also increases in REM sleep (Lenzi *et al.*, 1987; Zoccoli *et al.*, 1993), and in rats it decreases in NREM sleep with respect to quiet wakefulness (Zoccoli *et al.*, 1993). The similar trend of blood flow changes in brain and spinal cord indicates that the sleep process involves a modulation of the activity in the entire central nervous system. Direct data on spinal cord metabolism during sleep are still lacking.

Cerebral blood perfusion during sleep may change not only quantitatively but also qualitatively. On the basis of local brain temperature changes, Azzaroni and Parmeggiani (1993) suggested a carotid-vertebral shift in the quotas of CBF during REM sleep (Parmeggiani *et al.*, 2002). An intra-extracerebral carotid blood redistribution during REM sleep is suggested by a series of experiments on regional brain temperature changes in cat (Azzaroni and Parmeggiani, 1993) and rabbit (Parmeggiani *et al.*, 2002). In cat, a specific heat exchanger in the carotid system (carotid rete) results in a lower arterial blood temperature (T_{ab}) than that in the vertebral system, cooled only by systemic heat exchangers (ear pinna, upper airway mucosa). This T_{ab} gradient affects the corresponding anatomical structures; as a consequence, anterior hypothalamic temperature (T_{hy}) is lower than pontine temperature (T_p). In NREM sleep, a reduction in tonic vasoconstrictor sympathetic outflow produces an increased blood flow in systemic heat exchangers, and both T_{hy} and T_p decrease with respect to W. During

REM sleep brain temperature increases, and T_{hy} tends towards T_p values (Azzaroni and Parmeggiani, 1993). Experiments of bilateral short-term carotid occlusion performed in rabbits (Parmeggiani *et al.*, 2002) suggested that this is the result of a carotid-vertebral shift. In normal conditions a drop in vasomotor tone to extracerebral head structures during REM sleep (Parmeggiani *et al.*, 1977; Franzini *et al.*, 1982) produces the expansion of the extracerebral carotid territory. Carotid blood is "stolen" from the brain, and it is replaced by warmer vertebral blood.

Time Course of Cerebral Blood Flow Changes during Sleep

Continuous recording of CBF changes during sleep with flow probes was instrumental in addressing the following issues: (1) the analysis of tonic and phasic changes in cerebral perfusion determinants during sleep; (2) the temporal sequence of CBF and sleep-state modifications; and (3) the CBF time course during the night, and the comparison between pre- and post-sleep wakefulness levels.

1. In lambs, REM sleep is accompanied by a tonic increase in CBF with respect to NREM sleep and wakefulness, and by superimposed phasic blood flow transients (Grant *et al.*, 1995, 1998; Silvani *et al.*, 2004). The analysis of the temporal relationship between cerebral perfusion pressure (CPP) and CBF changes indicates that a fall in vascular resistance is the primary event which both underlies the tonic CBF increment and initiates the phasic CBF surges associated with transient BP increases. Moreover, this approach allows evaluating sleep-related changes in CBF regulation, by quantifying the extent to which variability in CBF is related to that of CPP in the different wake–sleep states (Silvani *et al.*, 2004). Results obtained suggest that in all states synchronised cerebral vasomotor fluctuations account for a quota of CBF variability not explained by CPP variability; their relative contribution to CBF variability differs among wake–sleep states, being highest during NREM sleep and lowest during REM sleep.
2. In rats, laser Doppler probes connected to an optical fibre were stereotaxically implanted in the hippocampus (Seno *et al.*, 1995; Osborne, 1997) or basal forebrain (Gerashenko and Matsumura, 1996), and relative increments in blood flow were recorded in the transition from NREM to REM sleep. However, the issue of the temporal relationship between circulatory and sleep-state changes remains unsolved: an early (Gerashenko and Matsumura, 1996), simultaneous (Seno *et al.*, 1995), or

late (Osborne, 1997) CBF change has been described with respect to the onset of the REM sleep episode. Regional, non-stereotyped differences in brain activation and blood flow rise with respect to the global state change might explain the different latencies reported.
3. In human adults (Droste *et al.*, 1993; Hajak *et al.*, 1994; Kuboyama *et al.*, 1997) CBF fluctuates from NREM to REM sleep within the same cycle, but decreases tonically throughout the night, and there are lower values in post-sleep wakefulness compared to pre-sleep wakefulness. This corresponds to results obtained with PET (Braun *et al.*, 1997) and reinforces the hypothesis of a "restorative" sleep function (see below).

Regulation of Cerebral Circulation during the Sleep–Wake Cycle

The regulation of cerebral circulation aims, on the one hand, to finely match blood flow to the metabolic needs of brain activity at a regional level (*flow–activity coupling*, see above), whereas, on the other hand, it protects the brain from systemic challenges ($PaO_2, PaCO_2$, pH changes, *chemical regulation*; BP fluctuations, *autoregulation*).

Chemical regulation

In NREM sleep, a slight hypercapnia develops (2–3 mmHg). This counteracts the circulatory effects of the decreased cerebral metabolic rate and accounts for the small increase in CBF in some species, e.g., goat (Santiago *et al.*, 1984). Madsen *et al.* demonstrated that if CBF is corrected for the vasodilatation induced by hypercapnia a strict flow–activity coupling is still present in this sleep state (Madsen and Vorstrup, 1991). The response to CO_2 at any rate is blunted by the decreased cerebral vascular reactivity to hypercapnia during NREM sleep (Meadows *et al.*, 2003). Recent data show that the cerebral vascular response to hypoxia is similarly reduced during NREM sleep (Meadows *et al.*, 2004). CBF response to isocapnic hypoxia results dramatically altered during this sleep state, and the blood flow increase recorded during wakefulness is substituted by a decrease during NREM sleep. The inability of the cerebral vasculature to respond to hypoxic stress during NREM sleep may represent a significant vulnerability for the brain in this state.

Hypocapnia decreases the amount of REM sleep in cats in normoxic conditions (Lovering *et al.*, 2003): one of the possible mechanisms is CO_2 effect on CBF and cerebral metabolism. $PaCO_2$ is also an important determinant of CBF changes during sleep in pathological conditions (e.g., sleep apnoea; Hajak *et al.*, 1996).

Autoregulation

During REM sleep, the tonic increase in CBF with respect to NREM sleep values is independent of blood pressure changes: a comparative study across species shows that the CBF increment occurs in the face of increases, decreases, or no changes in blood pressure (Franzini, 1992). Moreover, the range of variations of blood pressure during REM sleep is well within the limits of autoregulation, which has been shown to operate during sleep: in lambs cerebral vasodilatation in response to acute hypotension induced by brachiocephalic artery occlusion occurred in all behavioural states (W, NREM sleep, and REM sleep), albeit with reduced efficacy in REM sleep (Grant *et al.*, 1998). REM sleep, however, is characterised by a high metabolic rate, high CBF, and consequently reduced vasodilatatory reserve; this may place the brain at risk for ischaemic hypoxia during acute hypotension.

The independence of CBF from systemic haemodynamics is further supported by the lack of correlation between blood flow changes in the brain and in other peripheral circulations (kidney, muscle, skin, splanchnic): CBF is not affected by the redistribution of regional flows occurring in REM sleep (Lenzi *et al.*, 1986). Further, an independent regulation of CBF and extracerebral carotid circulation has been suggested during this sleep state in rats (Zoccoli *et al.*, 1994). Taken together, these data suggest a local regulation of CBF during REM sleep, and local factors remain the most probable candidates accounting for the CBF surge in REM sleep.

Conclusions and Implications for Future Research

The main conclusions from the reviewed data can be summarised as follows:

1. Flow–activity coupling currently appears to be the principal mechanism controlling CBF changes during sleep. Studies of brain microcirculation (Zoccoli *et al.*, 1996) and the low extraction coefficient of glucose describe this substrate as an improbable candidate for critical coupling factor of brain metabolism and blood flow. On the other hand, in the absence of capillary recruitment during sleep, an increase of CBF might be essential

to maintain the driving force for O_2 diffusion from plasma to brain. Future researches are to evaluate the role of O_2 in flow–activity coupling.

2. Brain activity and CBF mostly decrease during NREM sleep with respect to wakefulness, and rise again markedly in REM sleep. At a regional level centrencephalic structures manifest a stereotyped pattern of blood flow changes during sleep with decrements in NREM and increments in REM sleep (Maquet *et al.*, 1996, 1997; Braun *et al.*, 1997). Focal activation of these structures during REM sleep could bear different functional aspects of this sleep state in particular autonomic phenomenology and established role in consolidation of recent memory. The same structures are deactivated both in NREM sleep and anaesthesia (Alkire *et al.*, 2000) and are the most rapidly activated brain structures on awakening (Balkin *et al.*, 2002). These data suggest that functional unity of centrencephalic structures might also underlie conscious awareness itself.

3. Greater fluctuations characterise the cortical circulatory pattern; these may result from inter-individual variability in small sample populations. Alternatively, it might be a true feature of cortical activation, especially during REM sleep, and even intra-individual activation variability might become apparent when longitudinal studies in the same subject become methodologically feasible. In general terms, associative cortices seem to be more affected by sleep than primary sensory areas (Braun *et al.*, 1997; Maquet *et al.*, 1997; Andersson *et al.*, 1998).

4. The analysis of the temporal relationship between CPP and CBF changes indicates that in REM sleep a fall in vascular resistance is the primary event that underlies the CBF increment characteristic of this sleep state. The mechanisms producing resistance decrease remain to be investigated. They are independent of systemic haemodynamic changes, particularly the redistribution of blood flow in other peripheral beds.

5. Apart of quantitative global and regional change of CBF in different states of the wake–sleep cycle, a change in carotid-vertebrobasilar contribution to centrencephalic blood perfusion has been proposed (Azzaroni and Parmeggiani, 1993; Parmeggiani *et al.*, 2002).

6. An overall reduction of CBF occurs during the night, with post-sleep values significantly lower than pre-sleep values (Droste *et al.*, 1993; Hajak *et al.*, 1994; Braun *et al.*, 1997; Kuboyama *et al.*, 1997). This favours the long-held view of a "restorative" function of sleep: whatever specific needs sleep may fulfil, it may be surmised that, given the flow–activity coupling in the brain, the resumption of the operational level occurs at a lower metabolic cost in post-sleep wakefulness. It may be proposed

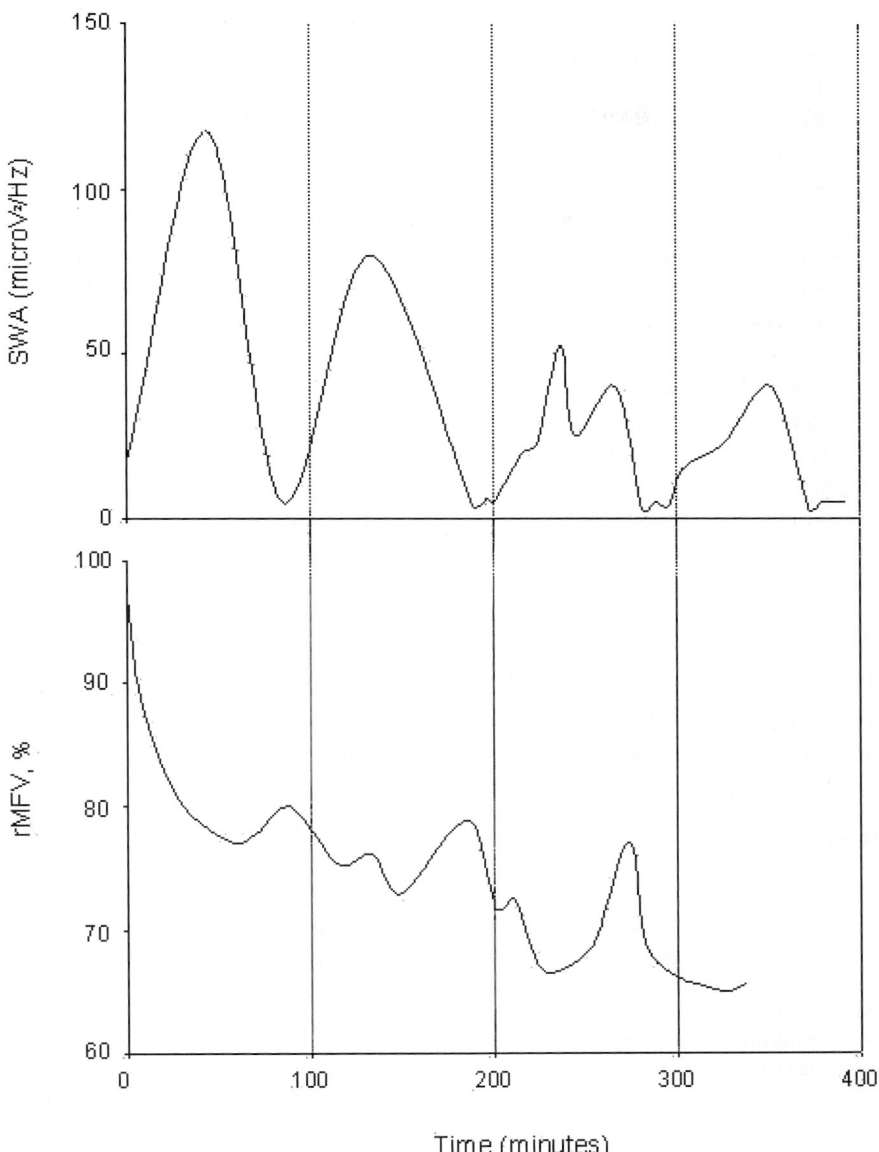

Figure 1. Recordings during baseline sleep: slow wave activity (SWA, redrawn from Dijk *et al.*, 1993, Top), and relative mean flow velocity in the middle cerebral artery (rMFV, redrawn from Hajak *et al.*, 1994, Bottom). A qualitative similarity in the decline of the two variables is apparent: this indicates that a recovery process may have occurred during the night.

that a "sleep debt" has been paid during sleep. The debt manifests itself as sleep propensity; a marker of this propensity is represented by EEG slow wave activity (SWA, 0.25–4.0 Hz) (Borbély and Achermann, 2000). In humans, SWA is highest at the beginning of the night and declines exponentially (Dijk *et al.*, 1993). The Doppler flowmeter data also reveal an exponential decline of CBF throughout the night (Hajak *et al.*, 1994). We may speculate on a possible link between these two variables (Figure 1). The payment of the debt entails a high metabolic cost; when during the night the debt is paid, SWA declines and the metabolic cost of sleep also declines, reaching the lowest values towards the morning hours. This trend is independent from the ultradian cycle. Thus, NREM sleep CBF value is always lower than the corresponding REM sleep value, but the absolute value of NREM sleep CBF at the beginning of the night can be higher than the REM sleep value at the end of the night. Thus, reduced SWA and reduced metabolic activity towards the end of sleep may suggest that some kind of "recovery" has occurred.

Acknowledgements

This work was supported by MIUR grants (Ministry of Education, Rome). The authors thank PhD students V. Asti, C. Berteotti, and V. Ferrari, who helped generously with comments and references.

References

Alkire, M.T., Haier, R.J., and Fallon, J.H. (2000). Toward a unified theory of narcosis: brain imaging evidence for a thalamocortical switch as the neuro-physiologic basis of anesthetic-induced unconsciousness. *Conscious Cogn.*, 9: 370–386.

Andersson, J.L.R., Onoe, H., Hetta, J., Lidstrom, K., Valind, S., Lilja, A., Sundin, A., Fasth, K.-J., Westerberg, G., Broman, J.-E., Watanabe, Y., and Langstrom, B. (1998). Brain networks affected by synchronized sleep visualized by positron emission tomography. *J. Cereb. Blood Flow Metab.*, 18: 701–715.

Attwell, D. and Iadecola, C. (2002). The neural basis of functional brain imaging signals. *Trends Neurosci.*, 25: 621–625.

Azzaroni, A. and Parmeggiani, P.L. (1993). Mechanisms underlying hypothalamic temperature changes during sleep in mammals. *Brain Res.*, 632: 136–142.

Baker, T.L. and McGinty, D.J. (1979). Sleep–waking patterns in hypoxic kitten. *Dev. Psychobiol.*, 12: 561–575.

Balkin, T.J., Braun, A.R., Wesensten, N.J., Jeffries, K., Varga, M., Baldwin, P., Belenky, G., and Herscovitch, P. (2002). The process of awakening: a PET study of regional brain activity patterns mediating the re-establishment of alertness and consciousness. *Brain,* 125: 2308–2319.

Borbély, A.A. and Achermann, P. (2000). Sleep homeostasis and models of sleep regulation. In: Kryger, M.H., Roth, T., and Dement, W.C. (Eds.). *Principles and Practice of Sleep Medicine.* Philadelphia: W. B. Saunders, pp. 377–390.

Bosinelli, M. (1995). Mind and consciousness during sleep. *Behav. Brain Res.,* 69: 195–201.

Boyle, P.J., Scott, J.C., Krentz, A.J., Nagy, R.J., Comstock, E., and Hoffman, C. (1994). Diminished brain glucose metabolism is a significant determinant for failing rates of systemic glucose utilization during sleep in normal humans. *J. Clin. Invest.,* 93: 529–535.

Braun, A.R., Balkin, T.J., Wesensten, N.J., Carson, R.E., Varga, M., Baldwin, P., Selbie, S., Belenky, G., and Herscovitch, P. (1997). Regional cerebral blood flow throughout the sleep–wake cycle. An $H_2^{15}O$ study. *Brain,* 120: 1173–1197.

Braun, A.R., Balkin, T.J., Wesensten, N.J., Gwadry, F., Carson, R.E., Varga, M., Baldwin, P., Belenky, G., and Herscovitch, P. (1998). Dissociated pattern of activity in visual cortices and their projections during human rapid eye movement sleep. *Science,* 279: 91–95.

Chao, C.R., Hohimer, A.R., and Bissonnette, J.M. (1989). The effect of electrocortical state on cerebral carbohydrate metabolism in fetal sheep. *Dev. Brain Res.,* 49: 1–5.

Clapp, J.F., Szeto, H.H., Abrams, R., Larrow, R., and Mann, L.I. (1980). Physiological variability and fetal electrocortical activity. *Am. J. Obstet. Gynecol.,* 136: 1045–1050.

Critchley, H.D., Corfield, D.R., Chandler, M.P., Mathias, C.J., and Dolan, R.J. (2000). Cerebral correlates of autonomic cardiovascular arousal: a functional neuroimaging investigation in humans. *J. Physiol.,* 523: 259–270.

Czisch, M., Wetter, T.C., Kaufmann, C., Pollmacher, T., Holsboer, F., and Auer, D.P. (2002). Altered processing of acoustic stimuli during sleep: reduced auditory activation and visual deactivation detected by a combined fMRI/EEG study. *Neuroimage,* 16: 251–258.

Dijk, D.-J., Hayes, B., and Czeisler, C.A. (1993). Dynamics of electroencephalographic sleep spindles and slow wave activity in men: effects of sleep deprivation. *Brain Res.,* 626: 190–199.

Droste, D.W., Berger, W., Schler, E., and Krauss, J.K. (1993). Middle cerebral artery blood flow velocity in healthy persons during wakefulness and sleep: a transcranial doppler study. *Sleep,* 16: 603–609.

Fiset, P., Paus, T., Daloze, T., Plourde, G., Meuret, P., Bonhomme, V., Hajj-Ali, N., Backman, S.B., and Evans, A.C. (1999). Brain mechanisms of propofol-induced loss of consciousness in humans: a positron emission tomographic study. *J. Neurosci.,* 19: 5506–5513.

Fox, P.T., Raichle, M.E., Mintun, M.A., and Dence, C. (1988). Nonoxidative glucose consumption during focal physiologic neural activity. *Science*, 241: 462–464.

Franzini, C. (1992). Brain metabolism and blood flow during sleep. *J. Sleep Res.*, 1: 3–16.

Franzini, C., Lenzi, P., Cianci, T., and Guidalotti, P.L. (1982). Neural control of vasomotion in rabbit ear is impaired during desynchronized sleep. *Am. J. Physiol.*, 243: 142–146.

Franzini, C., Zoccoli, G., Cianci, T., and Lenzi, P. (1996). Sleep-dependent changes in regional circulations. *News Physiol. Sci.*, 11: 274–280.

Gerashenko, D. and Matsumura, H. (1996). Continuous recording of brain regional circulation during sleep/wake state transitions in rats. *Am. J. Physiol.*, 270: 855–863.

Grant, D.A., Franzini, C., Wild, J., and Walker, A.M. (1995). Continuous measurement of blood flow in the superior sagittal sinus of the lamb. *Am. J. Physiol.*, 269: 274–279.

Grant, D.A., Franzini, C., Wild, J., and Walker, A.M. (1998). Cerebral circulation in sleep: vasodilatory response to cerebral hypothension. *J. Cereb. Blood Flow. Metab.*, 18: 639–645.

Hajak, G., Klingelhofer, J., Schulz-Varszegi, M., Matzander, G., Sander, D., Conrad, B., and Ruther, E. (1994). Relationship between blood flow velocities and cerebral electrical activity in sleep. *Sleep*, 17: 11–19.

Hajak, G., Klingelhofer, J., Schulz-Varszegi, M., Sander, D., and Ruther, E. (1996). Sleep apnea syndrome and cerebral hemodynamics. *Chest*, 110: 670–679.

Hofle, N., Paus, T., Reutens, D., Fiset, P., Gotman, J., Evans, A.C., and Jones, B.E. (1997). Regional cerebral blood flow changes as a function of delta and spindle activity during slow wave sleep in humans. *J. Neurosci.*, 17: 4800–4808.

Kajimura, N., Uchiyama, M., Takayama, Y., Uchida, S., Uema, T., Kato, M., Sekimoto, M., Watanabe, T., Nakajima, T., Horikoshi, S., Ogawa, K., Nishikawa, M., Hiroki, M., Kudo, Y., Matsuda, H., Okawa, M., and Takahashi, K. (1999). Activity of midbrain reticular formation and neocortex during the progression of human non-rapid eye movement sleep. *J. Neurosci.*, 19: 1065–1073.

Kjaer, T.W., Law, I., Wiltschiotz, G., Paulson, O.B., and Madsen, P.L. (2002). Regional cerebral blood flow during light sleep — a H(2)(15)O-PET study. *J. Sleep Res.*, 11: 201–207.

Kuboyama, T., Hori, A., Sato, T., Mikami, T., Yamaki, T., and Ueda, S. (1997). Changes in cerebral blood flow velocity in healthy young men during overnight sleep and while awake. *Electroenceph. Clin. Neurophysiol.*, 102: 125–131.

Lenzi, P., Cianci, T., Guidalotti, P.L., and Franzini, C. (1986). Regional spinal cord blood flow during sleep–waking cycle in rabbit. *Am. J. Physiol.*, 251: 957–960.

Lenzi, P., Cianci, T., Guidalotti, P.L., Leonardi, G.S., and Franzini, C. (1987). Brain circulation during sleep and its relation to extracerebral hemodynamics. *Brain Res.*, 415: 14–20.

Lenzi, P., Zoccoli, G., Walker, A.M., and Franzini, C. (1999). Cerebral blood flow regulation in REM sleep: a model for flow-metabolism coupling. *Arch. Ital. Biol.*, 137: 165–179.

Lenzi, P., Zoccoli, G., Walker, A.M., and Franzini, C. (2000). Cerebral circulation in REM sleep: is Oxygen a main regulating factor? *Sleep Res. Online*, 3: 77–85.

Loos, N., Grant, D.A., Wild, J., Paul, S., Barfield, C., Zoccoli, G., Franzini, C., and Walker, A.M. (2005). Sympathetic nervous control of the cerebral circulation in sleep. *J. Sleep Res.*, in press.

Lovering, A.T., Fraigne, J.J., Dunin-Barkowski, W.L., Vidruk, E.H., and Orem, J.M. (2003). Hypocapnia decreases the amount of rapid eye movement sleep in cats. *Sleep*, 26: 961–967.

Lugaresi, E., Medori, R., Montagna, M., Baruzzi, A., Cortelli, P., Lugaresi, A., Tinuper, P., Zucconi, M., and Gambetti, P.L. (1986). Fatal familial insomnia and dysautonomia with selective degeneration of thalamic nuclei. *New Engl. J. Med.*, 315: 997–1003.

Madsen, P.L. and Vorstrup, S. (1991). Cerebral blood flow and metabolism during sleep. *Cerebrovasc. Brain Metab. Rev.*, 3: 281–296.

Maquet, P. (2000). Functional neuroimaging of normal human sleep by positron emission tomography. *J. Sleep Res.*, 9: 207–231.

Maquet, P. (2001). The role of sleep in learning and memory. *Science*, 294: 1048–1052.

Maquet, P., Péters, J.-M., Aerts, J., Delfiore, G., Degueldre, C., Luxen, A., and Franck, G. (1996). Functional neuroanatomy of human rapid-eye-movement sleep and dreaming. *Nature*, 383: 163–166.

Maquet, P., Degueldre, C., Delfiore, G., Aerts, J., Péters, J.-M., Luxen, A., and Franck, G. (1997). Functional neuroanatomy of human slow wave sleep. *J. Neurosci.*, 17: 2807–2812.

Meadows, G.E., Dunroy, H.M., Morrell, M.J., and Corfield, D.R. (2003). Hypercapnic cerebral vascular reactivity is decreased, in humans, during sleep compared with wakefulness. *J. Appl. Physiol.* 94: 2197–2202.

Meadows, G.E., O'Driscoll, D.M., Simonds, A.K., Morrell, M.J., and Corfield, D.R. (2004). Cerebral blood flow response to isocapnic hypoxia during slow wave sleep and wakefulness. *J. Appl. Physiol.*, 97: 1343–1348.

Mizuno, K., Asano, K., and Okudaira, N. (1993). Sleep and respiration under acute hypobaric hypoxia. Japan. *J. Physiol.*, 43: 161–175.

Onoe, H., Watanabe, V., Tamura, M., and Hayaishi, O. (1991). REM-sleep associated hemoglobin oxygenation in the monkey forebrain studied using near-infrared spectrophotometry. *Neurosci. Lett.*, 129: 209–213.

Osborne, P.G. (1997). Hippocampal and striatal blood flow during behavior in rats: chronic laser doppler flowmetry study. *Physiol. Behav.*, 61: 485–492.

Pappenheimer, J.R. (1977). Sleep and respiration of rats during hypoxia. *J. Physiol.*, 266: 191–207.

Parmeggiani, P.L. (1980a). Behavioral phenomenology of sleep (somatic and vegetative). *Experientia*, 36: 6–11.

Parmeggiani, P.L. (1980b). Temperature regulation during sleep: a study in homeostasis. In: Orem, J. and Barnes, C.D. (Eds.). *Physiology in Sleep*. New York: Academic Press, pp. 97–143.

Parmeggiani, P.L., Zamboni, G., Cianci, T., and Calasso, M. (1977). Absence of thermoregulatory vasomotor responses during fast wave sleep in cats. *Electroenceph. Clin. Neurophysiol.*, 42: 372–380.

Parmeggiani, P.L., Azzaroni, A., and Calasso, M. (2002). Systemic hemodynamic changes raising brain temperature in REM sleep. *Brain Res.*, 940: 55–60.

Peigneux, P., Laureys, S., Fuchs, S., Destrebecqz, A., Collette, F., Delbeuck, X., Phillips, C., Aerts, J., Del Fiore, G., Degueldre, C., Luxen, A., Cleeremans, A., and Maquet, P. (2003). Learned material content and acquisition level modulate cerebral reactivation during posttraining rapid-eye-movements sleep. *Neuroimage*, 20: 125–134.

Phillipson, E.A. and Bowes, G. (1986). Control of breathing during sleep. In: Cherniack, N.S. and Widdicombe, J.G. (Eds.). *The Respiratory System. Control of Breathing*. Bethesda: Am. Physiol. Soc., pp. 649–689.

Roy, C.S. and Sherrington, C.S. (1890). On the regulation of the blood-supply of the brain. *J. Physiol.*, 11: 85–108.

Santiago, T.V., Guerra, E., Neubauer, J.A., and Edelman, N.H. (1984). Correlation between ventilation and brain blood flow during sleep. *J. Clin. Invest.*, 73: 497–506.

Santiago, T.V., Neubauer, J.A., and Edelman, N.H. (1986). Correlation between ventilation and brain blood flow during hypoxic sleep. *J. Appl. Physiol.*, 60: 295–298.

Seno, H., Sano, A., and Maita, Y. (1995). Cerebral local blood flow with a laser-Doppler flowmetry in rat sleep. *Tokushima J. Exp. Med.*, 42: 1–4.

Shinozuka, T., Nemoto, E.M., and Winter, P.M. (1989). Mechanisms of cerebrovascular O_2 sensitivity from hyperoxia to moderate hypoxia in the rat. *J. Cereb. Blood Flow Metab.*, 9: 187–195.

Silvani, A., Asti, V., Berteotti, C., Bojic, T., Cianci, T., Ferrari, V., Franzini, C., Lenzi, P., and Zoccoli, G. (2005). Sleep-related brain activation does not increase the permeability of the blood-brain barrier to glucose. *J. Cereb. Blood Flow Metab.*, doi: 10.1038/sj.jcbfm.9600100.

Silvani, A., Bojic, T., Franzini, C., Lenzi, P., Walker, A.M., Grant, D.A., Wild, J., and Zoccoli, G. (2004). Sleep-related changes in the regulation of cerebral blood flow in newborn lambs. *Sleep*, 27: 36–41.

Steriade, M., Contreras, D., and Amzica, F. (1994). Synchronized sleep oscillations and their paroxysmal developments. *Trends Neurosci.*, 17: 199–208.

Tassi, P. and Muzet, A. (2000). Sleep inertia. *Sleep Med. Rev.*, 4: 341–353.

Thomas, M., Sing, H., Belenky, G., Holcomb, H., Mayberg, H., Dannals, R., Wagner, H., Thorne, D., Popp, K., Rowland, L., Welsh, A., Balwinski, S., and Redmond, D. (2000). Neural basis of alertness and cognitive performance impairments during sleepiness. I. Effects of 24 h of sleep deprivation on waking human regional brain activity. *J. Sleep Res.*, 9: 335–352.

Tung, A. and Mendelson, W.B. (2004). Anesthesia and sleep. *Sleep Med. Rev.*, 8: 213–225.

West, J.B. (1995). Oxygen enrichment of room air to relieve the hypoxia of high altitude. *Respir. Physiol.*, 99: 225–232.

Wu, J.C., Gillin, J.C., Buchsbaum, M.S., Hershey, T., Hazlett, E., Sicotte, N., and Bunney, W.E. (1991). The effect of sleep deprivation on cerebral glucose metabolic rate in normal humans assessed with positron emission tomography. *Sleep*, 14: 155–162.

Zoccoli, G., Bach, V., Nardo, B., Cianci, T., Lenzi, P., and Franzini, C. (1993). Spinal cord blood flow changes during the sleep–wake cycle in rat. *Neurosci. Lett.*, 163: 173–176.

Zoccoli, G., Bach, V., Cianci, T., Lenzi, P., and Franzini, C. (1994). Brain blood flow and extracerebral carotid circulation during sleep in rat. *Brain Res.*, 641: 46–50.

Zoccoli, G., Lucchi, M.L., Andreoli, E., Bach, V., Cianci, T., Lenzi, P., and Franzini, C. (1996). Brain capillary perfusion during sleep. *J. Cereb. Blood Flow Metab.*, 16: 1312–1318.

Zoccoli, G., Grant, D.A., Wild, J., and Walker, A.M. (2001). Nitric oxide inhibition abolishes sleep–wake differences in cerebral circulation. *Am. J. Physiol.*, 280: H2598–H2606.

Zoccoli, G., Walker, A.M., Lenzi, P., and Franzini, C. (2002). The cerebral circulation during sleep: regulation mechanisms and functional implications. *Sleep Med. Rev.*, 6: 443–455.

Chapter 17

CENTRAL NEURAL MECHANISMS UNDERLYING DISORDERED BREATHING AND CARDIOVASCULAR CONTROL DURING SLEEP

Ronald M. Harper[1], Paul M. Macey, Mary A. Woo, Christopher A. Richard, Rajesh Kumar, and Luke A. Henderson

This chapter outlines structural and functional neural processes that are deficient in conditions associated with sleep-disordered breathing and elicit acute and chronic pathological cardiovascular patterns. These conditions are associated with damage or dysfunction of cerebellar cortex and deep nuclei, limbic structures, as well as cerebral cortical areas mediating sympathetic outflow. The damage can contribute to cardiovascular pathology and may continue even after appropriate therapeutic intervention, suggesting sustained neural injury.

Disorders of breathing and cardiovascular regulation during sleep in the human provide the opportunity to obtain insights into the nature of neural control of cardiovascular action that would be difficult to reveal solely from examination of animal or humans unaffected by pathology. These insights derive from the close interactions between breathing mechanisms and processes that control blood pressure and heart rate. Integration of these two vital systems is obvious from even casual physiological observation, as demonstrated by such phenomena as apnea or diminished

---

[1] rharper@ucla.edu

respiratory muscle effort resulting from transient increases in blood pressure or enhanced ventilation with lowered pressure (Trelease *et al.*, 1985; Ohtake and Jennings, 1992), and the moment-by-moment changes in heart rate from respiratory efforts. More severe stresses on vital systems, such as high-altitude exposure, result in substantial blood chemistry changes and major cardiovascular consequences, but these changes occur as expected compensatory mechanisms serving normal functions. Certain disorders in breathing control, however, such as loss of upper airway muscle tone in obstructive sleep apnea (OSA), lead to exaggerated patterns of blood pressure and heart rate change, as well as long-lasting cardiovascular and cognitive deficits. These lasting changes include heightened sympathetic activity and hypertension (Somers *et al.*, 1995; Narkiewicz and Somers, 1997) and memory deficits. The alterations persist even after mechanical restoration of ventilation (Naegele *et al.*, 1998), and suggest the normal neural compensatory mechanisms for cardiovascular control have been compromised, and in the case of cognitive processes, perhaps irreparably damaged. Moreover, nearly half of all patients with heart failure show either OSA (even without evidence of obesity or reduced airway dimensions) or Cheyne–Stokes breathing during sleep in addition to their characteristic high sympathetic and diminished parasympathetic tone (Bradley, 1992; Javaheri *et al.*, 1995). Other "experiments of nature" in which the primary complaint is disordered breathing during sleep also exert concurrent cardiovascular abnormalities; a primary example is Congenital Central Hypoventilation Syndrome (CCHS). This condition, characterized by a loss of drive to breathe during sleep and a diminished sensitivity to CO_2 and O_2 (Haddad *et al.*, 1978), is also distinguished by poor sympathetic and parasympathetic control and abolished influences of breathing on heart rate variation (Woo *et al.*, 1992). The co-existence of breathing and autonomic pathologies in all of these sleep-related syndromes suggests that common neural mechanisms may be failing, and that examination of structure and function of neural sites that mediate respiratory and cardiovascular action may demonstrate the means of failure.

Magnetic Resonance Imaging Procedures

Magnetic resonance imaging (MRI) procedures provide a noninvasive means to evaluate structural damage in brain areas mediating cardiovascular control and to assess the functional manner by which brain structures alter perfusion and breathing in syndromes with disordered vital functions in sleep. Structural damage can be shown with regional volume loss procedures.

These techniques assess regional volumes of brain tissue and compare those volumes with a database of healthy controls (Ashburner and Friston, 2000). Functional deficits can be assessed with noninvasive functional MRI procedures. The latter procedure commonly uses a technique that measures regional changes in magnetic properties of deoxygenated vs. oxygenated blood as activated or deactivated brain regions elicit local blood flow changes (Ogawa *et al.*, 1990) in response to a challenge.

Gray Matter Damage in Obstructive Sleep Apnea and Heart Failure

Structural studies that assess localized volumetric loss of gray matter in the brain have provided remarkable insights into common areas of damage across different sleep disordered breathing syndromes. Patients with OSA show severe gray matter loss in the cerebellar cortex and deep cerebellar "autonomic" nuclei, hippocampus, cingulate, temporal, and frontal cortices (Macey *et al.*, 2002). Heart failure patients show similar, or even more exaggerated damage in the cerebellum, and also show gray matter loss in the parahippocampal gyrus overlying the hippocampus, and the insular frontal, parietal, and cingulate cortices (Woo *et al.*, 2003; Figure 1).

The loss of gray matter in OSA and heart failure patients may partially result from repeated exposure to hypoxia or ischemia as a consequence of successive apneic episodes during sleep, the extreme changes in perfusion that may be associated with Cheyne–Stokes breathing, or inflammatory processes that apparently accompany sleep disordered breathing (Tauman *et al.*, 2004). Inflammatory effects are normally considered as playing a role in the etiology of atherosclerosis that may accompany OSA, and potentially alter perfusion of neural areas; neural processes may also be directly affected by inflammatory action.

Cerebellar cortical fibers and deep nuclei receive afferent information on blood pressure and respiratory-related stimuli partially from the inferior olive. Climbing fibers projecting from the inferior olive to Purkinje cells in the cerebellar cortex are exceptionally sensitive to hypoxia and ischemia, with the potential to damage these Purkinje cells through excitotoxic mechanisms (Welsh *et al.*, 2002). The repeated hypoxic episodes induced by successive apnea in OSA or the extremes in perfusion associated with cardiovascular sequaelae of Cheyne–Stokes breathing may provide such excessive excitation. A comparable excitotoxic action initiated by hypoxia may operate through perforant path neurons to selectively damage CA1 fibers in the hippocampus in OSA, in a fashion reminiscent of

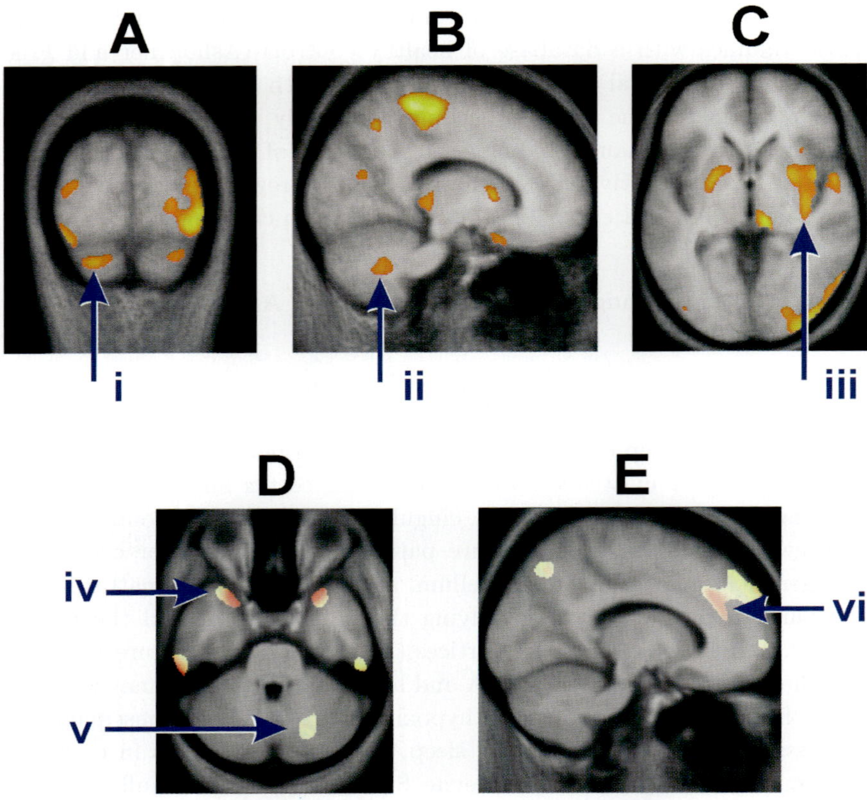

Figure 1. Areas of gray matter loss (arrows) within the cerebellar cortex (A, i), fastigial nucleus (B, ii), and insula (C, iii) of heart failure patients ($n = 9$) and hippocampus (D, iv), cerebellum (D, v), and cingulate cortex (E, vi) of OSA patients ($n = 21$); gray matter loss was calculated from structural MRI scans relative to controls. (A, B, and C from Woo *et al.*, 2003; D and E from Macey *et al.*, 2002.)

processes that operate in temporal lobe epilepsy to damage hippocampal neurons (Sloviter *et al.*, 1996).

Recruitment of cerebellar structures in mediating blood pressure and breathing responses has been recognized (Lutherer *et al.*, 1983; Xu and Frazier, 2002). Purkinje cells in the cerebellar cortex normally inhibit the cerebellar deep nuclei (Bao *et al.*, 2002), and thus the release of inhibition to deep cerebellar nuclei can "undampen" output from these deep nuclei. The fastigial nucleus, the "autonomic" nucleus of the cerebellum, has been shown to play a key role in regulating extremes of blood pressure, particularly during blood loss (Lutherer *et al.*, 1983; Chen *et al.*, 1994). A portion of the contribution of the cerebellum to blood pressure and breathing control appears to result from vestibular interactions with the cerebellum (Doba and Reis, 1974; Yates, 1996). During increases in blood pressure, functional MRI studies have demonstrated a widespread activation of neural sites including the deep cerebellar nuclei and cerebellar cortex, the cingulate, insula, and frontal cortices (Critchley *et al.*, 2000; Harper *et al.*, 2000). Since the deep nuclei constitute the major output from the cerebellum, medullary, and more rostral sites, which are also affected by changes in blood pressure, can be influenced by structural cerebellar damage.

Regional neural activity changes show that the areas affected by structural damage also have functional deficits. When brain areas are examined for responses to application of cold to the forehead, which elicits a rise in blood pressure and a sequence of breathing changes, multiple sites show aberrant responses in OSA, many of which overlap structural damage (Harper *et al.*, 2003a).

For example, the anterior cingulate, an area of consistent gray matter loss, shows a response pattern to a cold pressor challenge in the opposite direction in OSA to that of controls, as do areas within the cerebellar cortex and insula (Figure 2). Multiple procedures have shown that the cingulate cortex participates in cardiovascular regulation (Burns and Wyss, 1985; Frysinger and Harper, 1986; Critchley *et al.*, 2003). Further, where some structures in control subjects show little change to the challenge, such as the hippocampus, signal declines are found in OSA cases. With other challenges, such as loaded breathing, certain sites show little change in OSA patients, but are very responsive in controls (Macey *et al.*, 2003).

Distortions in Levels and Timing of Autonomic Outflow

Both OSA and heart failure patients show high sustained levels of sympathetic tone, a characteristic which has been suggested to underlie blood pressure control deficiencies found in both syndromes, and to contribute to the progression of pathology in heart failure (Packer, 1996). The focus of attention for altered sympathetic outflow has been on "resetting" of baroreceptor processes after repeated transient hypertensive episodes associated with each apneic event (Brooks *et al.*, 1999). Such influences may indeed be operating; however, other aberrant control mechanisms may participate. A substantial loss of gray matter occurs in the insula of heart failure patients, especially on the right side (Figure 1), and deficient insular

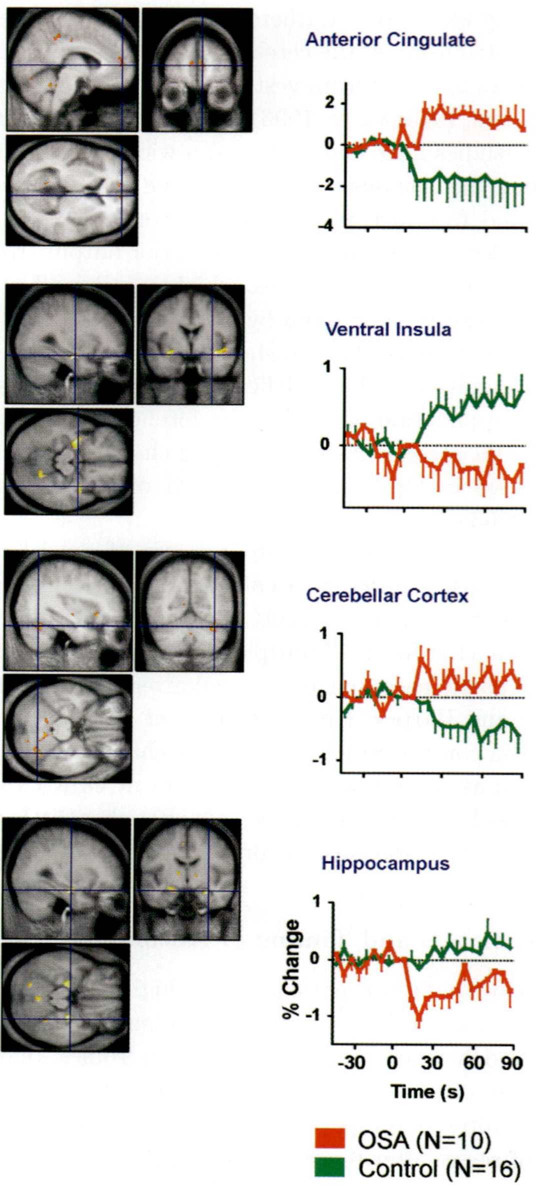

Figure 2. Four regions (anterior cingulate, ventral insula, cerebellar cortex, and hippocampus) exhibiting significant differences in signal intensity change between control and OSA subjects during a forehead cold pressor challenge. Time trends from the four regions are shown on the right. (From Harper *et al.*, 2003a.)

responses to pressor challenges occur both in OSA and heart failure (Harper *et al.*, 2003a,b). The insular cortex exerts substantial control over autonomic nervous action, with the right insula contributing to control of sympathetic outflow, and parasympathetic aspects principally mediated by the left insula (Oppenheimer and Cechetto, 1990; Oppenheimer, 2001). Those influences can be of an inhibitory or disfacilatory nature (Harper *et al.*, 2003a; Henderson *et al.*, 2003); damage to right insular tissue could have the effect of reducing the potential to inhibit sympathetic outflow, producing the high levels of sympathetic tone found in the two syndromes.

It is not just altered levels of sympathetic or parasympathetic outflow that are of concern in OSA and heart failure, but timing of that outflow. Since transient elevation of blood pressure suppresses respiratory muscle action, preferentially in the upper airway (Marks *et al.*, 1987), delayed or advanced release of a sympathetic surge could initiate premature suppression of upper airway tone, or desynchronize timing of diaphragmatic and upper airway action. Similarly, sympathetic and parasympathetic outflow expressed in conjunction with the initiation and cessation of breathing in Cheyne–Stokes respiration depends on central coordination of that release, and the insular cortex would participate in that regulation. The insular cortex shows a substantial phase delay on the right side to a Valsalva maneuver in both OSA and heart failure patients as measured by functional MRI (Harper *et al.*, 2003b; Henderson *et al.*, 2003; Figure 3). The delays are not trivial, with time periods of approximately 18 s apparent. The processes that are faulty in eliciting the delay are unclear; appropriate signals may be late in arriving from the cerebellum, or intrinsic processes of the insula may be deficient. Since the insula plays a significant role in sympathetic nervous system outflow, any autonomic responses to blood pressure manipulation in OSA and heart failure would be compromised.

Cerebellar Coordination of Autonomic and Respiratory Responses

The contributions of cerebellar structures to cardiovascular control should be viewed in the context of the usual perspective of that structure's role, which is that of motor coordination, the synchronization of sensory input to somatomotor output. The cerebellum has been especially implicated in timing roles, particularly for rapid compensation to deviation from motor paths. Although participation of certain cerebellar structures in cardiovascular control has been known for over half a century (Moruzzi, 1940),

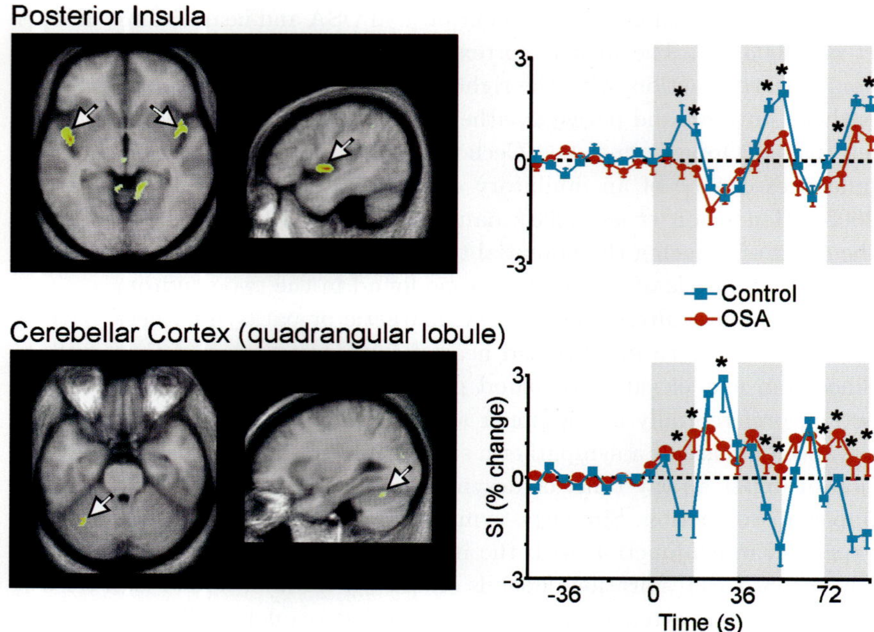

Figure 3. Left: Significant response differences between control and OSA subjects in cerebellar cortex and posterior insula during Valsalva maneuvers ($P < 0.05$; corresponding to $t > 2$). The averaged ($\pm$SE) time trends (Right) of functional MRI signal changes during the course of three Valsalva maneuvers (vertical shaded areas) are shown on the right. Both cerebellar cortex and posterior insula show muted and phase-shifted responses. *Significant difference ($P < 0.05$) between control and OSA groups. SI, signal intensity. (From Henderson et al., 2003.)

only recently has a role been recognized for compensation of extremes in blood pressure changes, coordinating appropriate timing of respiratory muscle patterning to assist autonomic outflow, and synchronization of afferent chemoreceptor and baroreceptor activities with appropriate respiratory and heart rate patterns (Xu and Frazier, 2002; Lutherer et al., 1983).

Deficient coordination of upper airway muscle activity with diaphragmatic action is a hallmark of OSA, since, instead of a sequence of action of upper airway muscles in a precise timing relationship with diaphragmatic muscle exertion, the upper airway muscles become hypotonic. The pattern of disordered breathing most frequently encountered in heart failure, Cheyne–Stokes breathing, is characterized by a reduction of breathing efforts followed by enhanced respiratory efforts repeated over a sustained period of time. The pattern may result from delayed circulatory stimulation of peripheral chemoreceptors with respect to central chemoreceptor action, i.e., a respiratory sequence based on timing incoordination of sensory information from multiple sources. The breathing sequence is accompanied by exaggerated cardiac rate swings occurring with each cycle of breathing and cessation of breathing. Figure 3 demonstrates a respiratory challenge that induces an autonomic/blood pressure sequence, the Valsalva maneuver, and results in a phase-reversed response in the cerebellar cortex of OSA cases.

Ventral Medullary Surface

Of all structures that have been classically associated with control of blood pressure, the ventral medullary surface (VMS) has been of particular interest, largely from the pioneering studies of the Bochum group (Loeschke *et al.*, 1970). The region has been extremely difficult to study during sleep–waking states, principally because of logistic issues related to access to the VMS in the intact animal; until recently, most of our information on the VMS has been derived from anesthetized preparations. Intrinsic optical imaging procedures, however, which measure reflected and scattered light changes accompanying neural discharge (Rector *et al.*, 1997), provide a means to examine the activity of large numbers of neurons in drug-free preparations. The technique has demonstrated that, in the waking state, the VMS shows activity declines to transient blood pressure elevation, and increases activity, often dramatically, to blood pressure lowering, especially if the hypotension is extreme (Harper *et al.*, 1999).

In contrast to the majority of neural sites, VMS activity declines during the state change to rapid eye movement (REM) sleep. This decline precedes the onset of the state by 5–60 s. The pattern of activity decline appears in the rostral VMS in the goat (Rector *et al.*, 1994), and extends to include the intermediate VMS of the cat (Richard *et al.*, 1999). The VMS joins a small number of other brain areas that decline in activity during REM sleep, including the dorsal raphe, locus coeruleus, ventromedial medulla, and histaminergic neurons (Chu and Bloom, 1974; McGinty and Harper, 1976; Sakai *et al.*, 1983, 1990). The REM-related activity decline may result in the VMS being unable to respond adequately to blood pressure challenges during that state, or to perform its regulatory functions in an entirely different fashion from other states. Blood pressure elevation, by phenylephrine, elicits an even larger VMS activity decline in REM sleep over quiet sleep and waking; a later activity rise occurs in all states (Figure 4). Arousals diminish

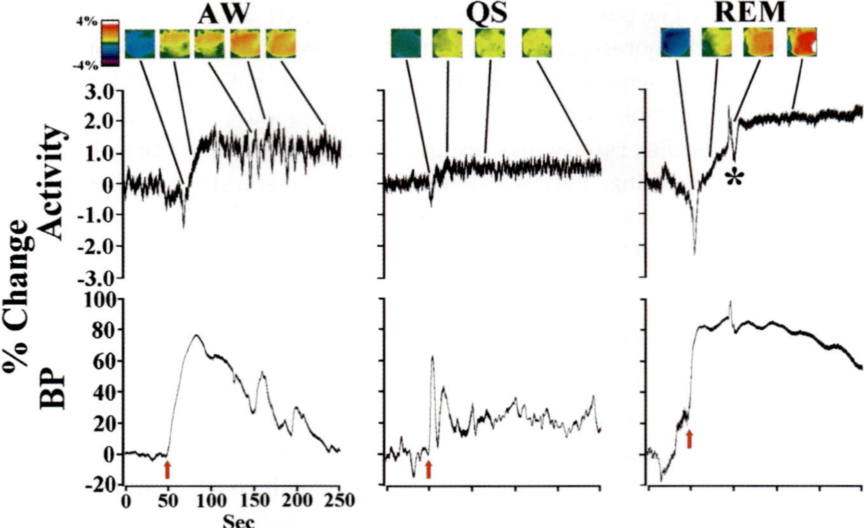

Figure 4. Plots of individual activity traces from the VMS (activity) of a single cat, together with selected images, averaged across 3-s segments, as well as accompanying blood pressure (BP) changes within (AW), quiet sleep (QS), and REM sleep during a 30 µg/kg phenylephrine challenge. Arrows indicate onset of phenylephrine action. A transient (asterisk) REM-related phasic event occurs on the optical trace. The decline to phenylephrine is much more enhanced during REM sleep. (From Rector *et al.*, 2000.)

this late rise, as does phasic REM activity (Richard *et al.*, 2003). Blood pressure lowering with sodium nitroprusside also results in greater VMS activity changes in REM sleep compared with quiet sleep, with the increase being even less in waking. The pattern of enhanced responses to blood pressure manipulations during REM sleep supports the suggestion that the VMS is less able to dampen evoked activity during that state. A dampening role for the VMS appears to be the case with ventilatory challenges as well, including simulated hypoxia with cyanide exposure (Carroll *et al.*, 1996). If the capability of the VMS to dampen responses to blood pressure varies with sleep, perhaps a portion of the state-related modification of baroreflex responses directly results from state-related VMS influences.

The contribution of the VMS to modulation of the baroreflex is a significant issue for the Sudden Infant Death Syndrome (SIDS). The marked bradycardia and hypotension that accompany a number of fatal sequences in SIDS (Meny *et al.*, 1994; Ledwidge *et al.*, 1998) suggest that inadequate compensation to a loss of blood pressure may contribute to a proportion

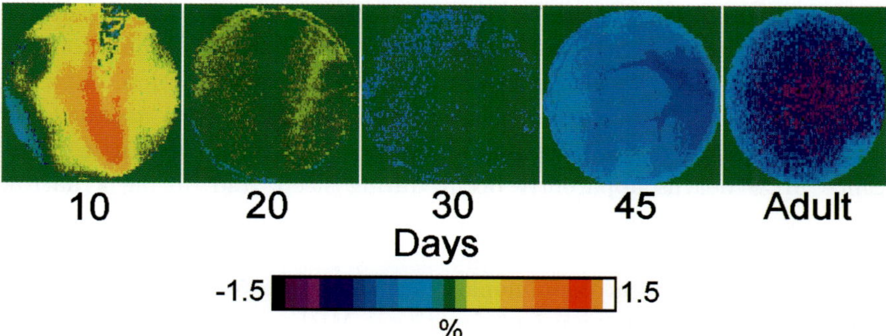

Figure 5. Averaged ($n = 60$) VMS images recorded by intrinsic optical procedures, calculated as differences from maximal peak of responses to 20 µg/kg phenylephrine and from control conditions in individual kittens at various postnatal ages and an adult cat. Green indicates no significant change in activity; black-to-blue colors represent activity declines, while yellow-to-white indicates increases in activity. The VMS response to blood pressure elevation reverses between 20 and 30 days. Percentage-change values represent corrections after compensation to maximize dynamic range of optical device. (From Gozal *et al.*, 1995.)

of SIDS deaths. The issue is of particular interest when viewed in the context of altered neurotransmitter receptors within the VMS in SIDS victims (Kinney *et al.*, 1995). The capability of the VMS to modulate baroreflex challenges in young human infants is unclear, but the immature (<25–30 days) feline preparation responds in the opposite fashion as adults to both blood pressure elevation and lowering, as assessed by optical imaging (Gozal *et al.*, 1995; Figure 5) and functional MRI procedures (Henderson *et al.*, 2004). Clearly, very young infants (and kittens) are able to compensate for blood pressure manipulations; the fMRI studies suggest that a network of cerebellar and forebrain areas contribute to mediating such compensatory responses. Sleep states can greatly modify the actions of these structures, and the interactions during development have yet to be defined for sleep conditions.

Cardiopulmonary Afferent Stimulation

A significant issue in cardiopulmonary disorders, especially those with increased breathing resistance, such as asthma, as well as those associated with coronary artery disease, is reflex responses to cardiopulmonary afferent stimulation. Marked stimulation of these afferents e.g., angina, can result in severe hypotension, bradycardia, and apnea, and thus is of considerable clinical interest. Loss of perfusion from the accompanying hypotension or induction of apnea with pulmonary afferent nociceptive stimulation can be life threatening. As in the case with impaired VMS function, damaged structures that mediate compensation to hypotension from activation of cardiopulmonary nociceptive afferents are of particular concern in SIDS. Since SIDS deaths apparently occur during sleep, and during a narrow time frame in early life, state modulation of the reflex, and ontology of its expression, are significant concerns.

Stimulation of cardiopulmonary afferents by 5-hydroxytryptamine results in rapid-onset, transient functional MRI signal intensity declines in medullary sites as well as the fastigial nucleus of the cerebellum. Slightly delayed phasic signal declines occur in other deep cerebellar nuclei and the pons, and even later signal changes develop in medullary and cerebellar sites with increases in the amygdala and hypothalamus (Henderson *et al.*, 2002). The responses indicate a participatory role of cerebellar structures, as well as rostral sites in overcoming the challenge. The study reflects responses in an anesthetized preparation; sleep state responses may vary, but the integrity of structures involved may be essential for effective recovery.

Summary

The close integration of breathing and cardiovascular systems provides a potential to reveal insights into central control of cardiovascular action by sleep-related breathing disorders. The demonstration of chronic modification to sympathetic outflow and impaired cardiovascular responses to the Valsalva maneuver in OSA and heart failure patients, and the presence of sleep disordered breathing in heart failure patients with anatomically not compromised airways, together with persistent cognitive deficits in both groups suggest central neural damage developing from the syndromes. Examination by structural MRI procedures demonstrate significant gray matter loss in cerebellar, hippocampal, and cortical areas in both groups and especially in insular cortex in heart failure patients, the latter a cortical region involved in autonomic outflow regulation. Functional MRI procedures demonstrate that areas of gray matter loss do not respond appropriately to manipulations of blood pressure by respiratory or cold pressor challenges, and show both muted and phase-shifted responses in cerebellar and insular cortices of both groups, and altered patterns in other brain areas. The VMS, which declines in activity to blood pressure elevation and increases activity to hypotension, shows substantial activity declines during REM sleep, with "undampened" responses to blood pressure manipulation during that state; responses in very early life are inverse to those of adults. The data suggest that neural areas that control both extent and timing of autonomic outflow are damaged in OSA and heart failure patients, and VMS, cerebellar, and insular areas play significant roles in cardiovascular control during sleep; SIDS risk may be particularly affected by VMS and cerebellar damage.

Acknowledgments

Supported by HD-22695, HL-22418, and HL-60296. We thank Rebecca Harper for assistance.

References

Ashburner, J. and Friston, K.J. (2000). Voxel-based morphometry — the methods. *Neuroimage*, 11: 805–821.

Bao, S., Chen, L., Kim, J.J., and Thompson, R.F. (2002). Cerebellar cortical inhibition and classical eyeblink conditioning. *Proc. Natl. Acad. Sci. USA*, 99: 1592–1597.

Brooks, D., Horner, R.L., Floras, J.S., Kozar, L.F., Render-Teixeira, C.L., and Phillipson, E.A. (1999). Baroreflex control of heart rate in a canine model of obstructive sleep apnea. *Am. J. Respir. Crit. Care Med.*, 159: 1293–1297.

Bradley, T.D. (1992). Right and left ventricular functional impairment and sleep apnea. *Clin. Chest Med.*, 13: 459–479.

Burns, S.M. and Wyss, J.M. (1985). The involvement of the anterior cingulate cortex in blood pressure control. *Brain Res.*, 340: 71–77.

Carroll, J.L., Gozal, D., Rector, D.M., Aljadeff, G., and Harper, R.M. (1996). Ventral medullary neuronal responses to peripheral chemoreceptor stimulation. *Neuroscience*, 73: 989–998.

Chen, C.H., Williams, J.L., and Lutherer, L.O. (1994). Cerebellar lesions alter autonomic responses to transient isovolaemic changes in arterial pressure in anaesthetized cats. *Clin. Auton. Res.*, 4: 263–272.

Chu, N.S. and Bloom, F.E. (1974). Activity patterns of catecholamine-containing pontine neurons in the dorso-lateral tegmentum of unrestrained cats. *J. Neurobiol.*, 5: 527–544.

Critchley, H.D., Corfield, D.R., Chandler, M.P., Mathias, C.J., and Dolan, R.J. (2000). Cerebral correlates of autonomic cardiovascular arousal: a functional neuroimaging investigation in humans. *J. Physiol.*, 523: 259–270.

Critchley, H.D., Mathias, C.J., Josephs, O., O'Doherty, J., Zanini, S., Dewar, B.-K., Cipolotti, L., Shallice, T., and Dolan, R.J. (2003). Human cingulate cortex and autonomic control: converging neuroimaging and clinical evidence. *Brain*, 126: 2139–2152.

Doba, N. and Reis, D.J. (1974). Role of the cerebellum and vestibular apparatus in regulation of orthostatic reflexes in the cat. *Circ. Res.*, 34: 9–18.

Frysinger, R.C. and Harper, R.M. (1986). Cardiac and respiratory relationships with neural discharge in the anterior cingulate cortex during sleep–waking states. *Exp. Neurol.*, 94: 247–263.

Gozal, D., Dong, X.-W., Rector, D.M., and Harper, R.M. (1995). Maturation of kitten ventral medullary surface activity during pressor challenges. *Dev. Neurosci.*, 192: 89–92.

Haddad, G.G., Mazza N.M., Defendini R., Blanc, W.A., Driscoll, J.M., Epstein, M.A., Epstein, R.A., and Mellins, R.B. (1978). Congenital failure of automatic control of ventilation, gastrointestinal motility and heart rate. *Medicine (Baltimore)*, 57: 517–526.

Harper, R.M., Richard, C.A., and Rector, D.M. (1999). Physiological and ventral medullary surface activity during hypovolemia. *Neuroscience*, 94: 579–586.

Harper, R.M., Bandler, R., Spriggs, D., and Alger, J.R. (2000). Lateralized and widespread brain activation during transient blood pressure elevation revealed by magnetic resonance imaging. *J. Comp. Neurol.*, 417: 195–204.

Harper, R.M., Macey, P.M., Henderson, L.A., Woo, M.A., Macey, K.E., Frysinger, R.C., Alger, J.R., Nguyen, K.P., and Yan-Go, F.L. (2003a). *F*MRI responses to cold pressor challenges in control and obstructive sleep apnea subjects. *J. Appl. Physiol.*, 94: 1583–1595.

Harper, R.M., Woo, M.A., Macey, P.M., Macey, K.E., Harper, R.K., Yan-Go, F., and Alger, J.R. (2003b). Heart failure patients show deficient heart rate and altered neural *f*MRI responses to Valsalva maneuvers. *Soc. Neurosci. Abstr.*, 768.12.

Henderson, L.A., Yu, P.L., Frysinger, R.C., Galons, J.-P., Bandler, R., and Harper, R.M. (2002). Neural responses to intravenous serotonin revealed by functional magnetic resonance imaging. *J. Appl. Physiol.*, 92: 331–342.

Henderson, L.A., Woo, M.A., Macey, P.M., Macey, K.E., Frysinger, R.C., Alger, J.R., Yan-Go, F., and Harper, R.M. (2003). Neural responses during Valsalva maneuvers in obstructive sleep apnea syndrome. *J. Appl. Physiol.*, 94: 1063–1074.

Henderson, L.A., Macey, P.M., Richard, C.A., Runquist, M.L., and Harper, R.M. (2004). Functional magnetic resonance imaging during hypotension in the developing animal. *J. Appl. Physiol.*, 97: 2248–2257.

Javaheri, S., Parker, T.J., Wexler, L., Michaels, S.E., Stanberry, E., Nishyama, H., and Roselle, G.A. (1995). Occult sleep-disordered breathing in stable congestive heart failure. *Ann. Intern. Med.*, 122: 487–492.

Kinney, H.C., Filiano, J.J., Sleeper, L.A., Mandell, F., Valdes-Dapena, M., and White, W.F. (1995). Decreased muscarinic receptor binding in the arcuate nucleus in sudden infant death syndrome. *Science*, 269: 1446–1450.

Ledwidge, M., Fox, G., and Matthews, T. (1998). Neurocardiogenic syncope: a model for SIDS. Arch. *Dis. Child*, 78: 481–483.

Loeschcke, H.H., de Lattre, J., Schläfke, M.E., and Trouth, C.O. (1970). Effects on respiration and circulation of electrically stimulating the ventral surface of the medulla oblongata. *Respir. Physiol.*, 10: 184–197.

Lutherer, L.O., Lutherer, B.C., Dormer, K.J., Janssen, H.F., and Barnes, C.D. (1983). Bilateral lesions of the fastigial nucleus prevent the recovery of blood pressure following hypotension induced by hemorrhage or administration of endotoxin. *Brain Res.*, 269: 251–257.

Macey, P.M., Henderson, L.A., Macey, K.E., Alger, J.R., Frysinger, R.C., Woo, M.A., Harper, R.K., Yan-Go, F.L., and Harper, R.M. (2002). Brain morphology associated with obstructive sleep apnea. *Am. J. Respir. Crit. Care Med.*, 166: 1382–1387.

Macey, P.M., Macey, K.M., Henderson, L.A., Alger, J.R., Frysinger, R.C., Woo, M.A., Yan-Go, F., and Harper, R.M. (2003). Functional magnetic resonance imaging responses to expiratory loading in obstructive sleep apnea. *Respir. Physiol. Neurobiol.*, 130: 275–290.

Marks, J.D., Frysinger, R.C., and Harper, R.M. (1987). State-dependent respiratory depression elicited by stimulation of the orbital frontal cortex. *Exp. Neurol.*, 95: 714–729.

McGinty, D.J. and Harper, R.M. (1976). Dorsal raphe neurons: depression of firing during sleep in cats. *Brain Res.*, 101: 569–575.

Meny, R.G., Carroll, J.L., Carbone, M.T., and Kelly, D.H. (1994). Cardiorespiratory recordings from infants dying suddenly and unexpectedly at home. *Pediatrics*, 93: 43–49.

Moruzzi, G. (1940). Paleocerebellar inhibition of vasomotor and respiratory carotid sinus reflexes. *J. Neurophysiol.*, 3: 20–32.

Naegele, B., Pepin, J.L., Levy, P., Bonnet, C., Pellat, J., and Feuerstein, C. (1998). Cognitive executive dysfunction in patients with obstructive sleep apnea syndrome (OSAS) after CPAP treatment. *Sleep*, 21: 392–397.

Narkiewicz, K. and Somers, V.K. (1997). The sympathetic nervous system and obstructive sleep apnea: implications for hypertension. *J. Hypertens.*, 15: 1613–1619.

Ogawa, S., Lee, T.M., Nayak, A.S., and Glynn, P. (1990). Oxygenation-sensitive contrast in magnetic resonance image of rodent brain at high magnetic fields. *Magn. Reson. Med.*, 14: 68–78.

Ohtake, P.J. and Jennings, D.B. (1992). Ventilation is stimulated by small reductions in arterial pressure in the awake dog. *J. Appl. Physiol.*, 73: 1549–1557.

Oppenheimer, S. (2001). Forebrain lateralization of cardiovascular function: physiology and clinical correlates. *Ann. Neurol.*, 49: 555–556.

Oppenheimer, S.M. and Cechetto, D.F. (1990). Cardiac chronotropic organization of the rat insular cortex. *Brain Res.*, 533: 66–72.

Packer, M. (1996). New concepts in the pathophysiology of heart failure: beneficial and deleterious interaction of endogenous haemodynamic and neurohormonal mechanisms. *J. Intern. Med.*, 239: 327–333.

Rector, D.M., Gozal, D., Forster, H.V., Ohtake, P.J., and Harper, R.M. (1994). Ventral medullary surface activity during sleep, waking and anesthetic states in the goat. *Am. J. Physiol.*, 267: 1154–1160.

Rector, D.M., Poe, G.R., and Harper, R.M. (1997). A miniature CCD video camera for high-sensitivity measurements in freely behaving animals. *J. Neurosci. Meth.*, 78: 85–91.

Rector, D.M., Richard, C.A., Staba, R.J., and Harper, R.M. (2000). Sleep states alter ventral medullary surface responses to blood pressure challenges. *Am. J. Physiol.*, 278: 1090–1098.

Richard, C.A., Rector, D.M., Harper, R.K., and Harper, R.M. (1999). Optical imaging of the ventral medullary surface across sleep–wake states. *Am. J. Physiol.*, 277: 1239–1245.

Richard, C.A., Rector, D.M., Macey, P.M., Ali, N., and Harper, R.M. (2003). Late-developing rostral ventral lateral medullary surface responses to cardiovascular challenges during sleep. *Brain Res.*, 985: 65–77.

Sakai, K., Vanni-Mercier, G., and Jouvet, M. (1983). Evidence for the presence of PS-OFF neurons in the ventromedial medulla oblongata of freely moving cats. *Exp. Brain Res.*, 49: 311–314.

Sakai, K., el Mansari, M., Lin, J.S., Zhang, J.G., and Vanni-Mercier, G. (1990). The posterior hypothalamus in the regulation of wakefulness and paradoxical sleep. In: Mancia, M. and Marini, G. (Eds.). *The Diencephalon and Sleep.* New York: Raven Press, pp. 171–198.

Sloviter, R.S., Dean, E., Sollas, A.L., and Goodman, J.H. (1996). Apoptosis and necrosis induced in different hippocampal neuron populations by repetitive perforant path stimulation in the rat. *J. Comp. Neurol.*, 366: 516–533.

Somers, V.K., Dyken, M.E., Clary, M.P., and Abboud, F.M. (1995). Sympathetic neural mechanisms in obstructive sleep apnea. *J. Clin. Invest.*, 96: 1897–1904.

Tauman, R., Ivanenko, A., O'Brein, L., and Gozal, D. (2004). Plasma C-reactive protein levels among children with sleep-disordered breathing. *Pediatrics*, 113: 564–569.

Trelease, R.B., Sieck, G.C., Marks, J.D., and Harper, R.M. (1985). Respiratory inhibition induced by transient hypertension during sleep. *Exp. Neurol.*, 90: 173–186.

Welsh, J.P., Yuen, G., Placantonakis, D.G., Vu, T.Q., Haiss, F., O'Hearn, E., Molliver, M.E., and Aicher, S.A. (2002). Why do Purkinje cells die so easily after global brain ischemia? Aldolase C, EAAT4, and the cerebellar contribution to posthypoxic myoclonus. *Adv. Neurol.*, 89: 331–359.

Woo, M.S., Woo, M.A., Gozal, D., Jansen, M.T., Keens, T.G., and Harper, R.M. (1992). Heart rate variability in congenital central hypoventilation syndrome. *Pediatr. Res.*, 31: 291–296.

Woo, M.A., Macey, P.M., Fonarow, G.C., Hamilton, M.A., and Harper, R.M. (2003). Regional brain gray matter loss in heart failure. *J. Appl. Physiol.*, 95: 677–684.

Xu, F. and Frazier, D.T. (2002). Role of the cerebellar deep nuclei in respiratory modulation. *Cerebellum*, 1: 35–40.

Yates, B.J. (1996). Vestibular influences on the autonomic nervous system. In: Highstein, S.M., Cohen, B., and Buttner-Ennever, J.A. (Eds.). *New Directions in Vestibular Research. Annals of the New York Academy of Sciences*, pp. 458–470.

Chapter 18

SLEEP BEHAVIOUR AND TEMPERATURE

Pier Luigi Parmeggiani[1]

Temperature is a physical variable which not only directly affects cellular activities (thermophysical and thermochemical effects), but also indirectly influences the somatic and autonomic activity of the organism by excitation of specific thermoreceptors. On this basis, temperature must be considered a signal of both physicochemical and biological relevance from the viewpoint of thermoregulation.

In mammals, thermoregulatory mechanisms are activated by the temperature signal to maintain a substantial homeothermy of the body core. This control stabilises the physicochemical effects of temperature according to the metabolic needs of body tissues within a wide range of ambient temperatures. However, thermoregulatory responses to the same temperature signal show a clear-cut behavioural state-dependence in sleep (Parmeggiani and Rabini, 1967), a fact which stresses the operative difference between a physical signal and a biological signal.

Biologically, temperature is a signal that ought to be regarded as both an endogenous and exogenous stimulus influencing the organism. The endogenous stimulus is compartmentalised by physiological mechanisms in the body core and the body periphery. Core temperature is further compartmentalised in the central nervous system by selective brain cooling in several

---

[1]pier.parmeggiani@unibo.it

species (Hayward and Baker, 1969; Parmeggiani *et al.*, 1998). The fact that selective brain cooling influences preoptic–hypothalamic thermoreceptors, but not thermoreceptive structures in the brain stem and spinal cord, is of relevance according to the hierarchical organisation of thermoregulatory integration (Satinoff, 1978). In the ambient thermal zone for vasomotor regulation of core temperature, namely under moderate positive (warm) or negative (cold) ambient thermal loads, selective brain cooling lowers the error signal of preoptic–hypothalamic temperature in comparison with brain stem temperature (Parmeggiani *et al.*, 1998). On this basis, selective brain cooling probably underlies a thermal load dependent graduation in the recruitment of preoptic–hypothalamic thermoregulatory responses optimising efficacy and energy cost of thermoregulation (Azzaroni and Parmeggiani, 1999; Parmeggiani *et al.*, 2000).

In conclusion, the physical temperature signal is so compartmentalised as an endogenous stimulus to assume varying regional intensity as a biological signal for thermoreceptive nervous structures influencing somatic and autonomic behaviour across the ultradian wake–sleep cycle (active wakefulness, AW; quiet wakefulness, QW; non-rapid eye movement sleep, NREM sleep; rapid eye movement sleep, REM sleep).

Thermoregulation

Before approaching the thermoregulatory peculiarities of sleep behaviour, it helps the untutored reader to summarise briefly the effector mechanisms of thermoregulation underlying the maintenance of thermal homeostasis in mammalian species.

The fact that the oscillations of body core temperature are small in mammals depends on the precise control of the balance between heat production and heat loss. A change in temperature may be quantitatively expressed as the ratio between the change in heat content and the mass of the tissue multiplied by the specific heat of the tissue ($\Delta T = \Delta Q/mc$). Cellular metabolism continuously produces heat which is transferred to the blood and carried to the systemic heat exchangers of the body where vasomotion controls heat dissipation helping to maintain the homeothermy of the body core. In theory, core temperature is constant when the heat content of the body is unchanged as the result of a perfect balance between heat production and heat loss to the environment. In reality, such a perfect homeothermy does not occur. A tachymetabolic organism is considered homeothermic when the cyclic variation in core temperature is maintained within arbitrarily defined limits ($\pm 2°C$) despite much wider variations in ambient temperature. From a mechanistic point of view, such a regulatory system entails a set range of core temperatures to define the error signal necessary to activate the thermoregulatory responses. Afferent discharges from superficial and deep thermoreceptors of the body act as inputs to control the activity of the central thermostat in the preoptic–hypothalamic area and of subordinate brain stem and spinal thermoregulatory mechanisms (Satinoff, 1978). Such structures are also equipped with thermoresponsive neurones, reacting selectively to central thermal stimuli, which are direct feedback inputs to them. The response gain of this feedback regulation shows that even the slightest preoptic–hypothalamic temperature deviations from set point temperature activate thermoregulation (Von Euler, 1964).

The thermoregulatory responses to external and internal positive (warm) and negative (cold) thermal loads are either behavioural or autonomic. The rationale of this distinction is that *behavioural thermoregulation* influences passive heat loss by means of changes in posture (e.g., curling or sprawling) and/or location (to increase or decrease exposure to sun, wind, humidity, etc.) of the body with respect to the thermal environment and *autonomic thermoregulation* actively influences both heat production (shivering, non-shivering thermogenesis) and heat loss (vasomotion of heat exchangers, piloerection, thermal tachypnea and panting, sweating). In other words, the first group of responses is aimed at establishing conditions appropriately affecting the heat exchange of the body with its environment and the second group at affecting the balance between the two variables underlying body core homeothermy, namely heat production and heat loss. Qualitative and quantitative changes in thermoregulatory responses occurring as a result of acclimatisation to low or high ambient temperature are not considered in this chapter.

The changes in somatic and autonomic activity underlying thermoregulation in relation to the ultradian sleep cycle are a specific and fundamental manifestation of sleep behaviour in mammalian species. The rationale of a hierarchical subordination of thermoregulation to sleep regulation is based on the fact that such regulations are not equivalent functional entities in terms of integrative complexity. Sleep is a global behaviour since it is characterised by changes in the somatic and autonomic functions of the whole organism. In contrast, thermoregulation is related to a group of other physiological functions (cardiovascular, respiratory, motor, and postural functions) sharing several effector mechanisms. A possible overlap of different synergistic or antagonistic executive controls on the same effectors is therefore possible and may result in central and/or peripheral facilitation or occlusion of effector responses. On this basis, the functional distinction between hierarchical levels of complexity in integrative physiological regulation guides this approach to the thermoregulatory aspects of sleep behaviour.

Specific Thermoregulatory Aspects of Sleep Behaviour

Mammals display an appetitive presomnic behaviour which is mainly characterised by motor and postural thermoregulatory features (Parmeggiani, 1968) elicited partly by the temperature signal, since such behaviour appears aimed at reducing the demand for autonomic temperature regulation during sleep. The motility is related to the search for a safe and thermally comfortable ecological niche and the preparation of the body for the natural sleep posture. This posture is basically characterised by decreased antigravity muscle activity, and curling up or sprawling, stretching and spreading the limbs in a cold or a warm environment, respectively (Parmeggiani and Rabini, 1970). Such postural attitudes, depending on ambient temperature, affect heat loss by decreasing or increasing the surface of the body which is exposed to open air or touching the ground. In particular, the intensity of abdominal thermal stimulation is effective in changing the sympathetic vasoconstrictor outflow to the heat exchangers of the body (skin, ear pinna, airway mucosa, tail) (Azzaroni and Parmeggiani, 1995a,b). Moreover, inspired air is thermally conditioned by placing the nose either close to or away from the body surface depending on the posture chosen by the animal under the influence of low or high ambient temperature. The thermal control of inspired air influences the temperature of the venous blood returning from the nasal mucosa to the venous plexus of the carotid rete or the basal venous lakes of the brain depending on the species (Hayward and Baker, 1969). This mechanism underlies selective brain cooling which in particular influences the temperature of the preoptic–hypothalamic thermostat (Hayward and Baker, 1969; Azzaroni and Parmeggiani, 1993, 1995a). Enumeration in detail of the many other measures devised by animals of different species, including humans, to achieve a behavioural defence against thermal loads during sleep is beyond the scope of this chapter. Whatever such behavioural defence may be, it is maintained throughout NREM sleep and provides practically a thermoneutral condition for the sleeping organism at low energetic cost also when ambient temperature does not correspond exactly to the ambient thermoneutral zone of the species (cf. Altman and Dittmer, 1966).

The thermal provisions of presomnic behaviour promote the occurrence of "normal" NREM sleep as the intrinsic metabolic and autonomic activity of this behaviour is characterised by a decrease in metabolic heat production (Brebbia and Altshuler, 1965; Webb and Heistand, 1975; Haskell *et al.*, 1981; Palca *et al.*, 1986) and an increase in heat loss (Azzaroni and Parmeggiani, 1995b) eventually resulting in a decrease in core temperature typical of this state of sleep. In particular, whatever the actual intensity of tonic vasoconstriction of heat exchangers may be in quiet wakefulness, there is always a decrease in this intensity during NREM sleep as a sleep-dependent event (Azzaroni and Parmeggiani, 1995b). The resulting vasodilatation is shown by an increase in heat exchanger temperature and a related increase in brain cooling that lowers preoptic–hypothalamic temperature during NREM sleep (Hayward and Baker, 1969; Parmeggiani *et al.*, 1975; Azzaroni and Parmeggiani, 1993, 1995a,b). A sharp decline of preoptic–hypothalamic temperature in cats, which is steeper at low ambient temperature than at neutral ambient temperature, has been observed when the head is lowered to assume the sleep posture (Parmeggiani *et al.*, 1975). The head-down posture (decrease in negative hydrostatic load raising the transmural pressure) contributes to the increase in heat exchanger vasodilatation and eventual brain cooling during NREM sleep (Azzaroni and Parmeggiani, 1995a). Under conditions of constant ambient temperature, the amount of NREM sleep-dependent heat loss is evidently due to both the increased thermal conductance (heat exchanger vasodilation) and the duration of such an increase, namely the duration of NREM sleep (Azzaroni and Parmeggiani, 1995b). In humans, thermal sweating (Sagot *et al.*, 1987) and skin vasodilatation in the lower extremities (Kräuchi *et al.*, 1997, 1999, 2000; Van Someren, 2000) are phenomena consistent with the down-regulation of body core temperature in NREM sleep. Skin vasodilatation in the lower extremities at the onset of NREM sleep, indicating a state-dependent change in the central regulation of sympathetic outflow, is characterised by both a decrease and an increase in vasoconstrictor and vasodilator sympathetic discharge, respectively (Noll *et al.*, 1994). In turn, the resulting increase in skin temperature, which may also be mimicked by artificial moderate warming, is a feedback acting on the central thermostat which positively influences sleep propensity (Krauchi *et al.*, 1997, 1999, 2000; Van Someren, 2000). This phenomenon, a result of the change in preoptic–hypothalamic drive on sympathetic outflow, is analogous to the systemic heat exchanger vasodilatation occurring in furry species and eliciting a decrease in preoptic–hypothalamic temperature during NREM sleep.

The fact that thermolysis is controlled by sleep mechanisms was evidenced by a study in cats (Parmeggiani *et al.*, 1975) showing that the decrease in preoptic–hypothalamic temperature with respect to wakefulness at the end of the NREM sleep episode depends not only on ambient temperature but is also related to the occurrence of either REM sleep or arousal (cf. Chapter 8). When NREM sleep is followed by REM sleep, the decrease in preoptic–hypothalamic temperature is greater at low (0°C) than at normal (20°C) ambient temperatures. Instead, when NREM sleep is followed by arousal the decrease is the same at both ambient temperatures. Therefore, the presence of a thermal load activating thermoregulation reveals that sleep processes interact with thermoregulation during NREM sleep to bring about REM sleep occurrence. That this is a controlled event is shown by the fact that only restricted ranges of preoptic–hypothalamic temperatures are compatible with REM sleep onset. Such different ranges evidence a functional REM sleep gate which constrains its occurrence more at 0°C than at 20°C ambient temperature (Figure 1). In conclusion, these results demonstrate that sleep processes may overrule strict homeothermy so as to induce heat loss probably by decreasing the

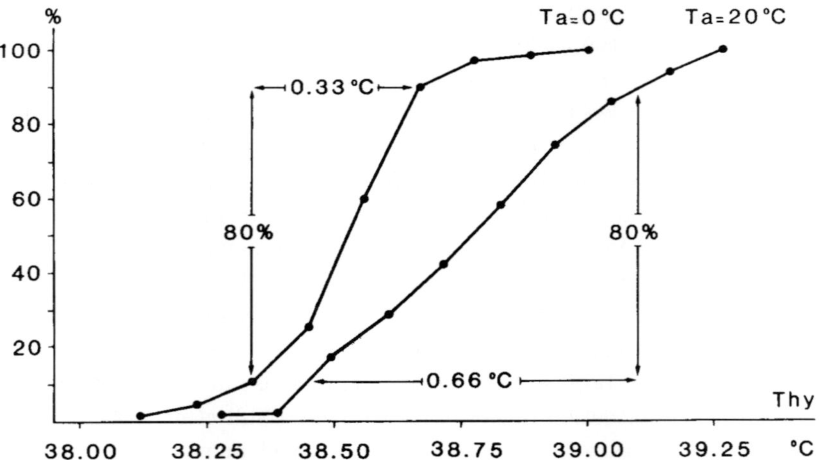

Figure 1. Cumulative relative frequency distributions of REM sleep episodes in the cat with respect to preoptic–anterior hypothalamic (PO-AH) temperature (Thy) at the end of preceding NREM sleep at 20°C and 0°C ambient temperature (Ta). The left shift of the distribution at low Ta shows the thermolytic adjustment of the PO-AH thermostat during NREM sleep. This thermoregulatory adjustment induces variable PO-AH cooling according to Ta. The PO-AH temperature gate of REM sleep occurrence is narrower at 0°C than at 20°C Ta (0.33 versus 0.66°C, respectively), and therefore the probability of such occurrence is reduced, apart from REM sleep pressure (Parmeggiani, 1987).

set temperature of the central thermostat regardless of ambient temperature. The probability of REM sleep occurrence is high at thermal neutrality since heat loss during NREM sleep is easily achieved lacking an antagonistic interaction between sleep processes and thermal influences. Under a substantial thermal load autonomic temperature regulation (vasomotion, piloerection, shivering, tachypnea, sweating) may be activated during NREM sleep (Table 1) (cf. Glotzbach and Heller, 2000; Parmeggiani, 2003) without eliciting immediate awakening from sleep, but the probability of REM sleep occurrence is decreased unless a consistent REM sleep pressure has been accumulated as a result of previous REM sleep suppression to meet thermoregulatory requirements (Parmeggiani *et al.*, 1969, 1980; Parmeggiani and Rabini, 1970).

The interaction between REM sleep and thermoregulation has features of a clear-cut functional antagonism (Parmeggiani, 1980). The thermoregulatory responses elicited by ambient thermal loads during NREM sleep are absent or depressed during REM sleep (cf. Glotzbach and Heller, 2000; Parmeggiani, 2003). The cat's posture clearly varies in relation to ambient temperature during NREM sleep, whereas the drop in postural muscle tonus during REM sleep is unrelated to ambient temperature (Parmeggiani and Rabini, 1970). Moreover, notwithstanding a positive thermal load, tachypnea in the cat (Parmeggiani and Rabini, 1967) and heat exchanger vasodilation in the cat (Parmeggiani *et al.*, 1977), rabbit (Franzini *et al.*, 1982), and rat (Alföldi *et al.*, 1990) disappear and sweating in humans is at first suppressed (Dewasmes *et al.*, 1997) and then depressed (Shapiro *et al.*, 1974; Henane *et al.*, 1977; Sagot *et al.*, 1987; Dewasmes *et al.*, 1997) during the episode of REM sleep. Likewise, under a negative thermal load,

Table 1. Thermoregulatory responses during wakefulness and sleep.

Responses		Wakefulness	NREM Sleep	REM Sleep
Specific				
	Behavioral	Locomotion		
		Posture	Posture	
	Autonomic	Vasomotion	Vasomotion	
		Piloerection	Piloerection	
		Shivering thermogenesis	Shivering thermogenesis	
		Non-shivering thermogenesis	Non-shivering thermogenesis	Non-shivering thermogenesis $(-)$
		Thermal tachypnea	Thermal tachypnea	
		Sweating	Sweating $(+)$	Sweating $(o,-)$
Unspecific		Vigilance	Arousal	Arousal

shivering in the cat (Parmeggiani and Rabini, 1967) and armadillo (Affanni *et al.*, 1972; Prudom and Klemm, 1973; Van Twyver and Allison, 1974), heat exchanger vasoconstriction in the cat (Parmeggiani *et al.*, 1977), rabbit (Franzini *et al.*, 1982), and rat (Alföldi *et al.*, 1990) and piloerection in the cat (Hendricks *et al.*, 1977; Hendricks, 1982) are suppressed during the REM sleep episode. In addition, the cold-defence function of interscapular brown adipose tissue is altered in rats during REM sleep (Calasso *et al.*, 1993).

None of the vasomotion phenomena observed during REM sleep is consistent with the paradigm of homeothermy control since the autonomic regulation of vascular transmural pressure and smooth muscle tonus is altered in several vascular beds (Cianci *et al.*, 1991; Parmeggiani, 1994). This alteration particularly affects heat exchanger vessels showing the prevalence of transmural pressure over the decreased tonus of smooth muscle fibres in a cold environment and the prevalence of residual tonus of smooth muscle fibres over the decreased transmural pressure in a warm environment. Therefore, on the transition from NREM to REM sleep, thermoregulatory vasoconstriction is replaced by vasodilatation at low ambient temperature and thermoregulatory vasodilatation by vasoconstriction at high ambient temperature (Parmeggiani *et al.*, 1977; Franzini *et al.*, 1982). Such paradoxical vasomotion is absent on the transition from NREM to REM sleep only within an intermediate range of ambient temperatures. This indifferent range of ambient temperatures, which varies in different species, reveals the persistence across the two behavioural states of a passive equilibrium between vascular transmural pressure and wall tension, as a result of proportional changes in such variables. During REM sleep, skin vasomotion in human adults is in general not inconsistent with thermoregulation except for forehead skin vasodilatation at 21°C ambient temperature in naked humans (Palca *et al.*, 1986).

The thermoregulatory responses elicited by positive and negative thermal loads applied directly to the thermoreceptive preoptic–hypothalamic area are dependent on the behavioural state. In the cat, warming elicits tachypnea (Parmeggiani *et al.*, 1973, 1976) and heat exchanger vasodilatation (Parmeggiani *et al.*, 1977) during NREM sleep but has no such effects during REM sleep. Likewise, in the kangaroo rat (Glotzbach and Heller, 1976) and marmot (Florant *et al.*, 1978), cooling increases oxygen consumption and metabolic heat production during NREM sleep, whereas it is ineffective during REM sleep.

The previous data show that an effective antagonism develops between REM sleep processes and thermoregulation in the control of somatic and autonomic effector mechanisms. Such interaction is also shown at the level of preoptic–hypothalamic thermoresponsive neurones by the changes in their thermal characteristics across the ultradian sleep cycle (Parmeggiani *et al.*, 1983, 1986, 1987; Glotzbach and Heller, 1984; Alam *et al.*, 1995a,b; 1997, 2002; McGinty *et al.*, 2001). In particular, the increase and decrease in responsiveness of warm- and cold-responsive neurones, respectively, to direct thermal stimulation in NREM sleep is consistent with the down-regulation of body and brain temperatures. In contrast, the state-dependent changes in neuronal firing rate during REM sleep are associated with depression or suppression of thermal responsiveness in a large number of thermoresponsive neurones (Figure 2). In conclusion, sleep processes,

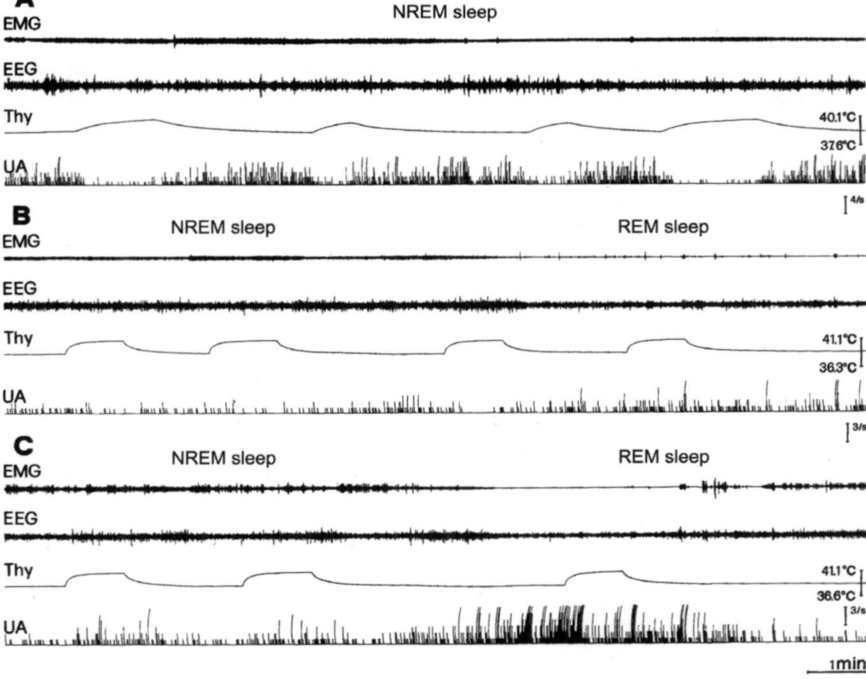

Figure 2. Responses of thermoresponsive neurones (UA) to preoptic–anterior hypothalamic (Thy) direct thermal stimulation during sleep. (A) A cold-responsive neurone is inhibited in relation to the duration and intensity of warming in NREM sleep. (B) A cold-responsive neurone is inhibited by warming in NREM sleep, whereas this effect disappears in REM sleep. (C) A warm-responsive neurone is excited by warming in NREM sleep, whereas this effect disappears in REM sleep as the result of state-dependent changes in neuronal firing. (Modified from Parmeggiani *et al.*, 1986.)

particularly in REM sleep, may completely override the specific activity of the preoptic–hypothalamic thermoreceptive network underlying thermoregulation. The result is that body temperature changes in REM sleep are positively correlated with ambient temperature, as expected in poikilothermic species (Parmeggiani *et al.*, 1971; Walker *et al.*, 1983). Table 1 summarises the thermoregulatory characteristics of the states of the ultradian wake–sleep cycle.

Influence of the Temperature Signal on Sleep Behaviour

The previous section of this chapter addressed the intrinsic thermoregulatory aspects of sleep behaviour. On this basis, it is now possible to approach the issue of the influence of the temperature signal, as both an endogenous and an exogenous stimulus, on the ultradian wake–sleep cycle.

The structure of the ultradian wake–sleep cycle at ambient temperature within thermoneutrality is conventionally considered the normal reference. Thermoneutrality, which varies in the different species (Altman and Dittmer, 1966), is defined as the range of ambient temperatures within which the metabolic rate decreases to the minimum at rest and temperature regulation is implemented by physical mechanisms alone. The amount of thermal load does not only depend on ambient temperature since other factors, like body size, thermal insulation, age, sexual cycle, feeding, season, humidity, etc., as well as differences in regional body sensitivity to temperature, consistently influence individual thermoregulatory responses. Acclimatisation to ambient temperatures beyond the limits of thermoneutrality induces shifts and/or modifications of the ambient temperature range well tolerated by the different species in terms of normal structure and duration of the ultradian wake–sleep cycle. The set of interacting variables, therefore, is complex from behavioural and physiological viewpoints. Figure 3 shows the influence of seasonal acclimatisation on the cumulative diurnal duration of wakefulness at different ambient temperatures.

Sleep time peaks around the upper limit of the ambient thermoneutrality range (Parmeggiani and Rabini, 1970; Schmidek *et al.*, 1972; Valatx *et al.*, 1973; Sakaguchi *et al.*, 1979; Obal *et al.*, 1983; Sichieri and Schmidek, 1984). Sleep time declines above and below such range but the rate of decline is larger above than below it. Deviations of ambient temperature from thermoneutrality not only increase the waking time but also modify the structure of sleep (Parmeggiani *et al.*, 1969; Parmeggiani and Rabini, 1970; Schmidek *et al.*, 1972; Sakaguchi *et al.*, 1979; Haskell *et al.*, 1981;

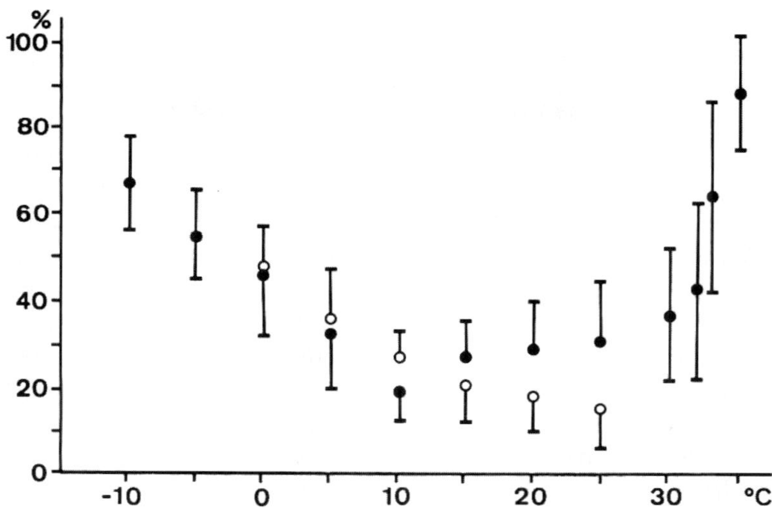

Figure 3. Relative duration (mean and SD) of wakefulness in the cat during the diurnal period (12 h) at different ambient temperatures. The filled and empty circles indicate autumn (November–December) and summer (June–July) experiments, respectively. Note that the minimal amount of wakefulness corresponds to an ambient temperature of 10°C in autumn and of 25°C in summer. (Parmeggiani, 1988.)

Sichieri and Schmidek, 1984; Sewitch *et al.*, 1986). In particular, NREM sleep and/or REM sleep may be selectively affected depending on the quality and intensity of the thermal load. Outside the thermoneutrality range in particular REM sleep is progressively depressed (Parmeggiani *et al.*, 1969, 1974; Parmeggiani and Rabini, 1970; Sakaguchi *et al.*, 1979; Szymusiak and Satinoff, 1981; Haskell *et al.*, 1981) and eventually suppressed until the accumulation of an increasing REM sleep debt produces a sufficient REM sleep pressure to overwhelm the thermoregulatory drive of the preoptic–hypothalamic thermostat (Parmeggiani *et al.*, 1969, 1974, 1980; Parmeggiani and Rabini, 1970; Parmeggiani, 1987; Zamboni *et al.*, 1997). In this case, brain stem effector mechanisms of REM sleep functionally escape from the normal preoptic–hypothalamic control and thermoregulatory responses are suppressed. Nevertheless, the organism is not endangered in REM sleep since the loss of the specific thermoregulatory effects of thermal stimuli is not associated with a loss of their non-specific arousing influence re-establishing full somatic and autonomic thermoregulatory functions (Table 1). Concerning the temporary suppression of REM sleep under negative thermal loads, two types of REM sleep episodes have been identified in rats: the "single episode," preceded and followed by a long interval without REM sleep, and the "sequential episode," occurring in clusters, namely in a sequence of REM sleep episodes separated by short intervals (Amici *et al.*, 1994). The "single episode" of REM sleep is less depressed by a negative thermal load than the "sequential episode" (Zamboni *et al.*, 1997). This result indicates the complexity of the interaction between thermoregulation and sleep even in a case of clear-cut antagonism. In addition, the importance of non-specific stress effects of ambient thermal loads ought to be considered concerning the changes in the structure of the ultradian wake–sleep cycle and particularly the decrease in REM sleep occurrence (Sakaguchi *et al.*, 1979; Haskell *et al.*, 1981; Szymusiak and Satinoff, 1981; Parmeggiani, 1987).

Experimentally induced changes in the preoptic–hypothalamic temperature affect the ultradian wake–sleep cycle. Cooling increases waking time (Sakaguchi *et al.*, 1979), and moderate warming promotes both NREM and REM sleep (Von Euler and Söderberg, 1957; Roberts and Robinson, 1969; Roberts *et al.*, 1969; Parmeggiani *et al.*, 1974, 1980; Sakaguchi *et al.*, 1979). Such effects depend on the specific thermoregulatory features of sleep behaviour. The thermoregulatory activity elicited by either ambient or preoptic–hypothalamic cooling is practically the opposite of the thermolytic adjustments induced by NREM sleep processes. In contrast, moderate ambient or preoptic–hypothalamic warming strengthens sleep promotion by inducing somatic effects, like muscle hypotonia and postural heat loss, and autonomic effects, like heat exchanger vasodilatation and sweating, that are synergistic with NREM sleep executive control on the same effector mechanisms (Figure 4). On the other hand, a balance between opposite ambient and preoptic–hypothalamic thermal loads influencing peripheral and central thermoreceptors, respectively, may be experimentally achieved so as to promote sleep. In particular, warming of the preoptic–hypothalamic region in a cold environment improves REM sleep onset and duration (Parmeggiani *et al.*, 1974, 1980; Sakaguchi *et al.*, 1979). The antagonistic interaction between warm- and cold-stimuli applied concomitantly at peripheral and central levels is also apparent in the activity of thermoresponsive-extrahypothalamic neurones during sleep (Cevolani and Parmeggiani, 1995). These results show how intimate the relation is between sleep processes and thermoregulation at high integration levels. In this respect, the changes in activity of preoptic–hypothalamic cold- and warm-responsive neurones across QW, NREM and REM sleep are also consistent with a direct involvement of

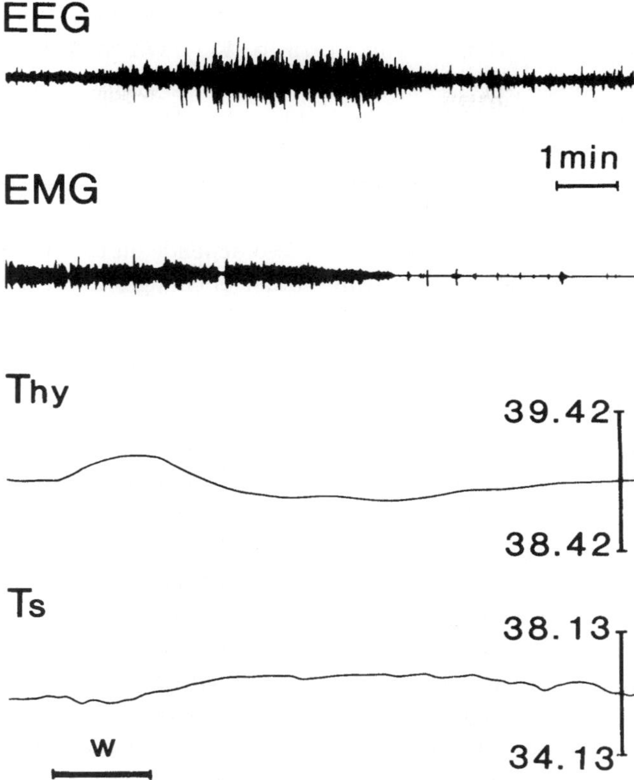

Figure 4. Sleep-promoting influence of preoptic–anterior hypothalamic (PO-AH) warming in the cat. The rise in PO-AH temperature (Thy) elicits an increase in ear pinna temperature (Ts), which is indicative of the central thermostat adjustment inducing heat loss. As a result, Thy decreases steeply after the end of warming (w) in concomitance with EEG synchronisation. A REM sleep episode ensues only when Thy reaches the lowest stable level in NREM sleep. Ambient temperature, 25°C. (Parmeggiani, 1987.)

such neurones in sleep regulation (Alam *et al.*, 1997; McGinty *et al.*, 2001; Szymusiak *et al.*, 2001). In particular, there are thermoresponsive neurones, also activated by peripheral thermoreceptors, which show increasing activity both at sleep onset and in response to increased core and/or skin temperatures. Such interactions at the level of preoptic–hypothalamic neurones may represent the neurophysiological basis for the sleep promoting influence of ambient or preoptic–hypothalamic moderate warming.

The decrease in sleep time without the thermoneutral range, characterised by a rate of change higher above than below it (cf. Figure 3), is inversely related to the rate of increase in energy expenditure for temperature regulation (Hensel *et al.*, 1973, p. 533). On the other hand, the correlation between body and brain weight and sleep cycle length is in general very high (Zepelin, 2000), when no exogenous factors (nutritional habit, ecological niche, predator–prey relationship) prevail over thermoregulation by affecting the survival conditions of the species. This suggests that the structure of the ultradian sleep cycle, particularly with regard to NREM sleep and REM sleep episode duration, also depends on the thermal inertia of the body which influences the time course of changes in the temperature signal affecting sleep processes.

Conclusion

The evidence that thermoregulatory and sleep processes interact antagonistically beyond ambient thermal neutrality points to the importance of behavioural thermoregulation for a normal development of the ultradian sleep cycle, that is the onset of an adequate presomnic behaviour in response to the ambient thermal load. As a result, the effective thermal load on the organism is reduced and maintained close to that of ambient thermoneutrality also in the presence of deviations of the actual ambient temperature signal from this range. At low energy cost, this behaviour protects the free occurrence of preoptic–hypothalamic temperature changes bound up with sleep processes. The passive defence of homeothermy during sleep is more effective the larger the thermal inertia of the body since the specific physiological changes of sleep can occur undisturbed by an imperative demand for autonomic temperature regulation. This demand would entail an increased energy expenditure in NREM sleep and an arousal in REM sleep to overcome the impairment of thermoregulation in this behavioural state. In conclusion, a successful constraint on energy expenditure for thermoregulation is a requisite for the normal development of the ultradian sleep cycle.

Acknowledgments

The author is indebted to his collaborators during many years of research. The studies carried out in the Institute of Physiology and later Department of Human and General Physiology of the University of Bologna were supported by grants of the Ministry of Education and the National Research Council of Italy.

References

Affanni, J.M., Lisogorsky, E., and Scaravilli, M. (1972). Sleep in the giant South American armadillo *Priodontes giganteus (Edentata, Mammalia)*. *Experientia*, 28: 1046–1047.

Alam, M.N., McGinty, D., and Szymusiak, R. (1995a). Neuronal discharge of preoptic/anterior hypothalamic thermosensitive neurons: relation to NREM sleep. *Am. J. Physiol.*, 269: R1240–R1249.

Alam, M.N., McGinty, D., and Szymusiak, R. (1995b). Preoptic/anterior hypothalamic neurons: thermosensitivity in rapid eye movement sleep. *Am. J. Physiol.*, 269: R1250–R1257.

Alam, M.N., McGinty, D., and Szymusiak R. (1997). Thermosensitive neurons of the diagonal band in rats: relation to wakefulness and non-rapid eye movement sleep. *Brain Res.*, 752: 81–89.

Alam, M.N., Gong, H., Alam, T., Jaganath, R., McGinty, D., and Szymusiak, R. (2002). Sleep-waking discharge patterns of neurons recorded in the rat perifornical lateral hypothalamic area. *J. Physiol.*, 538: 619–631.

Alföldi, P., Rubicsek, G., Cserni, G., and Obal, F., Jr. (1990). Brain and core temperatures and peripheral vasomotion during sleep and wakefulness at various ambient temperatures in the rat. *Pflügers Arch.*, 417: 336–341.

Altman, P.L. and Dittmer, D.S. (1966). *Environmental Biology*. Bethesda, MD: FASEB.

Amici, R., Zamboni, G., Perez, E., Jones, C.A., Toni, I., Culin, F., and Parmeggiani P.L. (1994). Pattern of desynchronized sleep during deprivation and recovery induced in the rat by changes in ambient temperature. *J. Sleep Res.*, 3: 250–256.

Azzaroni, A. and Parmeggiani, P.L. (1993). Mechanisms underlying hypothalamic temperature changes during sleep in mammals. *Brain Res.*, 632: 136–142.

Azzaroni, A. and Parmeggiani, P.L. (1995a). Postural and sympathetic influences on brain cooling during the ultradian wake–sleep cycle. *Brain Res.*, 671: 78–82.

Azzaroni, A. and Parmeggiani, P.L. (1995b). Synchronized sleep duration is related to tonic vasoconstriction of thermoregulatory heat exchangers. *J. Sleep Res.*, 4: 41–47.

Azzaroni, A. and Parmeggiani, P.L. (1999). Changes in selective brain cooling across the behavioral states of the ultradian wake–sleep cycle. *Brain Res.*, 844: 206–209.

Brebbia, D.R. and Altshuler, K.Z. (1965). Oxygen consumption rate and electroencephalographic stage of sleep. *Science*, 150: 1621–1623.

Calasso, M., Zantedeschi, E., and Parmeggiani, P.L. (1993). Cold-defense function of brown adipose tissue during sleep. *Am. J. Physiol.*, 265: R1060–R1064.

Cevolani, D. and Parmeggiani, P.L. (1995). Responses of extrahypothalamic neurons to short temperature transients during the ultradian wake–sleep cycle. *Brain Res. Bull.*, 37: 227–232.

Cianci, T., Zoccoli, G., Lenzi, P., and Franzini, C. (1991). Loss of integrative control of peripheral circulation during desynchronized sleep. *Am. J. Physiol.*, 261: R373–R377.

Dewasmes, G., Bothorel, B., Candas, V., and Libert, J.P. (1997). A short-term poikilothermic period occurs just after paradoxical sleep onset in humans: characterization changes in sweating effector activity. *J. Sleep Res.*, 6: 252–258.

Florant, G.L., Turner, B.M., and Heller, H.C. (1978). Temperature regulation during wakefulness, sleep, and hibernation in marmots. *Am. J. Physiol.*, 235: R82–R88.

Franzini, C., Cianci, T., Lenzi, P., and Guidalotti, P.L. (1982). Neural control of vasomotion in rabbit ear is impaired during desynchronized sleep. *Am. J. Physiol.*, 243: R142–R146.

Glotzbach, S.F. and Heller, H.C. (1976). Central nervous regulation of body temperature during sleep. *Science*, 194: 537–539.

Glotzbach, S.F. and Heller, H.C. (1984). Changes in the thermal characteristics of hypothalamic neurons during sleep and wakefulness. *Brain Res.*, 309: 17–26.

Glotzbach, S.F. and Heller, H.C. (2000). Temperature regulation. In: Kryger, M.H., Roth, T., and Dement, W.C. (Eds.). *Principles and Practice of Sleep Medicine.* Philadelphia: Saunders, pp. 289–304.

Haskell, E.H., Palca, J.W., Walker, J.M., Berger, R.J., and Heller, H.C. (1981). Metabolism and thermoregulation during stages of sleep in humans exposed to heat and cold. *J. Appl. Physiol.*, 51: 948–954.

Hayward, J.N. and Baker, M.A. (1969). A comparative study of the role of the cerebral arterial blood in the regulation of brain temperature in five mammals. *Brain Res.*, 16: 417–440.

Henane, R., Buguet, A., Roussel, B., and Bittel J. (1977). Variations in evaporation and body temperatures during sleep in man. *J. Appl. Physiol.*, 42: 50–55.

Hendricks, J.C. (1982). Absence of shivering in the cat during paradoxical sleep without atonia. *Exp. Neurol.*, 75: 700–710.

Hendricks, J.C., Bowker, R.M., and Morrison, A.R. (1977). Functional characteristics of cats with pontine lesions during sleep and wakefulness and their usefulness for sleep research. In: Koella, W.P. and Levin, P. (Eds.). *Sleep 1976.* Basel: Karger, pp. 6–10.

Hensel, H., Brück, K., and Raths, P. (1973). Homeothermic organisms. In: Precht, H., Christophersen, J., Hensel, H., and Larcher, W. (Eds.). *Temperature and Life.* Berlin: Springer Verlag, pp. 503–761.

Kräuchi, K., Cajochen, C., and Wirz-Justice, A. (1997). A relationship between heat loss and sleepiness: effects of postural change and melatonin administration. *J. Appl. Physiol.*, 83: 134–139.

Kräuchi, K., Cajochen, C., Werth, E., and Wirz-Justice, A. (1999). Warm feet promote the rapid onset of sleep. *Nature*, 401: 36–37.

Kräuchi, K., Cajochen, C., Werth, E., and Wirz-Justice, A. (2000). Functional link between distal vasodilation and sleep-onset latency. *Am. J. Physiol.*, 278: R741–R748.

McGinty, D., Alam, M.N., Szymusiak, R., Nakao, M., and Yamamoto, M. (2001). Hypothalamic sleep-promoting mechanisms: coupling to thermoregulation. *Arch. Ital. Biol.*, 139: 63–65.

Noll, G., Elam, M., Kunimoto, M., Karlsson, T., and Wallin, B.G. (1994). Skin sympathetic nerve activity and effector function during sleep in humans. *Acta Physiol. Scand.*, 151: 319–329.

Obal, F., Jr., Tobler, I., and Borbely, A. (1983). Effect of ambient temperature on the 24-hour sleep–wake cycle in normal and capsaicin-treated rats. *Physiol. Behav.*, 30: 425–430.

Palca, J.W., Walker, J.M., and Berger, R.J. (1986). Thermoregulation, metabolism, and stages of sleep in cold-exposed men. *J. Appl. Physiol.*, 61: 940–947.

Parmeggiani, P.L. (1968). Telencephalo-diencephalic aspects of sleep mechanisms. *Brain Res.*, 7: 350–359.

Parmeggiani, P.L. (1980). Temperature regulation during sleep: a study in homeostasis. In: Orem, J. and Barnes, C.D. (Eds.). *Physiology in Sleep. Research Topics in Physiology.* New York: Academic Press, pp. 97–143.

Parmeggiani, P.L. (1987). Interaction between sleep and thermoregulation: an aspect of the control of behavioral states. *Sleep*, 10: 426–435.

Parmeggiani, P.L. (1988). Physiological basis of the interaction between thermoregulation and vigilance. In: Leonard, J.P. (Ed.). *Vigilance: Methods, Models and Regulation.* Frankfurt am Main: Peter Lang, pp. 201–208.

Parmeggiani, P.L. (1994). The autonomic nervous system in sleep. In: Kryger, M.H., Roth, T., and Dement, W.C. (Eds.). *Principles and Practice of Sleep Medicine.* Philadelphia: Saunders, pp. 194–203.

Parmeggiani, P.L. (2003). Thermoregulation and sleep. *Front. Biosci.*, 8: s557–s567.

Parmeggiani, P.L. and Rabini, C. (1967). Shivering and panting during sleep. *Brain Res.*, 6: 789–791.

Parmeggiani, P.L. and Rabini, C. (1970). Sleep and environmental temperature. *Arch. Ital. Biol.*, 108: 369–387.

Parmeggiani, P.L., Rabini, C., and Cattalani, M. (1969). Sleep phases at low environmental temperature. *Arch. Sci. Biol. (Bologna)*, 53: 277–290.

Parmeggiani, P.L., Franzini, C., Lenzi, P., and Cianci, T. (1971). Inguinal subcutaneous temperature changes in cats sleeping at different environmental temperatures. *Brain Res.*, 33: 397–404.

Parmeggiani, P.L., Franzini, C., Lenzi, P., and Zamboni, G. (1973). Threshold of respiratory responses to preoptic heating during sleep in freely moving cats. *Brain Res.*, 52: 189–201.

Parmeggiani, P.L., Zamboni, G., Cianci, T., Agnati, L.F., and Ricci, C. (1974). Influence of anterior hypothalamic heating on the duration of fast-wave sleep episodes. *Electroencephalogr. Clin. Neurophysiol.*, 36: 465–470.

Parmeggiani, P.L., Agnati, L.F., Zamboni, G., and Cianci, T. (1975). Hypothalamic temperature during the sleep cycle at different ambient temperatures. *Electroencephalogr. Clin. Neurophysiol.*, 38: 589–596.

Parmeggiani, P.L., Franzini, C., and Lenzi, P. (1976). Respiratory frequency as a function of preoptic temperature during sleep. *Brain Res.*, 111: 253–260.

Parmeggiani, P.L., Zamboni, G., Cianci, T., and Calasso, M. (1977). Absence of thermoregulatory vasomotor responses during fast wave sleep in cats. *Electroencephalogr. Clin. Neurophysiol.*, 42: 372–380.

Parmeggiani, P.L., Cianci, T., Calasso, M., Zamboni, G., and Perez, E. (1980). Quantitative analysis of short term deprivation and recovery of desynchronized sleep in cats. *Electroencephalogr. Clin. Neurophysiol.*, 50: 293–302.

Parmeggiani, P.L., Azzaroni, A., Cevolani, D., and Ferrari, G. (1983). Responses of anterior hypothalamic–preoptic neurons to direct thermal stimulation during wakefulness and sleep. *Brain Res.*, 269: 382–385.

Parmeggiani, P.L., Azzaroni, A., Cevolani, D., and Ferrari, G. (1986). Polygraphic study of anterior hypothalamic–preoptic neuron thermosensitivity during sleep. *Electroencephalogr. Clin. Neurophysiol.*, 63: 289–295.

Parmeggiani, P.L., Cevolani, D., Azzaroni, A., and Ferrari, G. (1987). Thermosensitivity of anterior hypothalamic–preoptic neurons during the waking–sleeping cycle: a study in brain functional states. *Brain Res.*, 415: 79–89.

Parmeggiani, P.L., Azzaroni, A., and Calasso, M. (1998). A pontine-hypothalamic temperature difference correlated with cutaneous and respiratory heat loss. *Respir. Physiol.*, 114: 49–56.

Parmeggiani, P.L., Azzaroni, A., and Calasso, M. (2000). Behavioral state-dependent thermal feedback influencing the hypothalamic thermostat. *Arch. Ital. Biol.*, 138: 277–283.

Prudom, A.E. and Klemm, W.R. (1973). Electrographic correlates of sleep behavior in a primitive mammal, the armadillo *Dasypus novemcinctus. Physiol. Behav.*, 10, 275–282.

Roberts, W.W. and Robinson, T.C.L. (1969). Relaxation and sleep induced by warming of the preoptic region and anterior hypothalalmus in cats. *Exp. Neurol.*, 25: 282–294.

Roberts, W.W., Bergquist, E.H., and Robinson, T.C.L. (1969). Thermoregulatory grooming and sleep-like relaxation induced by local warming of preoptic area and anterior hypothalamus in opossum. *J. Comp. Physiol. Psychol.*, 67: 182–188.

Sagot, J.C., Amoros, C., Candas, V., and Libert, J.P. (1987). Sweating responses and body temperatures during nocturnal sleep in humans. *Am. J. Physiol.*, 252: R462–R470.

Sakaguchi, S., Glotzbach, S.F., and Heller, H.C. (1979). Influence of hypothalamic and ambient temperatures on sleep in kangaroo rats. *Am. J. Physiol.*, 294: R80–R88.

Satinoff, E. (1978). Neural organization and evolution of thermal regulation in mammals. *Science*, 201: 16–22.

Schmidek, W.R., Hoshino, K., Schmidek, M., and Timo-Iaria, C. (1972). Influence of environmental temperature on the sleep-wakefulness cycle in the rat. *Physiol. Behav.*, 8: 363–371.

Sewitch, D.E., Kittrell, E.M.W., Kupfer, D.J., and Reynolds, C.F., III. (1986). Body temperature and sleep architecture in response to a mild cold stress in women. *Physiol. Behav.*, 36: 951–957.

Shapiro, C.M., Moore, A.T., Mitchell, D., and Yodaiken, M.L. (1974). How well does man thermoregulate during sleep? *Experientia*, 30: 1279–1281.

Sichieri, R. and Schmidek, W.R. (1984). Influence of ambient temperature on the sleep-wakefulness cycle in the golden hamster. *Physiol. Behav.*, 33: 871–877.

Szymusiak, R. and Satinoff, E. (1981). Maximal REM sleep time defines a narrower thermoneutral zone than does minimal metabolic rate. *Physiol. Behav.*, 26: 687–690.

Szymusiak, R., Steiniger, T., Alam, M.N., and McGinty, D. (2001). Preoptic area sleep-regulating mechanisms. *Arch. Ital. Biol.*, 139: 77–92.

Valatx, J.L., Roussel, B., and Curé, M. (1973). Sommeil et température cérébrale du rat au cours de l'exposition chronique en ambiance chaude. *Brain Res.*, 55: 107–122.

Van Someren, E.J.W. (2000). More than a marker: interaction between the circadian regulation of temperature and sleep, age-related changes, and treatment possibilities. *Chronobiol. Int.*, 17: 313–354.

Van Twyver, H. and Allison, T. (1974). Sleep in the armadillo *Dasypus novemcinctus* at moderate and low ambient temperatures. *Brain Behav. Evol.*, 9: 107–120.

Von Euler, C. (1964). The gain of the hypothalamic temperature regulating mechanisms. In: Bargman, W. and Schadé, J.P. (Eds.). *Lectures on the Diencephalon*. Amsterdam: Elsevier, pp. 127–131.

Von Euler, C. and Söderberg, U. (1957). The influence of hypothalamic thermoceptive structures on the electroencephalogram and gamma motor activity. *Electroencephalogr. Clin. Neurophysiol.*, 42: 112–129.

Walker, J.M., Walker, L.E., Harris, D.V., and Berger R.J. (1983). Cessation of thermoregulation during REM sleep in the pocket mouse. *Am. J. Physiol.*, 244: R114–R118.

Webb, P. and Hiestand, M. (1975). Sleep metabolism and age. *J. Appl. Physiol.*, 38: 257–262.

Zamboni, G., Perez, E., and Amici, R. (1997). Biochemical approach to the wake–sleep cycle. In: Lugaresi, E. and Parmeggiani, P.L. (Eds.). *Somatic and Autonomic Regulation of Sleep*. Berlin: Springer, pp. 3–24.

Zepelin, H. (2000). Mammalian sleep. In: Kryger, M.H., Roth, T., and Dement, W.C. (Eds.). *Principles and Practice of Sleep Medicine*. Philadelphia: Saunders, pp. 82–92.

Chapter 19

THERMOREGULATION AND SLEEP IN THE HUMAN

Jean-Pierre Libert[1] and Véronique Bach

Numerous studies have shown that sleep is disturbed as soon as the ambient thermal conditions deviate from thermoneutrality, i.e., as soon as the thermoregulatory mechanisms that maintain homeothermy are activated by thermal loads. Thermoneutrality is defined as the range of air temperatures within which the metabolic rate decreases to a minimum where body temperature is mainly regulated by changing peripheral skin blood flow and behavioural responses. Above the thermoneutral zone, the body temperature rises slightly and sweating starts combating a further increase in body temperature. Below the thermoneutral zone, the body temperature falls slightly. Heat production as evidenced by oxygen consumption is increased through shivering in adults and non-shivering mechanims in neonates, and the body temperature reaches a new steady state.

The magnitude of the thermal load depends not only on air temperature, mean radiant temperature, air humidity, and velocity but also on the thermal insulation provided by clothing. Various other factors can also induce consistent shifts of several degrees in the thermoneutral temperature. For example, adaptation to ambient temperature modifies the thermal responses and the sleep debt. The limits of the thermoneutral zone are also sleep stage dependent and may fluctuate during the night. Thus,

---

[1]jean-pierre.libert@u-picardie.fr

pronounced sweating responses are observed in sleep stages 3 and 4 (slow wave sleep, SWS) whereas lower responses are seen in other sleep stages or in waking (Muzet and Libert, 1985). As a result, thermoneutrality is difficult to determine in sleeping adults.

The same difficulty holds for human neonates, determining the ambient temperature level at which neonates should be nursed is a complex problem in clinicial routine — thermoneutrality is known to decrease the risks for morbidity and mortality while body weight gain is optimal. Indeed, although neonates are homeotherms, the efficiency of their thermoregulatory processes is limited, whereas their body heat exchanges with the environment are greater. The high skin permeability of premature neonates enhances evaporative water loss while the high value of their skin surface area to body volume ratio increases heat losses to the environment. Therefore, neonates can rapidly become hypothermic, especially for preterm and low-birth-weight babies who therefore need more additional heat to maintain homeothermy. As a result, the lower limit of the thermoneutral zone may be as high as 35°C in small premature neonates (1000 g) and may change with postnatal development as body size increases. Moreover, during ontogenesis, there are strong inter-individual differences in the thermoregulatory responses to thermal loads: neonates of similar body size and mass exposed to similar air temperature can equilibrate at very different body temperatures (Telliez *et al.*, 1997). Owing to the multiplicity of factors reported above, it is very difficult to define a range of temperatures over which metabolic heat production and evaporative water loss are minimised (Azaz *et al.*, 1992). Other factors (such as thermal insulation, feeding, and local differences in skin sensitivity to air temperature variations) should also be taken into account. As a result, the high observed inter-study and inter-laboratory variations in sleep disturbances could be partly related to non-controlled differences in these various interacting variables.

Indeed, thermal challenges do influence sleep. For example, when the human adult is exposed to cold or heat, total sleep time diminishes, whereas the sleep onset latency increases and intra-sleep awakenings become more frequent. Rapid eye movement (REM, paradoxical sleep) sleep is particularly affected. The origin of these changes (which have been observed in all mammals studied to date) may result from a "clash" between thermoregulatory and hypnic processes. The neurophysiological basis of this conflict is not really known, and has been tackled using thermal regulatory models built on a variety of hypotheses — mainly those founded on animal data. The present review describes these models and presents the inter-species differences that prevent the formulation of a common model of thermoregulation capable of explaining the antagonistic interaction between sleep and thermoregulatory processes.

Thermal Effects on Sleep in the Adult

Influence of thermal loads on sleep

The effects on sleep of nocturnal, acute exposure to thermal loads were extensively studied in adults in the 1970s and 1980s but recent studies are lacking.

Sleep continuity parameters (reduced sleep efficiency, increased fragmentation) are particularly altered by ambient conditions (Figure 1).

High air temperatures increase the number and duration of awakenings after sleep onset (Kendel and Schmidt-Kessen, 1973). Using a blanket heated by a circulating fluid at a temperature of 49°C (producing a microclimate air temperature of 39°C inside the bed), Karacan *et al.* (1978) reported that the total sleep time decreased. Hénane *et al.* (1977) found that increasing air temperature to 35–39°C did not greatly change sleep structure (and in particular the progression and periodicity of the sleep stages), whereas awakening periods increased. In naked subjects, Okamoto-Mizuno *et al.* (1999) showed that humid heat exposure increased wakefulness and suppressed the intra-night decrease in rectal temperature. This can be explained by a high level of air humidity, which reduces evaporative skin cooling and increases heat storage by the body. Warm conditions increased the frequency of transient activation phases during SWS

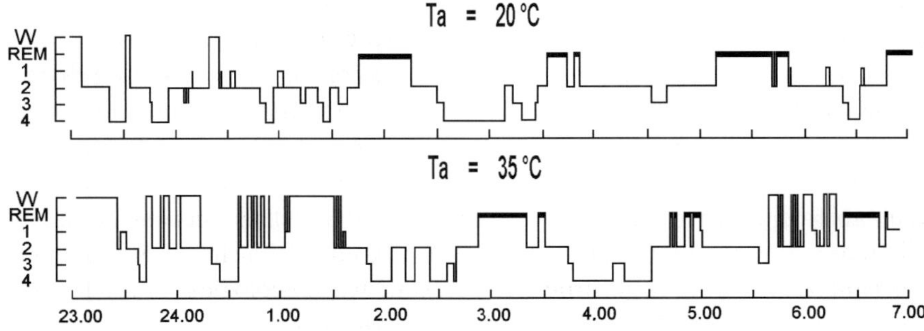

Figure 1. Hypnograms of one adult sleeping at 20°C or at 35°C of air temperature (unpublished data).

(Libert *et al.*, 1991). The activation phases described by Schieber *et al.* (1971) (characterised by concomitant and reversible modifications of electrophysiological data) were mostly accompanied by body movements, and thus reflected sleep pattern fragmentation.

Very few studies have been performed in acute cold environments. Buguet *et al.* (1979) pointed out that in subjects sleeping in tents in the Arctic winter, sleep was shortened and frequently interrupted by awakenings and body movements. Comparing the influence of high (34–37°C) and low (21°C) ambient temperatures on sleep, Haskell *et al.* (1981) pointed out that the durations of wakefulness and stage 1 sleep increased in cold exposure whereas that of stage 2 sleep decreased. They concluded that cold was more disruptive to sleep than heat.

Comparing five experimental conditions (room temperatures of 13, 16, 19, 22, and 25°C) with subjects clothed with a pyjama and covered with two cotton sheets and a woollen blanket, Muzet *et al.* (1979) reported that sleeping at 13°C induced more awakenings, whereas the lowest number and duration of awakenings after sleep onset was observed at an air temperature of 16°C: the latter thus appeared to be the most appropriate environment for the thermal comfort of a covered, sleeping adult. However, these authors pointed out that sleep disturbances were relatively small, since the air temperature inside the bed was nearly constant (26.1–30.9°C) and varied little with the actual air temperature in the room. The authors put forward the hypothesis that a sleeping human might build a microclimate inside the bed, by heat dissipation from the body to the air trapped between the skin surface area and the covering. This explanation was confirmed by the fact that the subjects who showed a large fall in rectal temperature slept in a hotter bed microclimate than those showing a smaller decrease. This emphasises that in sleeping, covered subjects, sleep disturbances should be discussed in terms of bed microclimate instead of room temperature.

As far as adult sleep architecture is concerned, the occurrence and rhythmicity of REM sleep are usually affected by ambient conditions, although this has not been reported in all cases (Kendel and Schmidt-Kessen, 1973; Hénane *et al.*, 1977; Muzet *et al.*, 1983; Libert *et al.*, 1988). Exposure to a high air temperature decreased the number of REM sleep episodes, whereas the mean duration and the mean length of REM sleep-intervals remained unchanged (Karacan *et al.*, 1978). In cold and warm exposures, Haskell *et al.* (1978, 1981) reported that the first REM sleep episode was delayed until later in the night but that the mean duration of the interval between two successive REM sleep episodes did not change. These modifications were more pronounced under cold stress. Thermal loads that activate thermoregulatory processes selectively depressed REM sleep by blocking its appearance in the first part of the night. These authors also found that REM sleep was depressed to a greater extent by low than by high air temperatures.

As a result, it is generally observed that the amount of REM sleep reaches a maximum in the thermoneutral zone, when compared to cold or hot conditions. In contrast to studies performed at high air temperatures, Muzet *et al.* (1983) reported that in environments near the thermoneutral zone, REM sleep latency and REM period duration did not change from one condition to another: only the average REM cycle length decreased when the ambient temperature increased from 13 to 19°C. These authors suggested that the mechanisms underlying REM rhythmicity are separate from those responsible for REM maintenance.

External heat load variations greatly affect the sleep stages (Candas *et al.*, 1982; Libert *et al.*, 1982). This is especially observed during REM sleep, since thermal transients (0.8–$1.6°C\,min^{-1}$) lead to interruption of the sleep episodes more often in REM sleep (about 70%) than in SWS sleep (about 40%). REM interruption always consists of awakenings, whereas SWS interruption lightens sleep by favouring sleep stages 1 and 2. Decreasing thermal transients are more disturbing than increasing ones. These alterations are not observed with less pronounced transient rates of temperature change ($0.02°C\,min^{-1}$; Dewasmes *et al.*, 1996). This suggests that REM sleep is more subject to thermal variations than SWS.

Several studies have investigated the effects of pre-sleep thermal exposures on sleep. After heat stress in a sauna, SWS increases during the first 2 h of sleep (Putkonen *et al.*, 1973). Immersion in a hot bath (Horne and Reid, 1985) increases SWS and reduces REM sleep durations. Similar findings were reported by Shapiro *et al.* (1989) for subjects exposed daily for 4 h to air temperatures of 35 or 45°C, as long as the thermal load ended 1.5 h before sleep onset. Bunnell *et al.* (1988) pointed out that heating the body late in the evening increased SWS during the first sleep cycle and decreased the first period of REM sleep. In contrast, early evening heating facilitated the subject's ability to fall asleep. Horne (1981) thus assumed that SWS was regulated by a waking factor that could be related to the cerebral metabolic rate and to serotoninergic activity (which increases with heat exposure).

In contrast to the range of studies performed in acute thermal environments, little attention has been paid to humans exposed to prolonged thermal loads. During 17 consecutive Arctic winter nights, Buguet *et al.* (1976) did not find large sleep disturbances during cold exposure of subjects in sleeping bags. A similar observation has been reported by Palca *et al.* (1986) for naked subjects exposed to five consecutive nights at 21°C: cold exposure increased wakefulness and decreased stage 2 sleep without any change in the other sleep stages.

In contrast, when looking at the effects of chronic exposure over five consecutive nights at an air temperature of 35°C preceded by a baseline period at 20°C, Libert *et al.* (1988) found that many sleep parameters (especially those concerning REM sleep) displayed alterations with heat exposure. The durations of REM sleep episodes and cycles were shortened. On return to thermoneutrality, a rebound effect was found for SWS, the duration of which increased above baseline values. In contrast, the REM sleep deprivation (8.3% below the baseline value) was not great enough to induce a cumulative REM sleep debt. This is in agreement with Parmeggiani and Rabini (1970), who, for cats exposed to cold, observed a recovery effect in REM sleep only when the debt fell below 30% of control values. Homeothermic adaptive mechanisms are not associated with a reduction of sleep disturbances in warm conditions (Libert *et al.*, 1988). Thermal adaptation reduces thermal strain without improving sleep quality. This suggests that the processes controlling thermal adaptation and sleep are dissociated.

Influence of sleep stages on thermoregulation

Except for the Tasmanian devil (Nicol and Maskrey, 1980) and the lamb in cold conditions (Fewell *et al.*, 1990), all the studies performed to date in sleeping mammals show that body temperature regulation is a discontinuous process. The control of body temperature is efficient and stable in synchronised sleep but is absent in desynchronised sleep. In contrast, thermal responses in the Tasmanian devil were impaired in cold conditions but persisted in warm ones, since thermal polypnea was observed in desynchronised sleep when the air temperature increased over 30°C. In lambs (with ages ranging between 10 and 24 days), decreasing the ambient temperature from 25 to 10°C increased the oxygen consumption by 25% in quiet sleep and 23% in active sleep. This result remains debatable, since Berger *et al.* (1989) did not find a similar increase of oxygen consumption during active sleep in 3- to 16-day-old lambs exposed to air temperatures of 10–15°C. Studies performed with cold-challenged cats have shown that shivering and increased metabolic heat production persisted during SWS but disappeared during REM sleep (Parmeggiani and Rabini, 1970). In the rabbit, Franzini *et al.* (1982) have equally demonstrated that the vaso-motor response observed in the course of REM sleep was ill-suited to the maintenance of homeothermy: in response to cold exposure, blood flow was redirected from the muscles towards cutaneous areas where body heat was lost, whereas in response to heat, the blood irrigating the skin was redirected towards splanchnic sites, thus limiting heat loss to the environment. In the absence of effective regulation, the organism's internal temperature passively follows fluctuations of the ambient temperature: REM sleep can thus be considered as a poikilothermic state where the conflict between thermoregulatory and hypnic mechanisms reaches its apogee.

According to Parmeggiani (1987), the alternation between SWS and REM sleep is subject to the body's homeothermy management, thus protecting it against hypo- or hyperthermia.

Data obtained from animal experiments cannot, however, be simply extrapolated to humans. Our thermoregulatory responses only show certain similarities with those observed in animals. In sleeping adults exposed to heat, Lenzi *et al.* (1990) reported that the mean body temperature calculated from mean skin and oesophageal temperatures was significantly correlated with air temperature during REM sleep, whereas no correlation was found during SWS. This positive correlation indicates that mean body temperature passively drifts under the effect of the thermal load during REM sleep. This was also reported by Hashizume (1997), who suggested that rectal and tympanic temperatures were influenced by air temperatures in hot exposure, since rectal and tympanic temperatures increased during the last part of the night (during which REM sleep is predominant). On this basis, the animal paradigm could be applied to humans, since REM sleep and thermoregulation negatively interact with each other. However, in humans faced with a cold or a heat challenge, thermoregulation is not abolished but is merely depressed. During exposure to cold, humans vasoconstrict in REM sleep, thus decreasing body cooling (Buguet *et al.*, 1979). Work by Haskell *et al.* (1981) showed that metabolic heat production in naked adults was greater at an air temperature of 21°C than at 34 or 37°C. They reported that this increase in oxygen consumption could not be attributed to a behavioural component but rather to an activation of non-shivering thermogenesis. Shapiro *et al.* (1974) pointed out that evaporation was depressed during REM sleep periods, while the metabolic heat production increased.

After investigating the thermal balance in sleeping humans exposed to neutral and warm environments ranging from 32 to 39.5°C,

Hénane *et al.* (1977) emphasised that evaporative skin cooling decreased by 70% in REM sleep — explaining the observation that rectal temperature showed cyclical waves occurring rhythmically with REM periods. In hot conditions, our own work (Libert *et al.*, 1982) showed that when heat burden on the body was specifically loaded during REM sleep and SWS, the sweating reaction (recorded using a sweat-collection capsule stuck on the skin of the right pectoral region) persisted in REM sleep, albeit at a lower level than in SWS (Figure 2). Moreover, in REM sleep, thermoregulatory mechanisms were able to elicit a proportional response. However, the sweating onset time was longer in REM sleep than in SWS, and was observed at higher body temperatures — thus evidencing the lower reactivity of the thermoregulatory system during this sleep stage. When transient thermal loads were performed during SWS, sweating started in concomitance with

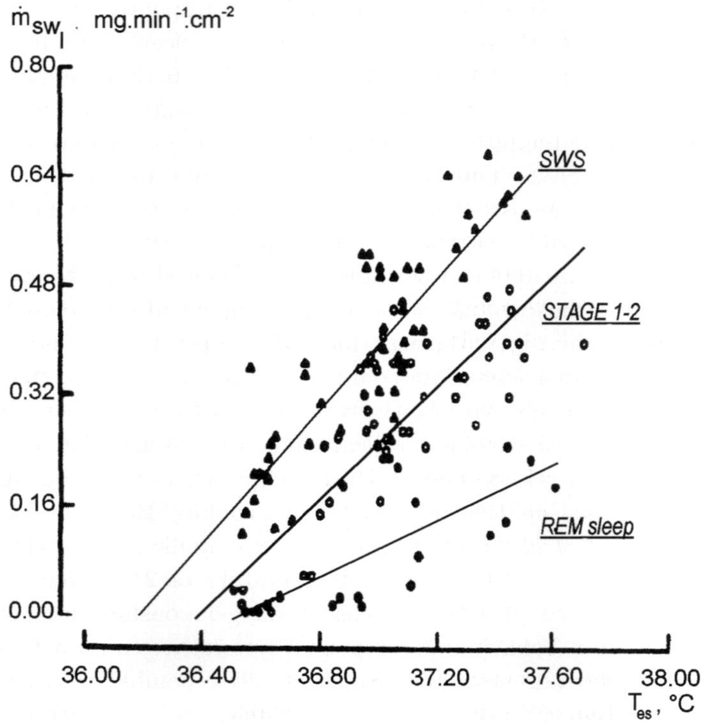

Figure 2. Relationship between local sweating rate (m_{sw}, $\mathrm{mg\,min^{-1}\,cm^{-2}}$) and esophageal temperature (T_{es}, °C) during slow wave sleep (SWS), sleep stage 2, and rapid eye movement (REM) sleep in adult humans (unpublished data).

an increased mean skin temperature and a decreased oesophageal temperature, showing the dominant role of peripheral thermal inputs as a determinant of sweating initiation in humans. During SWS, the sweat rate was particularly high and was greater than that observed during sleep stages 1 and 2. Thus, for a naked adult exposed to a near-thermoneutral environment, a sweating activity was only observed during SWS, which thus promotes body cooling. This heat-loss function linked to SWS may also explain the increase in the duration of this sleep stage seen when subjects are exposed to diurnal thermal charges. This augmentation may help to optimise body cooling by facilitating an initial fall in internal temperature during the first part of the night. This is reinforced by the fact that the increase in SWS is not observed when the body heating is prevented by cooling the subject with a fan (Horne and Staff, 1983).

Thus, several observations suggest that the impairment of thermoregulation in REM sleep is less dramatic in humans than in animals. However, for all these species, it appears that the only appropriate way to endure a heavy thermal load is to cut down REM sleep, since thermoregulatory responses are fully preserved in SWS and depressed or abolished in REM sleep. REM sleep interruptions during exposures to thermal loads can thus be interpreted as being an adaptive mechanism for the maintenance of body homeothermia, preventing body temperature deviations from normal values. In thermoneutral environments, the transition of SWS towards REM sleep is driven by the debt in this sleep stage, whereas under thermal loads, the need for homeothermia maintenance prevails over REM sleep debt.

The SWS–REM sleep alternation may thus be driven by thermal signals. When considering parts of consecutive 3 and 4 sleep stages in terms of whether or not they were followed by REM sleep, Lenzi *et al.* (1990) showed that during heat exposure, the duration of SWS was higher and the drop in mean body temperature was longer when REM sleep ensued. In a warm environment, the occurrence of REM sleep is thus favoured by a prior decrease in body temperature. Two hypotheses could explain this observation. The first refers to the fact that in order to avoid any risk of hypo- or hyperthermia during REM sleep, thermal signals provoke a change towards a state better suited to the maintenance of homeothermy (SWS or wakefulness). The second supposes that peripheral thermal information prevents the transition from SWS to REM sleep, by explaining that when faced with a thermal challenge, the frequency of occurrence of short-duration REM sleep episodes (i.e., abortive episodes) initially increases, rather than lower average episode lengths. The thermal fluctuations observed during SWS would appear to determine the distribution of the different sleep stages over the course of a night.

Thermal Effects on Sleep in the Neonate

In contrast to the data reported above, most studies of neonates are performed in cold environments: the likelihood of body cooling is present at birth and imposes extra metabolic energy requirements which endanger body weight gain and can even threaten the infant's very survival.

Specific aspects of sleep thermoregulation in the neonate

The preoptic anterior hypothalamic structure appears to play a key role in managing the interaction between sleep and thermoregulatory processes by integrating information from telencephalic sources and peripheral and internal thermosensors and sending signals to thermoregulatory effectors. The preoptic–hypothalamic region drives not only subordinate brainstem and spinal mechanisms controlling thermal responses (Satinoff, 1978) but also other autonomic functions, such as cardiorespiratory regulation. This structure might therefore be a comparator that measures the difference between a "set-point value" (for which the thermal response is nil) and the actual body temperature as measured by the thermosensors (error signal). The more the air temperature deviates from thermoneutrality, the stronger the thermal signals activating hypothalamic thermoregulatory structures. Modifications in hypothalamic sensitivity could be due to changes in the set-point value as a function of skin temperature variation or sleep state changes. Other results underline the importance of the gain of the thermoregulatory system: hypothalamic sensitivity could vary through a change in the gain (i.e., the slope value of the thermal response vs. body temperature relationship) rather than a shift in the set-point value's threshold. However, in contrast to adults, the role of internal temperature is thought to be of less importance in neonates (Mestyan *et al.*, 1964). Inhaled, cool air also induces a thermal response, indicating that cold thermoreceptors are present in the mucus membrane of the upper respiratory tract (Pribylova, 1971; San't Ambrogio and Widdicombe, 2001). Certain specific, thermoreceptive areas seem to play an important role in thermoregulation. Thus, facial cooling increases metabolic heat production in premature and full-term neonates.

The body temperature of the neonate shows more fluctuations than that of the adult, since the efficiency of the neonate's thermoregulatory processes are restricted and the body heat exchanges with the environment are larger. The likelihood of body cooling is thus augmented.

Sweating appears to be poorly developed in neonates born 3 weeks before term, whereas those born more than 8 weeks before term seem unable to sweat. In neonates born after a short gestation, limitation of the sweat function is due to immaturity of the sweat glands (Foster *et al.*, 1969; Nessmann and Baverel, 1972). Although the density of sweat glands per unit of surface area is greater in full-term neonates than in adults, their maximal response is only one-third of the latter (Foster *et al.*, 1969), thus reducing the capability to lose heat in warm conditions. In cold stress, metabolic heat production can increase through non-shivering thermogenesis in order to maintain a nearly constant body temperature. It was reported that the oxygen consumption recorded in cold exposure was $13\,\mathrm{ml\,min^{-1}\,kg^{-1}}$ when the neonate's rectal temperature was 34°C, i.e., double the resting rate. The largest value was $15.2\,\mathrm{ml\,min^{-1}\,kg^{-1}}$ for a neonate weighing 3800 g with a postnatal age of 2.5 h exposed to an ambient temperature of 15°C. These maximal metabolic values are comparable to those seen in adults exposed to extreme cold stress. The main component of this metabolic heat production is due to the oxidation of triglycerides in the brown adipose tissue, the lipolytic activity of which is controlled by the sympathetic nervous system. Moreover, low-birth-weight premature neonates are able to regulate heat production at a lower set-point level (Brück, 1968; Perlstein *et al.*, 1974). A set-point fall can explain the rapid adaptation to mild cold stress occurring over the first 3 days of life (Perlstein *et al.*, 1974). Similarly, the threshold temperature for sweating is probably not kept constant but there is only a little experimental evidence to suggest that it falls progressively with postnatal development (Sulyok, 1973). Vasomotor responses to ambient temperature changes vary regionally, and have been observed in premature as well as in full-term neonates. However, since the extent of tissue insulation and the difference between core and mean skin temperatures are lower in the neonate than in the adult, neonatal cold defence reactions are elicited at higher mean skin temperatures. The threshold for eliciting vasoconstriction and an increase in metabolic heat production is shifted to a higher level in the infant. Shivering (which is controlled by the somatomotor system) is seldom observed in neonates, and is never seen before non-shivering thermogenesis has reached its maximal level. The shivering threshold is displaced to a lower body temperature compared to the adult. There is evidence that the shivering process is developed at birth but is suppressed by non-shivering thermogenesis, which is the most important mechanism of heat production. The inhibition of shivering disappears progressively with advancing age and could occur via cervicospinal warmth receptors (Brück, 1992), probably as long as sufficient heat is provided by the brown adipose tissue.

In contrast to adults, it appears that a strong behavioural component linked to body movement is involved in the maintenance of homeothermy in neonates. In many species, behavioural thermoregulation precedes autonomic thermoregulation and is also elicited by peripheral and internal temperature changes integrated at the hypothalamic level (although the involvement of other subordinate structures at spinal level cannot be excluded). It seems that peripheral inputs are more important than internal ones in terms of eliciting a behavioural response — suggesting that the process activity is an anticipatory response to thermal stress and intervenes only when external, thermal loads are moderate. Similar observations have been reported in human adults by Franck *et al.* (1999), who demonstrated that mean skin temperature served to initiate behavioural thermoregulation responses before the autonomic ones. The behavioural response increases metabolic heat production through muscular activity but also modifies thermal insulation by changing the skin surface area exchanging heat with the environment. The exposed surface affects convective, radiative, conductive, and evaporative heat exchanges. For a reclining infant, Leblanc (1983), reported that the radiating surface area was 55.5% of total body surface area, whereas Bell and Rios (1983), published a figure of 50%. This value can be reduced by one-quarter in the case of a tight crouch. Using a manikin with movable joints, Wheldon (1982) reported that the body surface area exchanging radiant heat increased from 48% (foetal posture) to 76% (spread-eagle posture).

According to bioelectrical criteria, active sleep (AS) and quiet sleep (QS) in the neonate are often considered to be immature forms of adult REM sleep and SWS, respectively. As in SWS, QS is characterised by the absence of eye movements, while respiratory and heart rates are regular. AS (preponderant in the neonate) only partly corresponds to REM sleep, since there is no muscle atonia. Moreover, AS only precedes QS if there is no thermal stress — otherwise waking occurs instead (Bach *et al.*, 2001).

Influence of thermal load on sleep

As in the adult, warm exposure produces less disruption of sleep stages than cold exposure. The few studies performed in moderately hot environments did not reveal any disruption of sleep architecture (Brück *et al.*, 1962;

Bach *et al.*, 1994). This could be explained by the small body temperature increases (in the order of 0.2–0.3°C) induced by the thermal loads. However, sleep is less interrupted by body movements than at thermoneutrality (Bach *et al.*, 1994).

In a cold environment, the sleep onset latency and the number of intra-sleep awakenings and body movements increase (Azaz *et al.*, 1992), while total sleep time decreases (Bach *et al.*, 1994). Enhanced awakening is somewhat specific to older neonates, and can be related to the increase in body activity observed at this age (Azaz *et al.*, 1992). Indeed, body activity is an important component of the behavioural response to cold. Fleming *et al.* (1988) and Azaz *et al.* (1992) observed increases in small movements, which were more pronounced in 1- to 3-month-old babies (Azaz *et al.*, 1992), whatever the sleep stage. Other authors have reported increased body activity during AS only (Bach *et al.*, 1994).

QS duration is often reduced (or even totally suppressed) during cold exposure (Brück *et al.*, 1962; Fleming *et al.*, 1988; Azaz *et al.*, 1992; Telliez *et al.*, 1997, 1998; Bach *et al.*, 2000), whereas that of AS increases (Fleming *et al.*, 1988; Bach *et al.*, 1994). Preferential switching into AS is also found (Fleming *et al.*, 1988; Azaz *et al.*, 1992). The neonates who exhibited the greatest increase in oxygen consumption during QS following a thermoneutral to cool transition (+41%) did not switch into AS (Fleming *et al.*, 1988). These observations suggest that thermal signals do not serve to arouse the infant but rather facilitate the transition to AS. This agrees with the results of Sakaguchi *et al.* (1979) who showed that the sleep stage distribution of the kangaroo rat was partly determined by thermal inputs and particularly those elicited from peripheral temperature receptors. This needs to be confirmed in the human.

Only one study has dealt with the effect of continuous thermal load on sleep in neonates (Telliez *et al.*, 1998). As shown in Figure 3, as cool exposure progresses (75 h, 2°C below thermoneutrality), sleep disturbances persist (increased levels of AS at the expense of QS) or even increase (increasing percentage of wakefulness after sleep onset), although cold resistance is improved (heat production increases constantly from the beginning to the end of the acclimation period).

Influence of sleep states on autonomic thermoregulation

Active sleep and QS are also characterised by basic differences in autonomic activity. Thermal studies performed on neonates reveal a wide range of

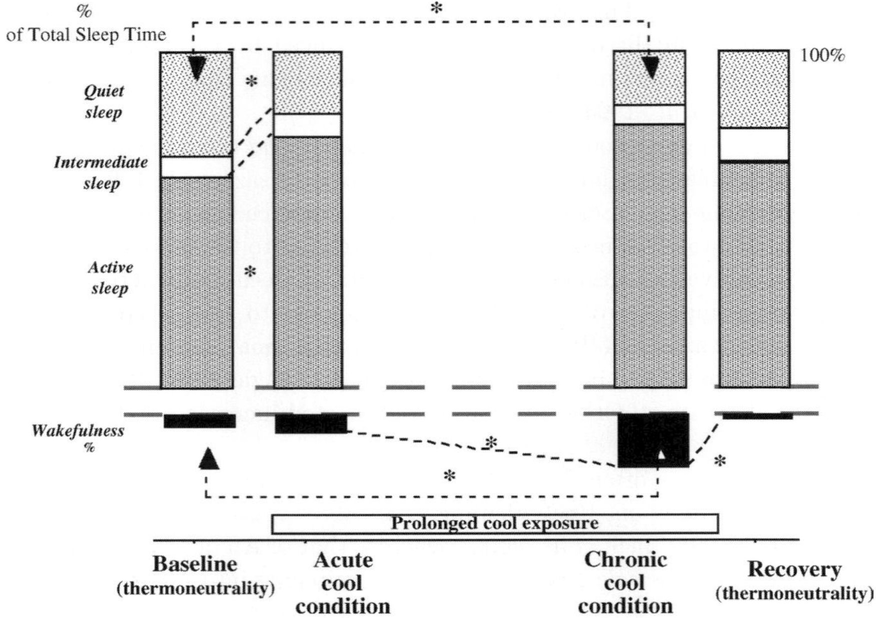

Figure 3. Wakefulness and sleep stage relative durations during thermoneutral, acute, and chronic cool condition (75 h, 2°C below thermoneutrality) measured on preterm neonates.*: Significant difference. (From Telliez, F. *et al.*, *Neurosci. Lett.*, 1998, 245: 25–28, modified.)

differences compared to the situation in the adult. Active sleep is a state that is particularly suited to the maintenance of homeothermy.

Since, in practice, neonates are more often subjected to cold than to heat stress, very few studies involving a heat challenge have been reported. A very dated publication (Day, 1941) on children aged from 5 months to 4 years found that the sweat rate at sleep onset was higher than during wakefulness. Unfortunately, this work did not include a sleep stage analysis. Only one study (Bach *et al.*, 1994) has dealt with this subject: it showed that sweating activity (measured in the trunk area using a sweat-collection capsule) did not differ between the various sleep stages. During AS, Bach *et al.* showed that there was a positive relationship between sweating rate and oesophageal temperature.

In cold conditions, the duration of AS increases, metabolic heat production rises proportionately with the fall in internal temperature, and intense peripheral vasoconstriction is observed. The metabolic response to cooling varies widely between neonates but is always higher in AS than in QS (Darnal and Ariagno, 1982; Stothers and Warner, 1984; Dane *et al.*, 1985; Azaz *et al.*, 1992). Thermogenesis is elicited through the brown adipose tissue, which is an important cold-defence process in the neonate. Mestyan *et al.* (1964) assumed that the rise in oxygen consumption followed a decrease in mean skin temperature, suggesting that closed-loop regulation operates during this sleep stage. Compared to QS, this more intense energy metabolism may be explained by a change in the thermoregulatory central controller's set-point value (rather than its gain). The maintenance of efficient thermal responses in these two sleep stages (especially in AS, episodes of which can last up to 1 h) protects the neonate from long periods of poikilothermy (Darnal and Ariagno, 1982).

Influence of sleep on behavioural responses

By using sedative drugs, Hey (1969) observed that the increase in heat production in neonates exposed to cold conditions was reduced when compared with controls — highlighting a behavioural component in the thermoregulatory response to cold exposure.

Most studies report that body activity increases during cool exposure, either in all sleep stages (Fleming *et al.*, 1988; Azaz *et al.*, 1992) or during AS only (Bach *et al.*, 1994): these observations show that there is no central inhibitory influence on muscles during this sleep stage.

In the same study (Bach *et al.*, 1994), the authors reported that from one individual to another, the thermal response to cold during AS could be either an increase in non-shivering thermogenesis (i.e., a negative relationship between heat production and body temperature) or a preferential increase in the frequency of body movements (i.e., increased thermogenesis through muscular activity; Figure 4). This latter response was described by a positive relationship between heat production and internal temperature. The decrease in mean skin temperature was a determinant factor in controlling an increase in body mobility. Sleep mechanisms must receive information from peripheral thermoreceptors which potentiate thermal stress and serve to elicit behavioural, thermoregulatory responses, suggesting that this behavioural response participates in the maintenance of homeothermia. The process spares brown adipose tissue and could reflect a thermoregulatory mechanism for neonates with a deficit of this tissue.

Another aspect of the behavioural response involves the body position. In cool environments, the neonate adopts a crouched position, thus reducing

                    J.-P. Libert and V. Bach

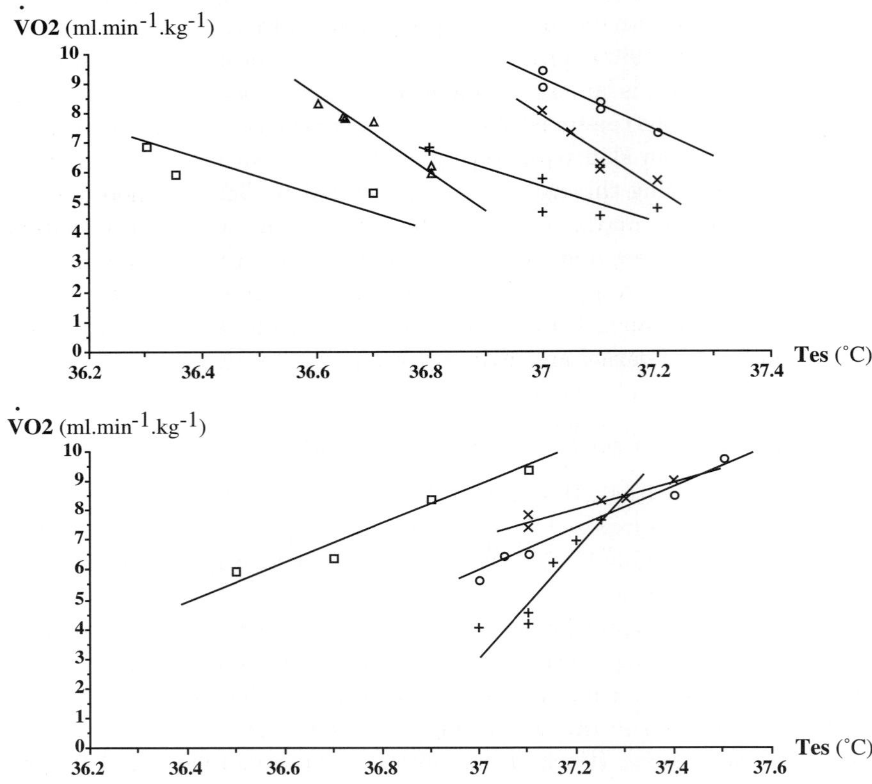

Figure 4. Individual relationships between oxygen consumption (V_{O2}, $ml\,min^{-1}\,kg^{-1}$) and esophageal temperature (T_{es}, °C) during active sleep in 10 neonates. Active sleep episodes were collected during thermoneutral or cool conditions, and lasted more than 5 min. In the cool environment, two different strategies for thermoregulation can be observed: an increased V_{O2} induced by a fall in oesophageal temperature (non-shivering thermogenesis) or an increased V_{O2} with increased oesophageal temperature (behavioural response). (Modified from Bach *et al.*, 1994, *Pediatrics*, 93: 789–796.)

body heat losses from the skin surface to the environment (Stothers *et al.*, 1984). In 3-month-old-neonates, thermographic imaging has shown that the uncovered skin surface area of the head is the main route of heat exchange, and that upper limbs may be used to regulate body temperature when necessary (Anderson *et al.*, 1990). A thermoregulatory behavioural component from flexion to extension also appeared when the incubator air temperature was progressively increased (Harpin *et al.*, 1983).

All these results indicate that behavioural, thermoregulatory responses persist in AS, in contrast to adults: in adult REM sleep, a drop in postural muscle tone impairs this process.

As a result, the neonate favours the maintenance of homeothermy in cold environments, despite an increase in metabolic energy expenditure — thus demonstrating the importance of the nutritional state in hypotrophic neonates, since a rise in energy expenditure is prejudicial to body growth. The thermoregulatory function overcomes the need for energy conservation.

In the neonate, the significant proportion of active sleep (about 60–80% of the total sleep time) and the fact that thermoregulation is particularly efficient emphasise that regulatory conflicts between thermoregulatory and hypnic processes are less significant than in the adult human or the animal. Active sleep appears to be a state where homeothermia can be more fully guaranteed, thus favouring the neural maturation process ascribed to this sleep state (Tolaas, 1978).

Thermoregulation and Sleep Interaction: What Type of Model?

Work by Glotzbach and Heller (1976) in kangaroo rats exposed to a 30°C air temperature indicated that the absence of a metabolic response in REM sleep is due to a significant increase in the set-point value of the central controller, coupled with a nil gain. Hence, the autonomic responses resulted from an open-loop mode of regulation. The difference between the thermal responses observed during SWS and awakening is supposedly due to a change in the thermoregulatory system's gain.

In REM sleep, the hypothalamus' responsiveness to thermal stimuli is depressed, and control mechanisms are released from the hypothalamic regulatory influences that are active during SWS and wakefulness. The nature of this temporary suspension of thermal regulation is an open question and is not completely understood. Studies performed in the cat (Parmeggiani *et al.*, 1983) and the kangaroo rat (Glotzbach *et al.*, 1984) showed that there is a loss of thermosensitivity in the anterior hypothalamic neurons in desynchronised sleep, compared to wakefulness and synchronised sleep. Similar findings have been reported by Parmeggiani and Sabattini (1972) with regard to thermal responses such as shivering and panting in the cat. A model for the functional organisation of neural structures has been proposed by Parmeggiani (1988) according to which central nervous system structures such as the telecephalon, diencephalon, and rhomboencephalon are organised into a functional hierarchy (depending on the sleep stage) where upstream structures control those downstream. Hence, wakefulness is characterised by a telencephalon → diencephalon → rhombencephalon functional dominance. Thermoregulation is coordinated by diencephalic influences modulated by cortical stimulation. During SWS, cephalic dominance decreases, thus establishing a diencephalon → rhombencephalon hierarchy. The diencephalon plays a preponderant role, and thermoregulation is particularly stable and efficient — fitting the idea of neural control of homeostasis via a close-loop regulation mode. In contrast, during REM sleep, thermoregulation is only under the control of the rhombencephalon, and the inactivation of the diencephalic structures containing the hypothalamus is at the origin of thermoregulatory responses ill-suited to the maintenance of homeothermy. The regulation of autonomic functions is highly unstable. Passage from one sleep stage to another (and thus from one functional dominance to another) can only occur when the dominant structure is not strongly stimulated. Hence, entry into SWS can occur if cortical activity decreases. Likewise, activation of the hypothalamus renders a transition to REM sleep impossible.

Changes in functional dominance could explain the modifications in hypothalamic reactivity, notably the nil gain of the thermoregulatory system during REM sleep.

The theory described above cannot therefore be applied to the adult human — unless one considers that thermoregulatory mechanisms are under the control of extra-hypothalamic centres. The control processes of body temperature regulation are widely distributed and are probably not only dependent on integrative mechanisms located in the hypothalamus. This is supported by various studies suggesting that the thermal information is integrated lower down in the structures of the neuroaxis, the activity of which is coordinated by the preoptic anterior hypothalamic area (Satinoff, 1978; Berner and Heller, 1998). In rabbits, Murakami and Sakata (1980) demonstrated the existence of thermosensitive neurons at the spinal cord level, which seems to be a very thermosensitive area (Jessen, 1985). In animals, cooling or warming this region does indeed elicit thermoregulatory responses, although large local temperature changes are required. The thermoreceptors of the spinal cord are connected to hypothalamic structures via afferent anterolateral pathways. The fact that (i) sweating is only depressed in REM sleep in human adults and that (ii) panting persists in cats exposed to heavy warm loads (Parmeggiani and Rabini, 1970) suggests that activation of warm-responsive preoptic hypothalamic neurons is not necessary, since activation of the subordinate brain stem and spinal process is possible. In animals, the impairment of thermoregulation (which mainly depends on hypothalamic structures) is thus more evident than in humans. During REM sleep, the sweat rate would thus be controlled by simple reflex mechanisms, comparable to those described by Parmeggiani (1980) for functions such as respiration or blood circulation. However, the results obtained by Sagot *et al.* (1987) during REM sleep show that the local sweat rate measured in the trunk area augments linearly with increasing oesophagus temperature, thus indicating that sweating activity is a regulated phenomenon that cannot easily be compared to a reflex mechanism. The increased hypothalamic sensitivity in stages 1–2 compared to REM sleep is due to a change in the thermoregulatory system's gain, whereas the sensitivity increase observed when passing from stages 1–2 into SWS is due to a decrease in the set-point value.

Peripheral factors (such as a release of neuroglandular transmitter substances for each neural impulse arriving at the sweat gland level) or decreased cholinergic sensitivity of the gland could decrease the thermal response in REM sleep — an initial period during which complex disturbances in sympathetic influences occur at the autonomic effector level. The sweat glands are innervated by postganglionic sympathetic fibres, and the depression of the sweating response in REM sleep is consistent with the change in tonic sympathetic outflow occurring during this sleep stage. This, however, is not an explanation that is consistent with the data obtained by Amoros *et al.* (1986).

In the neonate, active sleep — often considered as the "precursor" of REM sleep — happens to be a state that is particularly well-suited to the maintenance of homeothermy. There are some doubts that the models of thermoregulation described in animals and human adults can be extrapolated to the human neonate. The differences may be related to the changes in the hierarchical control of central nervous system structures but also to the various thermal effectors that differ as a function of maturity and from one species to another. Compared with human adults or animals who primarily utilise shivering (absent during AS in animals) to increase heat production during cold exposure, sleep may affect thermogenesis differently in neonates since the latter utilise non-shivering thermogenesis to maintain body homeothermia during exposure to cold. Moreover, the increased metabolism observed in the human adult or neonate exposed to cold may also depend on the extent of their brain activity, which accounts for 20% of total metabolic activity. During REM sleep, the brain's neural activity increases and is associated with increased cerebral blood flow in humans (Towsend *et al.*, 1973). Finally, in premature neonates (and even though the cerebral blood flow-metabolism coupling is present), active sleep does not show the increased cerebral blood flow and metabolism seen at a later age (Greisen *et al.*, 1985). This finding (together with the fact that the wake–sleep shift pattern differs from that of adults) suggests that the sleep states during this early period are still not fully developed. In terms of the neurovegetative mechanisms of thermoregulation, it is not therefore possible to suggest that active sleep and quiet sleep are the direct precursors of REM sleep and SWS, respectively. This observation concurs in part with recent studies. Thus, Frank and Heller (1997) suggest that behaviourally determined AS in the rat could be an immature, undifferentiated state with SWS properties. Vogel *et al.* (2000) indicated that the loss of active sleep during development is mainly replaced by wakefulness, whereas quiet sleep is at the origin of SWS. Taking into account the results for thermoregulation appears to plead in favour of these hypotheses — adult thermoregulation is particularly efficient during SWS and wakefulness, just as in active sleep in the neonate. Let us assume that the classification of sleep stages cannot be based only on electrophysiological and behavioural criteria but also on those related to the operation of autonomic functions.

References

Amoros, C., Sagot, J.C., Libert, J.P., and Candas, V. (1986). Sweat gland response to local heating during sleep in man. *J. Physiol. (Paris)*, 81: 209–215.

Anderson, E.S., Wailoo, M.P., and Petersen, S.A. (1990). Use of thermographic imaging to study babies sleeping at home. *Arch. Dis. Child*, 65: 1266–1267.

Azaz, Y., Fleming, PJ., Levine, M., McCabe, R., Stewart, A., and Johnson, P. (1992). The relationship between environmental temperature, metabolic rate, sleep stage, and evaporative water loss in infants from birth to three months. *Pediatr. Res.*, 32: 417–423.

Bach, V., Bouferrache, B., Kremp, O., Maingourd, Y., and Libert, J.P. (1994). Regulation of sleep and body temperature in response to exposure to cool and warm environments in neonates. *Pediatrics*, 93: 789–796.

Bach, V., Telliez, F., Zoccoli, G.P., Lenzi, P., Léké, A., and Libert, J.P. (2000). Interindividual differences in the thermoregulatory response to cool exposure in sleeping neonates. *Eur. J. Appl. Physiol.*, 81: 455–462.

Bach, V., Telliez, F., Léké, A.A., Chiorri, A., and Libert, J.P. (2001). Interaction between body temperatures and the direction of sleep stage transition in neonates. *Sleep Res. Online*, 4: 43–49.

Bell, E.F. and Rios, G.R. (1983). A double-walled incubator alters the partition of body heat loss of premature infants. *Pediatr. Res.*, 17: 135–140.

Berger, P.J., Horne, R.S.C., and Walker, A.M. (1989). Cardiorespiratory responses to cool ambient temperature differ with sleep state in neonatal lambs. *J. Physiol.*, 412: 351–363.

Berner, N.J. and Heller, H.C. (1988). Does the preoptic anterior hypothalamus receive thermo afferent information? *Am. J. Physiol., Regul. Integr. Comp. Physiol.*, 43: R9–R18.

Brück, K. (1968). Which environmental temperature does the premature infant prefer? *Pediatrics*, 41: 1027–1030.

Brück, K. (1992). Neonatal thermal regulation. In: Polin, R.A. and Fox, W.W. (Eds.). *Fetal and Neonatal Physiology*. Philadelphia: Saunders W.B., pp. 488–515.

Brück, K., Parmelee, A.H., and Brück, M. (1962). Neutral temperature range and range of "thermal comfort" in premature infants. *Biol. Neonate*, 4: 32–51.

Buguet, A.G.C., Linvingstone, S.D., Reed, L.D., and Limmer, R.E. (1976). EEG patterns and body temperatures in man during sleep in Arctic winter nights. Int. *J. Biometeorol.*, 20: 61–69.

Buguet, A.G.C., Livingstone, S.D., and Reed, L.D. (1979). Skin temperature changes in paradoxical sleep in man in the cold. *Aviat. Space Environ. Med.*, 50: 567–570.

Bunnell, D.E., Agnew, J.A., Horwath, S.M., and Wills, M. (1988). Passive body heating and sleep: influence of proximity to sleep. *Sleep*, 11: 210–219.

Candas,V., Libert, J.P., and Muzet, A. (1982). Heating and cooling stimulations during SWS and REM sleep in man. *J. Therm. Biol.*, 7: 155–158.

Dane, H.J., Sauer, P.J.J., and Visser, H.K.A. (1985). Oxygen consumption and CO_2 production of low-birth-weight infants in two sleep states. *Biol. Neonate*, 47: 205–210.

Darnall, R.A. and Ariagno, R.L. (1982). The effects of sleep state on active thermoregulation in the premature infant. *Pediatr. Res.*, 16: 512–514.

Day, R. (1941). Regulation of body temperature during sleep. *Am. J. Dis. Child.*, 61: 734–746.

Dewasmes, G., Signoret, P., Nicolas, A., Ehrhart, J., and Muzet, A. (1996). Advances of human core temperature minimum and maximal paradoxical sleep propensity by ambient thermal transients. *Neurosci. Lett.*, 215: 25–28.

Fewell, J.E., Kondo, C.S., and Dascalu, V. (1990). Influence of sleep on the cardiovascular and metabolic responses to a decrease in ambient temperature in lambs. *J. Dev. Physiol.*, 13: 223–230.

Fleming, P.J., Levine, M.R., Azaz, Y., and Johnson, P. (1988). The effect of sleep state on the metabolic response to cold stress in newborn infants. In: Jones, C.T. (Ed.). *Fetal and Neonatal Development*. Ithaca, NY: Perinatology Press, pp. 635–639.

Foster, K.G., Hey, E.N., and Katz, G. (1969). The response of the sweat glands of the newborn baby to thermal stimuli and to intradermal acetycholine. *J. Appl. Physiol.*, 203: 13–19.

Franck, S.M., Raja, S.N., Bulcao, C.F., and Golstein, D.S. (1999). Relative contribution of core and cutaneous temperatures to thermal comfort and automatic responses in humans. *J. Appl. Physiol.*, 80: 1588–1593.

Frank, M.G. and Heller, H.C. (1997). Development of REM and slow wave sleep in the rat. *Am. J. Physiol.*, 41: 1792–1799.

Franzini, C., Cianci, T., Lenzi, P., and Guidallotti, P.L. (1982). Neural control of vasomotion in rabbit ear is impaired during desynchronized sleep. *Am. J. Physiol.*, 243: 142–144.

Glotzbach, S.F. and Heller, H.C. (1976). Central nervous regulation of body temperature during sleep. *Science*, 194: 537–539.

Glotzbach, S.F. and Heller., H.C. (1984). Changes in the thermal characteristics of hypothalanic neurons during sleep and wakefulness. *Brain Res.*, 309: 17–26.

Greisen, G., Hellström-Vestas, L., Lou, H., Rosen, I., and Sevenningsen, N. (1985). Sleep waking shifts and cerebral blood flow in stable preterm-infants. *Pediatr. Res.*, 19: 1156–1159.

Harpin, V.A., Chellappah, G., and Rutter, N. (1983). Responses of the newborn infant to overheating. *Biol. Neonate*, 44: 65–75.

Hashizume, Y. (1997). Fluctuations of rectal and tympanic temperatures with changes of ambient temperature during night sleep. *Psychiatry Clin. Neurosci.*, 51: 129–133.

Haskell, E.H., Palca, J.W., Walker, J.M., Berger, R.J., and Heller, H.C. (1978). The influence of ambient temperatures on electrophysiological sleep in humans. *Sleep Res.*, 7: 169.

Haskell, E.H., Palca, J.W., Walker, J.M., Berger, J., and Heller, H.C. (1981). Metabolism and thermoregulation during stages of sleep in humans exposed to heat and cold. *J. Appl. Physiol: Respirat. Environ. Exercise Physiol.*, 51: 948–954.

Hénane, R., Buguet, A., Roussel, B., and Bittel, J. (1977). Variations in evaporation and body temperatures during sleep in man. *J. Appl. Physiol.*, 42: 50–55.

Hey, E.N. (1969). The relation between environmental temperature and oxygen consumption in the newborn baby. *J. Physiol. (Lond.)*, 200: 589–603.

Horne, J.A. (1981). The effects of exercise on sleep: a critical review. *Biol. Psychol.*, 12: 241–290.

Horne, J.A. and Staff, L.H.E. (1983). Exercise and sleep: body heating effects. *Sleep*, 6: 36–46.

Horne, J.A. and Reid, A.J. (1985). Night-time sleep EEG changes following body heating in a warm bath. *Electoencephalogr. Clin. Neurophysiol.*, 60: 154–157.

Jessen, C. (1985). Thermal afferents in the control of body temperature. *Pharmacol. Ther.*, 28: 107.

Karacan, I., Thornby, J.I., Anch, M., Williams, R.L., and Perkins, H.M. (1978). Effects of high ambient temperature on sleep in young men. *Aviat. Space Environ. Med.*, 49: 855–860.

Kendel, K. and Schmidt-Kessen, W. (1973). The influence of room temperature on nigth sleep in man (polygraphic-night sleep recordings in the climatic chamber). In: Koella, W.P. and Levin, P. (Eds.). *Sleep.* Basel: Krager, pp. 423–425.

Leblanc, M.H. (1983). Oxygen consumption in premature infants in an incubator of proven clinical efficiency. *Biol. Neonate,* 44: 76–84.

Lenzi, P., Libert, J.P., Cianci, T., and Franzini, C. (1990). Comparative aspects of the interaction between sleep and thermoregulation. In: Horne, J. (Ed.). *Sleep'90.* Bochum: Pontenagel Press, pp. 388–390.

Libert, J.P., Candas, V., Muzet, A., and Ehrhart, J. (1982). Thermoregulatory adjustements to thermal transients during slow wave sleep and REM sleep in man. *J. Physiol. (*Paris*),* 78: 251–257.

Libert, J.P., Di Nisi, J., Fukuda, H., Muzet, A., Ehrhart, J., and Amoros, C. (1988). Effect of continuous heat exposure on sleep stages in humans. *Sleep,* 11: 195–209.

Libert, J.P., Bach, V., Johnson, L.C., Ehrhart, J., Wittersheim, G., and Keller, D. (1991). Relative and combined effects of heat and noise exposure on sleep in humans. *Sleep,* 14: 24–31.

Mestyan, J., Jarai, I., Bata, G., and Fekete, M. (1964). Surface temperature versus deep body temperature and metabolic response to cold of hypothermic premature infants. *Biol. Neonate,* 7: 230–242.

Mestyan, J., Jarai, I., Bata, G., and Fekete, M. (1964). The significance of facial skin temperature in the chemical heat regulation of premature infants. *Biol. Neonate,* 7: 243–254.

Murakami, N. and Sakata, Y. (1980). Convergence of thermal inputs at medullary temperature responsive neurons in rabbits. *J. Therm. Biol.,* 5: 83–88.

Muzet, A., Ehrhart, J., Libert, J.P., and Candas, V. (1979). The effect of thermal environment on sleep stages. In: Fanger, P.O. and Valbjorn, O. (Eds.). *Indoor Climate: Effects on Human Comfort, Performance and Health.* Copenhagen: Danish Building Research Institute, pp. 753–761.

Muzet, A., Ehrhart, J., Candas, V., Libert, J.P., and Vogt, J.J. (1983). REM sleep and ambient temperature in man. *Int. J. Neurosci.,* 18: 117–126.

Muzet, A. and Libert, J.P. (1985). Effects of ambient temperature on sleep in man in sleep 84. In: Koella, W.P., Rüther, E., and Schulz H. (Eds.). Basel: Karger, pp. 74–76.

Nicol, S.C. and Maskrey, M. (1980). Thermoregulation, respiration and sleep in the Tasmanian devil, *Sarcophilus havrissii (Marsupialia: Dasyvriade). J. Comp. Physiol.,* 140: 241–248.

Nessmann, C. and Baverel, F. (1972). Le développement de la peau chez l'embryon et le fœtus humain. *Biol. Reprod.,* 1: 527–550.

Okamoto-Mizuno, K., Mizuno, K., Michie, S., Maeda, A., and Lizuka, S. (1999). Effects of humid heat exposure on human sleep stages and body temperature. *Sleep,* 22: 767–773.

Palca, J.W., Walker, J.M., and Berger, R.J. (1986). Thermoregulation, metabolism and stages of sleep in cold-exposed men. *J. Appl. Physiol.,* 61: 940–947.

Parmeggiani, P.L. (1980). Temperature regulation during sleep: a study in homeostasis. In: Orem, J. and Barnes, C. (Eds.). *Physiology in Sleep. Topics in Physiology.* New York: Academic Press, pp. 97–143.

Parmeggiani, P.L. (1987). Interaction between sleep and thermoregulation: an aspect of the control of behavioral states. *Sleep*, 10: 426–435.

Parmeggiani, P.L. (1988). Thermoregulation during sleep from the view point of homeostasis. In: Lydic, R.L. and Biebuyk, R.L. (Eds.).*Clinical Physiology of Sleep*. Bethesda: American Physiology Society, Vol. 3, pp. 159–169.

Parmeggiani, P.L. and Rabini, C. (1970). Sleep and environmental temperature. *Arch. Ital. Biol.*, 108: 369–387.

Parmeggiani, P.L. and Sabattini, L. (1972). Electromyographic aspects of postural, respiratory and thermoregulatory mechanisms in sleeping cats. *Electroencephalogr. Clin. Neurophysiol.*, 33: 1–13.

Parmeggiani, P.L., Azzaroni, A., Cevolani, D., and Ferrari, D. (1983). Responses of anterior hypothalanic-preoptic neurons to direct thermal stimulation during wakefulness and sleep. *Brain Res.*, 269: 382–385.

Perlstein, P.H., Hersh, C., Glück, C.J., and Sutherland, J.M. (1974). Adaptation to cold in the first three days of life. *Pediatrics*, 54: 411–416.

Pribylova, H. (1971). Effect of temperature of inspired air on the metabolic response of the neonate. *Rev. Czech. Med.*, 17: 133–136.

Putkonen, P.T.S., Elomaa, E., and Kotilainen, P.V. (1973). Increase in delta (3+4) sleep after heat stress in sauna. *Scand. J. Clin. Lab. Invest.*, 31(suppl. 130): 19.

San't Ambrogio, G. and Widdicombe, J. (2001). Reflexes from airway rapidly adapting receptors. *Respir. Physiol.*, 125: 33–45.

Sagot, J.C., Amoros, C., Candas, V., and Libert, J.P. (1987). Sweating responses and body temperatures during nocturnal sleep in humans. *Am. J. Physiol.*, 252: R462–R470.

Sakaguchi, S., Glotzbach, S.F., and Heller, H.C. (1979). Influence of hypothalamic and ambient temperatures on sleep in kangaroo rats. *Am. J. Physiol.*, 273: R80–R88.

Satinoff, E. (1978). Neural organization and evolution of thermal regulation in mammals. *Science*, 201: 16–22.

Schieber, J.P., Muzet, A., and Ferrière, P.J.R. (1971). Les phases d'activation transitoire spontanées au cours du sommeil normal chez l'homme. *Arch. Sci. Physiol.*, 25: 443–465.

Shapiro, C.M., Moore, A.T., Mitchell, D., and Yodaiken, M.L. (1974). How well does man thermoregulate during sleep? *Experientia*, 30: 1279–1281.

Shapiro, C.M., Allan, M., Driver, H., and Mitchell, D. (1989). Thermal load alters sleep. *Biol. Psychiatry*, 26: 733–736.

Stothers, J.K. and Warner, R.M. (1984). Thermal balance and sleep state in the newborn. *Early Human Develop.*, 9: 313–322.

Sulyok, E., Jéquier, E., and Prod'hom, L.S. (1973). Thermal balance of the newborn infant in a heat-gaining environment. *Pediatr. Res.*, 7: 888–900.

Telliez, F., Bach, V., Delanaud, S., Bouferrache, B., and Libert, J.P. (1997). Skin derivative control of thermal environment in closed incubators. *Med. Biol. Eng. Comput.*, 35: 516–520.

Telliez, F., Bach, V., Dewasmes, G., Léké, A., and Libert, J.P. (1998). Sleep modifications during cool acclimation in human neonates. *Neurosci. Lett.*, 245: 25–28.

Tolaas, J. (1978). REM sleep and concept of vigilance. *Biol. Psychiatry*, 13: 135–147.

Towsend, R.E., Prinz, P.N., and Obrist, W.D. (1973). Human cerebral blood flow during sleep and waking. *J. Appl. Physiol.*, 35: 620–625.

Vogel, G.W. Feng, P., and Kinney, G.G. (2000). Ontogeny of REM sleep in rats: possible implications for endogenous depression. *Physiol. Behav.*, 63: 432–461.

Wheldon, A.E. (1982). Energy balance in the newborn baby: use of a manikin to estimate radiant and convective heat loss. *Phys. Med. Biol.*, 27: 285–296.

Chapter 20

ENDOCRINE CORRELATES OF SLEEP IN HUMANS

Gabrielle Brandenberger[1]

Sleep and wakefulness are thought to be regulated by three basic processes: (1) the timing control of the circadian clock resulting in alternating 24-h cycles of high and low sleep propensity, (2) a homeostatic process derived from the time course of slow wave activity during normal sleep and after sleep deprivation, and (3) an ultradian process within sleep which defines the cycles of the two basic sleep states of non-rapid eye movement (NREM) and REM sleep and the corresponding oscillations in slow wave activity. Various mathematical models have been proposed to account for the circadian, homeostatic, and ultradian aspects of sleep regulation (Borbély and Achermann, 1992, 1999; Dijk and Kronauer, 1999). Circadian models (Process C) assume that multiple oscillators cause the differences in periods and entrainment properties of the sleep–wake cycle. Homeostatic models propose that a sleep–wake-dependent process (Process S) underlies the rise in sleep pressure during waking and its decay during sleep. The interaction of Process S with Process C can account for multimodal sleep–wake patterns, internal desynchronisation, and the time course of daytime sleepiness. Ultradian models simulate the cyclic alternation of NREM sleep and REM sleep.

---

[1] brandenberger.gabrielle@medecine.u-strasbg.fr

Molecularly, the circadian rhythm of sleep involves interlocking positive and negative feedback mechanisms of circadian genes and their protein products in cells of the suprachiasmatic nucleus (SCN) that are entrained to ambient conditions by light (for a review, see Pace-Schott and Hobson, 2002). A homeostatic sleep need is integrated with circadian information in nuclei of the anterior hypothalamus. These nuclei interact with arousal systems in the posterior hypothalamus, basal forebrain, and brainstem. An ultradian oscillator in the mesopontine brainstem controls the alternation of NREM and REM sleep by a reciprocal interaction between aminergic REM-on and cholinergic REM-off cell populations (Hobson *et al.*, 1975; McCarley and Massaquoi, 1992).

The endocrine regulation during sleep and wakefulness has become an important facet in the science of sleep regulation. In humans, a prominent feature of the hormonal system is its high degree of temporal organisation, the overall 24-h wave shape reflecting circadian, sleep-related, or ultradian influences. A complex temporal organisation underlies the secretion of each hormone, with well-characterised 24-h profiles and well-defined secretory pulses demonstrating a high degree of reproducibility in their relationship with sleep stages. In this chapter, we attempt to integrate the endocrine system in the models of sleep regulation, and highlight recent evidence against the classic concept on the relationship between sleep and certain endocrine systems. We present advances in knowledge of the link between hormone pulses and oscillations in sleep electroencephalographic (EEG) activity, estimated by spectral analysis of sleep EEG using a fast Fourier transform which allows a dynamic description of sleep processes.

Circadian Control of Hormone Release

Evidence from animal studies has shown that the SCN is the major component of the biological clock that generates and coordinates a wide variety of physiological, endocrine, and behavioural rhythms, including the sleep–wake cycle. Local versions of the SCN clockwork are also active in peripheral, non-neural tissues, driving the tissue-specific cycles of gene expression that underpin circadian organisation (Hastings *et al.*, 2003). In recent years, the hypothalamic structures through which the SCN signal is translated into an hormonal pattern have been identified in rats. As proposed by Buijs and Kalsbeek (2001), the SCN uses four important means to organise hormonal secretion: first, by direct contact with neuroendocrine neurons; second, by contact with neuroendocrine neurons via intermediate neurones; third, by projections to the autonomic paraventricular nucleus which act on the autonomic nervous system, preparing the endocrine organs for the arrival of hormones; and fourth, by influencing its own feedback. One example is the regulation of the melatonin rhythm which is generated via a multisynaptic neural pathway from the SCN to the pineal gland. The rhythm of adrenal corticosterone secretion is under the control of SCN by direct contact with neurons containing corticotropin-releasing hormone.

In humans, immunocytochemical post mortem neuronal tracing experiments have shown that hypothalamic projections of human SCN are identical to those observed in the rat brain (Dai *et al.*, 1998a,b). However, it is not clear how the activity of the SCN is transformed into a signal that induces activity instead of inactivity in diurnal animals and simultaneously reverses the endocrine profiles. More frequently, several experimental strategies have been used in man (i.e., acute or repeated shifts in the timing of sleep, selective or total sleep deprivation), together with specific methods of measurement, including frequent blood sampling, sensitive hormone assays, and appropriate mathematical analysis to differentiate between the circadian and the sleep-related influences on the hormone profiles. As a result, it has become well established that melatonin represents the best example of an endogenous circadian rhythm, widely studied in the most prestigious laboratories (Arendt *et al.*, 1995; Czeisler, 1997; Czeisler and Klermann, 1999; Weaver, 1999). Melatonin, unlike core body temperature rhythm (Figure 1), is little influenced by acute shifts in the sleep period or by total sleep deprivation (Weibel *et al.*, 1997). Thus, melatonin is well recognised as a reliable circadian clock output (Rosenthal, 1992), and the dim light melatonin onset is a convenient way to assess circadian phase in humans (Lewy and Sack, 1989).

Adrenocorticotropin (ACTH) and cortisol rhythms, which arise from a succession of secretory pulses, are also primarily driven by the endogenous circadian pacemaker, but might not be entirely independent of sleep influences. Early studies led to the concept of an inhibitory effect of sleep on plasma cortisol levels (Weitzman *et al.*, 1983). Furthermore, one night of sleep deprivation has been described to be followed by elevated cortisol levels the following evening (Leproult *et al.*, 1997), although another study has found higher cortisol levels only in the second 24-h period of sleep deprivation (Ho *et al.*, 2001). During sleep, an inverse relation between cortisol secretory pulses and oscillations in slow wave activity has been reported both during nocturnal and diurnal sleep (Gronfier *et al.*, 1998). When the 24-h cortisol patterns are considered with regard to the oscillations in slow wave activity (Figure 2), three important points should be emphasised: (1) cortisol pulses occur independently of slow waves, as observed during

                    G. Brandenberger

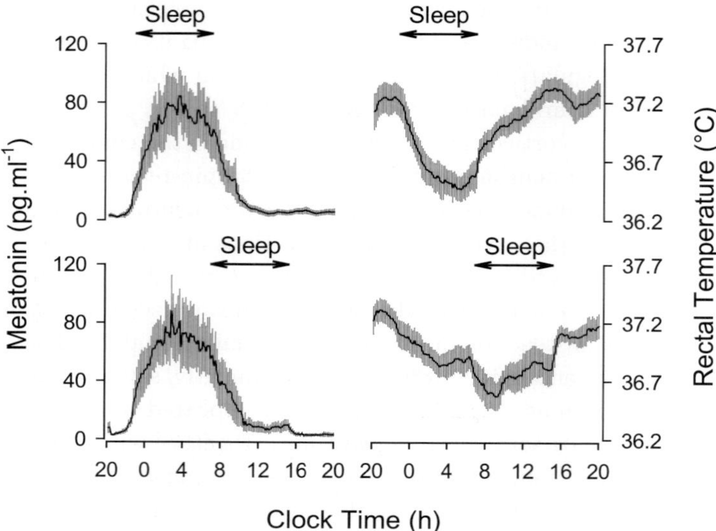

Figure 1. Mean (±SE) plasma melatonin and rectal temperature profiles in eight day-active subjects, sleeping alternately once at night and once during the day. The acute 8-h shift in the sleep period does not affect the melatonin rhythm but it induces a biphasic curve for the temperature which reveals the dual influence of sleep and circadian processes on temperature regulation.

waking states and sleep deprivation; (2) oscillations in slow waves can occur without any concomitant cortisol pulses, as observed at the beginning of night sleep; (3) when cortisol secretory pulse and oscillations in slow waves are simultaneously present, as observed at the end of nocturnal sleep and during daytime sleep, both rhythms are synchronised in phase opposition. It has then been proposed that cortisol and slow waves might have independent generators, oscillating independently of each other, and may be coupled in phase opposition at certain times of the day. The time advance observed for cortisol pulses, which precede oscillations in slow wave activity by about 10 min, supports the view that endocrine processes adjust in anticipation of sleep events and that low corticotropic activity is a prerequisite for the increase in slow waves. However, the reverse situation, described previously (Weitzman *et al.*, 1983) whereby endocrine processes are influenced by sleep cannot be totally excluded. Future studies are needed to find further support for one or the other of the views that the temporal organisation of cortisol pulses is independent of sleep with the requirement

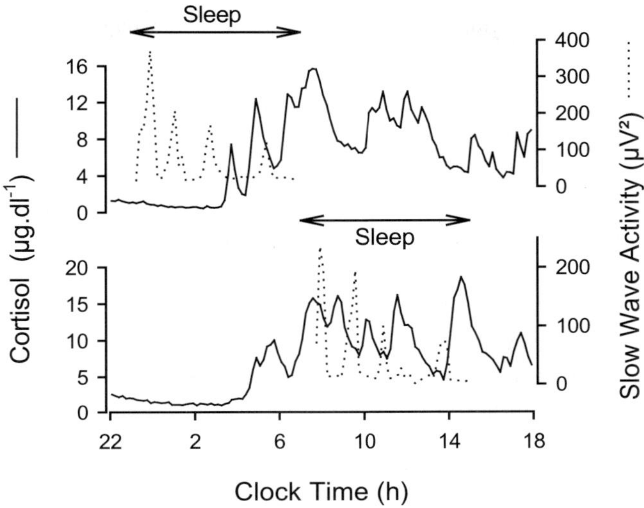

Figure 2. Twenty-four-hour profiles of plasma cortisol and slow wave activity in one subject, during nocturnal sleep (top) and during diurnal sleep (bottom). When slow wave activity and cortisol pulses were simultaneously present (at the end of night sleep and during diurnal sleep), they oscillated in phase opposition. Note the quiescent period of cortisol secretion between 2200 and 0300 hours: the first cortisol secretory pulse occurs during the night, without any identifying signal on the electroencephalogram or the electrocardiogram.

of low cortisol secretion for slow wave enrichment, or alternatively, that sleep processes exert an inhibitory effect on cortisol release.

Homeostatic Control of Hormone Release

Growth hormone (GH), a major regulator of protein anabolism and tissue growth, is thought to fit into the homeostatic model of sleep regulation. The time course of the homeostatic variable S was derived from EEG slow wave activity which results from the progressive hyperpolarisation of thalamocortical neurons (Steriade *et al.*, 1993, 1994; McCormick and Bal, 1997) and constitutes an index of sleep intensity and changes as a function of prior sleep and waking (Borbély *et al.*, 1981; Dijk *et al.*, 1990).

In humans, under usual night sleep and daytime wake routine, a major GH pulse occurs after sleep onset in temporal association with the first slow wave sleep (SWS) episode (Takahashi *et al.*, 1968; Sassin *et al.*, 1969). This pulse is correlated with SWS duration (Van Cauter *et al.*,

1992) and with the oscillations in slow wave activity during normal sleep (Gronfier *et al.*, 1996), and during recovery sleep demonstrating a rebound of GH secretion following low levels during forced waking periods (for a review, see Van Cauter *et al.*, 1998). Additional evidence for the existence of a homeostatic control of GH release has been obtained in studies using pharmacological stimulation of SWS. Administration of ritanserin, a selective 5HT2 receptor antagonist (Gronfier *et al.*, 1996), and of gamma-hydroxybutyrate provokes reliable increases in SWS in normal subjects and a corresponding stimulation in GH secretion during the same period (Van Cauter *et al.*, 1997).

Nevertheless, the notion of a high sleep dependence of GH release has been questioned in recent studies. In sleep-deprived persons, the reduction of the normal sleep-related pulse is compensated for during the day by the emergence of large individual pulses (Figure 3) so that the amount of GH

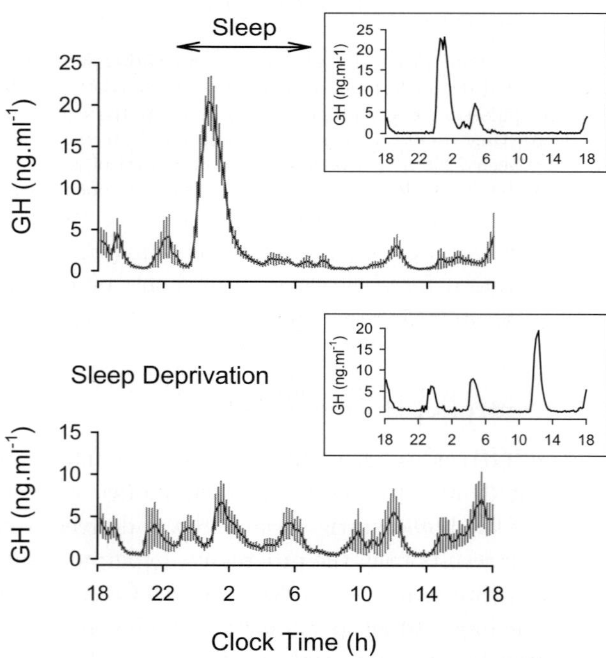

Figure 3. Effect of sleep deprivation on mean (±SE) 24-h growth hormone (GH) profiles in 10 subjects. In sleep-deprived persons, the reduction of the sleep-related pulse is compensated for by the emergence of large individual pulses during the day, so that the amount of GH secreted over 24 h is similar whether or not a person had slept during the night. Insets give typical examples of individual profiles.

secreted over 24 h is similar whether or not a person has slept during the night (Brandenberger *et al.*, 2000). Also, during chronic sleep debt, the GH profiles were found to be biphasic (Spiegel *et al.*, 2000), which does not conform with predictions of previous sleep deprivation studies.

Finally, in night workers, who form a model challenging sleep and circadian processes, the sleep-related GH pulse too was lowered, and again this reduction was counteracted by a compensatory mechanism promoting GH pulses during wakefulness. These results support findings in the rat that NREM sleep promotion and GH stimulation are independent outputs of hypothalamic GH-releasing hormone neurons (Obal and Krueger, 2001) and may explain the temporal dissociation between GH pulses and SWS often seen in previous studies (Steiger *et al.*, 1987; Saini *et al.*, 1993). Therefore sleep processes, whatever the conditions, do not play the dominating role on GH release that many have ascribed to it. It is suggested that sleep exerts a strong effect on GH release when it occurs in phase angle with the circadian pacemaker such as in day-active people. When sleep and circadian influences are misaligned, GH surges occur unpredictably throughout the 24 h. Corroboration for this view could stem from previous results in other situations, such as short or long night conditions (Wehr, 1996) or forced desynchrony, which also revealed constant 24-h GH production despite a lowered sleep-related pulse in entrained conditions (Gronfier *et al.*, 2001). Re-examination of these data may lead to new thinking on the relationship between sleep, circadian processes, and GH pulsatility.

Ultradian Control of Hormone Release

The ultradian component of sleep regulation is evident from the 80–120-min period of the NREM–REM sleep cycles and the time courses of slow wave activity that oscillates with a similar period. In addition to the homeostatic parameters of sleep, the rhythmic occurrence of the NREM–REM sleep cycles is considered as a salient feature of good sleep quality. Poor sleep is attributed to irregular and fragmented sleep cycles. In humans, included in this period is the time of recurrence of the episodic pulses of many hormones under control of their hypothalamic releasing factors, as well as a number of rhythms of apparently unrelated physiological and behavioural processes, such as the rate of urine flow, gastric motility, and cognitive variables.

The functional significance of most of these ultradian rhythms is still unknown. However, based on early findings of Knobil (1980) and of Leyendecker *et al.* (1980), the crucial role of pulsatile hormone secretion has been recognised for the endocrine reproductive system and has led to important therapeutic applications with the demonstration of the absolute requirement for gonadotropin-releasing hormone (GnRH) administration to be pulsatile. Given at a frequency of 90–120 min, which approximates that of endogenous GnRH secretion during the follicular phase, GnRH has been proved capable of ripening a follicle and inducing ovulation in women with hypothalamic amenorrhoea and congenital GnRH deficiency (Homburg *et al.*, 1989; Martin *et al.*, 1990), while numerous attempts employing continuous infusions of GnRH to induce ovulation have failed. Generated by episodic GnRH release, LH pulses are under the multifactorial influence of ultradian, sleep-related, circadian, and infradian (menstrual, seasonal) rhythms which interact continually depending on the maturation of the reproductive system (Filicori *et al.*, 1986).

The demonstration of a such an important physiological role and important therapeutic application of pulsatility has not been made for other hormonal systems. The present state of knowledge is limited to the identification of certain ultradian rhythms, without knowing either their production mechanisms or their physiological functions. Only the diversity and robustness of the relationship between sleep and pituitary hormones have been reported. For example, mean prolactin (PRL) levels increase during sleep irrespective of the time of day (Sassin *et al.*, 1972; Spiegel *et al.*, 1994; Van Cauter and Spiegel, 1999), whereas thyreotropin (TSH) has been described as reacting in a distinctive manner. In the case of sleep deprivation, the amplitude of the circadian TSH surge markedly increases, so that it is generally assumed that sleep exerts an inhibitory effect on the circadian TSH rhythm (Brabant *et al.*, 1990). Surprisingly, following sleep debt (Figure 4), TSH levels were low compared to sleep recovery conditions (Spiegel *et al.*, 1999), which does not fit into the notion that sleep inhibits TSH release. Within sleep, slow wave activity develops with increasing PRL levels (Spiegel *et al.*, 1995), and decreasing TSH levels (Gronfier *et al.*, 1995) (Figure 5). Earlier, SWS had been found to be consistently associated with a descending slope of plasma TSH levels (Goichot *et al.*, 1992), while discrepant results emerged from the analysis of PRL pulses in regard with sleep stages (Parker *et al.*, 1974; Van Cauter *et al.*, 1982) due possibly to the small variations of high PRL levels in the second sleep cycle. These relations persist remarkably well despite a disruption of 24-h hormonal profiles observed for example in night workers not fully adapted to the night work schedule (Weibel *et al.*, 1996) or in sleeping sickness patients who present

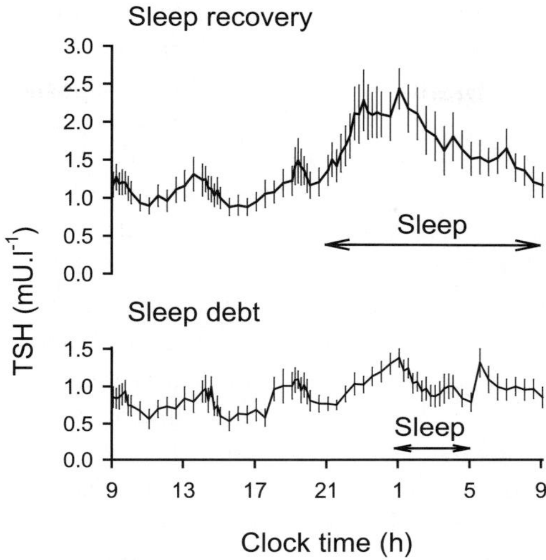

Figure 4. Thyreotropin (TSH) concentrations in sleep debt and sleep recovery conditions. These data do not fit into the classic notion that sleep inhibits TSH release. (Adapted with permission from Spiegel *et al.*, 1999.)

a disruption of their sleep–wake cycle accompanied by profound modifications in their 24-h hormonal rhythms (Brandenberger *et al.*, 1996). In these patients, hormone pulsatility is preserved. Compared to normal subjects, the difference lies in the temporal distribution of hormone pulses within the 24-h period. But despite such alterations, the relationship between hormone pulses and specific sleep stage persists, which emphasises the strength of the processes linking hormone release and internal sleep structure.

Together with the prominent rhythm of the NREM–REM sleep cycles, an ultradian rhythm emerges, the renin–angiotensin–aldosterone system, which is closely coupled to oscillations in slow wave activity. This system is of pivotal importance for the appropriate regulation of sodium balance and extracellular fluid volume. Renin activation is a major component of the homeostatic responses that maximise sodium conservation and maintain blood pressure and extracellular fluid volume. Aldosterone, the most potent mineralocorticoid hormone which is under the multifactorial control of three main factors, i.e., potassium, ACTH, and angiotensin II, acts on the collecting duct to stimulate sodium reabsorption, as well as potassium and hydrogen ion excretion.

     G. Brandenberger

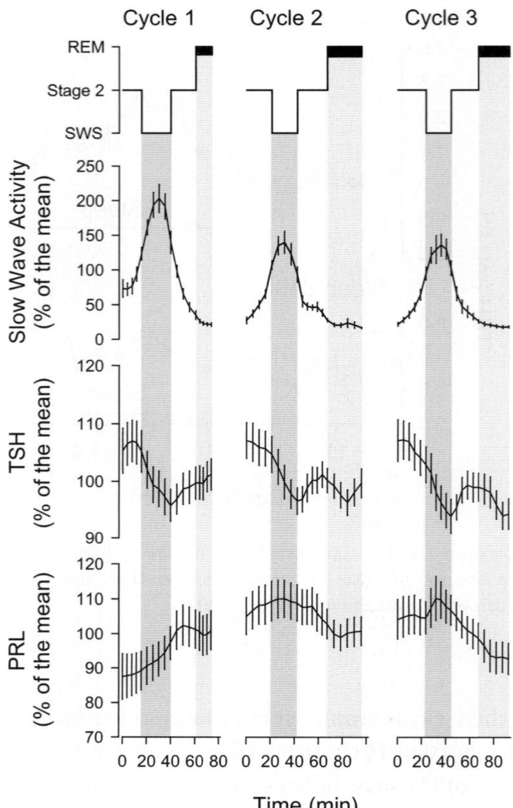

Figure 5. Mean ($\pm$SE) time courses of slow wave activity (0.5–3.5 Hz) and concomitant profiles of plasma levels of thyreotropin (TSH) and prolactin (PRL) during the NREM–REM sleep cycles in 22 subjects. In this figure, the individual differences in the occurrence and duration of sleep stages are normalised according to a method derived from Achermann *et al.* (1993). For each individual, the unequal time spent in sleep stage 2, SWS, and REM sleep was subdivided into equal parts so that EEG and hormonal data could be averaged over subjects. This procedure somewhat distorts the hormonal profiles but shows clearly the relationship between hormones and specific sleep stages.

Several studies have demonstrated that the 24-hour rhythm of the renin–angiotensin–aldosterone system is generated by sleep processes, with high renin and aldosterone levels during the sleep period whenever it occurs, and blunted levels during waking periods or sleep deprivation (Brandenberger *et al.*, 1988; 1994). During sleep, a well-defined ultradian rhythm in plasma renin activity (PRA), reflecting renin release, was found closely linked

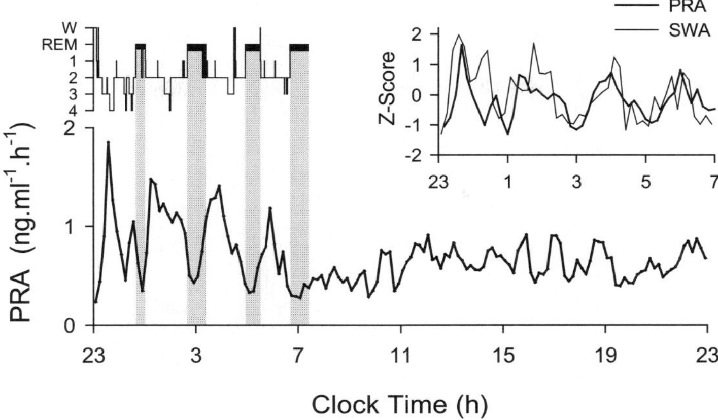

Figure 6. Individual 24-h profile of plasma renin activity (PRA) together with the hypnogram. The close relationship between nocturnal PRA oscillations and slow wave activity is illustrated in the inset.

to sleep stage alternation, with increasing levels during NREM sleep and decreasing levels during REM sleep (Figure 6). Overnight PRA oscillations strongly correlate with slow wave activity in normal subjects (Luthringer *et al.*, 1995). Converting enzyme inhibitors, beta-blockers, diuretics, and low sodium diet modulate the amplitude of these oscillations but do no abolish the relationship between PRA and sleep structure (Brandenberger *et al.*, 1990). In patients with sleep disorders, PRA reflects the disorganisation of the internal sleep structure (Schulz *et al.*, 1992; Brandenberger *et al.*, 1996). These findings led to the hypothesis that common central mechanisms, possibly involving the serotoninergic system (Van de Kar *et al.*, 1981, 1987), control both the increase in SWA and renin release from the juxtaglomerular cells. However, a recent study involving the simultaneous analysis of arterial blood pressure, activity of the autonomic nervous system as inferred from heart rate variability (HRV), of slow wave activity and renin release (Figure 7) lends support to the view that nocturnal oscillations in renin are possibly linked to blood pressure regulation rather than to direct sleep-related processes controlling both the generation of slow waves and the release of renin from the kidney (Charloux *et al.*, 2002).

The 24-h aldosterone rhythm is classically thought to be under circadian influence (Katz *et al.*, 1972; Armbruster *et al.*, 1975; Lightman *et al.*, 1981). However, recent results based on sleep deprivation (Figure 8) or on acute shift of sleep from nighttime to daytime demonstrate a major influence of

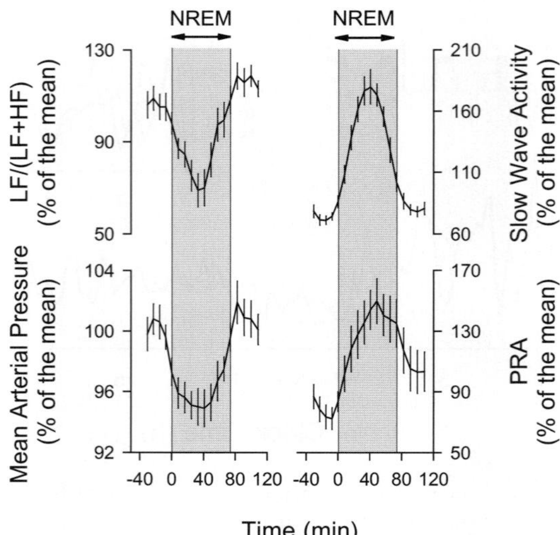

Figure 7. Cascade of events leading to increased renin release during non-rapid eye movement (NREM) sleep in eight subjects. Sympathetic tone as inferred from the LF/(LF+HF) ratio [low frequency (LF); high frequency (HF)] and mean arterial blood pressure decrease concomitantly, with a subsequent increase in slow wave activity (SWA) and in plasma renin activity (PRA). Values are expressed as percentages of the mean overnight values.

sleep processes on aldosterone release (Charloux *et al.*, 1999; 2001). Aldosterone pulses are related mainly to renin oscillations during sleep periods, following them by about 10–20 min, whereas they are related to cortisol pulses during waking. Such a dual control on aldosterone pulses depending on the vigilance state, by the renin-angiotensin system during sleep, and by the adrenocorticotropic system during wakefulness, has not been described for any other endocrine system.

One model for examining the physiological action of the renin–angiotensin–aldosterone system is represented by sleep apnea patients who have fragmented sleep, increased urine and sodium excretion, increased atrial natriuretic peptide (ANP) release and decreased activity of the renin–angiotensin system (Follenius *et al.*, 1991).

The treatment with nasal positive airways pressure immediately restores the sleep cycles, diminishes ANP levels, and restores the nocturnal oscillations in renin and aldosterone which contribute to normalising urine and sodium output.

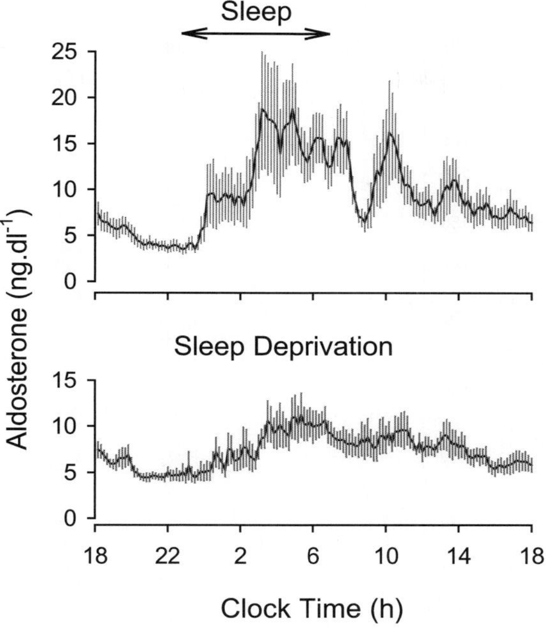

Figure 8. Effect of sleep deprivation on mean (±SE) 24-h aldosterone profiles in eight subjects. This figure demonstrates the major influence of sleep on aldosterone rhythm.

Coupling with the Activity of the Autonomic Nervous System: Duality of Sleep Stage 2

The autonomic nervous system seems to play a decisive role for the coordination among ultradian, hormonal and sleep phenomena. Using either time or frequency domain indexes of HRV which provide information on the activity of the autonomic nervous system, many studies have reported that HRV varies according to sleep stages, switching from vagally dominated SWS to sympathetic dominated REM sleep (Zemaitytë *et al.*, 1984; Berlad *et al.*, 1993; Baharav *et al.*, 1995; Vanoli *et al.*, 1995; Vaughn *et al.*, 1995; Otzenberger *et al.*, 1998; Brandenberger *et al.*, 2001). One example of the harmonious coordination of ultradian rhythms already described by Shannahoff-Khalsa *et al.* (1996) is given in Figure 9, which illustrates the increases in slow wave activity during NREM sleep, associated with low adrenocorticotropic activity and low sympathetic activity, whereas sleep stage 2 clearly reveals its hormonal and autonomic duality, depending on

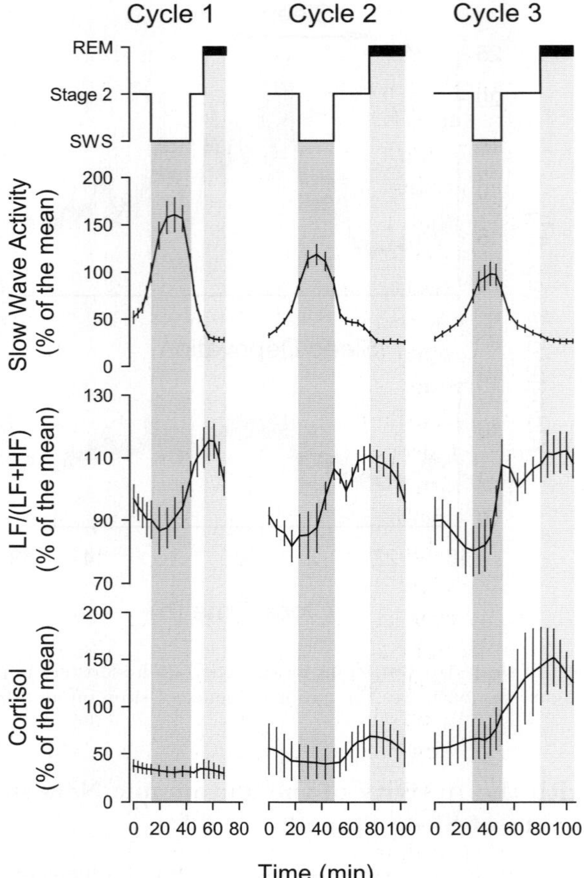

Figure 9. Coupling of slow wave activity, adrenocorticotropic activity, and autonomic nervous system activity as inferred from the LF/(LF+HF) ratio in 13 subjects (means ± SE). The time advance between cortisol pulses and LF/(LF+HF) oscillations which precede oscillations in slow wave activity supports the view that low sympathetic and adrenocorticotropic activity are prerequisites for the increase in slow waves. Note the autonomic and hormonal duality in sleep stage 2 whether it precedes SWS or REM sleep.

whether it prepares SWS or REM sleep. It is tempting to propose that sleep disorders might result from an alteration of the autonomic nervous system activity, or from inadequate coupling between endocrine, autonomic, and EEG ultradian rhythms.

Summary

The purpose of this review was to integrate the endocrine system into the processes combining circadian, homeostatic, and ultradian aspects that underlie sleep regulation. Within this framework, it is clearly apparent that melatonin is a reliable marker of circadian clock output, basically independent of sleep and waking, whereas ACTH and cortisol rhythms, albeit dominated by the circadian pacemaker, might not be entirely independent of sleep influences. GH fits into the homeostatic model of sleep regulation. Indeed, GH secretion has often been reported to be linked to SWS duration or to the amount of slow wave activity. However, recent studies in sleep-deprived persons challenged the notion of a high sleep-dependence of GH release whatever the conditions, and propose new thinking of the relationship between its pulsatile release, sleep, and circadian processes. The ultradian component of sleep regulation is reflected in the time courses of pituitary and adrenal hormones. Well-defined secretory pulses demonstrate a high degree of reproducibility in their relationship with sleep stages. A prominent ultradian rhythm emerges for the renin–angiotensin–aldosterone system which parallels slow wave activity, so that renin can been considered as a humoral marker of ultradian sleep processes. The aldosterone rhythm, previously thought to be under circadian influence, has recently been recognised as being sleep-dependent. Aldosterone pulses are under a dual control, depending on the vigilance state, by the renin–angiotensin system during sleep and by the adrenocorticotropic system during wakefulness. The activity of the autonomic nervous system underlies the coupling between hormones and EEG activity, switching from vagally dominated SWS to sympathetically dominated REM sleep. Currently, these highly coordinated systems have not revealed all the mysteries of their origin, interactions, and causal connections. They may constitute the functional basis of living organisms.

Acknowledgments

The results presented in this chapter are based mainly on the work of Claude Gronfier, Karine Spiegel, Laurence Weibel, and Anne Charloux, who are former PhD students in the laboratory. The expert assistance of Michèle Siméoni with data analysis and graphic presentations is gratefully acknowledged. The author is indebted to Jean Ehrhart and Daniel Joly for sleep recordings and analysis. We thank Marguerite Follenius Chantal Simon and François Piquard for their invaluable collaboration.

References

Achermann, P., Dijk, D.J., Brunner, D.P., and Borbély, A.A. (1993). A model of human sleep homeostasis based on EEG slow-wave activity: quantitative comparison of data and simulations. *Brain Res. Bull.*, 31: 97–113.

Arendt, J., Deacon, S., English, J., Hampton, S., and Morgan, L. (1995). Melatonin and adjustment to phase shift. *J. Sleep Res.*, 4: 74–79.

Armbruster, H., Vetter, W., Beckerhoo, R., Nussberger, J., Vetter, H., and Siegenthaler, W. (1975). Diurnal variations of plasma aldosterone in supine man: relation to plasma renin activity and plasma cortisol. *Acta Endocrinol.*, 80: 95–103.

Baharav, A., Kotagal, S., Gibbons, V., Rubin, B.K., Pratt, G., Karin, J., and Akselrod, S. (1995). Fluctuations in autonomic nervous activity during sleep displayed by power spectrum analysis of heart rate variability. *Neurology*, 45: 1183–1187.

Berlad, I., Shlitner, A., Ben-Haims, S., and Lavie, P. (1993). Power spectrum analysis and heart rate variability in stage 4 and REM sleep: evidence for state-specific changes in autonomic dominance. *J. Sleep Res.*, 2: 88–90.

Borbély, A.A. and Achermann, P. (1992). Concepts and models of sleep regulation: an overview. *J. Sleep Res.*, 1: 63–79.

Borbély, A.A. and Achermann, P. (1999). Sleep homeostasis and models of sleep regulation. *J. Biol. Rhythms*, 14: 557–568.

Borbély, A.A., Baumann, F., Brandeis, D., Strauch, I., and Lehmann, D. (1981). Sleep deprivation: effects on sleep stages and EEG power density in man. *Electroencephalogr. Clin. Neurophysiol.*, 51: 483–493.

Brabant, G., Prank, K., Ranft, U., Schuermeyer, T., Wagner, T.O., Hausser, H., Kummer, B., Feistner, H., Hesch, R.D., and von zur Muhlen, A. (1990). Physiological regulation of circadian and pulsatile thyrotropin secretion in normal man and woman. *J. Clin. Endocrinol. Metab.*, 70: 403–409.

Brandenberger, G., Follenius, M., Simon, C., Ehrhart, J., and Libert. J.P. (1988). Nocturnal oscillations in plasma renin activity and REM–NREM sleep cycles in humans: a common regulatory mechanisms? *Sleep*, 11: 242–250.

Brandenberger, G., Krauth, M.O., Ehrhart, J., Libert, J.P., Simon, C., and Follenius, M. (1990). Modulation of episodic renin release during sleep in humans. *Hypertension*, 15: 370–375.

Brandenberger, G., Follenius, M., Goichot, B., Saini, J., Spiegel, K., Ehrhart, J., and Simon, C. (1994). Twenty-four-hour profiles of plasma renin activity in relation to sleep–wake cycle. *J. Hypertens.*, 12: 277–283.

Brandenberger, G., Buguet, A., Spiegel, K., Stanghellini, A., Muanga, G., Bogui, P., and Dumas, M. (1996). Disruption of endocrine rhythms in sleeping sickness with preserved relationship between hormonal pulsatility and the REM–NREM sleep cycles. *J. Biol. Rhythms*, 11: 258–267.

Brandenberger, G., Gronfier, C., Chapotot, F., Simon, C., and Piquard, F. (2000). Effect of sleep deprivation on overall 24 h growth hormone secretion. *Lancet*, 356: 1408.

Brandenberger, G., Ehrhart, J., Piquard, F., and Simon, C. (2001). Inverse coupling between ultradian oscillations in delta wave activity and heart rate variability during sleep. *Clin. Neurophysiol.*, 112: 992–996.

Buijs, R. and Kalsbeek, A. (2001). Hypothalamic integration of central and peripheral clocks. *Nat. Rev.*, 2: 521–526.

Charloux, A., Gronfier, C., Lonsdorfer-Wolf, E., Piquard, F., and Brandenberger, G. (1999). Aldosterone release during the sleep–wake cycle in humans. *Am. J. Physiol.*, 276: 43–49.

Charloux, A., Gronfier, C., Chapotot, F., Ehrhart, J., Piquard, F., and Brandenberger, G. (2001). Sleep deprivation blunts the nighttime increase in aldosterone release in humans. *J. Sleep Res.*, 10: 27–33.

Charloux, A., Piquard, F., Ehrhart, J., Mettauer, B., Geny, B., Simon, C., and Brandenberger, G. (2002). Time-courses in renin and blood pressure during sleep in humans. *J. Sleep Res.*, 11: 73–79.

Czeisler, C.A. (1997). Commentary: evidence for melatonin as a circadian phase-shifting agent. *J. Biol. Rhythms*, 12: 618–623.

Czeisler, C.A. and Klermann, E.B. (1999). Circadian and sleep-dependent regulation of hormone release in humans. *Recent Prog. Horm. Res.*, 54: 94–130.

Dai, J.P., Swaab, D.F., and Buijs, R.M. (1998a). Recovery of axonal transport in "dead neurons". *Lancet*, 351: 499–500.

Dai, J.P., Swaab, D.F., Van der Viet, J., and Buijs, R.M. (1998b). Post-mortem tracing reveals the organization of hypothalamic projections of the suprachiasmatic nucleus in the human brain. *J. Comp. Neurol.*, 400: 87–102.

Dijk, D.J. and Kronauer, R.E. (1999). Commentary: models of sleep regulation: successes and continuous challenges. *J. Biol. Rhythms*, 14: 569–573.

Dijk, D.J., Brunner, D.P., Beersma, D.G.M., and Borbély, A.A. (1990). Slow wave sleep and electroencephalogram power density as a function of prior waking and circadian phase. *Sleep*, 13: 430–440.

Filicori, M., Santoro, N., Merriam, G.R., and Crowley, W.F. (1986). Characterization of the physiological pattern of episodic gonadotropin secretion throughout the human menstrual cycle. *J. Clin. Endocrinol. Metab.*, 62: 1136–1144.

Follenius, M., Krieger, J., Krauth, M.O., Sforza, F., and Brandenberger, G. (1991). Obstructive sleep apnea treatment: peripheral and central effects on plasma renin activity and aldosterone. *Sleep*, 14: 211–217.

Goichot, B., Brandenberger, G., Saini, Y., Wittersheim, G., and Follenius, M. (1992). Nocturnal plasma thyrotropin variations are related to slow-wave sleep. *J. Sleep Res.*, 1: 186–190.

Gronfier, C., Luthringer, R., Follenius, M., Schaltenbrand, N., Macher, J.P., Muzet, A., and Brandenberger, G. (1995). Temporal link between plasma thyrotropin levels and electroencephalographic activity in man. *Neurosci. Lett.*, 200: 97–100.

Gronfier, C., Luthringer, R., Follenius, M., Schaltenbrand, N., Macher, J.P., Muzet, A., and Brandenberger, G. (1996). A quantitative evaluation of the relationship between growth hormone secretion and delta wave electroencephalographic activity during normal sleep and after enrichment in delta waves. *Sleep*, 19: 817–824.

Gronfier, C., Chapotot, F., Weibel, L., Jouny, C., Piquard, F., and Brandenberger, G. (1998). Pulsatile cortisol secretion and EEG delta waves are controlled by two independent but synchronized generators. *Am. J. Physiol. Endocrinol. Metab.*, 275: 94–100.

Gronfier, C., Wright, K.P., and Czeisler, C.A. (2001). Growth hormone secretion during entrained and non-entrained conditions in humans. *Sleep*, 24: 89–90.

Hastings, M.H., Reddy, A.B., and Maywood, E.S. (2003). A clockwork web: circadian timing in brain and periphery, in health and disease. *Nat. Rev. Neurosci.*, 4: 649–661.

Ho, A.W., Gronfier, C., and Czeisler, C.A. (2001). Effect of prolonged sleep deprivation on cortisol secretion. *Sleep*, 24: A251–A252.

Hobson, J.A., McCarley, R.W., and Wyzincki, P.W. (1975). Sleep cycle oscillation: reciprocal discharge by two brainstem neuronal groups. *Science*, 189: 55–58.

Homburg, R., Eshel, A., Armar, N.A., Tucker, M., Mason, P.W., Adams, J., Kilborn, J., Sutherland, I.A., and Jacobs, H.S. (1989). One hundred pregnancies after treatment with pulsatile luteinising hormone releasing hormone to induce ovulation. *Br. Med. J.*, 298: 809–812.

Katz, F.H., Romfh, P., and Smith, J. (1972). Episodic secretion of aldosterone in supine man: relationship to cortisol. *J. Clin. Endocrinol. Metab.*, 35: 178–181.

Knobil, E. (1980). The neuroendocrine control of the menstrual cycle. *Recent Prog. Horm. Res.*, 36: 53–88.

Leproult, R., Copinschi, G., Buxton, O., and Van Cauter, E. (1997). Sleep loss results in an elevation of cortisol levels the next evening. *Sleep*, 20: 865–870.

Lewy, A.J. and Sack, R.L. (1989). The dim light melatonin onset as a marker for circadian phase position. *Chronobiol. Int.*, 6: 93–102.

Leyendecker, G., Struve, T., and Plotz, E.J. (1980). Induction of ovulation with chronic intermittent (pulsatile) administration of LH-RH in women with hypothalamic and hyperprolactinemic amenorrhea. *Arch. Gynecol.*, 229: 177–190.

Lightman, S.L., James, V.H.T., Linsell, C., Mullen, P.E., Peart, W.S., and Sever, P.S. (1981). Studies of diurnal changes in plasma renin activity and plasma noradrenaline, aldosterone and cortisol concentrations in man. *Clin. Endocrinol.*, 14: 213–223.

Luthringer, R., Brandenberger, G., Schaltenbrand, N., Muller, G., Spiegel, K., Macher, J.P., Muzet, A., and Follenius, M. (1995). Slow wave electroencephalographic activity parallels renin oscillations during sleep in humans. *Electroencephalogr. Clin. Neurophysiol.*, 95: 318–322.

Martin, K.A., Hall, J.E., Adams, J.M., and Crowley, W.F. (1990). Management of disorders with pulsatile gonadotropin-releasing hormone. *J. Clin. Endocrinol. Metab.*, 71: 1081R–1081G.

McCarley, R.W. and Massaquoi, S.G. (1992). Neurobiological structure of the revised limit cycle reciprocal interaction model of REM cycle control. *J. Sleep Res.*, 1: 132–137.

McCormick, D.A. and Bal, T. (1997). Sleep and arousal: thalamocortical mechanisms. *Annu. Rev. Neurosci.*, 20: 185–215.

Obal, F. and Krueger, J.M. (2001). The somatotropic axis and sleep. *Rev. Neurol. (Paris)*, 157: S12–S15.

Otzenberger, H., Gronfier, C., Simon, C., Charloux, A., Ehrhart, J., Piquard, F., and Brandenberger, G. (1998). Dynamic heart rate variability: a tool for exploring sympathovagal balance continuously during sleep in men. *Am. J. Physiol.*, 275: 946–950.

Pace-Schott, E. and Hobson, J. (2002). The neurobiology of sleep: genetics, cellular physiology and subcortical networks. *Nat. Rev.*, 3: 591–605.

Parker, D.C., Rossman, L.G., and Vanderlaan, E.F. (1974). Relation of sleep-entrained human prolactin release to REM–non-REM cycles. *J. Clin. Endocrinol. Metab.*, 38: 646–651.

Rosenthal, N.E. (1992). Editorial: plasma melatonin as measure of the human clock. *J. Clin. Endocrinol. Metab.*, 73: 225–226.

Saini, J., Krieger, J., Brandenberger, G., Wittersheim, G., Simon, C., and Follenius, M. (1993). Continuous positive airway pressure treatment. Effects on growth hormone, insulin and glucose profiles in obstructive sleep apnea patients. *Horm. Metab. Res.*, 25: 375–381.

Sassin, J.F., Parker, D.C., Mace, J.W., Grotlin, R.W., Johnson, L.C., and Rossman, L.G. (1969). Human growth hormone release: relation to slow-wave sleep and sleep–waking cycles. *Science*, 165: 513–515.

Sassin, J.F., Frantz, A.G., Kapen, S., and Weitzman, E.D. (1972). Human prolactin: 24 hour pattern with increased release during sleep. *Science*, 177: 1205–1207.

Schulz, H., Brandenberger, G., Gudewill, S., Hasse, D., Kiss, E., Löhr, K., Pollmächer, T., and Follenius, M. (1992). Plasma renin activity and sleep–wake structure of narcoleptic patients and control subjects under continuous bedrest. *Sleep*, 15: 423–429.

Shannahoff-Khalsa, D.S., Kennedy, B., Yates, F.E., and Ziegler, M.G. (1996). Ultradian rhythms of autonomic, cardiovascular, and neuroendocrine systems are related in humans. *Am. J. Physiol.*, 270: 873–887.

Spiegel, K., Follenius, M., Simon, C., Saini, J., Ehrhart, J., and Brandenberger, G. (1994). Prolactin secretion and sleep. *Sleep*, 17: 20–27.

Spiegel, K., Luthringer, R., Follenius, M., Schaltenbrand, N., Macher, J.P., Muzet, A., and Brandenberger, G. (1995). Temporal relationships between prolactin secretion and slow-wave electroencephalic activity during sleep. *Sleep*, 18: 543–548.

Spiegel, K., Leproult, R., and Van Cauter, E. (1999). Impact of sleep debt on metabolic and endocrine function. *Lancet*, 354: 1435–1439.

Spiegel, K., Leproult, R., Colecchia, E.F., L'Hermite-Baleriaux, M., Nie, Z., Copinschi, G., and Van Cauter, E. (2000). Adaptation of the 24-hr growth hormone profile to a state of sleep debt. *Am. J. Physiol.*, 279: 874–883.

Steiger, A., Herth, T., and Holsboer, F. (1987). Sleep-electroencephalography and the secretion of cortisol and growth hormone in normal controls. *Acta Endocrinol.*, 116: 36–42.

Steriade, M., McCormick, D.A., and Sejnowski, T.J. (1993). Thalamocortical oscillations in the sleeping and aroused brain. *Science*, 262: 679–685.

Steriade, M., Contreras, D., and Amzica, F. (1994). Synchronized sleep oscillations and their paraoxysmal developments. *Trends Neurosci.*, 17: 199–208.

Takahashi, Y., Kipnis, D.M., and Daughaday, W.H. (1968). Growth hormone secretion during sleep. *J. Clin. Invest.*, 47: 2079–2090.

Van Cauter, E. and Spiegel, K. (1999). Circadian and sleep control of hormonal secretion. In: Turek, F.W. and Zee, Ph.C. (Eds.). *Regulation of Sleep and Circadian Rhythms.* New York: Marcel Dekker, pp. 397–425.

Van Cauter, E., Désir, D., Refetoff, S., Spirc, J.P., Noel, P., L'Hermite, M., Robyn, C., and Copinschi, G. (1982). The relationship between episodic variations of plasma prolactin and REM–non-REM cyclicity is an artefact. *J. Clin. Endocrinol. Metab.*, 54: 70–75.

Van Cauter, E., Kerkhofs, M., Caufriez, A., Van Onderbergen, A., Thorner, M.O., and Copinschi, G. (1992). A quantitative estimation of growth hormone secretion in normal man: reproducibility and relation to sleep and time of day. *J. Clin. Endocrinol. Metab.*, 74: 1441–1450.

Van Cauter, E., Plat, L., Scharf, M.B., Leproult, R., Cespedes, S., L'Hermite-Balériaux, M., and Copinschi, G. (1997). Simultaneous stimulation of slow-wave sleep and growth hormone secretion by gamma-hydroxybutyrate in normal young men. *J. Clin. Invest.*, 100: 745–753.

Van Cauter, E., Plat, L., and Copinschi, G. (1998). Interrelations between sleep and the somatotropic axis. *Sleep*, 21: 553–566.

Van de Kar, L., Wilkinson, C.W., and Ganong, W.F. (1981). Pharmacological evidence for a role of brain serotonin in the maintenance of plasma renin activity in unanesthetized rats. *J. Pharmacol. Exp. Ther.*, 219: 85–90.

Van de Kar, L., Urban, J.H., Brownfield, M.S., and Simmons, W.H. (1987). Partial characterization of a renin-releasing factor from plasma and hypothalamus. *Hypertension*, 9: 598–606.

Vanoli, E., Adamson, P.B., Ba-Lin, M.S., Pinna, G.D., Lozzara, R., and Orr, W.C. (1995). Heart rate variability during specific sleep stages, a comparison of healthy subjects with patients after myocardial infarction. *Circulation*, 91: 1918–1922.

Vaughn, B.V., Quint, S.R., Messenheimer, J.A., and Robertson, K.R. (1995). Heart rate variability in sleep. *Electroencephalogr. Clin. Neurophysiol.*, 94: 155–162.

Weaver, D.R. (1999). Melatonin and circadian rhythmicity in vertebrates. In: Turek, F.W. and Zee, Ph.C. (Eds.). *Regulation of Sleep and Circadian Rhythms.* New York: Marcel Dekker, pp. 397–425.

Wehr, T.A. (1996). A "clock for all seasons" in the human brain. In: Buijs, R.M., Kalsbeek, A., Romihn, J.H., Pennartz, C.M.A., and Mirmiran, M. (Eds.). *Progress in Brain Research.* Amsterdam: Elsevier, pp. 91–104.

Weibel, L., Spiegel, K., Follenius, M., Ehrhart, J., and Brandenberger, G. (1996). Internal dissociation of the circadian markers of the cortisol rhythm in regular night workers. *Am. J. Physiol. Endocrinol. Metab.*, 270: 608–613.

Weibel, L., Spiegel, K., Gronfier, C., Follenius, M., and Brandenberger, G. (1997). 24-hour melatonin and core body temperature rhythms: their adaptation in night workers. *Am. J. Physiol.*, 272: 948–954.

Weitzman, E.D., Zimmerman, J.C., Czeisler, C.A., and Ronda, J. (1983). Cortisol secretion is inhibited during sleep in normal man. *J. Clin. Endocrinol. Metab.*, 56: 352–358.

Zemaitytë, D., Varoneckas, G., and Sokolov, E. (1984). Heart rhythm control during sleep. *Psychophysiology*, 2: 279–289.

Chapter 21

THE USE OF MELATONIN AS A CHRONOBIOTIC-CYTOPROTECTIVE AGENT IN SLEEP DISORDERS

Daniel P. Cardinali[1]

Melatonin is produced in most organisms from algae to mammals, and its role varies considerably across the phylogenetic spectra (Reiter *et al.*, 2001). In humans it plays a major function in the coordination of circadian rhythmicity, remarkably the sleep–wake cycle (Cardinali and Pevet, 1998; Kennaway and Wright, 2002). The circadian rhythm of melatonin is generated by the central pacemaker located in the suprachiasmatic nuclei (SCN) of the hypothalamus, and like many other circadian rhythms, it is synchronized to a 24-h period largely by cues from the light–dark cycle received via the retino-hypothalamic pathway to the SCN.

The evening increase in melatonin secretion is associated with an increase in the propensity for sleep (Lavie, 2001). Secretion of melatonin during the day, as occurs in diverse pathological or occupational health situations, is strongly associated with daytime sleepiness or napping, and the administration of melatonin during the day induces sleepiness (Zhdanova *et al.*, 2001).

Melatonin Acts as an Endocrine Arm of the Circadian Clock

Melatonin secretion is an "arm" of the biologic clock in the sense that it responds to signals from the SCN and in that the timing of the melatonin

---

[1] dcardinali@fmed.uba.ar

rhythm indicates the status of the clock, both in terms of phase (i.e., internal clock time relative to external clock time) and amplitude. From another point of view, melatonin is also a chemical code of night: the longer the night, the longer the duration of its secretion. In many species, this pattern of secretion serves as a time cue for seasonal rhythms (Cardinali and Pevet, 1998).

Daily timed administration of melatonin to rats shifts the phase of the circadian clock, and this phase shifting may partly explain melatonin effect on sleep in humans, or "chronobiotic effect" (Dawson and Armstrong, 1996). Indirect support for such a physiological role derived from clinical studies on blind subjects showing free running of their circadian rhythms while a more direct support for this hypothesis was provided by the demonstration that the phase response curve for melatonin was opposite (i.e., 180° out of phase) to that of light (Lewy *et al.*, 1998; Kennaway and Wright, 2002).

Melatonin (in a dose of 3–5 mg daily, timed to advance the phase of the internal clock) can maintain synchronization of the circadian rhythm to a 24-h cycle in sighted persons who are living in conditions likely to induce a free-running rhythm, and it synchronizes the rhythm in some persons after a short period of free-running. In blind subjects with free-running rhythms, it has been possible to stabilize, or entrain, the sleep–wake cycle to a 24-h period by giving melatonin, with resulting improvements in sleep and mood (Skene *et al.*, 1999). In normal aged subjects (Cardinali *et al.*, 2002c) and in demented patients with desynchronization of sleep–wake cycle (Cardinali *et al.*, 2002b) melatonin administration is helpful to reduce the variation of onset time of sleep. The phase shifting effects of melatonin were also sufficient to explain its effectivity as a treatment for circadian-related sleep disorders such as jet lag or the delayed phase sleep syndrome (Cardinali *et al.*, 2002a; Arendt, 2003; Beaumont *et al.*, 2004).

Melatonin Administration Induces Sleep in Healthy Subjects

The promoting effect of exogenous melatonin administration on sleep and sedation has been known since long. Shortly after the isolation and characterization of melatonin, Lerner and Case (1960) established that the intravenous administration of 80 mg of melatonin increased self-reported sleepiness in two young adults. Initial studies addressing the effect of melatonin on sleep made use of the i.v. or the intranasal route (Anton-Tay, 1974; Cramer *et al.*, 1974; Vollrath *et al.*, 1981) or administered very large doses of the methoxyindole by the oral route (Anton-Tay, 1974; Lieberman *et al.*, 1984). From these early studies it was concluded that melatonin reduces sleep latency and induces sleepiness and fatigue. Such effect of melatonin is probably the consequence of increasing sleep propensity (by inducing a fall in body temperature) and of the synchronizing effect on the circadian clock above mentioned (chronobiotic effect). A dose of 5 mg of melatonin at 14:00 hours significantly reduced sleep onset latency and reduced core body temperature, the decline being due to an increase in peripheral heat loss and a reduction in heat production (Holmes *et al.*, 2002). Typically, the thermoregulatory effect of melatonin arises immediately after melatonin administration while the second one needs some days (or weeks) to develop.

More recently, the effect of lower doses of melatonin were examined. These studies included young normal volunteers and patients with insomnia of different origins. In most instances melatonin significantly improved subjective and/or objective sleep parameters. Melatonin 0.3 or 1 mg p.o. significantly reduced sleep latency and increased sleep efficiency in normal volunteers (Zhdanova *et al.*, 1995, 1996). In contrast, a 5-mg dose did not modify sleep induction or maintenance (James *et al.*, 1987). In healthy nocturnal young subjects, oral administration of exogenous melatonin before going to bed increased stage 2 sleep significantly, with slight hypothermic action (Shirakawa *et al.*, 2001). The effect of a high melatonin dose (80 mg p.o.), when tested in subjects with insomnia induced by exposure to recorded traffic noise, was a reduction of sleep latency and of the number of awakening episodes and the increase of stage 2 sleep and sleep efficiency (Waldhauser *et al.*, 1990).

Administered during the day to normal volunteers melatonin (1–40 mg) significantly reduced sleep latency and increased total sleep time (Nave *et al.*, 1995; Badia *et al.*, 1996; Reid *et al.*, 1996). In addition, sleep-onset latency, oral temperature, and the number of correct responses on the Wilkinson vigilance task decreased significantly (Dollins *et al.*, 1994). Administration of melatonin previous to the nap in subjects who were partially sleep deprived and allowed a 4-h nap starting at 13:00 hours did not significantly modify sleep induction or maintenance (Dijk *et al.*, 1995).

After the administration of a 5-mg dose of melatonin p.o. at either 13:00 or 18:00 hours sleepiness increased significantly as well as theta/alpha frequencies of waking EEG (Cajochen *et al.*, 1996). Alertness and performance decreased following the morning melatonin administration to healthy young individuals, an effect that lasted for 6 h (Graw *et al.*, 2001). Melatonin (0.1, 0.5, and 5 mg p.o.) decreased wake time after sleep onset and increased feelings of sleepiness and fatigue in the late afternoon (17:00–21:00 hours) in healthy volunteers (Terlo *et al.*, 1997). When melatonin (0.1–10 mg) was administered at 11:45 hours all doses significantly increased sleep duration and self-reported sleepiness and fatigue.

Assessment of the hypnotic action of melatonin during daytime administration and its comparison with triazolam indicated that a 6-mg dose of melatonin had hypnotic effects that were nearly equal to those of 0.125 mg of triazolam. Rectal temperature was significantly decreased by melatonin (Satomura *et al.*, 2001). In another placebo-controlled and double-blind study with a cross-over design including temazepam (20 mg), the hypnotic activity of melatonin at early evening (presumably in the absence of endogenous melatonin) was similar to that of temazepam (Gilbert *et al.*, 1999; Stone *et al.*, 2000). These data in humans reproduced previous findings in rodents (Golombek *et al.*, 1993).

It has been contended that high pharmacological doses of melatonin are needed to improve sleep of normal volunteers during nighttime (Lavie, 1997). However, an important question, not yet adequately solved, concerns as to what "physiological" means in terms of intracerebral melatonin levels (Reiter and Tan, 2003) The levels of a lipophilic substance like melatonin reaching neurons under physiological conditions may differ considerably from circulating hormone concentration. In sheep, third ventricle cerebrospinal fluid (CSF) melatonin concentration was 20-fold higher than concomitant plasma values (Skinner and Malpaux, 1999; Tricoire *et al.*, 2002, 2003). In 12-month old mice 6-sulphatoxymelatonin concentration was approximately 1000-fold greater than that of melatonin in the cerebral cortex (Lahiri *et al.*, 2004b).

Exogenous Melatonin is Useful to Improve Slow Wave Sleep in Aged Subjects Suffering Insomnia

Melatonin levels in the pineal gland declines with age, such that in elderly humans the levels of melatonin available to the organism are a fraction of that of young individuals (Iguchi *et al.*, 1982). Hence a feasible situation in which melatonin may have a beneficial effect is age-related insomnia.

The effect of melatonin on the polysomnographic sleep of insomniac patients was assessed in a number of studies. Melatonin (1 or 5 mg, 15 min before bedtime for one night) did not modify variables related to sleep induction and maintenance (James *et al.*, 1990; Ellis *et al.*, 1996). It must be noted that in these studies subject population under placebo showed low sleep efficiency (about 85%); hence any possible effect of melatonin could have been limited by a ceiling effect.

In middle-aged and elderly insomniacs who made use of immediate-release (0.5 mg) and controlled release (0.5 mg) preparations of melatonin 30 min before bedtime, polysomnographic recordings and sleep actigraphy showed that melatonin shortened latencies to persistent sleep (Hughes *et al.*, 1998). There was no correlation between prior melatonin production and responsiveness to melatonin replacement.

Administration of a 3-mg dose of melatonin during 14 nights to elderly patients with chronic primary insomnia brought about a significant reduction in wake time after sleep onset while total sleep time and sleep efficiency increased, with an increase of stage 2 sleep (Monti *et al.*, 1999). No correlation was found between prior 6-sulphatoxymelatonin levels in urine and subsequent sleep improvement after receiving melatonin.

Although, in general, the urinary excretion of 6-sulphatoxymelatonin correlated negatively and significantly with age, but not with intensity of sleep disorder or outcome of treatment, a recent observation in 517 insomniac patients did indicate a reduction in urinary 6-sulphatoxymelatonin as compared to controls (Leger *et al.*, 2004). Those patients with the lowest melatonin production were those more responsive to exogenous melatonin treatment (Leger *et al.*, 2004). Diminished melatonin secretion in the elderly has been associated with insufficient environmental illumination (Mishima *et al.*, 2001).

In studies monitoring sleep quality by wrist actigraphy in elderly insomniacs, controlled-release melatonin (2 mg) taken 2 h before the desired bedtime during 3 weeks reduced sleep latency and wake time after sleep onset and increased total sleep time and sleep efficiency (Garfinkel *et al.*, 1995). Melatonin (3 mg) administered 30 min before the expected bedtime for 21 nights to patients with chronic insomnia significantly improved sleep quality and decreased the number of awakenings from day 2–3 of treatment (Fainstein *et al.*, 1997). A sustained-release preparation of melatonin (2 mg) improved sleep initiation, with further improvement of sleep initiation and sleep maintenance after 2 months (Haimov and Lavie, 1995). Insomniac patients receiving 75 mg melatonin at 22:00 hours for seven consecutive nights reported improved subjective sleep time and subjective daytime alertness (MacFarlane *et al.*, 1991). Low amounts of melatonin (0.3 mg) given during three nights to middle-aged and elderly patients with chronic insomnia reduced sleep latency, the number of nocturnal awakenings and body movements per night, whereas core temperature remained unchanged (Zhdanova *et al.*, 2001). In medically ill persons with initial insomnia receiving 5.4 mg melatonin or placebo, double-blind assessments of aspects of sleep indicated that melatonin significantly hastened sleep onset, improved quality and depth of sleep, and increased sleep duration (Andrade *et al.*, 2001). In a study aimed to explore the effects of melatonin on sleep, waking up and well being in subjects with varying degrees of seasonal or weather-associated changes in mood and behavior, 2 mg of sustained-release melatonin significantly improved the quality of sleep and vitality in seasonal affective disorder patients but attenuated the improvement of atypical symptoms and physical parameters of quality of life compared to placebo in the subjects with weather-associated changes (Leppamaki *et al.*, 2003). Melatonin was recently shown to be very effective to restore rapid eye movement (REM) sleep in patients with REM sleep deficiency (Kunz *et al.*, 2004).

It must be noted that melatonin effects on sleep are not universally seen. In a double blind randomized placebo controlled cross-over trial in healthy older volunteers (20 normal and 20 problem sleepers), 5 mg of melatonin or matching placebo were given at bedtime for 4 weeks, separated by a 4-week washout period (Baskett *et al.*, 2003). Sleep quality was measured using sleep diaries, the Leeds Sleep Evaluation Questionnaire, and actigraphy. There was a significant difference between the groups in self-reported sleep quality indicators at entry, but no difference in melatonin secretion. Melatonin did not significantly improve any sleep parameter measured in either group (Baskett *et al.*, 2003). Another negative observation was recently published in 10 patients who met the DSM-IV criteria for primary insomnia received using 0.3 or 1.0 mg of melatonin for 7 days or placebo 60 min before bedtime (Almeida Montes *et al.*, 2003). There were no significant differences in sleep EEG, the amount or subjective quality of sleep or side effects between the placebo and melatonin. The very short time of melatonin administration should be considered in interpreting these observations (Almeida Montes *et al.*, 2003).

Administration of melatonin (3 mg p.o.) for up to 6 months did not affect circulating prolactin, follicle-stimulating hormone (FSH), thyroid-stimulating hormone (TSH) or estradiol, nor were any indications of hematological or blood biochemistry alteration found, in elderly insomniac females (Siegrist *et al.*, 2001). In a study assessing the acute effect of melatonin (1 mg) on serum PRL, luteinizing hormone, FSH, growth hormone (GH), and TSH, only levels of PRL were stimulated (Ninomiya *et al.*, 2001). Melatonin augmented sleep quality and duration, and decreased sleep latency and the number of awakening episodes; estimates of next-day function also improved significantly (Siegrist *et al.*, 2001). The urinary excretion of 6-sulphatoxymelatonin before starting administration of melatonin correlated negatively and significantly with age but not with intensity of sleep disorder or outcome of treatment. In another study blood parameters were not affected by a dose of 10 mg of melatonin for 28 days (Seabra *et al.*, 2000).

It is interesting to note that melatonin can facilitate discontinuation of benzodiazepine therapy while maintaining good sleep quality. This can be helpful in the elderly in view of the contraindications for a prolonged use of benzodiazepine at this age. In aged subjects, sleep disturbance is complex and often difficult to relieve because the physiologic parameters of sleep normally change with age (Pandi-Perumal *et al.*, 2002). Since any long-term use of benzodiazepines should be avoided, particularly in the elderly, appropriate strategies to decrease or to halt benzodiazepine use should be welcome. A number of animal studies indicated that several behavioral effects of melatonin can be suppressed by inhibiting central benzodiazepine receptors (Golombek *et al.*, 1992, 1996; Wang *et al.*, 2003). Indeed melatonin and benzodiazepines share several properties, remarkable anxiolytic effects, and therefore melatonin could be useful to help patients to discontinue benzodiazepine treatment. In one study, 14 out of 18 subjects under benzodiazepine therapy receiving melatonin (2 mg in a controlled-release formulation) discontinued benzodiazepine therapy and after a 6-month follow-up assessment of the 24 patients who discontinued benzodiazepine and received melatonin therapy, 19 maintained good sleep quality (Garfinkel *et al.*, 1999). In another study, 13 of 20 patients taking benzodiazepines together with melatonin, benzodiazepine use could be stopped, and in another four patients, benzodiazepine dose could be decreased to 25–66% of the initial dose (Siegrist *et al.*, 2001).

Many times, old patients with minor or none sleep disturbance received, on a long-term basis, anxiolytic benzodiazepines in low doses for relief of a disturbance that has numerous, often concurrent etiologies, including medical conditions, medication or poor sleep hygiene (Pandi-Perumal *et al.*, 2002). Recently we carried out a study to assess whether melatonin could be useful to reduce low benzodiazepine dosage in this group of patients, as it is in insomniac patients treated with hypnotic benzodiazepines (Cardinali *et al.*, 2002c). A double blind-placebo controlled study on the efficacy of a 3 mg melatonin dose p.o. was undertaken. The possible correlation of urinary excretion of 6-sulphatoxymelatonin before starting treatment and outcome of treatment was also examined. The results indicated that melatonin lacked to affect subjective assessment of wakefulness or sleep in this group of patients with minor sleep disturbance. The only effect that melatonin had in this group of patients was to advance sleep onset and to decrease significantly the variability of sleep onset time as compared to placebo (Cardinali *et al.*, 2002c). Indeed, melatonin efficacy to reduce variability of the sleep onset time was first described in demented patients exhibiting sundowning (Fainstein *et al.*, 1997) and is the basis for the indication of melatonin as an effective therapy of sundowning in Alzheimer's disease (AD), as discussed below.

Melatonin is Useful in Other Types of Insomnia

Melatonin was found helpful in sleep disturbance liked to restless legs syndrome (Kunz and Bes, 2001) and Gilles de la Tourette syndrome (Ayalon *et al.*, 2002) as well as in parasomnia-like REM sleep behavior disorder (Kunz and Bes, 1999; Takeuchi *et al.*, 2001). Typically, circadian sleep disorders like delayed sleep phase syndrome and non-24-h sleep–wake syndromes can be treated with melatonin (Kamei *et al.*, 2000; Lockley *et al.*, 2000; Nagtegaal *et al.*, 2000; Yang *et al.*, 2001). Melatonin is regarded as the most beneficial therapy to treat sleep disturbances found in mucopolysaccharidosis type III (Sanfilippo syndrome) (Dijk and Lockley, 2002; Fraser *et al.*, 2002) and in the Angelman syndrome (Zhdanova *et al.*, 1999; Galvan *et al.*, 2002), as well as in postoperative delirium (Hanania and Kitain, 2002).

Melatonin improves sleep quality of patients with treatment-resistant depression (Dalton *et al.*, 2000). However, as it was observed previously (Fainstein *et al.*, 1997), depression itself is not modified by melatonin treatment. Melatonin can be also useful for sleep disturbances in manic patients with treatment resistant insomnia (Bersani and Garavini, 2000) and in patients with fibromyalgia (Citera *et al.*, 2000). Melatonin improved sleep in intensive care patients (Shilo *et al.*, 2000), a finding that is correlated with data indicating that patients with coronary disease had a low melatonin production rate, with higher decreases in those with higher risk of cardiac infarction (Girotti *et al.*, 2000).

Another promising field of application for melatonin is that of sleep disorders in children. There is a high prevalence of chronic sleep–wake cycle disorders in developmentally and neurologically disabled children. Such disorders are often resistant to hypnotic and psychotropic drugs. Administration of exogenous melatonin can have an effect upon the circadian rhythm and establish a normal sleep–wake cycle. Reported results generally indicate that melatonin improves sleep–wake cycle disorders in children. Observations included patients with childhood sleep onset insomnia (Jan *et al.*, 2001; Smits *et al.*, 2001; Wassmer *et al.*, 2001), children with attention deficit/hyperactivity disorder (Tjon Pian Gi *et al.*, 2003) and children with sleep disorders linked to developmental disabilities (Zhdanova *et al.*, 1999; Hayashi, 2000; Jan *et al.*, 2000; Pillar *et al.*, 2000; Ross *et al.*, 2002; Paavonen *et al.*, 2003). Melatonin has been reported recently to reduce oxidative stress in neonates with sepsis, asphyxia, and respiratory distress (Gitto *et al.*, 2004). It must be noted that majority of studies were open, and knowledge about side effects and long-term effects is limited.

A meta-analysis on the efficacy of melatonin to prevent and treat jet-lag indicated that melatonin, taken close to the target bedtime at the destination, decreased effectively jet-lag from flights crossing five or more time zones (Herxheimer and Petrie, 2001). We recently demonstrated that a combination of melatonin treatment, an appropriate environmental light schedule and timely applied physical exercise was useful to help elite athletes to overcome the consequences of jet-lag after a transmeridian flight of 12 time zones (Cardinali *et al.*, 2002a).

Melatonin Curtails Major Processes in Neuronal Damage

Neurons are selectively vulnerable to injury and death due to their high energy demand and their specific chemical composition. The neuronal death or damage often leads to the loss and/or disruption of the subjects' behaviors and/or physiological functions crucial to normal living. Many acute conditions, e.g., hypoxia, stroke, physical trauma, hypoglycemia, drug neurotoxicity, viruses, radiation, or noxious stimuli, are sufficient to produce neuronal damage. Similar mechanisms are also likely to be involved in neurodegenerative disorders, a group of chronic and progressive diseases that are characterized by selective and symmetric loss of neurons in motor, sensory, or cognitive systems. Clinically relevant examples of these disorders are AD, Parkinson's disease, amyotrophic lateral sclerosis and Huntington's chorea (Martin, 1999).

Although the origin of neurodegenerative diseases mostly remained undefined, three major processes — glutamate excitotoxicity, free radical-mediated nerve injury and apoptosis — have been identified as common physiopathological mechanisms leading to neuronal death (Reiter, 1998). Melatonin is an oxygen radical scavenger and lipid antioxidant and on these bases it has been proposed as a neuroprotective agent against excitotoxicity. Studies employing kainate, an agonist of ionotropic glutamate receptors, gave support to the hypothesis that melatonin prevents neuronal death induced by glutamate (Giusti *et al.*, 1995, 1996).

It has also been reported that administration of melatonin reduces the injury of hippocampal CA1 neurons caused by transient forebrain ischemia (Cho *et al.*, 1997; Kilic *et al.*, 1999). In addition, there is a more severe brain damage and neurodegeneration after stroke or excitotoxic seizures in melatonin-deficient rats (Manev *et al.*, 1996), suggesting that melatonin deficiency potentiates neuronal damage.

The reactive oxygen species (free radicals), e.g., $O_2^{\bullet-}$ (superoxide anion radical), $^\bullet OH$ (hydroxyl radical), $^\bullet NO_2$ (peroxynitrite anion radical), can damage lipid, protein, and DNA, and can result ultimately in injury and cellular death (Reiter *et al.*, 2002). Normally, free radicals exhibit a very short life and are processed enzymatically or scavenged before they can inflict damage to the cell. Endogenous antioxidant defenses include the antioxidant enzyme superoxide dismutase, which dismutates $O_2^{\bullet-}$ to H_2O_2, and the enzymes glutathione peroxidase and catalase, which clear H_2O_2. A condition of "oxidative stress" occurs when there is an imbalance in favor of free radical generation relative to elimination, such that an increase in oxidative damage may occur. This condition occurs during a variety of brain insults in which free radical are generated and/or antioxidant defenses are impaired. For example, under conditions of neural trauma, iron released from stores may catalyze oxygen radical reactions leading to increased generation of $^\bullet OH$, a potent initiator of lipid peroxidation (Reiter *et al.*, 2002).

In the context of oxidative stress, the brain is particularly vulnerable to injury since it is enriched with phospholipids and proteins that are sensitive to oxidative damage, and may not possess high levels of antioxidant defence enzymes. Furthermore, the iron content of certain brain regions, e.g., substantia nigra, is high relative to other tissues. Indeed, free radical-mediated injury may not be a causative factor in some brain disorders, but it certainly plays a permissive role in the severity of the disease (Reiter, 1998).

Melatonin protects against focal cerebral ischemia mainly via its potent direct and indirect antioxidant effects. Melatonin scavenges the highly toxic hydroxyl radical, the peroxynitrite anion, and possibly the peroxyl radical. Also, secondarily, it reportedly scavenges the superoxide anion radical and it quenches singlet oxygen. Additionally, melatonin stimulates mRNA levels for superoxide dismutase and the activities of glutathione peroxidase, glutathione reductase and glucose-6-phosphate dehydrogenase (all of which are antioxidative enzymes) (Reiter *et al.*, 2002; Rodriguez *et al.*, 2004). Likewise, melatonin inhibits nitric oxide synthase, a pro-oxidative enzyme. In both *in vivo* and *in vitro* experiments, melatonin has been shown to reduce lipid peroxidation and oxidative damage to nuclear DNA. Melatonin also possesses other beneficial effects, e.g., it improves electron transport chain, reduces mitochondrial oxidative damage, increases ATP production, and modulates mitochondrial energy metabolism (Acuna-Castroviejo *et al.*, 2001; Reyes Toso *et al.*, 2003).

Overproduction of free radicals is an important mechanism of the ischemic necrosis typical of stroke. Melatonin has been found to have protective effects in various models of brain ischemia (Pei *et al.*, 2002, 2003). The efficacy of melatonin in inhibiting oxidative damage has also been tested in a variety of neurological disease models where free radicals have been implicated as being in part causative of the condition. Thus, melatonin has been shown to reduce amyloid β protein toxicity of AD (Pappolla *et al.*, 1997), to reduce oxidative damage in several models of Parkinson's disease (Jin *et al.*, 1998; Dabbeni-Sala *et al.*, 2001; Zisapel, 2001; Chuang and Chen, 2004), to protect against glutamate excitotoxicity (Giusti *et al.*, 1995, 1996; Yalcin *et al.*, 2004), to lower neural damage due to δ-aminolevulinic acid (porphyria) (Carneiro and Reiter, 1998; Tomas-Zapico *et al.*, 2002), hyperbaric hyperoxia (Shaikh *et al.*, 1997), brain trauma (Beni *et al.*, 2004), γ-radiation (Erol *et al.*, 2004), focal ischemia (Dupuis *et al.*, 2004; Lee *et al.*, 2004; Torii *et al.*, 2004) and a variety of neural toxins (Reiter, 1998).

Concerning the third mechanism leading to neuronal death, i.e., apoptosis, it is defined by a programmed cell death that does not involve necrosis, inflammation, or reactive gliosis. Apoptotic neuronal death needs RNA and protein synthesis, and depletion of trophic factors. Apoptosis also involves breaks of unique DNA strands, which is probably caused by increased oxidative stress. Neurotrophic factors have been found to rescue neurons from this type of death. They may act via cellular anti-apoptotic components, like the B cell lymphoma proto-oncogene protein (Bcl-2). In the central nervous system, the neuroprotective function of Bcl-2 is particularly well demonstrated in naturally occurring or experimentally induced neuronal death, that can be prevented by overexpression of Bcl-2 (Dubois-Dauphin *et al.*, 1994). Bcl-2 may be an antioxidant and is capable of blocking the apoptotic pathway by preventing the release of the mitochondrial enzyme cytochrome *c* (Kluck *et al.*, 1997). *In vitro* studies indicate that melatonin enhances expression of Bcl-2 and prevents apoptosis (Shen *et al.*, 2002; Yoo *et al.*, 2002; Jiao *et al.*, 2004).

Therefore, data have been collected indicating that melatonin may curtail all three major processes in neuronal damage, i.e., glutamate excitotoxicity, free radical-mediated nerve injury and apoptosis. In addition, melatonin acting as an endocrine arm of the circadian clock, promotes the restorative phases of sleep, a situation associated with neurotrophic effects. Thus melatonin may constitute a unique chronobiotic-cytoprotective agent.

Clinical Application: Melatonin, Sleep, and Alzheimer's Disease

Approximately 4.5–5 million Argentines (13–15% of the national population) are 65 years or older. Approximately 450,000 Argentines are currently afflicted with AD and this number is expected to increase three- to four-fold over the next 50 years. Cross-sectional studies report that about 40% of AD patients have disruptions in their sleep (Carpenter *et al.*, 1995; McCurry *et al.*, 2000). Indeed, older people with dementia at some point in their illness develop behavioral disturbances such as wandering, sleep disturbance and agitation. Collectively, these are termed "behavioral symptoms of dementia."

AD patients show a greater breakdown of the circadian sleep–wake cycle compared to similarly aged, non-demented controls. Demented patients spend their nights in a state of frequent restlessness and their days in a state of frequent sleepiness. These sleep–wake disturbances become increasingly more marked with progression of the disease. The sleep–wake disturbances in elderly people and particularly AD patients may result from changes at different levels: reduction of environmental synchronizers or their perception, lack of mental and physical activity, and age- or disease-related anatomical changes with loss of functionality of the circadian clock.

When sleep disturbances do occur, they constitute a significant physical and psychological stress for the caregiver and are frequently related to patient institutionalization. A very fragmented sleep–wake pattern occurs in AD. Increased duration and frequency of awakenings and daytime napping and decreased non-REM and to a less extent REM sleep, characterize the sleep of AD patients (Vitiello *et al.*, 1990). Cross-sectional studies have shown that sleep disturbances are associated with increased memory impairment in AD patients, as well as with more rapid cognitive decline (McCurry *et al.*, 2000). For these reasons, optimization in management of sleep disturbances is a treatment priority for AD patients.

In AD patients with disturbed sleep–wake rhythms, there is a higher degree of irregularities in melatonin secretion (Mishima *et al.*, 1999). An impairment of melatonin secretion is present that is related to both age and severity of mental impairment. The suppressed nocturnal GH and the increase of both the mean levels and nadir values of plasma cortisol are also related to mental impairments (Magri *et al.*, 1997, 2004). Shifts in the basic circadian sleep wake rhythm of dementia patients can be severe, and in extreme cases may lead to complete day/night sleep pattern reversals.

After excluding treatable causes such as concurrent infections, non-pharmacological approaches are the recommended first line intervention in AD patients with sleep disturbances. In AD patients, controlling sleep–wake disturbances with sedative drugs often increases both sleep disturbance and cognitive dysfunction. In practice, however, drugs such as neuroleptics and other sedatives are often prescribed in an attempt to control what can be an alarming situation (McCurry *et al.*, 2000). However, the chronic use of benzodiazepines to treat sleep in AD patients is associated with risk, since the use of sedative hypnotics can result in habituation and drug-induced insomnia, without significant improvements in daytime function (Kripke, 2000). Therefore, new developments in pharmacological strategies to treat sleep disorder in AD are needed.

Clinical findings strongly argue in favor of disruption of the circadian timing system in AD (Hoogendijk *et al.*, 1996; Giubilei *et al.*, 2001; Harper *et al.*, 2001). Dementia is associated with circadian rhythm disturbances expressed in several dimensions including body temperature, hormonal concentrations and rest–activity cycles. Circadian alterations are detectable at an advanced stage of AD, with large acrophases between rest activity and core body temperature rhythms and reduced rhythm amplitudes and nocturnal rest, indicating a diminished capacity to synchronize body rhythms with behavior (Satlin *et al.*, 1995). Loss or damage of neurons in the hypothalamic SCN and other parts of the circadian timing system have been implicated in the circadian disturbances of demented patients (Swabb *et al.*, 1985; van Someren, 2000; Skene and Swaab, 2003). There are reports that the expression of vasopressin is preferentially lost from the SCN in AD (Liu *et al.*, 2000) and that light therapy prevents the age-related loss of vasopressin expressing neurons in the rat (Lucassen *et al.*, 1995). The SCN of AD patients have tangles (Stopa *et al.*, 1999) indicating that the SCN is affected by AD. However, diffuse amyloid plaques are only seldom noted in this nucleus. The data mentioned above support the idea that damage to the SCN may be the underlying anatomical substrate for the disturbances in circadian rhythmicity observed in AD. A substantial proportion of both nursing home residents with nighttime incontinence and frail geriatric patients experience a reversal of the normal diurnal pattern of urine excretion (Ouslander *et al.*, 1998). The circadian rhythm in blood pressure has been reported to be preserved in the early stages of AD, but is disrupted in advanced or institutionalized patients (Cugini *et al.*, 1999).

The decreased secretion of melatonin with aging is well documented (Iguchi *et al.*, 1982; Dori *et al.*, 1994; Girotti *et al.*, 2000; Mishima *et al.*,

2000, 2001; Luboshitzky *et al.*, 2001; Siegrist *et al.*, 2001) and more profound reductions are reported in populations with dementia (Skene *et al.*, 1990; Uchida *et al.*, 1996; Liu *et al.*, 1999; Mishima *et al.*, 1999; Ohashi *et al.*, 1999; Ferrari *et al.*, 2000). Moreover, a significantly positive correlation between the abnormalities of rest-activity cycle and decrease in melatonin secretion occurs (Mishima *et al.*, 2000), although not uniformly (Baskett *et al.*, 2001). An increased melatonin MT1 receptor immunoreactivity signal was reported in the hippocampus of AD patients and was attributed to the up-regulation of the receptor as a compensatory response to impaired melatonin levels (Savaskan *et al.*, 2002). In a recent study, melatonin levels were determined in ventricular postmortem CSF of 121 subjects (Zhou *et al.*, 2003). Melatonin levels were significantly decreased in the aged individuals with early neuropathological changes in the temporal cortex, where the AD process starts. Indeed, the decrease in CSF melatonin levels may be an early event in the development of AD, possibly occurring even before the clinical symptoms (Zhou *et al.*, 2003).

In patients who lack serum melatonin rhythms, clinical symptoms of delirium and sleep–wake disturbance were frequently but not always observed (Uchida *et al.*, 1996). Thus, an impairment of melatonin secretion is present that is related to both age and severity of mental impairment. Although AD patients appear to have diminished pineal function, no evidence has been observed in this structure of neurofibrillary tangles, the accumulation of neurofilaments, tau, hyperphosphorylated tau or β amyloid deposition in pinealocytes (Pardo *et al.*, 1990).

A chronobiological phenomenon in AD related to the sleep disturbances is "sundowning." Symptoms of sundowning agitation include a reduced ability to maintain attention to external stimuli, disorganized thinking and speech, a variety of motor disturbances including agitation, wandering and repetitious physical behaviors, and perceptual and emotional disturbances (Taylor *et al.*, 1997). The delirium-like symptoms associated with sundowning are usually more prevalent in the late afternoon to early evening. Medication toxicity, infection, electrolytic disturbance, or environmental factors can all be triggers for sundowning. A chronobiological approach with bright-light therapy, restricted time in bed, and diurnal activity may be an interesting therapeutic alternative in the management of sleep–wake disorders in AD patients. The aim of these therapeutics is to improve sleep and diurnal activity and consequently to increase the quality of life in AD patients (McGaffigan and Bliwise, 1997; Mishima *et al.*, 2000). However, there is a very significant risk of retinal damage from repetitious exposure to the high intensities of visible light provided by bright-light units in this population since a substantial number of studies have indicated that age related macular degeneration is the result of natural aging processes exacerbated by the cumulative effects of photo-oxidative damage (Beatty *et al.*, 2000; Cai *et al.*, 2000; Barron *et al.*, 2001; Boulton and Dayhaw-Barker, 2001; Roberts, 2001; Hall and Gale, 2002). Indeed, age-related maculopathy is associated with AD (Klaver *et al.*, 1999) and the optic nerve also shows degenerative changes in AD (Blanks *et al.*, 1996). A recent development in phototherapy is the demonstration that the spectral sensitivity of the circadian system is very different than the spectral sensitivity of the retina used in visual activities such as reading and used to measure light in illuminating engineering (Brainard *et al.*, 2001). Very short wavelength (blue) light is maximally effective at affecting the circadian system whereas middle wavelengths (yellow-green) are maximally effective for visual performance. By restricting light emission to wavelengths between 480 and 515 nm, one can reduce the intensity of light to levels normally used in artificially illuminated environments, thus providing effective stimulation in a comfortable environment and without the risk of retinal damage from high intensity light. In addition, the associate use of an antioxidant substance like melatonin may be useful to reduce potential photo-oxidative damage in AD patients.

As mentioned above, a number of studies have shown that melatonin levels are lower in AD patients compared with aged matched controls (Skene *et al.*, 1990; Uchida *et al.*, 1996; Liu *et al.*, 1999; Mishima *et al.*, 1999; Ohashi *et al.*, 1999; Ferrari *et al.*, 2000). Based on this evidence the supplementary administration of melatonin to treat sleep and behavior disorders in AD patients seemed to be a logical therapeutic approach. Indeed, initial studies of melatonin therapy in AD have had positive results. However, the majority of studies are open, and knowledge about side effects and long-term effects of melatonin is still limited.

In a first examination of the sleep-promoting action of melatonin (3 mg p.o. for 21 days) in a small non-homogenous group of elderly patients with primary insomnia and with insomnia associated with dementia or depression, 7 out of 10 dementia patients having sleep disorders and treated with melatonin (3 mg p.o. at bed time) showed a decreased sundowning and reduced variability of sleep onset time (Fainstein *et al.*, 1997). In another study, 10 individuals with mild cognitive impairment were given 6 mg of melatonin before bedtime. Improvement was found in sleep, mood, and memory (Jean-Louis *et al.*, 1998a).

Other studies include daily administration of 6–9 mg melatonin for longer periods of time to AD patients with sleep disorders and sundowning agitation. The retrospective account of 14 AD patients after a 2–3-year period of treatment with melatonin indicated that all improved sleep quality (Brusco *et al.*, 1998a). Sundowning, diagnosed clinically in all patients examined, was not longer detectable in 12 of them, and persisted attenuated in the other two patients. Another significant observation in this study was the halted evolution of the cognitive and mnesic alterations expected in comparable populations of patients not receiving melatonin. This should be contrasted with the significant deterioration of clinical conditions of the disease expected from patients after 1–3 years of evolution of AD. Further support to the hypothesis that melatonin is useful in AD patients was given by a case report study which included two 79-year-old male monozygotic twins with AD diagnosed 8 years earlier (Brusco *et al.*, 1998b).

Other studies also support the efficacy of melatonin treatment in AD patients. Mishima and co-workers administered a 6 mg dose of melatonin for 4 weeks to seven in-patients with AD who exhibited irregular sleep-waking cycle (Mishima *et al.*, 2000). Melatonin significantly reduced percentage of nighttime activity compared to placebo. Cohen-Mansfield *et al.* (2000) reported the efficacy of melatonin (3 mg/day at bed time) for improving sleep and alleviating sundowning in 11 elderly AD patients. Analysis revealed a significant decrease in agitated behavior and a significant decrease in daytime sleepiness. In a case report observation on two AD patients, melatonin administration enhanced and stabilized the circadian rest–activity rhythm in one of them along with reduction of daytime sleepiness and improvement in mood (Jean-Louis *et al.*, 1998b). Likewise, another observation on two AD patients given 6 mg melatonin daily for one year indicated appreciable improvement of the Mini-Mental score (Pappolla *et al.*, 2000). The capacity of melatonin to improve sleep in 45 AD patients with sleep disturbances after 4 months of treatment with 6–9 mg melatonin/day was recently assessed (Cardinali *et al.*, 2002b). A significant effect of treatment on global subjective evaluation of sleep was detected in this group. Moreover, sundowning, clinically diagnosed in all patients disappeared after 4 months of treatment with melatonin. The effect of melatonin was seen regardless of any concomitant medication employed to treat cognitive or behavioral signs of disease. In a double-blind study to examine the effects of melatonin on the sleep–wake rhythm, cognitive and non-cognitive functions in AD type of dementia it was observed that a 3 mg melatonin dose for 4 weeks significantly prolonged actigraphically evaluated sleep time, decreased activity at the night and inproved cognitive function (Asayama *et al.*, 2003).

Observations in AD patients, however, are not always consistent. In a double-blind randomized placebo-controlled trial on the effect of

6 mg/day of melatonin for 2 weeks in demented patients with sleep disorders melatonin had no effect on median total time asleep, number of awakenings, or sleep efficiency (Serfaty *et al.*, 2002). It must be noted that the doses employed and, particularly, the short term of observation might account for this discrepancy with earlier results. As noted above, melatonin effect in synchronizing the circadian clock needs sometimes weeks to develop.

In a multi-centre, randomized, placebo-controlled clinical trial of two-dose formulations of oral melatonin 157 subjects with AD and nighttime sleep disturbance were randomly assigned to one of three treatment groups: placebo, 2.5-mg slow-release melatonin, or 10-mg melatonin given daily for 2 months (Singer *et al.*, 2003). When sleep was defined by an automated algorithmic analysis of wrist actigraphy, trends for increased nocturnal total sleep time and decreased wake after sleep onset in the melatonin groups, for a greater percentage of subjects having more than a 30-min increase in nocturnal total sleep time in the 10-mg melatonin group and for a decline in the day–night sleep ratio in the 2.5-mg sustained-release melatonin group were observed. On subjective measures, caregiver ratings of sleep quality showed improvement in the 2.5-mg sustained-release melatonin group relative to placebo. There were no significant differences in the number or seriousness of adverse events between the placebo and melatonin groups (Singer *et al.*, 2003).

Since there was no published study on the circadian consequences of injecting β-amyloid peptide in experimental animals we recently assessed whether melatonin had the ability to protect against the circadian changes produced by β-amyloid peptide 25–35 microinjections in SCN of golden hamsters (Furio *et al.*, 2002). Melatonin was given in the drinking water $(25\,\mu g/ml)$ starting 15 days in advance to the microinjection of β-amyloid peptide into SCN. β-amyloid-treated hamsters exhibited a significant phase advance of onset of running activity as compared to saline-injected animals. They also showed a significantly greater variability in onset time of wheel running activity, mainly evident from 6 to 15 days of treatment. Melatonin administration prevented the phase advance of onset time and the increased variability of onset time brought about by β-amyloid peptide. These results underlie the circadian consequences of injecting β-amyloid peptide 25–35 microinjections in the SCN of hamsters (Furio *et al.*, 2002). The "fixing" effect of melatonin on onset time reported in hamsters administered with β-amyloid peptide in their SCN somewhat resembles the reduction in variability of sleep onset time reported in demented (Fainstein *et al.*, 1997) and non-demented patients (Cardinali *et al.*, 2002c).

The mechanisms accounting for the therapeutic effect of melatonin in AD patients remain unknown. Melatonin treatment promotes mainly

non-REM sleep in the elderly (Monti *et al.*, 1999), and can be beneficial
in AD by augmenting the restorative phases of sleep, including the augmented secretion of GH (van Coevorden *et al.*, 1991) and neurotrophins.
In addition, *in vitro* experiments indicated that melatonin protects neurons against β-amyloid toxicity (Pappolla *et al.*, 1997, 2002), prevents
β-amyloid-induced lipid peroxidation (Daniels *et al.*, 1998) and alters the
metabolism of the β-amyloid precursor protein (Song and Lahiri, 1997).
Melatonin given orally to rats was very effective to reduce β-amyloid-
induced oxidative stress, and the neuroinflammatory response in the CNS
(Rosales-Corral *et al.*, 2003). In addition, melatonin was able to reduce
the free radical formation which follows the interaction between transition
metal ions and β-amyloid (Zatta *et al.*, 2003).

AD is considered a part of an emerging complex group of chronic and
progressive neurodegenerative entities collectively known as disorders of
protein folding (Martin, 1999). In these diseases, normal molecules or their
genetic variants self-assemble to form aggregates and/or fibrils that deposit
in the cerebral vessels and/or brain parenchyma and that are associated
with cognitive deficits, dementia, and cerebellar and extrapyramidal signs.
Among them, the most pathological conformer is rich in the β-sheet con-
formation which can be stabilized by aggregation.

Thus melatonin may have two different ways of action to prevent pro-
amyloidogenic environment that leads to AD amyloidosis: (1) anti-amyloi-
dogenic and (2) antioxidant properties. The former causes the reduction of
the β-sheet-rich conformer which becomes aggregated and neurotoxic, contributing to neuroprotection. Using AD transgenic mice the possibility that
increases in microaggregated amyloid may be sufficient to produce oxidative stress was put forth (Pappolla *et al.*, 1998). Increased lipid peroxidation
precedes amyloid plaque formation in transgenic mice, suggesting that brain
oxidative stress contributes to amyloidosis before its deposition in affected
brain (Pratico *et al.*, 2001). The demonstration of the direct relationship
between melatonin and the biochemical pathology of AD was recently made
in a transgenic mouse model of Alzheimer's amyloidosis by monitoring the
effects of administering melatonin on brain levels of β-amyloid abnormal
protein nitration and survival of the mice. The administration of melatonin partially inhibited the expected time-dependent elevation of β-amyloid,
reduced abnormal nitration of proteins and increased survival in the treated
transgenic mice (Matsubara *et al.*, 2003). Several recent publications endorse
the view that melatonin interferes very efficiently with β-amyloid formation

and toxicity (Lahiri *et al.*, 2004a; Li *et al.*, 2004; Louzada *et al.*, 2004; Wang *et al.*, 2004; Zhang *et al.*, 2004).

Since there is information indicating that supplementation with antioxidants delayed development of AD (Sano *et al.*, 1997; Kontush *et al.*, 2001), melatonin treatment may constitute a selection therapy to slow evolution of cognitive impairment in AD patients because it combines a potent neuroprotective activity with the amelioration of sundowning, the latter not observed with the use of regular antioxidants. Moreover, the combined treatment of melatonin together with bright light has the potential advantage of a preventing antioxidant effect of melatonin on harmful photooxidative processes at the retinal level.

Concluding Remarks

Melatonin may provide an innovative neuroprotective strategy against at least three known mechanism of neuronal death: oxyradical-mediated damage, apoptosis and glutamate excitotoxicity (Figure 1). Melatonin has also

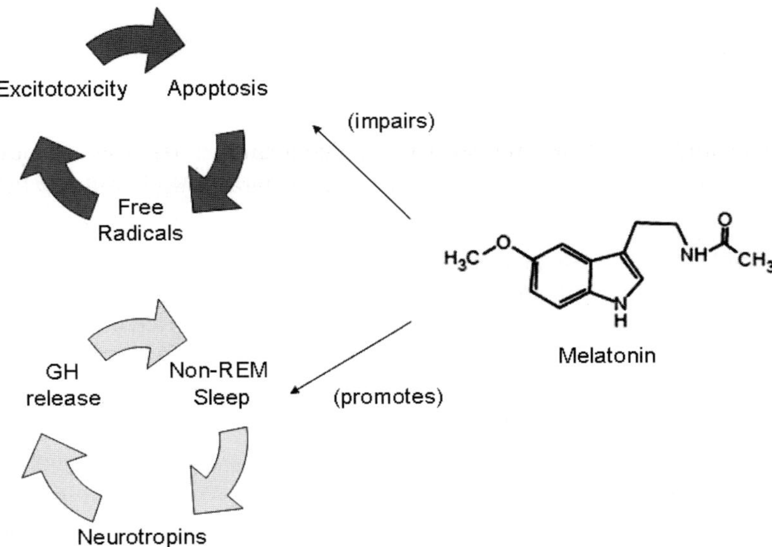

Figure 1. As discussed in the text, melatonin gives neuroprotection against three mechanisms of neuronal death: free-radical-mediated damage, apoptosis and glutamate excitotoxicity. In addition, and through restoration of non-REM sleep, melatonin presumably results in neurotropin synthesis and GH release.

very strong cytoprotective activity in a number of situations including ischemia-reperfusion of peripheral organs or osteoporosis (Cardinali *et al.*, 2003).

Through restoration of slow wave sleep melatonin treatment can result in better regulation of neuronal metabolism (Figure 1). Indeed a better sleep must be considered as a neuroprotective strategy that can potentially improve the course and outcome of several brain disorders, and thus the quality of life of the affected individuals and their family members. To promote and protect an appropriate sleep can substantially reduce the costs of treatment and management, in particular, the enormous costs of lifetime treatment of some neuropsychiatric disorders.

Acknowledgments

Studies in the author's laboratory were supported by the University of Buenos Aires, the Consejo Nacional de Investigaciones Científicas y Técnicas, Argentina, the Agencia Nacional de Promoción Científica y Tecnológica, Argentina (PICT 6153), and Fundación Bunge y Born, Buenos Aires.

References

Acuña-Castroviejo, D., Martin, M., Macias, M., Escames, G., Leon, J., Khaldy, H., and Reiter, R.J. (2001). Melatonin, mitochondria, and cellular bioenergetics. *J. Pineal Res.*, 30: 65–74.

Almeida Montes, L.G., Ontiveros Uribe, M.P., Cortes, S.J., and Heinze, M.G. (2003). Treatment of primary insomnia with melatonin: a double-blind, placebo-controlled, crossover study. *J. Psychiatry Neurosci.*, 28: 191–196.

Andrade, C., Srihari, B.S., Reddy, K.P., and Chandramma, L. (2001). Melatonin in medically ill patients with insomnia: a double-blind, placebo-controlled study. *J. Clin. Psychiatry*, 62: 41–45.

Anton-Tay, F. (1974). Melatonin: effects on brain function. *Adv. Biochem. Psychopharmacol.*, 11: 315–324.

Arendt, J. (2003). Importance and relevance of melatonin to human biological rhythms. *J. Neuroendocrinol.*, 15: 427–431.

Asayama, K., Yamadera, H., Ito, T., Suzuki, H., Kudo, Y., and Endo, S. (2003). Double blind study of melatonin effects on the sleep–wake rhythm, cognitive and non-cognitive functions in Alzheimer type dementia. *J. Nippon Med. Sch.*, 70: 334–341.

Ayalon, L., Hermesh, H., and Dagan, Y. (2002). Case study of circadian rhythm sleep disorder following haloperidol treatment: reversal by risperidone and melatonin. *Chronobiol. Int.*, 19: 947–959.

Badia, P., Hughes, R., Murphy, B.D., Myers, B.L., and Wright, K. (1996). Effects of exogenous melatonin on memory, sleepiness, and performance after a 4-hr nap. *J. Sleep. Res.*, 5(suppl. 1): 11.

Barron, M.J., Johnson, M.A., Andrews, R.M., Clarke, M.P., Griffiths, P.G., Bristow, E., He, L.P., Durham, S., and Turnbull, D.M. (2001). Mitochondrial abnormalities in ageing macular photoreceptors. *Invest. Ophthalmol. Vis. Sci.*, 42: 3016–3022.

Baskett, J.J., Wood, P.C., Broad, J.B., Duncan, J.R., English, J., and Arendt, J. (2001). Melatonin in older people with age-related sleep maintenance problems: a comparison with age matched normal sleepers. *Sleep*, 24: 418–424.

Baskett, J.J., Broad, J.B., Wood, P.C., Duncan, J.R., Pledger, M.J., English, J., and Arendt, J. (2003). Does melatonin improve sleep in older people? A randomised crossover trial. *Age Ageing*, 32: 164–170.

Beatty, S., Koh, H., Phil, M., Henson, D., and Boulton, M. (2000). The role of oxidative stress in the pathogenesis of age-related macular degeneration. *Surv. Ophthalmol.*, 45: 115–134.

Beaumont, M., Batejat, D., Pierard, C., Van Beers, P., Denis, J.B., Coste, O., Doireau, P., Chauffard, F., French, J., and Lagarde, D. (2004). Caffeine or melatonin effects on sleep and sleepiness after rapid eastward transmeridian travel. *J. Appl. Physiol.*, 96: 50–58.

Beni, S.M., Kohen, R., Reiter, R.J., Tan, D.X., and Shohami, E. (2004). Melatonin-induced neuroprotection after closed head injury is associated with increased brain antioxidants and attenuated late-phase activation of NF-kappa B and AP-1. *FASEB J.*, 18: 149–151.

Bersani, G. and Garavini, A. (2000). Melatonin add-on in manic patients with treatment resistant insomnia. *Prog. Neuropsychopharmacol. Biol. Psychiatry*, 24: 185–191.

Blanks, J.C., Schmidt, S.Y., Torigoe, Y., Porrello, K.V., Hinton, D.R., and Blanks, R.H. (1996). Retinal pathology in Alzheimer's disease. II. Regional neuron loss and glial changes in GCL. *Neurobiol. Aging*, 17: 385–395.

Boulton, M. and Dayhaw-Barker, P. (2001). The role of the retinal pigment epithelium: topographical variation and ageing changes. *Eye*, 15: 384–389.

Brainard, G.C., Hanifin, J.P., Greeson, J.M., Byrne, B., Glickman, G., Gerner, E., and Rollag, M.D. (2001). Action spectrum for melatonin regulation in humans: evidence for a novel circadian photoreceptor. *J. Neurosci.*, 21: 6405–6412.

Brusco, L.I., Marquez, M., and Cardinali, D.P. (1998a). Melatonin treatment stabilizes chronobiologic and cognitive symptoms in Alzheimer's disease. *Neuroendocrinol. Lett.*, 19: 111–115.

Brusco, L.I., Marquez, M., and Cardinali, D.P. (1998b). Monozygotic twins with Alzheimer's disease treated with melatonin: case report. *J. Pineal Res.*, 25: 260–263.

Cai, J., Nelson, K.C., Wub, M., Sternberg, P., and Jones, D.P. (2000). Oxidative damage and protection of the RPE. *Prog. Retin. Eye Res.*, 19: 205–221.

Cajochen, C., Krauchi, K., von Arx, M.A., Mori, D., Graw, P., and Wirz-Justice, A. (1996). Daytime melatonin administration enhances sleepiness and theta/alpha activity in the waking EEG. *Neurosci. Lett.*, 207: 209–213.

Cardinali, D.P. and Pevet, P. (1998). Basic aspects of melatonin action. *Sleep Med. Rev.*, 2: 175–190.

Cardinali, D.P., Bortman, G.P., Liotta, G., Perez, L.S., Albornoz, L.E., Cutrera, R.A., Batista, J., and Ortega, G.P. (2002a). A multifactorial approach employing melatonin to accelerate resynchronization of sleep–wake cycle after a 12 time-zone westerly transmeridian flight in elite soccer athletes. *J. Pineal Res.*, 32: 41–46.

Cardinali, D.P., Brusco, L.I., Liberczuk, C., and Furio, A.M. (2002b). The use of melatonin in Alzheimer's disease. *Neuroendocrinol. Lett.*, 23: 26–29.

Cardinali, D.P., Gvozdenovich, E., Kaplan, M.R., Fainstein, I., Shifis, H.A., Pérez Lloret, S., Albornoz, L.E., and Negri, A. (2002c). A double blind-placebo controlled study on melatonin efficacy to reduce anxiolytic benzo-diazepine use in the elderly. *Neuroendocrinol. Lett.*, 23: 55–60.

Cardinali, D.P., Ladizesky, M.G., Boggio, V., Cutrera, R.A., and Mautalen, C.A. (2003). Melatonin effects on bone: experimental facts and clinical perspectives. *J. Pineal Res.*, 34: 81–87.

Carneiro, R.C. and Reiter, R.J. (1998). Melatonin protects against lipid peroxidation induced by delta-aminolevulinic acid in rat cerebellum, cortex and hippocampus. *Neuroscience*, 82: 293–299.

Carpenter, B.D., Strauss, M.E., and Patterson, M.B. (1995). Sleep disturbances in community-dwelling patients with Alzheimer's disease. *Clin. Gerontol.*, 16: 35–49.

Cho, S., Joh, T.H., Baik, H.H., Dibinis, C., and Volpe, B.T. (1997). Melatonin administration protects CA1 hippocampal neurons after transient forebrain ischemia in rats. *Brain Res.*, 755: 335–338.

Chuang, J.I. and Chen, T.H. (2004). Effect of melatonin on temporal changes of reactive oxygen species and glutathione after MPP(+) treatment in human astrocytoma U373MG cells. *J. Pineal Res.*, 36: 117–125.

Citera, G., Arias, M.A., Maldonado-Cocco, J.A., Lazaro, M.A., Rosemffet, M.G., Brusco, L.I., Scheines, E.J., and Cardinali, D.P. (2000). The effect of melatonin in patients with fibromyalgia: a pilot study. *Clin. Rheumatol.*, 19: 9–13.

Cohen-Mansfield, J., Garfinkel, D., and Lipson, S. (2000). Melatonin for treatment of sundowning in elderly persons with dementia. *Arch. Gerontol. Geriatr.*, 31: 65–76.

Cramer, H., Rudolph, J., Consbruch, U., and Kendel, K. (1974). On the effects of melatonin on sleep and behavior in man. *Adv. Biochem. Psychopharmacol.*, 11: 187–191.

Cugini, P., Gori, M.C., Petrangeli, C.M., Tisei, P., and Giubilei, F. (1999). Preserved blood pressure and heart rate circadian rhythm in early stage Alzheimer's disease. *J. Gerontol. A Biol. Sci. Med. Sci.*, 54: M304–M308.

Dabbeni-Sala, F., Di Santo, S., Franceschini, D., Skaper, S.D., and Giusti, P. (2001). Melatonin protects against 6-OHDA-induced neurotoxicity in rats: a role for mitochondrial complex I activity. *FASEB J.*, 15: 164–170.

Dalton, E.J., Rotondi, D., Levitan, R.D., Kennedy, S.H., and Brown, G.M. (2000). Use of slow-release melatonin in treatment-resistant depression. *J. Psychiatry Neurosci.*, 25: 48–52.

Daniels, W.M., van Rensburg, S.J., van Zyl, J.M., and Taljaard, J.J. (1998). Melatonin prevents beta-amyloid-induced lipid peroxidation. *J. Pineal Res.*, 24: 78–82.

Dawson, D. and Armstrong, S.M. (1996). Chronobiotics — drugs that shift rhythms. *Pharmacol. Ther.*, 69: 15–36.

Dijk, D.J. and Lockley, S.W. (2002). Integration of human sleep–wake regulation and circadian rhythmicity. *J. Appl. Physiol.*, 92: 852–862.

Dijk, D.J., Roth, C., Landolt, H.P., Werth, E., Aeppli, M., Achermann, P., and Borbely, A.A. (1995). Melatonin effect on daytime sleep in men: suppression of EEG low frequency activity and enhancement of spindle frequency activity. *Neurosci. Lett.*, 201: 13–16.

Dollins, A.B., Zhdanova, I.V., Wurtman, R.J., Lynch, H.J., and Deng, M.H. (1994). Effect of inducing nocturnal serum melatonin concentrations in daytime on sleep, mood, body temperature, and performance. *Proc. Natl. Acad. Sci. USA*, 91: 1824–1828.

Dori, D., Casale, G., Solerte, S.B., Fioravanti, M., Migliorati, G., Cuzzoni, G., and Ferrari, E. (1994). Chrono-neuroendocrinological aspects of physiological aging and senile dementia. *Chronobiologia*, 21: 121–126.

Dubois-Dauphin, M., Frankowski, H., Tsujimoto, Y., Huarte, J., and Martinou, J.C. (1994). Neonatal motoneurons overexpressing the bcl-2 protooncogene in transgenic mice are protected from axotomy-induced cell death. *Proc. Natl. Acad. Sci. USA*, 91: 3309–3313.

Dupuis, F., Regrigny, O., Atkinson, J., Liminana, P., Delagrange, P., Scalbert, E., and Chillon, J.M. (2004). Impact of treatment with melatonin on cerebral circulation in old rats. *Br. J. Pharmacol.*, 141: 399–406.

Ellis, C.M., Lemmens, G., and Parkes, J.D. (1996). Melatonin and insomnia. *J. Sleep Res.*, 5: 61–65.

Erol, F.S., Topsakal, C., Ozveren, M.F., Kaplan, M., Ilhan, N., Ozercan, I.H., and Yildiz, O.G. (2004). Protective effects of melatonin and vitamin E in brain damage due to gamma radiation. An experimental study. *Neurosurg. Rev.*, 27: 65–69.

Fainstein, I., Bonetto, A., Brusco, L.I., and Cardinali, D.P. (1997). Effects of melatonin in elderly patients with sleep disturbance. A pilot study. *Curr. Ther. Res.*, 58: 990–1000.

Ferrari, E., Arcaini, A., Gornati, R., Pelanconi, L., Cravello, L., Fioravanti, M., Solerte, S.B., and Magri, F. (2000). Pineal and pituitary-adrenocortical function in physiological aging and in senile dementia. *Exp. Gerontol.*, 35: 1239–1250.

Fraser, J., Wraith, J.E., and Delatycki, M.B. (2002). Sleep disturbance in mucopolysaccharidosis type III (Sanfilippo syndrome): a survey of managing clinicians. *Clin. Genet.*, 62: 418–421.

Furio, A.M., Cutrera, R.A., Castillo Thea, V., Pérez Lloret, S., Riccio, P., Caccuri, R.L., Brusco, L.I., and Cardinali, D.P. (2002). Effect of melatonin on changes in locomotor activity rhythm of Syrian hamsters injected with beta amyloid peptide 25–35 in the suprachiasmatic nuclei. *Cell. Mol. Neurobiol.*, 22: 699–709.

Galvan, M.M., Campistol, J., Monros, E., Poo, P., Vernet, A.M., Pineda, M., Sans, A., Colomer, J., Conill, J.J., and Sanmarti, F.X. (2002). Angelman syndrome: physical characteristics and behavioural phenotype in 37 patients with confirmed genetic diagnosis. *Rev. Neurol.*, 35: 425–429.

Garfinkel, D., Laudon, M., Nof, D., and Zisapel, N. (1995). Improvement of sleep quality in elderly people by controlled-release melatonin. *Lancet*, 346: 541–544.

Garfinkel, D., Zisapel, N., Wainstein, J., and Laudon, M. (1999). Facilitation of benzodiazepine discontinuation by melatonin: a new clinical approach. *Arch. Intern. Med.*, 159: 2456–2460.

Gilbert, S.S., Van Den Heuvel, C.J., and Dawson, D. (1999). Daytime melatonin and temazepam in young adult humans: equivalent effects on sleep latency and body temperatures. *J. Physiol. (Lond.)*, 514: 905–914.

Girotti, L., Lago, M., Ianovsky, O., Carbajales, J., Elizari, M.V., Brusco, L.I., and Cardinali, D.P. (2000). Low urinary 6-sulphatoxymelatonin levels in patients with coronary artery disease. *J. Pineal Res.*, 29: 138–142.

Gitto, E., Romeo, C., Reiter, R.J., Impellizzeri, P., Pesce, S., Basile, M., Antonuccio, P., Trimarchi, G., Gentile, C., Barberi, I., and Zuccarello, B. (2004). Melatonin reduces oxidative stress in surgical neonates. *J. Pediatr. Surg.*, 39: 184–189.

Giubilei, F., Patacchioli, F.R., Antonini, G., Sepe, M.M., Tisei, P., Bastianello, S., Monnazzi, P., and Angelucci, L. (2001). Altered circadian cortisol secretion in Alzheimer's disease: clinical and neuroradiological aspects. *J. Neurosci. Res.*, 66: 262–265.

Giusti, P., Gusella, M., Lipartiti, M., Milani, D., Zhu, W., Vicini, S., and Manev, H. (1995). Melatonin protects primary cultures of cerebellar granule neurons from kainate but not from N-methyl-D-aspartate excitotoxicity. *Exp. Neurol.*, 131: 39–46.

Giusti, P., Lipartiti, M., Franceschini, D., Schiavo, N., Floreani, M., and Manev, H. (1996). Neuroprotection by melatonin from kainate-induced excitotoxicity in rats. *FASEB J.*, 10: 891–896.

Golombek, D.A., Escolar, E., Burin, L.J., De Brito, S., Fernandez, D.D., and Cardinali, D.P. (1992). Chronopharmacology of melatonin: inhibition by benzodiazepine antagonism. *Chronobiol. Int.*, 9: 124–131.

Golombek, D.A., Martini, M., and Cardinali, D.P. (1993). Melatonin as an anxiolytic in rats: time-dependence and interaction with the central gabaergic system. *Eur. J. Pharmacol.*, 237: 231–236.

Golombek, D.A., Pevet, P., and Cardinali, D.P. (1996). Melatonin effects on behavior: possible mediation by the central GABAergic system. *Neurosci. Biobehav. Rev.*, 20: 403–412.

Graw, P., Werth, E., Krauchi, K., Gutzwiller, F., Cajochen, C., and Wirz-Justice, A. (2001). Early morning melatonin administration impairs psychomotor vigilance. *Behav. Brain Res.*, 121: 167–172.

Haimov, I. and Lavie, P. (1995). Potential of melatonin replacement therapy in older patients with sleep disorders. *Drugs Aging*, 7: 75–78.

Hall, N.F. and Gale, C.R. (2002). Prevention of age related macular degeneration. *Br. Med. J.* 325: 1–2.

Hanania, M. and Kitain, E. (2002). Melatonin for treatment and prevention of postoperative delirium. *Anesth. Analg.*, 94: 338–339.

Harper, D.G., Stopa, E.G., McKee, A.C., Satlin, A., Harlan, P.C., Goldstein, R., and Volicer, L. (2001). Differential circadian rhythm disturbances in men with Alzheimer disease and frontotemporal degeneration. *Arch. Gen. Psychiatry*, 58: 353–360.

Hayashi, E. (2000). Effect of melatonin on sleep-wake rhythm: the sleep diary of an autistic male. *Psychiatry Clin. Neurosci.*, 54: 383–384.

Herxheimer, A. and Petrie, K.J. (2001). Melatonin for preventing and treating jet lag (Cochrane Review). *Cochrane Database Syst. Rev.* 1, CD001520.

Holmes, A.L., Gilbert, S.S., and Dawson, D. (2002). Melatonin and zopiclone: the relationship between sleep propensity and body temperature. *Sleep*, 25: 301–306.

Hoogendijk, W.J., van Someren, E.J., Mirmiran, M., Hofman, M.A., Lucassen, P.J., Zhou, J.N., and Swaab, D.E. (1996). Circadian rhythm-related behavioral disturbances and structural hypothalamic changes in Alzheimer's disease. *Int. Psychogeriatr.*, 8: 245–252.

Hughes, R.J., Sack, R.L., and Lewy, A.J. (1998). The role of melatonin and circadian phase in age-related sleep-maintenance insomnia: assessment in a clinical trial of melatonin replacement. *Sleep*, 21: 52–68.

Iguchi, H., Kato, K.I., and Ibayashi, H. (1982). Age-dependent reduction in serum melatonin concentrations in healthy human subjects. *J. Clin. Endocrinol. Metab.*, 55: 27–29.

James, S.P., Mendelson, W.B., Sack, D.A., Rosenthal, N.E., and Wehr, T.A. (1987). The effect of melatonin on normal sleep. *Neuropsychopharmacology*, 1: 41–44.

James, S.P., Sack, D.A., Rosenthal, N.E., and Mendelson, W.B. (1990). Melatonin administration in insomnia. *Neuropsychopharmacology*, 3: 19–23.

Jan, J.E., Hamilton, D., Seward, N., Fast, D.K., Freeman, R.D., and Laudon, M. (2000). Clinical trials of controlled-release melatonin in children with sleep–wake cycle disorders. *J. Pineal Res.*, 29: 34–39.

Jan, J.E., Tai, J., Hahn, G., and Rothstein, R.R. (2001). Melatonin replacement therapy in a child with a pineal tumor. *J. Child Neurol.*, 16: 139–140.

Jean-Louis, G., von Gizycki, H., and Zizi, F. (1998a). Melatonin effects on sleep, mood, and cognition in elderly with mild cognitive impairment. *J. Pineal Res.*, 25: 177–183.

Jean-Louis, G., Zizi, F., von Gizycki, H., and Taub, H. (1998b). Effects of melatonin in two individuals with Alzheimer's disease. *Percept. Mot. Skills*, 87: 331–339.

Jiao, S., Wu, M.M., Hu, C.L., Zhang, Z.H., and Mei, Y.A. (2004). Melatonin receptor agonist 2-iodomelatonin prevents apoptosis of cerebellar granule neurons via K(+) current inhibition. *J. Pineal Res.*, 36: 109–116.

Jin, B.K., Shin, D.Y., Jeong, M.Y., Gwag, M.R., Baik, H.W., Yoon, K.S., Cho, Y.H., Joo, W.S., Kim, Y.S., and Baik, H.H. (1998). Melatonin protects nigral dopaminergic neurons from 1-methyl-4- phenylpyridinium (MPP+) neurotoxicity in rats. *Neurosci. Lett.*, 245: 61–64.

Kamei, Y., Hayakawa, T., Urata, J., Uchiyama, M., Shibui, K., Kim, K., Kudo, Y., and Okawa, M. (2000). Melatonin treatment for circadian rhythm sleep disorders. *Psychiatry Clin. Neurosci.*, 54: 381–382.

Kennaway, D.J. and Wright, H. (2002). Melatonin and circadian rhythms. *Curr. Top. Med. Chem.*, 2: 199–209.

Kilic, E., Ozdemir, Y.G., Bolay, H., Kelestimur, H., and Dalkara, T. (1999). Pinealectomy aggravates and melatonin administration attenuates brain damage in focal ischemia. *J. Cereb. Blood Flow Metab.*, 19: 511–516.

Klaver, C.C., Ott, A., Hofman, A., Assink, J.J., Breteler, M.M., and de Jong, P.T. (1999). Is age-related maculopathy associated with Alzheimer's disease? The Rotterdam Study. *Am. J. Epidemiol.*, 150: 963–968.

Kluck, R.M., Bossy-Wetzel, E., Green, D.R., and Newmeyer, D.D. (1997). The release of cytochrome c from mitochondria: a primary site for Bcl-2 regulation of apoptosis. *Science*, 275: 1132–1136.

Kontush, A., Mann, U., Ant, S., Ujeyl, A., Lürs, C., Müller-Thomsen, T., and Beisiegel, U. (2001). Influence of vitamin E and C supplementation on lipoprotein oxidation in patients with Alzheimer's disease. *Free Radic. Biol. Med.*, 31: 345–354.

Kripke, D.F. (2000). Chronic hypnotic use: deadly risks, doubtful benefit. *Sleep Med. Rev.*, 4: 5–20.

Kunz, D. and Bes, F. (1999). Melatonin as a therapy in REM sleep behavior disorder patients: an open-labeled pilot study on the possible influence of melatonin on REM-sleep regulation. *Mov. Disord.*, 14: 507–511.

Kunz, D. and Bes, F. (2001). Exogenous melatonin in periodic limb movement disorder: an open clinical trial and a hypothesis. *Sleep*, 24: 183–187.

Kunz, D., Mahlberg, R., Muller, C., Tilmann, A., and Bes, F. (2004). Melatonin in patients with reduced REM sleep duration: two randomized controlled trials. *J. Clin. Endocrinol. Metab.*, 89: 128–134.

Lahiri, D.K., Chen, D., Ge, Y.W., Bondy, S.C., and Sharman, E.H. (2004a). Dietary supplementation with melatonin reduces levels of amyloid beta-peptides in the murine cerebral cortex. *J. Pineal Res.*, 36: 224–231.

Lahiri, D.K., Ge, Y.W., Sharman, E.H., and Bondy, S.C. (2004b). Age-related changes in serum melatonin in mice: higher levels of combined melatonin and 6-hydroxymelatonin sulfate in the cerebral cortex than serum, heart, liver and kidney tissues. *J. Pineal Res.*, 36: 217–223.

Lavie, P. (1997). Melatonin: role in gating nocturnal rise in sleep propensity. *J. Biol. Rhythms*, 12: 657–665.

Lavie, P. (2001). Sleep–wake as a biological rhythm. *Annu. Rev. Psychol.*, 52: 277–303.

Lee, E.J., Wu, T.S., Lee, M.Y., Chen, T.Y., Tsai, Y.Y., Chuang, J.I., and Chang, G.L. (2004). Delayed treatment with melatonin enhances electrophysiological recovery following transient focal cerebral ischemia in rats. *J. Pineal Res.*, 36: 33–42.

Leger, D., Laudon, M., and Zisapel, N. (2004). Nocturnal 6-sulfatoxymelatonin excretion in insomnia and its relation to the response to melatonin replacement therapy. *Am. J. Med.*, 116: 91–95.

Leppamaki, S., Partonen, T., Vakkuri, O., Lonnqvist, J., Partinen, M., and Laudon, M. (2003). Effect of controlled-release melatonin on sleep quality, mood, and quality of life in subjects with seasonal or weather-associated changes in mood and behaviour. *Eur. Neuropsychopharmacol.*, 13: 137–145.

Lerner, A.B. and Case, M.D. (1960). Melatonin. *Fed. Proc.*, 19: 590–592.

Lewy, A.J., Bauer, V.K., Ahmed, S., Thomas, K.H., Cutler, N.L., Singer, C.M., Moffit, M.T., and Sack, R.L. (1998). The human phase response curve (PRC) to melatonin is about 12 hours out of phase with the PRC to light. *Chronobiol. Int.*, 15: 71–83.

Li, S.P., Deng, Y.Q., Wang, X.C., Wang, Y.P., and Wang, J.Z. (2004). Melatonin protects SH-SY5Y neuroblastoma cells from calyculin A-induced neurofilament impairment and neurotoxicity. *J. Pineal Res.*, 36: 186–191.

Lieberman, H.R., Waldhauser, F., Garfield, G., Lynch, H.J., and Wurtman, R.J. (1984). Effects of melatonin on human mood and performance. *Brain Res.*, 323: 201–207.

Liu, R.Y., Zhou, J.N., vanHeerikhuize, J., Hofman, M.A., and Swaab, D.F. (1999). Decreased melatonin levels in postmortem cerebrospinal fluid in relation to aging, Alzheimer's disease, and apolipoprotein E-epsilon 4/4 genotype. *J. Clin. Endocrinol. Metab.*, 84: 323–327.

Liu, R.Y., Zhou, J.N., Hoogendijk, W.J., van Heerikhuize, J., Kamphorst, W., Unmehopa, U.A., Hofman, M.A., and Swaab, D.F. (2000). Decreased vasopressin gene expression in the biological clock of Alzheimer disease patients with and without depression. *J. Neuropathol. Exp. Neurol.*, 59: 314–322.

Lockley, S.W., Skene, D.J., James, K., Thapan, K., Wright, J., and Arendt, J. (2000). Melatonin administration can entrain the free-running circadian system of blind subjects. *J. Endocrinol.*, 164: R1–R6.

Louzada, P.R., Lima, A.C., Mendonca-Silva, D.L., Noel, F., De Mello, F.G., and Ferreira, S.T. (2004). Taurine prevents the neurotoxicity of beta-amyloid and glutamate receptor agonists: activation of GABA receptors and possible implications for Alzheimer's disease and other neurological disorders. *FASEB J.*, 18: 511–518.

Luboshitzky, R., Shen-Orr, Z., Tzischichinsky, O., Maldonado, M., Herer, P., and Lavie, P. (2001). Actigraphic sleep–wake patterns and urinary 6-sulfatoxymelatonin excretion in patients with Alzheimer's disease. *Chronobiol. Int.*, 18: 513–524.

Lucassen, P.J., Hofman, M.A., and Swaab, D.F. (1995). Increased light intensity prevents the age related loss of vasopressin-expressing neurons in the rat suprachiasmatic nucleus. *Brain Res.*, 693: 261–266.

MacFarlane, J.G., Cleghorn, J.M., Brown, G.M., and Streiner, D.L. (1991). The effects of exogenous melatonin on the total sleep time and daytime alertness of chronic insomniacs: a preliminary study. *Biol. Psychiatry*, 30: 371–376.

Magri, F., Locatelli, M., Balza, G., Molla, G., Cuzzoni, G., Fioravanti, M., Solerte, S.B., and Ferrari, E. (1997). Changes in endocrine circadian rhythms as markers of physiological and pathological brain aging. *Chronobiol. Int.*, 14: 385–396.

Magri, F., Sarra, S., Cinchetti, W., Guazzoni, V., Fioravanti, M., Cravello, L., and Ferrari, E. (2004). Qualitative and quantitative changes of melatonin levels in physiological and pathological aging and in centenarians. *J. Pineal Res.*, 36: 256–261.

Manev, H., Uz, T., Kharlamov, A., and Joo, J.Y. (1996). Increased brain damage after stroke or excitotoxic seizures in melatonin-deficient rats. *FASEB J.*, 10: 1546–1551.

Martin, J.B. (1999). Molecular basis of the neurodegenerative disorders. *N. Engl. J. Med.*, 340: 1970–1980.

Matsubara, E., Bryant-Thomas, T., Pacheco, Q.J., Henry, T.L., Poeggeler, B., Herbert, D., Cruz-Sanchez, F., Chyan, Y.J., Smith, M.A., Perry, G., Shoji, M., Abe, K., Leone, A., Grundke-Ikbal, I., Wilson, G.L., Ghiso, J., Williams, C., Refolo, L.M., and Pappolla, M.A. (2003). Melatonin increases survival and inhibits oxidative and amyloid pathology in a transgenic model of Alzheimer's disease. *J. Neurochem.*, 85: 1101–1108.

McCurry, S.M., Reynolds, C.F., Ancoli-Israel, S., Teri, L., and Vitiello, M.V. (2000). Treatment of sleep disturbance in Alzheimer's disease. *Sleep Med. Rev.*, 4: 603–628.

McGaffigan, S. and Bliwise, D.L. (1997). The treatment of sundowning. A selective review of pharmacological and nonpharmacological studies. *Drugs Aging*, 10: 10–17.

Mishima, K., Tozawa, T., Satoh, K., Matsumoto, Y., Hishikawa, Y., and Okawa, M. (1999). Melatonin secretion rhythm disorders in patients with senile dementia of Alzheimer's type with disturbed sleep-waking. *Biol. Psychiatry*, 45: 417–421.

Mishima, K., Okawa, M., Hozumi, S., and Hishikawa, Y. (2000). Supplementary administration of artificial bright light and melatonin as potent treatment for disorganized circadian rest-activity and dysfunctional autonomic and neuroendocrine systems in institutionalized demented elderly persons. *Chronobiol. Int.*, 17: 419–432.

Mishima, K., Okawa, M., Shimizu, T., and Hishikawa, Y. (2001). Diminished melatonin secretion in the elderly caused by insufficient environmental illumination. *J. Clin. Endocrinol. Metab.*, 86: 129–134.

Monti, J.M., Alvarino, F., Cardinali, D., Savio, I., and Pintos, A. (1999). Polysomnographic study of the effect of melatonin on sleep in elderly patients with chronic primary insomnia. *Arch. Gerontol. Geriatr.*, 28: 85–98.

Nagtegaal, J.E., Laurant, M.W., Kerkhof, G.A., Smits, M.G., van der Meer, Y.G., and Coenen, A.M. (2000). Effects of melatonin on the quality of life in patients with delayed sleep phase syndrome. *J. Psychosom. Res.*, 48: 45–50.

Nave, R., Peled, R., and Lavie, P. (1995). Melatonin improves evening napping. *Eur. J. Pharmacol.*, 275: 213–216.

Ninomiya, T., Iwatani, N., Tomoda, A., and Miike, T. (2001). Effects of exogenous melatonin on pituitary hormones in humans. *Clin. Physiol.*, 21: 292–299.

Ohashi, Y., Okamoto, N., Uchida, K., Iyo, M., Mori, N., and Morita, Y. (1999). Daily rhythm of serum melatonin levels and effect of light exposure in patients with dementia of the Alzheimer's type. *Biol. Psychiatry*, 45: 1646–1652.

Ouslander, J.G., Buxton, W.G., Al Samarrai, N.R., Cruise, P.A., Alessi, C., and Schnelle, J.F. (1998). Nighttime urinary incontinence and sleep disruption among nursing home residents. *J. Am. Geriatr. Soc.*, 46: 463–466.

Paavonen, E.J., Nieminen-Von Wendt, T., Vanhala, R., Aronen, E.T., and Von Wendt, L. (2003). Effectiveness of melatonin in the treatment of sleep disturbances in children with asperger disorder. *J. Child Adolesc. Psychopharmacol.*, 13: 83–95.

Pandi-Perumal, S.R., Seils, L.K., Kayumov, L., Ralph, M.R., Lowe, A., Moller, H., and Swaab, D.F. (2002). Senescence, sleep, and circadian rhythms. *Ageing Res. Rev.*, 1: 559–604.

Pappolla, M.A., Sos, M., Omar, R.A., Bick, R.J., Hickson-Bick, D.L., Reiter, R.J., Efthimiopoulos, S., and Robakis, N.K. (1997). Melatonin prevents death of neuroblastoma cells exposed to the Alzheimer amyloid peptide. *J. Neurosci.*, 17: 1683–1690.

Pappolla, M.A., Chyan, Y.J., Omar, R.A., Hsiao, K., Perry, G., Smith, M.A., and Bozner, P. (1998). Evidence of oxidative stress and *in vivo* neurotoxicity of beta-amyloid in a transgenic mouse model of Alzheimer's disease: a chronic oxidative paradigm for testing antioxidant therapies *in vivo*. *Am. J. Pathol.*, 152: 871–877.

Pappolla, M.A., Chyan, Y., Poeggeler, B., Frangione, B., Wilson, G., Ghiso, J., and Reiter, R.J. (2000). An assessment of the antioxidant and the antiamyloidogenic properties of melatonin: implications for Alzheimer's disease. *J. Neural Transm.*, 107: 203–231.

Pappolla, M.A., Simovich, M.J., Bryant-Thomas, T., Chyan, Y.J., Poeggeler, B., Dubocovich, M., Bick, R., Perry, G., Cruz-Sanchez, F., and Smith, M.A. (2002). The neuroprotective activities of melatonin against the Alzheimer beta-protein are not mediated by melatonin membrane receptors. *J. Pineal Res.*, 32: 135–142.

Pardo, C.A., Martin, L.J., Troncoso, J.C., and Price, D.L. (1990). The human pineal gland in aging and Alzheimer's disease: patterns of cytoskeletal antigen immunoreactivity. *Acta Neuropathol. (Berl).*, 80: 535–540.

Pei, Z., Pang, S.F., and Cheung, R.T. (2002). Pretreatment with melatonin reduces volume of cerebral infarction in a rat middle cerebral artery occlusion stroke model. *J. Pineal Res.*, 32: 168–172.

Pei, Z., Pang, S.F., and Cheung, R.T. (2003). Administration of melatonin after onset of ischemia reduces the volume of cerebral infarction in a rat middle cerebral artery occlusion stroke model. *Stroke*, 34: 770–775.

Pillar, G., Shahar, E., Peled, N., Ravid, S., Lavie, P., and Etzioni, A. (2000). Melatonin improves sleep-wake patterns in psychomotor retarded children. *Pediatr. Neurol.*, 23: 225–228.

Pratico, D., Uryu, K., Leight, S., Trojanoswki, J.Q., and Lee, V.M. (2001). Increased lipid peroxidation precedes amyloid plaque formation in an animal model of Alzheimer amyloidosis. *J. Neurosci.*, 21: 4183–4187.

Reid, K., Van den Heuvel, C., and Dawson, D. (1996). Day-time melatonin administration: effects on core temperature and sleep onset latency. *J. Sleep Res.*, 5: 150–154.

Reiter, R.J. (1998). Oxidative damage in the central nervous system: protection by melatonin. *Prog. Neurobiol.*, 56: 359–384.

Reiter, R.J. and Tan, D.X. (2003). What constitutes a physiological concentration of melatonin? *J. Pineal Res.*, 34: 79–80.

Reiter, R.J., Tan, D.X., Burkhardt, S., and Manchester, L.C. (2001). Melatonin in plants. *Nutr. Rev.*, 59: 286–290.

Reiter, R.J., Tan, D., and Burkhardt, S. (2002). Reactive oxygen and nitrogen species and cellular and organismal decline: amelioration with melatonin. *Mech. Ageing Dev.*, 123: 1007–1019.

Reyes Toso, C., Ricci, C., de Mignone, I.R., Reyes, P., Linares, L.M., Albornoz, L.E., Cardinali, D.P., and Zaninovich, A.A. (2003). *In vitro* effect of melatonin on oxygen consumption in liver mitochondria of rats. *Neuroendocrinol. Lett.*, 24: 341–344.

Roberts, J.E. (2001). Ocular phototoxicity. *J. Photochem. Photobiol.*, 64: 136–143.

Rodriguez, C., Mayo, J.C., Sainz, R.M., Antolin, I., Herrera, F., Martin, V., and Reiter, R.J. (2004). Regulation of antioxidant enzymes: a significant role for melatonin. *J. Pineal Res.*, 36: 1–9.

Rosales-Corral, S., Tan, D.X., Reiter, R.J., Valdivia-Velázquez, M., Martínez-Barboza, G., Pablo Acosta-Martínez, J., and Ortiz, G.G. (2003). Orally administered melatonin reduces oxidative stress and proinflammatory cytokines induced by amyloid-beta peptide in rat brain: a comparative, *in vivo* study versus vitamins C and E. *J. Pineal Res.*, 35: 80–84.

Ross, C., Davies, P., and Whitehouse, W. (2002). Melatonin treatment for sleep disorders in children with neurodevelopmental disorders: an observational study. *Dev. Med. Child Neurol.*, 44: 339–344.

Sano, M., Ernesto, C., Thomas, R.G., Klauber, M.R., Schafer, K., Grundman, M., Woodbury, P., Growdon, J., and Corman, C.W. (1997). A controlled trial of selegiline, alpha-tocopherol, or both as treatment for Alzheimer's disease. *N. Engl. J. Med.*, 336: 1216–1222.

Satlin, A., Volicer, L., Stopa, E.G., and Harper, D. (1995). Circadian locomotor activity and core-body temperature rhythms in Alzheimer's disease. *Neurobiol. Aging*, 16: 765–771.

Satomura, T., Sakamoto, T., Shirakawa, S., Tsutsumi, Y., Mukai, M., Ohyama, T., Uchimura, N., and Maeda, H. (2001). Hypnotic action of melatonin during daytime administration and its comparison with triazolam. *Psychiatry Clin. Neurosci.*, 55: 303–304.

Savaskan, E., Olivieri, G., Meier, F., Brydon, L., Jockers, R., Ravid, R., and Wirz-Justice, A. (2002). Increased melatonin 1a-receptor immunoreactivity in the hippocampus of Alzheimer's disease patients. *J. Pineal Res.*, 32: 59–62.

Seabra, M.L.V., Bignotto, M., Pinto, L.R., and Tufik, S. (2000). Randomized, double-blind clinical trial, controlled with placebo, of the toxicology of chronic melatonin treatment. *J. Pineal Res.*, 29: 193–200.

Serfaty, M., Kennell-Webb, S., Warner, J., Blizard, R., and Raven, P. (2002). Double blind randomised placebo controlled trial of low dose melatonin for sleep disorders in dementia. *Int. J. Geriatr. Psychiatry*, 17: 1120–1127.

Shaikh, A.Y., Xu, J., Wu, Y., He, L., and Hsu, C.Y. (1997). Melatonin protects bovine cerebral endothelial cells from hyperoxia-induced DNA damage and death. *Neurosci. Lett.*, 229: 193–197.

Shen, Y.X., Xu, S.Y., Wei, W., Wang, X.L., Wang, H., and Sun, X. (2002). Melatonin blocks rat hippocampal neuronal apoptosis induced by amyloid beta-peptide 25–35. *J. Pineal Res.*, 32: 163–167.

Shilo, L., Dagan, Y., Smorjik, Y., Weinberg, U., Dolev, S., Komptel, B., and Shenkman, L. (2000). Effect of melatonin on sleep quality of COPD intensive care patients: a pilot study. *Chronobiol. Int.*, 17: 71–76.

Shirakawa, S.I., Sakamoto, T., Uchimura, N., Tsutsumi, Y., Tanaka, J., and Maeda, H. (2001). Effect of melatonin on sleep and rectal temperature of young healthy evening types. *Psychiatry Clin. Neurosci.*, 55: 301–302.

Siegrist, C., Benedetti, C., Orlando, A., Beltran, J.M., Tuchscherr, L., Noseda, C.M., Brusco, L.I., and Cardinali, D.P. (2001). Lack of changes in serum prolactin, FSH, TSH, and estradiol after melatonin treatment in doses that improve sleep and reduce benzodiazepine consumption in sleep-disturbed, middle-aged, and elderly patients. *J. Pineal Res.*, 30: 34–42.

Singer, C., Tractenberg, R.E., Kaye, J., Schafer, K., Gamst, A., Grundman, M., Thomas, R., and Thal, L.J. (2003). A multicenter, placebo-controlled trial of melatonin for sleep disturbance in Alzheimer's disease. *Sleep*, 26: 893–901.

Skene, D.J. and Swaab, D.F. (2003). Melatonin rhythmicity: effect of age and Alzheimer's disease. *Exp. Gerontol.*, 38: 199–206.

Skene, D.J., Vivien-Roels, B., Sparks, D.L., Hunsaker, J.C., Pevet, P., Ravid, D., and Swaab, D.F. (1990). Daily variation in the concentration of melatonin and 5-methoxytryptophol in the human pineal gland: effect of age and Alzheimer's disease. *Brain Res.*, 528: 170–174.

Skene, D.J., Lockley, S.W., and Arendt, J. (1999). Melatonin in circadian sleep disorders in the blind. *Biol. Signals Recept.*, 8: 90–95.

Skinner, D.C. and Malpaux, B. (1999). High melatonin concentrations in third ventricular cerebrospinal fluid are not due to Galen vein blood recirculating through the choroid plexus. *Endocrinology*, 140: 4399–4405.

Smits, M.G., Nagtegaal, E.E., van der, H.J., Coenen, A.M., and Kerkhof, G.A. (2001). Melatonin for chronic sleep onset insomnia in children: a randomized placebo-controlled trial. *J. Child Neurol.*, 16: 86–92.

Song, W. and Lahiri, D.K. (1997). Melatonin alters the metabolism of the beta-amyloid precursor protein in the neuroendocrine cell line PC12. *J. Mol. Neurosci.*, 9: 75–92.

Stone, B.M., Turner, C., Mills, S.L., and Nicholson, A.N. (2000). Hypnotic activity of melatonin. *Sleep*, 23: 663–669.

          D. P. Cardinali

Stopa, E.G., Volicer, L., Kuo-Leblanc, V., Harper, D., Lathi, D., Tate, B., and Satlin, A. (1999). Pathologic evaluation of the human suprachiasmatic nucleus in severe dementia. *J. Neuropathol. Exp. Neurol.*, 58: 29–39.

Swabb, D.F., Fliers, E., and Partiman, T.S. (1985). The suprachiasmatic nucleus of the human brain in relation to sex, age and senile dementia. *Brain Res.*, 342: 37–44.

Takeuchi, N., Uchimura, N., Hashizume, Y., Mukai, M., Etoh, Y., Yamamoto, K., Kotorii, T., Ohshima, H., Ohshima, M., and Maeda, H. (2001). Melatonin therapy for REM sleep behavior disorder. *Psychiatry Clin. Neurosci.*, 55: 267–269.

Taylor, J.L., Friedman, L., Sheikh, J., and Yesavage, J.A. (1997). Assessment and management of "sundowning" phenomena. *Semin. Clin. Neuropsychiatry*, 2: 113–122.

Terlo, L., Laudon, M., Tarasch, R., Schatz, T., Caine, Y.G., and Zisapel, N. (1997). Effects of low doses of melatonin on late afternoon napping and mood. *Biol. Rhythms Res.*, 28: 2–15.

Tjon Pian Gi, C.V., Broeren, J.P., Starreveld, J.S., and FG, A.V. (2003). Melatonin for treatment of sleeping disorders in children with attention deficit/hyperactivity disorder: a preliminary open label study. *Eur. J. Pediatr.*, 162: 554–555.

Tomás-Zapico, C., Martínez-Fraga, J., Rodríguez-Colunga, M.J., Tolivia, D., Hardeland, R., and Coto-Montes, A. (2002). Melatonin protects against delta-aminolevulinic acid-induced oxidative damage in male Syrian hamster Harderian glands. *Int. J. Biochem. Cell Biol.*, 34: 544–553.

Torii, K., Uneyama, H., Nishino, H., and Kondoh, T. (2004). Melatonin suppresses cerebral edema caused by middle cerebral artery occlusion/reperfusion in rats assessed by magnetic resonance imaging. *J. Pineal Res.*, 36: 18–24.

Tricoire, H., Locatelli, A., Chemineau, P., and Malpaux, B. (2002). Melatonin enters the cerebrospinal fluid through the pineal recess. *Endocrinology*, 143: 84–90.

Tricoire, H., Malpaux, B., and Moller, M. (2003). Cellular lining of the sheep pineal recess studied by light-, transmission-, and scanning electron microscopy: morphologic indications for a direct secretion of melatonin from the pineal gland to the cerebrospinal fluid. *J. Comp. Neurol.*, 456: 39–47.

Uchida, K., Okamoto, N., Ohara, K., and Morita, Y. (1996). Daily rhythm of serum melatonin in patients with dementia of the degenerate type. *Brain Res.*, 717: 154–159.

van Coevorden, A., Mockel, J., Laurent, E., Kerkhofs, M., L'Hermite-Baleriaux, M., Decoster, C., Neve, P., and Van Cauter, E. (1991). Neuroendocrine rhythms and sleep in aging men. *Am. J. Physiol.*, 260: 651–661.

van Someren, E.J.W. (2000). Circadian rhythms and sleep in human aging. *Chronobiol. Int.*, 17: 233–243.

Vitiello, M.V., Prinz, P.N., Williams, D.E., Frommlet, M.S., and Ries, R.K. (1990). Sleep disturbances in patients with mild-stage Alzheimer's disease. *J. Gerontol. Med. Sci.*, 45: M131–M138.

Vollrath, L., Semm, P., and Gammel, G. (1981). Sleep induction by intranasal administration of melatonin. *Adv. Biosci.*, 29: 327–329.

Waldhauser, F., Saletu, B., and Trinchard-Lugan, I. (1990). Sleep laboratory investigations on hypnotic properties of melatonin. *Psychopharmacology (Berl).* 100: 222–226.

Wang, F., Li, J., Wu, C., Yang, J., Xu, F., and Zhao, Q. (2003). The GABA(A) receptor mediates the hypnotic activity of melatonin in rats. *Pharmacol. Biochem. Behav.*, 74: 573–578.

Wang, Y.P., Li, X.T., Liu, S.J., Zhou, X.W., Wang, X.C., and Wang, J.Z. (2004). Melatonin ameliorated okadaic-acid induced Alzheimer-like lesions. *Acta Pharmacol. Sin.*, 25: 276–280.

Wassmer, E., Quinn, E., Whitehouse, W., and Seri, S. (2001). Melatonin as a sleep inductor for electroencephalogram recordings in children. *Clin. Neurophysiol.*, 112: 683–685.

Yalcin, A., Kanit, L., and Sozmen, E.Y. (2004). Altered gene expressions in rat hippocampus after kainate injection with or without melatonin pretreatment. *Neurosci. Lett.*, 359: 65–68.

Yang, C.M., Spielman, A.J., D'Ambrosio, P., Serizawa, S., Nunes, J., and Birnbaum, J. (2001). A single dose of melatonin prevents the phase delay associated with a delayed weekend sleep pattern. *Sleep*, 24: 272–281.

Yoo, Y.M., Yim, S.V., Kim, S.S., Jang, H.Y., Lea, H.Z., Hwang, G.C., Kim, J.W., Kim, S.A., Lee, H.J., Kim, C.J., Chung, J.H., and Leem, K.H. (2002). Melatonin suppresses NO-induced apoptosis via induction of Bcl-2 expression in PGT-beta immortalized pineal cells. *J. Pineal Res.*, 33: 146–150.

Zatta, P., Tognon, G., and Carampin, P. (2003). Melatonin prevents free radical formation due to the interaction between beta-amyloid peptides and metal ions [Al(III), Zn(II), Cu(II), Mn(II), Fe(II)]. *J. Pineal Res.*, 35: 98–103.

Zhang, Y.C., Wang, Z.F., Wang, Q., Wang, Y.P., and Wang, J.Z. (2004). Melatonin attenuates beta-amyloid-induced inhibition of neurofilament expression. *Acta Pharmacol. Sin.*, 25: 447–451.

Zhdanova, I.V., Wurtman, R.J., Lynch, H.J., Ives, J.R., Dollins, A.B., Morabito, C., Matheson, J.K., and Schomer, D.L. (1995). Sleep-inducing effects of low doses of melatonin ingested in the evening. *Clin. Pharmacol. Ther.*, 57: 552–558.

Zhdanova, I.V., Wurtman, R.J., Morabito, C., Piotrovska, V.R., and Lynch, H.J. (1996). Effects of low oral doses of melatonin, given 2–4 hours before habitual bedtime, on sleep in normal young humans. *Sleep*, 19: 423–431.

Zhdanova, I.V., Wurtman, R.J., and Wagstaff, J. (1999). Effects of a low dose of melatonin on sleep in children with Angelman syndrome. *J. Pediatr. Endocrinol. Metab.*, 12: 57–67.

Zhdanova, I.V., Wurtman, R.J., Regan, M.M., Taylor, J.A., Shi, J.P., and Leclair, O.U. (2001). Melatonin treatment for age-related insomnia. *J. Clin. Endocrinol. Metab.*, 86: 4727–4730.

Zhou, J.N., Liu, R.Y., Kamphorst, W., Hofman, M.A., and Swaab, D.F. (2003). Early neuropathological Alzheimer's changes in aged individuals are accompanied by decreased cerebrospinal fluid melatonin levels. *J. Pineal Res.*, 35: 125–130.

Zisapel, N. (2001). Melatonin–dopamine interactions: from basic neurochemistry to a clinical setting. *Cell. Mol. Neurobiol.*, 21: 605–616.

Chapter 22

WHAT INDIVIDUAL NEURONES TELL US ABOUT ENCODING AND SENSORY PROCESSING IN SLEEP

Marisa Pedemonte[1] and Ricardo A. Velluti

The precise understanding of the brain's functions is at the initial stages, and the future is full of promises. The neuroscientific and general physiological knowledge of sleep is one of the important subjects lacking elucidation and is under close research scrutiny. Only by revealing the underlying mechanisms and the description/explanation of several pathologies will we be able to maintain healthier brains for a longer time. Further, only by using every available methodology, approach, and viewpoint can real advances will be achieved in this matter.

The brain as a whole is functionally involved in sleep as well as during wakefulness, although in quite a different way. Many brain functional shifts exhibited on passing to sleep will, in addition, influence the general physiology showing significant changes in every function and, perhaps, in pathological processes.

Our assessment will contribute to examine the results related to how auditory sensory information is worked out by the waking and sleeping brain. The firing rate, its temporal discharge distribution, and the relationship to hippocampal theta rhythm of the auditory system neurones will be

---

[1] mpedemon@fmed.edu.uy

considered, together, as components of information processing (Velluti and Pedemonte, 2002; Pedemonte and Velluti, 2005). Furthermore, considering the auditory sensory system activity as an important piece of the sleep neurophysiology enigma, the influence of incoming sensory information is postulated as an active contributor intended for the development of sleep processes.

The Auditory System and Sleep

Several reasons support the notion that the auditory system is specially related to sleep: (1) It is a tele-receptor system that is continuously open and facilitates the central nervous system (CNS) being aware of the environment during wakefulness and sleep. (2) The blood flow in the auditory brainstem nuclei and the auditory cortex increases on passing to sleep. In particular, the cochlear nucleus during paradoxical sleep (PS) increases its blood flow to ~170% in comparison to a waking state (Reivich *et al.*, 1968). (3) The human oneiric activity shows auditory "images" in 65% of the dream contents just second to the visual 100% and far above other sensory modalities that amount to no more than 8% or less each (Whiton Calkins, cited by Sante de Sanctis, 1899; McCarley and Hoffman, 1981). (4) A noisy night may reduce total sleep time and produce several awakenings in humans (Vallet, 1982; Pearson *et al.*, 1995) and in rodents (Rabat *et al.*, 2004). (5) Experimental deafening increases sleep time, particularly PS, while wakefulness (W) is reduced (Pedemonte *et al.*, 1996a; Cutrera *et al.*, 2000). Further, human deaf patients with intra-cochlear implants, which permit them to hear again, exhibit differences in percentages of sleep stages when recorded with the cochlear implant turned on or off (Velluti *et al.*, 2003).

The overall importance of the sensory input in general was demonstrated when animals experimentally deprived of most of their sensory input exhibited a totally different pattern of brain activity. The *quasi-*total deafferentation in cat, performed by Vital-Durand and Michel (1971), revealed a sleep–waking cycle with the following changes: (a) the W time was reduced (from 44 to 18%); (b) the time spent in slow wave sleep (SWS) was also reduced from 41 to 29%, while the total amount of PS was not significantly reduced (13 to 11%); (c) regarding behaviour, the above-mentioned experiment presented a *quasi-*constant "somnolence" in a sphinx position and different bioelectrical activities at the amygdala and the hippocampus level. The concept that a new behavioural state developed after the sensory deprivation experimental approach was then suggested by Velluti (1997). Furthermore, animal recordings of cortical auditory local field evoked responses representing a neuronal population at different cortical depths, in the medial geniculate body, the thalamic reticular formation, and the hippocampus, showed all components of the averaged evoked potentials being larger during SWS than in W and PS (Hall and Borbély, 1970). Human far-field evoked activity supports the view that sophisticated auditory information processing persists during sleep while the evoked activity is present in all sleep phases (Bastuji and García-Larrea, 1999; Bastuji *et al.*, 2002; Bastuji and García-Larrea, 2005, Chapter 23).

The hippocampal theta rhythm

The hippocampus produces a high-amplitude transient theta rhythm when a cat is looking itself in a mirror; this observation by Grastyán *et al.* (1959) connected this rhythm to a sensory input, the vision, and to higher processes such as, perhaps, conspecific recognition. At the same time, recordings carried out in primary auditory cortex showed evoked neuronal firing shifts elicited by electrical stimulation of the hippocampus, indicating that these brain regions are interconnected and exhibit a functional relationship. These results support the notion that an auditory–hippocampal shared functional interaction, although unknown in detail, may be present (Cazard and Buser, 1963; Redding, 1967; Parmeggiani and Rapisarda, 1969; Parmeggiani *et al.*, 1982).

The ultradian hippocampal theta rhythm, within the wakefulness–sleep circadian cycle, may modulate the sensory neuronal activity. It has been one of the conspicuous time givers postulated as an internal *zeitgeber*, a temporal organiser for auditory sensory processing (Pedemonte *et al.*, 1996b; Velluti *et al.*, 2000; Velluti and Pedemonte, 2002; Pedemonte and Velluti, 2005). The theta waves, 4–10 cycles per second (cps), may affect spatially distant neurones by inducing fluctuations of the cellular excitability due to membrane potential oscillations (García-Austt, 1984; Kocsis and Vertes, 1992). Although more prominent in active W and PS, the theta rhythm is always present in the brain, e.g., the hippocampal theta frequencies can also be observed during SWS when analysed in the frequency domain, the Fourier transform (Komisariuk, 1970; Gaztelu *et al.*, 1994).

This particular hippocampal rhythm has been related to several brain processes; it was found involved in motor activities during both W and PS (Buño and Velluti, 1977; García-Austt, 1984; Lerma and García-Austt,

1985), as well as in the sensory processing related to a motor context (Grastyan *et al.*, 1959; Kramis *et al.*, 1975). It was also found involved in spatio-temporal learning (Winson, 1978; O'Keefe and Recce, 1993), associating distant, discontiguous events (Wallestein *et al.*, 1998) and learning of temporal sequences (Mehta *et al.*, 2002). The role of the theta rhythm in learning and memory has been proposed from different viewpoints (Adey *et al.*, 1960; Burgess and Gruzelier, 1997; Doppelmayr *et al.*, 1998; Klimesch, 1999; Kahana *et al.*, 1999; Vinogradova, 2001), and has also been linked to modulation of autonomic processes such as the heart rate (Pedemonte *et al.*, 1999, 2003).

As previously stated, auditory neurones exhibit phase locking, i.e., temporal correlation with theta rhythm at different levels of the auditory pathway, from the brainstem — the cochlear nucleus, the superior olive, the inferior colliculus — to the primary cortical region (Velluti and Pedemonte, 2002; Pedemonte and Velluti, 2005). The processing in other sensory modalities has also been associated to the theta rhythm, e.g., touch (Nuñez *et al.*, 1991), pain (Vertes and Kocsis, 1997), vision (Gambini *et al.*, 2002), and olfaction (Margrie and Schaefer, 2003; Affani and Cervino, 2005, Chapter 25).

Thus, it is our tenet that the theta rhythm of the hippocampus contributes, in the time domain, to the complex problem of the central auditory information processing in sleep and waking.

Coding

For any kind of neural processing, and particularly for auditory data processing, a basic code is needed. In general, it is likely that this basic code is a cell assembly one; i.e., the assembled activity of a population of neurones (Sakurai, 1999). We may assume that the code is similar during the dissimilar brain states considered herein, i.e., the quiet wakefulness and sleep stages. The differences between states would then be based on the configuration of the active regions of the newly organised neuronal networks/cell assemblies. The final result of the processing during W or sleep will be different taking into account that the regions now involved have changed. That is, the brain is to a large part functionally different upon passing to sleep phases.

A dynamic modulation of the correlated neuronal firing may occur; i.e., a neurone that participates in a certain functional cell assembly/network may later on become associated with another activated and perhaps competing neuronal assembly, e.g., on passing from W into sleep. The partial overlapping of neurones among assemblies is due to the ability of one neurone to participate in different types of information processing (Sakurai, 1999). Moreover, this condition may be repeated during the many and diverse W states, during human stage 1 or 2, and SWS, and also during phasic or tonic epochs of PS.

Cochlear Microphonics and the Activity of the Auditory Nerve and Central Neurones in Sleep and Wakefulness

Actions of sleep on the auditory nerve and receptor potential

In hearing, as well as in other sensory modalities, there are different types of mechanisms to control the sensory input: (i) Pre-receptorial actions that indirectly regulate the stimulus energy through voluntary or reflex motor activities. Head and animal's pinna movements and contractions of the stapedius and tensor tympani muscles are examples of these regulating actions. (ii) The efferent system. The auditory system is composed of ascending and descending pathways. The latter originates at cortical level and ends, through the olivo-cochlear bundle, onto the external and internal hair cells and on the initial part of the auditory nerve fibres at the base of the internal hair cells. These anatomical facts bestow the system with a wide range of interaction possibilities, e.g., the CNS may control, select, or condition its auditory input, while auditory input may affect the CNS in diverse ways (Velluti *et al.*, 1989, 2003; Pedemonte *et al.*, 1996a, 2004).

The central influence begins to be exerted at the receptor itself as demonstrated by the changes imposed on the auditory nerve compound action potential (cAP) and the cochlear microphonic (CM) recordings by habituation to a tone-burst (Buño *et al.*, 1966) and by the shift from W to sleep as well (Velluti *et al.*, 1989). Figure 1 is an example exhibiting significant amplitude changes of cAP and CM on passing from W to SWS and PS. The averaged amplitude increases during SWS and decreases in PS to levels similar to quiet W. These field potentials were recorded in freely moving guinea pigs with the pre-receptorial mechanisms removed or avoided.

Sleep changes the neuronal activity in brainstem auditory nuclei and auditory cortex

Table 1 presents the firing rate changes of auditory neurones recorded in partially restrained guinea pigs recorded through a glass micropipette, during W and sleep phases. The extracellularly recorded unitary response

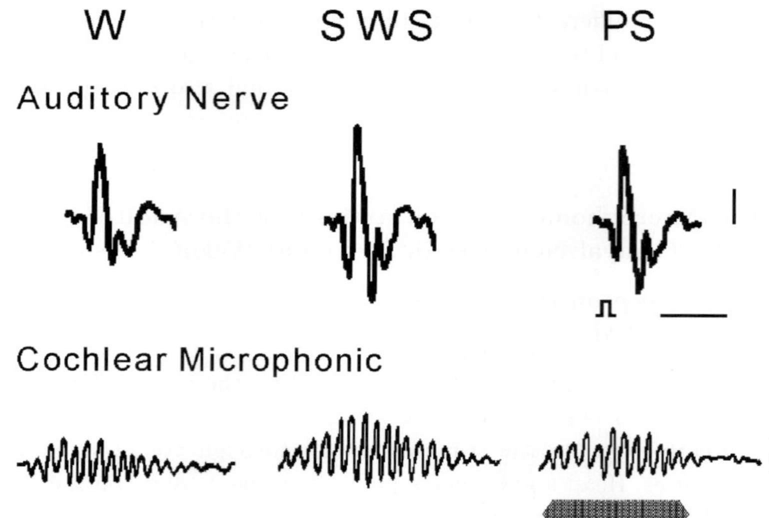

Figure 1. Auditory nerve compound action potential (cAP) and cochlear microphonic (CM) during wakefulness (W), slow wave sleep (SWS), and paradoxical sleep (PS) in the guinea pig. Both signals were recorded from the round window with an implanted macro-electrode. The CM was evoked by a pure tone-burst (1000 Hz) and the cAP by a click (0.15 ms). CM and cAP were averaged ($n = 30$) and in both cases the amplitude increases during SWS and decreases during PS in comparison with a quiet waking period. Calibration bars are: cAP, 5 ms, 50 μV; CM, 5 ms, 200 μV. (Modified from Velluti *et al.*, 1989.)

in each nucleus and in the primary cortex was grouped according to the firing rate changes upon passing to sleep. Neurones could decrease, increase, or exhibit no significant shifts in their discharge. However, there were never completely silent neurones detected when entering into sleep, SWS, or PS (Peña *et al.*, 1992, 1999; Pedemonte *et al.*, 1994, 2001, 2004; Morales-Cobas *et al.*, 1995; Velluti *et al.*, 2000; Velluti and Pedemonte, 2002; Pedemonte and Velluti, 2005). Thus, it is concluded that the afferent input to the primary auditory cortex is not interrupted during any sleep phase, i.e., there is no deafferentation.

Neurones of the medial geniculate nucleus, the auditory thalamus, showed evoked firing shifts mainly decreasing on passing from W to SWS, while the spatial receptive field was preserved indicating that the information sent to cortical cells may carry significant content (Edeline *et al.*, 2000; Edeline, 2003).

Approximately one-half of the auditory cortical neurones responding to a characteristic frequency tone-burst maintained a firing rate equal to that

Table 1. Neuronal firing during the sleep–waking cycle.

	Firing increment (% of neurons)			Firing decrement (% of neurons)			No firing change (% of neurons)		
	W→SWS	SWS→PS	PS→W control	W→SWS	SWS→PS	PS→W control	W→SWS	SWS→PS	PS→W control
Auditory cortex	18	25	22	24	25	22	58	50	56
Inferior colliculus	29	32		36	36		35	32	
Lateral superior olive	33	44		47	42		20	14	
Cochlear nucleus	47	50		29	20		24	30	

W, wakefulness; SWS, slow wave sleep; PS, paradoxical sleep. (Data from: Peña *et al.*, 1992, 1999; Pedemonte *et al.*, 1994; Morales-Cobas *et al.*, 1995.)

observed in a previous or subsequent W. We assume that this set of units is performing a continuous monitoring of the environment. The other $\sim 50\%$ of the neurones is divided into neurones that increase or decrease their discharge. This particular set of neurones may be part of neuronal networks that, in some unknown way, could actively participate in sleep processes. Further, we support the notion that the incoming sensory information is functionally active in sleep processes, not only a passive participant (Velluti, 2005, Chapter 11).

To further demonstrate how the auditory neuronal firing changes at the cortical level on passing from W to SWS to PS, and back from PS to W, the PS to W (last row in Table 1) shows, after a sleep cycle, a return to the initial W–SWS percentages. This is an indication of a neatly reversible process, being also another experimental demonstration that the afferent input to the auditory cortex is dynamic, although predictable, and that the cortex is not deafferented during sleep.

Four examples of changes in the unitary response on passing from W to SWS and PS are shown in Figure 2. A cochlear nucleus neurone that exhibits a "primary-like" post-stimulus time histogram increased its firing during SWS and PS. The control W periods, pre- and post-sleep epochs, showed a remarkable pattern and firing similarities.

The lateral superior olive example presents a different situation: the unit progressively decreases its discharge rate when passing to sleep phases while the pattern of discharge is neatly changed. The neurone that initially, during W, was an "on-sustained" unit is transformed into an "onset" one during PS, i.e., discharging only at the beginning of the stimulus.

The example neurone of the inferior colliculus changes the pattern, that is, the temporal distribution of the neuronal discharge, in spite of a non-significant firing rate shift, on passing from W to sleep phases.

In the primary auditory cortex (AI), a continuously decreasing unitary firing rate during sleep shows a recovered pattern in the subsequent W epoch after a sleep cycle is completed.

Temporal correlation between auditory neuronal firing and hippocampal theta rhythm in sleep and wakefulness

> El movimiento, ocupación de sitios distintos en instantes distintos, es inconcebible sin tiempo; asimismo lo es la inmovilidad, ocupación de un mismo lugar en distintos puntos del tiempo.
>
> *Historia de la Eternidad. Jorge Luis Borges (1936)**

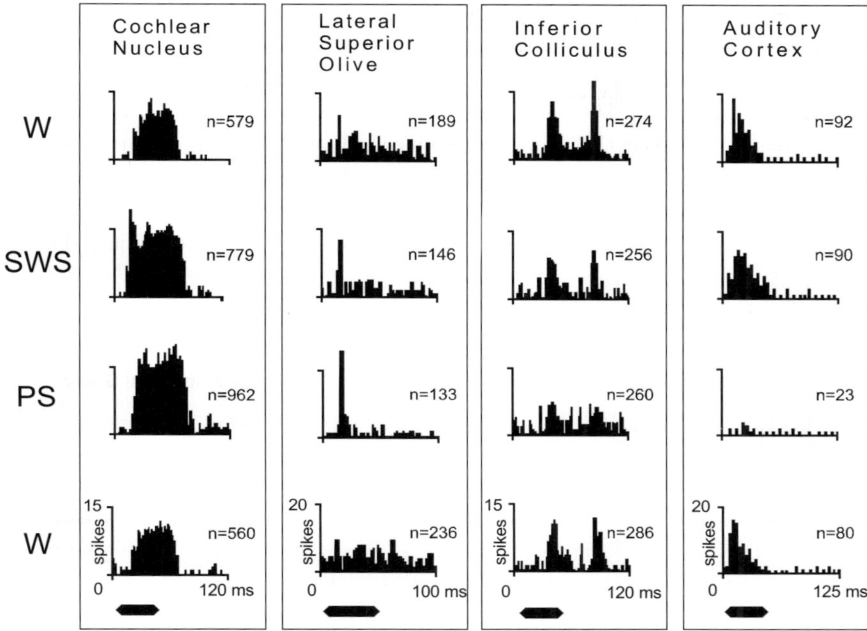

Figure 2. Four representatives auditory neurones recorded at different auditory loci (cochlear nucleus, lateral superior olive, inferior colliculus, and auditory cortex) during the sleep–waking cycle are shown. Post-stimulus time histograms exhibit changes in the pattern and/or in the frequency of discharge on passing from wakefulness (W) to slow wave sleep (SWS) and paradoxical sleep (PS). In these examples the cochlear nucleus recorded neurone increases the firing rate during sleep maintaining the same pattern of discharge; the lateral superior olive shows both a change in pattern and a decrease in firing during sleep. The inferior colliculus neurone exhibits a changed pattern but not significant variation in firing rate. The auditory cortex neurone significantly decreases its firing only during PS, recovering it in the following W epoch. Stimuli: tone-burst (50 ms, 5 ms rise-decay time, at the unit characteristic frequency). (Data from Peña *et al.*, 1992, 1999; Pedemonte *et al.*, 1994; Morales-Cobas *et al.*, 1995.)

**Movement, that is occupying different positions at successive points in time, is inconceivable without time; likewise, immobility is occupying the same position at successive points in time (Free translation).

Historia de la Eternidad. Jorge Luis Borges (1936)

The hippocampus is involved in the neural coding of spatial positions (O'Keefe and Recce, 1993; Wallestein *et al.*, 1998; Best *et al.*, 2001) and is necessarily associated with sensory processing. As an experimental animal traverses space, the phase of neurones firing progressively changes to an earlier phase of the ongoing theta rhythm (Skaggs *et al.*, 1996; Magee, 2003). In agreement with Borges (1936), it is our tenet that, "Movement, that is occupying different positions... is unconceivable without time; ...." Time is the other variable that may be controlled by the hippocampus and is represented by the field activity, the theta rhythm, which is postulated as a meaningful factor in the temporal processing of auditory signals. The temporal correlation phenomenon (phase locking) was described during

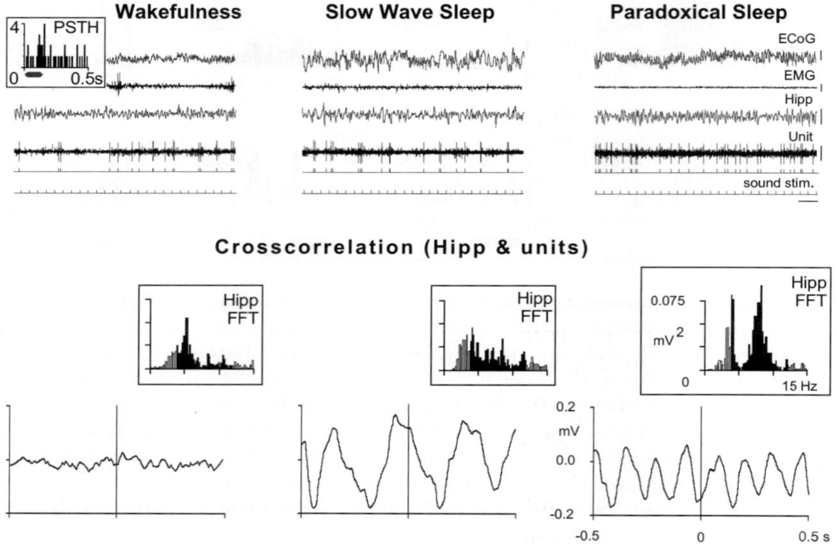

Figure 3. Temporal correlation between the evoked discharges of a primary auditory cortex neurone and hippocampus (Hipp) theta rhythm, during the sleep–wakefulness cycle. Top, raw recordings of the electrocorticogram (ECoG), electromyogram (EMG), Hippocampal (Hipp) field activity, and neuronal discharge (unit) during wakefulness, slow wave, and paradoxical sleep. Digitised units and acoustic stimuli are shown below. The left corner inset shows the post-stimulus time histogram (PSTH) in response to a pure tone-burst stimulus at the unit characteristic frequency. Bottom, the cross-correlation between Hipp field activity and auditory units obtained by spike-triggered averaging. The insets show the Hipp power spectra (FFT) with the theta range in black. The neuronal discharge is phase-locked with the Hipp theta rhythm during slow wave and paradoxical sleep whereas no temporal correlation appears in the wakefulness epoch. Cals.: ECoG, 0.5 mV; EMG, 0.1 mV; Hipp, 0.5 mV; Unit, 0.1 mV; time, 1 s. (Modified from Velluti and Pedemonte, 2002.)

W as well as in both sleep phases, SWS and PS (Figure 3; Pedemonte *et al.*, 1996b, 2001; Velluti *et al.*, 2000; Velluti and Pedemonte, 2002). Furthermore, it is not a fixed phenomenon; it changes because of known and unknown factors. For instance, when a different sensory stimulation is introduced, a shift in phase locking may occur, in W as well as during sleep. Besides, a cyclic on and off temporal correlation to the theta rhythm of about 5 s has been reported (Vinogradova, 2001; Velluti and Pedemonte, 2002).

Vinogradova (2001) classifies the modulator influence of theta rhythm into two systems: (1) a regulatory system, linking the hippocampus to the brain-stem structures, which senses the attention level, introducing primary information about the changes in the environment and, (2) an informational system that holds reciprocal interactions with the neocortex. Moreover, human intracranial recording has revealed theta oscillations in cortical places, suggesting the existence of theta generators in the brain surface (Kahana *et al.*, 2001).

Unitary level processing of complex sound in the guinea pig

When guinea pigs were stimulated with their own call, part of a "whistle" of 700 ms duration, the response of auditory cortex neurones was different when recorded during W or asleep. Furthermore, when the natural call was played backwards, i.e., inverted in time, the neuronal firing changed in W as well as during SWS. As depicted in Figure 4, the response to a "whistle" in W decreased when the same vocalisation was reversed in time.

The same cortical auditory neurone recorded during an SWS epoch exhibited a totally different evoked response. The PSTH with normally played stimulus showed a peak in close temporal correlation with the largest part of the "whistle." On the other hand, when the natural call was played back inverted in time, the evoked unit firing and latency decreased. Perhaps, the PSTH unit peak discharges was relevant in relation to the highest part of the stimulus; however, it is evident that the cortical processing of complex sounds continues to be carried out in SWS.

The reported relationship between the auditory neurones and the hippocampal theta waves, phase locking, was present when the natural call stimulation was used. The neurones studied exhibited phase locking in the cross-correlation during W, SWS, and PS (Pérez-Perera *et al.*, 2001; Pérez-Perera, 2002).

Auditory Cortex Neuron

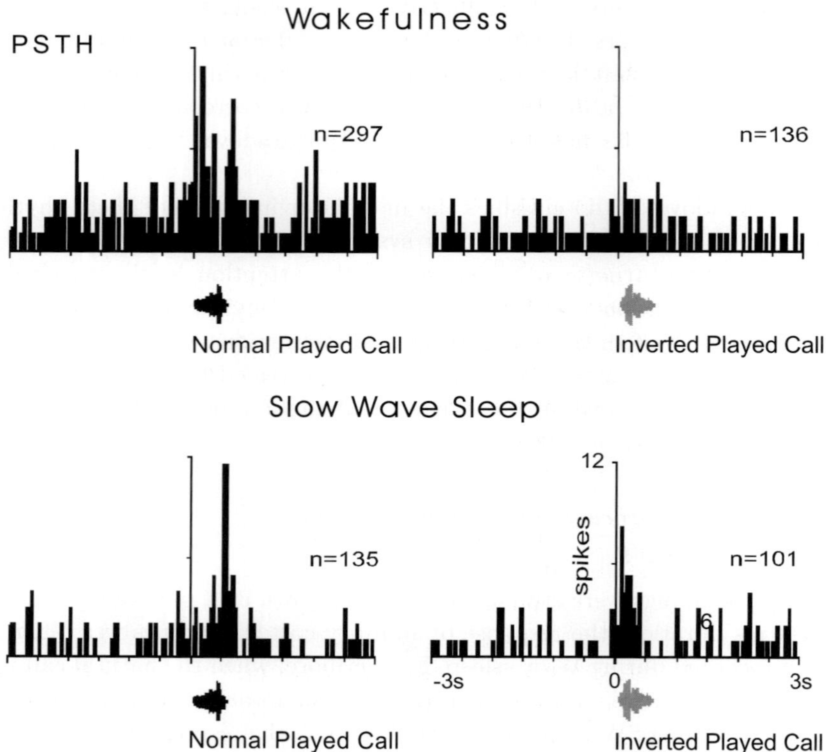

Figure 4. Response of an auditory cortex (AI) neurone evoked by a guinea pig recorded natural call ("whistle") presented in its natural form and reversed in time, during wakefulness and slow wave sleep. Peri-stimulus time histograms (PSTH) analysed during a wakefulness epoch shows that the unit's response to the natural call decreases to about half when the same sound was played backwards. During slow wave sleep these changes also depend on whether the sound reversed or not, but the response does not disappear. The response to the stimulus that is inverted in time in slow wave sleep is smaller and has shorter latency. A relation to the highest part of the stimulus appears as possible (Pérez-Perera *et al.*, 2001; Pérez-Perera, 2002).

Conclusions

The three experimental approaches shown — the auditory neurone's firing rate, the discharge pattern, and the temporal correlation with the theta rhythm — represent evidence of the changes of different aspects of sensory processing that occur in sleep and waking. This also gives an insight into how sensory information processing and sleep mechanisms reciprocally affect each other, participating in the processing and/or in a postulated active promotion of sleep functions. Our main remarks are:

The changes in neuronal discharge rate and pattern in response to constant stimuli indicate that the CNS modulates the incoming auditory information according to the behavioural state, from the auditory nerve to the auditory cortex. Likewise, somatosensory (Pompeiano, 1970; Soja *et al.*, 1998) and visual neurones (Livingstone and Hubel, 1981; McCarley *et al.*, 1983) exhibit changes in their firing rates in correlation with stages of sleep and wakefulness (review, Velluti, 1997). This is consistent with the hypothesis that a general shift in the neuronal network/cell assembly's organisation involved in sensory processing occurs during sleep. This assumption is supported by magnetoencephalographic study of auditory stimulation during sleep performed in humans. The dipole location changed in the auditory cortex on passing to SWS, thus demonstrating the existence of a functional/anatomical network/cell assembly shift upon passing to sleep (Kakigi *et al.*, 2003).

A number of neurones at different auditory *loci*, from the brainstem to the cortex itself, exhibited significant quantitative and qualitative changes in their evoked firing rate and pattern of discharge on passing to sleep. Most important, no neurone belonging to any auditory pathway level or cortex was observed to stop firing on passing to sleep. In addition, our results indicate that the responsiveness of the auditory system during sleep can be considered preserved. Those neurones that continue to fire equal to their firing during W ($\sim 50\%$ at the AI primary cortex) are probably related to a continuous monitoring of the environment, whereas the units that increase or decrease their evoked discharge would participate in sleep-related functions, probably associated with different sleep-related active neuronal networks. We cannot advance what their involvement in sleep neurophysiology could be, but it is our hypothesis that they are actively involved in sleep processes, e.g., sleep organisation, maintenance, and mechanisms of arousal. Functional magnetic resonance imaging (fMRI) in humans has provided evidences that the sleeping brain can process auditory stimuli and detect meaningful events (Portas *et al.*, 2000).

The temporal correlation between hippocampal theta rhythm and the firing of sensory units was shown at several stages in the auditory pathway, and in visual neurones of the thalamus (Gambini *et al.*, 2002). At a neuronal population scale, this phase locking may result in a composite final signal that could be used in processes like attention, movements, and, in particular, auditory sensory processing of incoming information. Furthermore, we propose that the phase locking to the hippocampal theta adds a temporal dimension to the sensory processing, perhaps necessary for time-related perception. Every auditory stimulus develops in time, which is why the CNS must have a functional possibility to encode this parameter. The hippocampus theta waves, being one of the most regular brain-generated low-frequency rhythms, may participate as an internal low-frequency clock acting as a time giver (Pedemonte *et al.*, 1996b, 2001; Velluti *et al.*, 2000; Velluti and Pedemonte, 2002; Pedemonte and Velluti, 2005).

Furthermore, discrimination of significant auditory signals from a background noise is a result of the enhancing of excitatory and inhibitory periods in the unit responses to the acoustic stimulus under hippocampal theta influences (Parmeggiani *et al.*, 1982). The phase precession of CA1 cell and theta waves that occur when the rat is approaching a specific place — i.e., the unit appears earlier in relation to theta waves — constitutes an example of a temporal coding in the mammalian (Magee, 2003). This precession phenomenon has also been associated with non-spatial behaviours such as PS (REM sleep; Buzsaki, 2002).

The temporal relationship between the neuronal firing and the hippocampus field activity is a varying phenomenon in the time domain and may be dependent on the interaction of sets of signals: (i) the hippocampal rhythm amplitude and/or frequency; (ii) the current state of the brain, awake or asleep; and (iii) the characteristics of the incoming sensory information.

The response of auditory neurones to vocalisations supports the experimental results obtained by using artificial sound (tone bursts). In general, the population of cortical neurones stimulated with natural sounds showed the same W and SWS firing shifts and hippocampal theta phase locking as in response to artificial stimuli. Furthermore, during SWS both responses were present and different, perhaps representing a component of another processing category in a different neuronal network/cell assembly. In addition, it has been suggested that AI might serve a general purpose hub of the auditory pathway for the representation of complex sound features to be later complemented with higher auditory centres that further process high-level properties (Griffiths *et al.*, 2004).

The corollaries of these findings are: (a) The units responding during both sleep and W are probably related to the environment monitoring; (b) The neurones that increase or decrease firing during sleep — as well as those units that exhibit theta phase locking — support the notion that the auditory input is part of an active process in sleep neurophysiology. This concept is also supported by human fMRI studies; (c) The changes in the response to natural "whistle" as stimulus may be indicative of a different processing although present during SWS; (d) It is further suggested that the activity-dependent development of the brain during early life may not only occur during wakefulness (Marks *et al.*, 1995) but also during the long physiological sleep periods of newborns and infants. During early ontogenetic development, and maybe also in adulthood, the sensory information that reaches the CNS during sleep may "sculpt" the brain and participate in the adaptation to novel conditions; (e) The first step towards an auditory learning process is the demonstration that the incoming corresponding information may be differentially processed in sleep and therefore could be learned. This is consistent with recent reports of learning during sleep in human newborns (Cheour *et al.*, 2002), consolidation of perceptual learning of spoken language in sleep (Fenn *et al.*, 2003), and visual discrimination improved after sleep (Stickgold *et al.*, 2000) observed in different sensory systems.

Acknowledgments

We are grateful to Dr José L. Peña (Caltech, USA), Prof P.L. Parmeggiani, and Prof G. Zamboni, from the Università di Bologna (Italy), for reading the manuscript and their valuable suggestions. Partially supported by the Program for Basic Sciences Development (PEDECIBA, Uruguay).

References

Adey, W.R., Dunlop, C.W., and Hendrix, C.E. (1960). Hippocampal slow waves distribution and phase relations in the course of approach learning. *Arch. Neurol.*, 3: 74–90.

Affani, J.M. and Cervino, C.O. (2005). Interactions between sleep, wakefulness and the olfactory system. In: Parmeggiani, P.L. and Velluti, R.A. (Eds.). *The Physiological Nature of Sleep*. London: Imperial College Press.

Bastuji, H. and García-Larrea, L. (1999). Evoked potentials as a tool for the investigation of human sleep. *Sleep Med. Rev.*, 3: 23–45.

Bastuji, H. and García-Larrea, L. (2005). Human auditory information processing during sleep assessed with evoked potentials. In: Parmeggiani, P.L. and Velluti, R.A. (Eds.). *The Physiological Nature of Sleep*. London: Imperial College Press.

Bastuji, H., Perrin, F., and García-Larrea, L. (2002). Semantic analysis of auditory input during sleep: studies with event related potentials. *Int. J. Psychophysiol.*, 46: 243–255.

Best, P.J., White, A.M., and Minai, A. (2001). Spatial processing in the brain: the activity of hippocampal place cells. *Ann. Rev. Neurosci.*, 24: 459–486.

Buño, W. and Velluti, J.C. (1977). Relationship of hippocampal theta cycle with bar pressing during self-stimulation. *Physiol. Behav.*, 19: 615–621.

Buño, W., Velluti, R., Handler, P., and García-Austt, E. (1966). Neural control of the cochlear input in the wakeful free guinea pig. *Physiol. Behav.*, 1: 23–35.

Burgess, A.P. and Gruzelier, J.H. (1997). Short duration synchronization of human theta rhythm during recognition memory. *Neurol. Rep.*, 8: 1039–1042.

Buszaki, G. (2002). Theta oscillations in the hippocampus. *Neuron*, 33: 325–340.

Cazard, P. and Buser, P. (1963). Modification des résponses sensorielles corticales par stimulation de l'hippocampe dorsal chez le lapin. *Electroenceph. Clin. Neurophysiol.*, 15: 413–425.

Cheour, M., Martynova, O., Naatanen, R., Erkkola, R., Sillanpaa, M., Kero, P., Raz, A., Kaipio, M.-L., Hiltunen, J., Aaltonen, O., Savela, J., and Hamalainen, H. (2002). Speech sounds learned by sleeping newborns. *Nature*, 415: 599–600.

Cutrera, R., Pedemonte, M., Vanini, G., Goldstein, N., Savorini, D., Cardinali, D.P., and Velluti, R.A. (2000). Auditory deprivation modifies biological rhythms in the golden hamster. *Arch. Ital. Biol.*, 138: 285–293.

Doppelmayr, M., Klimesch, W., Schwaiger, J., Auinger, P., and Winkler, T. (1998). Theta synchronization in the human EEG and episodic retrieval. *Neurosci. Lett.*, 257: 41–44.

Edeline, J.-M. (2003). The thalamo-cortical auditory receptive fields: regulation by the sates of vigilance, learning and neuromodulatory systems. *Exp. Brain Res.*, 153: 554–572.

Edeline, J.-M., Manunta, Y., and Hennevin, E. (2000). Auditory thalamus neurones during sleep: changes in frequency selectivity, threshold, and receptive field size. *J. Neurophysiol.*, 84: 934–952.

Fenn, K.M., Nusbaum, H.C., and Margoliash, D. (2003). Consolidation during sleep of perceptual learning of spoken language. *Nature*, 425: 614–616.

Gambini, J.P., Velluti, R.A., and Pedemonte, M. (2002). Hippocampal theta rhythm synchronized visual neurones in sleep and waking. *Brain Res.*, 926: 137–141.

García-Austt, E. (1984). Hippocampal level of neural integration. In: Ajmone-Marsan, E. and Reinoso-Suárez, F. (Eds.). *Cortical Integration Basic Archicortical and Cortical Association Levels of Neuronal Integrations.* IBRO Monograph Series. New York: Raven Press, pp. 91–104.

Gaztelu, J.M., Romero-Vives, M., Abraira, V., and García-Austt, E. (1994). Hippocampal EEG theta power density is similar during slow-wave sleep and paradoxical sleep. A long-term study in rats. *Neurosci. Lett.*, 172: 31–34.

Grastyán, E., Lissák, K., and Madarász, I. (1959). Hippocampal activity during the development of conditioned reflex. *Electroenceph. Clin. Neurophysiol.*, 11: 409–430.

Griffiths, T.D., Warren, J.D., Scott, S.K., Nelken, I., and King, A.J. (2004). Cortical processing of complex sound: a way forward? *Trends Neurosci.*, 27: 181–185.

Hall, R.D. and Borbély, A.A. (1970). Acoustically evoked potentials in the rat during sleep and waking. *Exp. Brain Res.*, 11: 93–110.

Kahana, M.J., Sekuler, R., Caplan, J.B., Kirschen, M., and Madsen, J.R. (1999). Human theta oscillations exhibit task dependence during virtual maze navigation. *Nature*, 399: 781–784.

Kahana, M.J., Seelig, D., and Madsen, J.R. (2001). Theta returns. *Curr. Opin. Neurobiol.*, 11: 739–744.

Kakigi, R., Naka, D., Okusa, T., Wang, X., Inui, K., Qiu, Y., Tran, T.D., Miki, K., Tamura, Y., Nguyen, T.B., Watanabe, S., and Hoshiyama, M. (2003). Sensory perception during sleep in humans: a magnetoencephalographic study. *Sleep Med.*, 4: 493–507.

Klimesch, W. (1999). EEG alpha and theta oscillations reflect cognitive and memory performance: a review and analysis. *Brain Res. Rev.*, 29: 169–195.

Kramis, R., Vanderwolf, C.H., and Bland, B.H. (1975). Two types of hippocampal rhythmical slow activity in both the rabbit and the rat: relations to behaviour and effects atropine, diethyl ether, urethane and pentobarbital. *Exp. Neurol.*, 49: 58–85.

Kocsis, B. and Vertes, R.P. (1992). Dorsal raphe neurones: synchronous discharge with theta rhythm of the hippocampus in the freely behaving rat. *J. Neurophysiol.*, 68: 1463–1467.

Komisariuk, B. (1970). Synchrony between limbic system theta activity and rhythmical behaviour in rats. *J. Comp. Physiol. Psychol.*, 10: 482–492.

Lerma, J. and García-Austt, E. (1985). Hippocampal theta rhythm during paradoxical sleep. Effects of afferent stimuli and phase-relationships with phasic events. *Electroenceph. Clin. Neurophysiol.*, 60: 46–54.

Livingstone, M.S. and Hubel, D.H. (1981). Effects of sleep and arousal on the processing of visual information in the cat. *Nature*, 291: 554–561.

Magee, J.C. (2003). A prominent role for intrinsic neuroneal properties in temporal coding. *Trends Neurosci.*, 26: 14–16.

Margrie, T.W. and Schaefer, A.T. (2003). Theta oscillation coupled spike latencies yield computational vigour in a mammalian sensory system. *J. Physiol.*, 546: 363–374.

Marks, G.A., Shaffery, J.P., Oksenberg, A., Speciale, S.G., and Roffwarg, H.P. (1995). A functional role for REM sleep in brain maturation. *Behav. Brain Res.*, 69: 1–11.

McCarley, R.W. and Hoffman, E.A. (1981). REM sleep dreams and the activation-synthesis hypothesis. *Am. J. Psychiatry*, 138: 904–912.

McCarley, R., Benoit, O., and Barrionuevo, G. (1983). Lateral geniculate nucleus unitary discharge in sleep and waking: state- and rate-specific aspects. *J. Neurophysiol.*, 50: 798–817.

Mehta, M.R., Lee, A.K., and Wilson, M.A. (2002). Role of experience and oscillations in transforming a rate code into a temporal code. *Nature*, 417: 741–746.

Morales-Cobas, G., Ferreira, M.I., and Velluti, R.A. (1995). Sleep and waking firing of inferior colliculus neurons in response to low frequency sound stimulation. *J. Sleep Res.*, 4: 242–251.

Nuñez, A., de Andrés, I., and García-Austt, E. (1991). Relationships of nucleus reticularis pontis oralis neuroneal discharge with sensory and carbachol evoked hippocampal theta rhythm. *Exp. Brain Res.*, 87: 303–308.

O'Keefe, J. and Recce, M.L. (1993). Phase relationship between hippocampal place units and EEG theta rhythm. *Hippocampus*, 3: 317–330.

Parmeggiani, P.L. and Rapisarda, C. (1969). Hippocampal output and sensory mechanisms. *Brain Res.*, 14: 387–400.

Parmeggiani, P.L., Lenzi, P., Azzaroni, A., and D'Alessandro, R. (1982). Hippocampal influence on unit responses elicited in the cat's auditory cortex by acoustic stimulation. *Exp. Neurol.*, 78: 259–274.

Pearson, K.S., Berber, D.S., Tabachnick, B.G., and Fidell, S. (1995). Predicting noise-induced sleep disturbances. *J. Acoust. Soc. Am.*, 97: 331–338.

Pedemonte, M. and Velluti, R.A. (2005). Sleep hippocampal theta rhythm and sensory processing. In: Lader, M., Cardinali, D.P., and Pandi-Perumal, S.R. (Eds.). *Sleep and Sleep Disorders: A Neuropsycho-Pharmacological Approach*. Georgetown, TX: Landes Biosciences, pp. 8–12.

Pedemonte, M., Peña, J.L., Morales-Cobas, G., and Velluti, R.A. (1994). Effects of sleep on the responses of single cells in the lateral superior olive. *Arch. Ital. Biol.*, 132: 165–178.

Pedemonte, M., Peña, J.L., Torterolo, P., and Velluti, R.A. (1996a). Auditory deprivation modifies sleep in the guinea-pig. *Neurosci. Lett.*, 223: 1–4.

Pedemonte, M., Peña, J.L., and Velluti, R.A. (1996b). Firing of inferior colliculus auditory neurone is phase-locked to the hippocampus theta rhythm during paradoxical sleep and waking. *Exp. Brain Res.*, 112: 41–46.

Pedemonte, M., Rodríguez, A., and Velluti, R.A. (1999). Hippocampal theta waves as an electrocardiogram rhythm timer in paradoxical sleep. *Neurosci. Lett.*, 276: 5–8.

Pedemonte, M., Pérez-Perera, L., Peña, J.L., and Velluti, R.A. (2001). Sleep and wakefulness auditory processing: cortical units vs. hippocampal theta rhythm. *Sleep Res. Online*, 4: 51–57.

Pedemonte, M., Goldstein-Daruech, N., and Velluti, R.A. (2003). Temporal correlation between heart rate, medullary units and hippocampal theta rhythm in anesthetized, sleeping and awake guinea pigs. *Auton. Neurosci.: Basic Clin.*, 107: 99–104.

Pedemonte, M., Drexler, D.G., and Velluti, R.A. (2004). Cochlear microphonic changes after noise exposure and gentamicin administration during sleep and waking. *Hearing Res.*, 194: 25–30.

Pérez-Perera, L. (2002). Actividad unitaria de la corteza auditiva: ritmo theta del hipocampo y respuesta a vocalizaciones en el ciclo vigilia-sueño. Master Thesis, Montevideo, Uruguay.

Pérez-Perera, L., Bentancor, C., Pedemonte, M., and Velluti, R.A. (2001). Auditory cortex unitary activity correlated to sleep–wakefulness and theta rhythm in response to natural sounds. *Acta Fsiología*, 7: 187.

Peña, J.L., Pedemonte, M., Ribeiro, M.F., and Velluti, R.A. (1992). Single unit activity in the guinea pig cochlear nucleus during sep and wakefulness. *Arch. Ital. Biol.*, 130: 179–189.

Peña, J.L., Pérez-Perera, L., Bouvier, M., and Velluti, R.A. (1999). Sleep and wakefulness modulation of the neuronal firing in the auditory cortex of the guinea-pig. *Brain Res.*, 816: 463–470.

Pompeiano, O. (1970). Mechanisms of sensorimotor integration during sleep. In: Stellar, E. and Sprague, J.M. (Eds.). *Progress in Physiological Psychology.* New York: Academic Press, pp. 1–179.

Portas, C.M., Krakow, K., Allen, P., Josephs, O., Armony, J.L., and Frith, C.D. (2000). Auditory processing across the sep-wake cycle: simultaneous EEG and fMRI monitoring in human. *Neuron*, 28: 991–999.

Rabat, A., Bouyer, J.J., Aran, J.M., Courtiere, A., Mayo, W., and LeMoal, M. (2004). Deleterious effects of an environmental noise on sleep and contribution of its physical components in a rat model. *Brain Res.*, 1009: 88–97.

Redding, F.K. (1967). Modification of sensory cortical evoked potentials by hippocampal stimulation. *Electroenceph. Clin. Neurophysiol.*, 22: 74–83.

Reivich, M., Isaacs, G., Evarts, E., and Kety, S.S. (1968). The effects of slow wave sleep and REM sleep on regional cerebral blood flow in cats. *J. Neurochem.*, 15: 301–306.

Sakurai, Y. (1999). How do cell assemblies encode information in the brain? *Neurosci. Biobehav. Rev.*, 23: 785–796.

Sante de Sanctis (1899). *I sogni.* Torino: Fratelli Bocca.

Skaggs, W.E., McNaughton, B.L., Wilson, M.A., and Barnes, C. (1996). Theta phase precession in hippocampal neuroneal populations and the compression of temporal sequences. *Hippocampus*, 6: 149–172.

Soja, P.J., Cairns, B.E., and Kristensen, M.P. (1998). Transmission through ascending trigeminal and lumbar sensory pathways: dependence on behavioral state. In: Lydic, R. and Baghdoyan, H.A. (Eds.). *Handbook of Behavioral State Control.* CRC Press, Boca Raton, FL: pp. 521–544.

Stickgold, R., James, L., and Hobson, J.A. (2000). Visual discrimination learning requires sleep after training. *Nat. Neurosci.*, 3: 1237–1238.

Vallet, M. (1982). La perturbation du sommeil par le bruit. *Soz. Praventivmed.*, 27: 124–131.

Velluti, R.A. (1997). Interactions between sleep and sensory physiology. *J. Sleep Res.*, 6: 61–77.

Velluti, R.A. (2005). Remarks on sensory neurophysiologic mechanisms participating in active sleep processes. In: Parmeggiani, P.L. and Velluti, R.A. (Eds.). *The Physiological Nature of Sleep.* London: Imperial College Press.

Velluti, R.A. and Pedemonte, M. (2002). In vivo approach to the cellular mechanisms for sensory processing in sleep and wakefulness. *Cell Mol. Neurobiol.*, 22: 501–516.

Velluti, R.A., Pedemonte, M., and García-Austt, E. (1989). Correlative changes of auditory nerve and microphonic potentials throughout sleep. *Hearing Res.*, 39: 203–208.

Velluti, R.A., Peña, J.L., and Pedemonte, M. (2000). Reciprocal actions between sensory signals and sleep. *Biol. Signals Receptors*, 9: 297–308.

Velluti, R.A., Pedemonte, M., Suárez, H., Inderkum, A., Rodríguez-Servetti, Z., and Rodríguez-Alvez, A. (2003). Human sleep architecture shifts due to auditory sensory input. *Sleep*, 26(Suppl): A19.

Vertes, R.P. and Kocsis, B. (1997). Brainstem-diencephalo-septohippocampal systems controlling the theta rhythm of the hippocampus. *Neuroscience*, 81: 893–926.

Vital-Durand, F. and Michel, F. (1971). Effets de la desafferentation periphérique sur le cicle veille-sommeil chez le chat. *Arch. Ital. Biol.*, 109: 166–186.

Vinogradova, O.S. (2001). Hippocampus as comparator: role of the two input and two output systems of the hippocampus in selection and registration of information. *Hippocampus*, 11: 578–598.

Wallestein, G.W., Eichenbaum, H., and Hasselmo, M.E. (1998). The hippocampus as an associator of discontiguous events. *Trends Neurosci.*, 21: 317–323.

Winson, J. (1978). Loss of hippocampal theta rhythm results in spatial memory deficit in the rat. *Science*, 201: 160–163.

Chapter 23

HUMAN AUDITORY INFORMATION PROCESSING DURING SLEEP ASSESSED WITH EVOKED POTENTIALS

Hélène Bastuji[1] and Luis García-Larrea

The question whether auditory information processing is or not preserved during sleep has been the subject of considerable controversy. On one hand, absence of behavioural responsiveness to auditory stimuli and of memory recollection during sleep has led to postulate a functional disconnection between the cerebral cortex and external auditory input (Horne, 1989; Jones, 1991; Steriade, 1994). This hypothesis has been supported by electrophysiological results in animal studies suggesting a strong decrease of sensory information processing during sleep, at least at the thalamic level (Pompeiano, 1970; Steriade *et al.*, 1990). On the other hand, awakening may be induced by meaningful stimuli of very low intensity, and sensory information can be incorporated into the sleeper's dreams; these well-known phenomena clearly indicate that sensory integration is not abolished by sleep (Aristotle trad., 1955; Burdach, 1830; Maury, 1878; Formby, 1967; Burton *et al.*, 1988; Halász, 1988; Hobson, 1990). Even if conscious perception is decreased during sleep, the brain needs to be permanently active, not only to control internal functions, but also to induce possible behavioural responses to external information (Halász *et al.*, 2004). Evoked potentials (EPs) to sensory stimuli represent a very effective tool to study sensory information processing in the absence of overt behaviour. Accordingly, they

---

[1] Helene.Bastuji@univ-lyon1.fr

offer a powerful, yet non-invasive means to assess the extent and limits of sensory integration during human sleep. After a brief summary of this specific technique, a review of the literature on this topic will be presented.

Principles and Terminology of Evoked Potentials

The neural electrophysiological responses to sensory stimulation from peripheral to cortical structures can be extracted from scalp EEG activity to obtain evoked potentials. They are recorded by electronic summation or averaging of consecutive responses, a technique that attenuates activities that are independent from the stimulus (i.e., background EEG) but enhances those time-locked to it (i.e., EPs). The number of consecutive stimuli needed to obtain sizeable EPs ranges from a few tens in the case of high amplitude late cortical potentials, to several thousands for low amplitude brainstem responses (for a review of EP technical aspects see Osselton *et al.*, 1995). The different components of EPs are usually labelled N or P according to their negative or positive polarity, followed by a number indicating either their approximate latency in milliseconds (e.g., N100, P150) or their order of occurrence (e.g., N1, P2).

Two kinds of responses are usually distinguished, commonly labelled "sensory" and "cognitive" (or "event-related") EPs. Sensory potentials reflect the activation of peripheral and subcortical afferent pathways and of cortical receiving areas. Accordingly, they arise after short delays following sensory stimulation (1–50 ms), and are strongly dependent on the physical characteristics of the stimulus (intensity, location, sensory modality). They are also described as "obligatory" responses since they are systematically present in normal subjects, and their absence, excessive delay or distortion indicate organic abnormality in sensory transmission or in cortical reception (see Osselton *et al.*, 1995). On the other hand, the "cognitive" (also called "endogenous" or "event-related") EPs are mainly cortical responses related to the processing of the information conveyed by the stimulus, rather than the stimulus itself. They reflect cognitive processes such as attention, memory and response preparation. The generators of these potentials, still imperfectly known, include several cortical associative areas and medial temporal lobe structures such as hippocampus, parahippocampus, and amygdala (for reviews, see Picton, 1992; Hansenne, 2000a). While sensory potentials are obtained by simple repetition of monotonous stimuli, recording of endogenous responses requires the subject to be involved in some stimulus-related cognitive task, such as the active detection of one particular class of stimulus in a stream of irrelevant inputs.

Sensory Evoked Potentials

Peripheral and brainstem responses

The so-called brainstem auditory evoked potentials (BAEPs), recorded within the first 10 ms after the stimulus, reflect the activation of the auditory nerve (wave I) and brainstem auditory structures up to in the upper pons, near the pontomesencephalic junction (wave V). Although early investigators reported sleep-related latency delays of wave V (Amadeo and Shagass, 1973; Osterhammel *et al.*, 1985), no significant effect of sleep was observed in later studies (Campbell and Bartoli, 1986; Bastuji *et al.*, 1988). Small BAEP latency changes during nocturnal sleep were found to correlate with the circadian night fall of body temperature, rather than with sleep stages (Bastuji *et al.*, 1988), and it is now generally accepted that BAEP latencies and amplitudes are insensitive to physiological sleep. These results are consistent with those obtained using sedative drugs, since neither barbiturates nor benzodiazepines modify brainstem EPs at doses inducing general anaesthesia (Sohmer *et al.*, 1978; García-Larrea *et al.*, 1992).

Scalp EP studies in humans have been so far limited to either brainstem or cortical responses, while no EP component has been found to reflect thalamic activation after sensory stimuli, probably due to the "closed field" characteristics of the thalamus preventing far-field recording of local potentials.

Early cortical responses

The study of the earliest cortical components during sleep yielded for several years somewhat conflicting reports. For instance, the "Pa" wave (25–30 ms) reflecting activation of the primary auditory cortex was attenuated during stage 2 and slow wave sleep for Mendel and Goldstein (1971) but remained unmodified in the study of Erwin and Buchwald (1986). Campbell (1992) suggested that early cortical auditory waves were attenuated only for relatively fast stimulation rates (16 stimuli per second). Using stimulus rates of 3–5 Hz, Deiber *et al.* (1989) reported a triphasic behaviour of wave Pa during the sleep cycle, whereby this component was first *enhanced* relative to waking in stage 2, then progressively attenuated during stages 3–4, and became again similar to waking during paradoxical sleep (PS). Reports concerning later cortical waves peaking between 35 and 50 ms (Nb and Pb) have been more uniform, and consistently described amplitude reduction during stages 2–4 (Mendel and Goldstein, 1971; Osterhammel *et al.*, 1985;

Erwin and Buchwald, 1986; Deiber *et al.*, 1989) with partial or total recovery in PS (Mendel and Goldstein, 1971; Erwin and Buchwald, 1986; Deiber *et al.*, 1989).

In summary, synchronised auditory inputs from the outside world give rise to peripheral and brainstem responses which, when recorded from the scalp, remain unaffected by the sleep cycle. Conversely, sleep exerts significant attenuating effects in all cortical responses, and this is consistent with the powerful inhibition exerted over sensorial afferents at the thalamic level, mainly via the nucleus reticularis thalami (Steriade, 1997). Interestingly, thalamic sensory inhibition in animal models partially disappears during paradoxical sleep (Paré and Llinás, 1995; Steriade, 1997), thus providing support for the reversion of sleep effects on evoked potentials during this stage in human. However, the stronger reduction of late cortical responses relative to primary cortical potentials suggests that thalamo-cortical loops may not be the only responsible for these changes, and that intracortical mechanisms and/or diffuse projection systems should also be postulated.

Long Latency Evoked Potentials

The N1–P2 complex

In wakefulness, long latency auditory potentials are formed by a diphasic, negative–positive complex peaking at 100–150 ms post-stimulus and usually labelled "N1–P2," after which the response becomes essentially flat. Although the precise neural generators of the N1–P2 responses are imperfectly known, both mathematical modelling data and intracranial recordings have implicated sources in secondary auditory cortical areas.

Sleep onset is characterised by an immediate latency delay and amplitude attenuation of the N1, associated to a somewhat surprising enhancement of P2 (for a review, see Campbell, 1992). This dissociated behaviour of N1 and P2 components has been interpreted as the progressive disappearance during sleep onset of a slow negative wave, which during wakefulness would be superimposed to N1 and P2. Attenuation or disappearance of this negative wave would reflect tonic decreased cortical excitability (de Lugt *et al.*, 1996). Changes in N1–P2 during sleep onset are so fast and time-locked to sleep entrance that their occurrence has been proposed as a reliable marker of sleep onset (Ogilvie *et al.*, 1991; Campbell, 1992; de Lugt *et al.*, 1996). After sleep entrance, the N1 and P2 modifications persist with little change during both slow wave and paradoxical sleep (for a review, see Bastuji and García-Larrea, 1999).

The evoked K-complex

The most impressive effect of sleep on EPs, observed exclusively in stage 2 and slow wave sleep (SWS), is an *increased complexity* of the response due to the appearance of a sequence of waves never observed during waking or PS. Thus, in stage 1b auditory stimuli evoke a high-amplitude negative wave peaking at about 350 ms post-stimulus (N350 or "N2"), which in stages 2–4 develops into a sequence of several high-amplitude waves persisting for more than 1 s. When fully developed, this complex incorporates four consecutive components with two negativities (N350 and N550) and two positivities (P450 and P900), the amplitude of which may exceed 20 μV (as a reference, the first cortical response Pa is only 2–5 μV).

Loomis *et al.* (1939) and Davis *et al.* (1939) were the first to suggest that the complex auditory late response recorded in humans during sleep stages 2–4 corresponded to *summed K-complexes* evoked by sensory stimulation. This was later verified also in other sensory modalities (mainly visual and somatosensory) and has been since confirmed by many other studies (for a review, see Bastien *et al.*, 2002). However, the K-complex is not systematically elicited by all sensory stimuli (Halász and Ujszászi, 1988; Sallinen *et al.*, 1994) and its different components are neither constant nor invariant in their combination (Ujszászi and Halász, 1986, 1988). The functional heterogeneity of evoked K-complex sub-components has been underscored by studies showing that, when auditory stimuli fail to evoke a full K-complex, an isolated "N350" can often still be recorded (Bastien and Campbell, 1992; Sallinen *et al.*, 1994; Niiyama *et al.*, 1995). The different components are also differentially sensitive to habituation, the N550 wave showing a much stronger decrease with stimulus repetition (i.e., habituation) than the late "P900" (Bastien and Campbell, 1992).

Amzica and Steriade (1998) have shown that K complexes result from a synchronised cortical network that "imposes periodic excitatory and inhibitory actions on cortical neurons," thus creating a cortically generated slow oscillation which spreads through the cortex and is transferred to the thalamus. Evoked K-complexes, although sharing similar features with the ones triggered by the slow oscillation, are for these authors rather the exception than the rule. A different view has been sustained by a number of other investigators, namely that all K-complexes, including the "spontaneous" ones, are in fact *induced* by some exteroceptive or — more often — interoceptive stimuli (for a review, see Halász, 1998). This notion has been supported by data comparing spontaneous and auditory-evoked

K-complexes in humans (Niiyama *et al.*, 1996). These authors observed *in both* types the presence of N1–P2 components preceding the characteristic sequence of K-complex waves, suggesting that even "spontaneous" K-complexes may be triggered by recurrent (maybe periodic) internal stimuli giving rise to early sensory potentials.

In summary, long latency EPs show profound changes during NREM sleep, which revert completely in PS. The N1 component is attenuated, while P2 is enhanced concomitant with sleep onset. A high-amplitude, complex waveform follows the P2 and dominates the response during sleep stages 2–4. This late response is unanimously considered as the result of summed K-complexes evoked by the sensory stimulus. Some components of the evoked K-complexes (N350 and N550) show habituation in response to repetitive stimuli, while habituation is less clear for others (P900).

Event-Related Potentials

Event-related potentials (ERPs) are usually recorded by introducing rare, deviant and/or intrinsically meaningful stimuli within a stimulus train. During wakefulness, these ERPs reflect some cognitive process such as attention, memory, motivation and event discrimination. The use of similar protocols during sleep has been therefore advocated to evaluate the possibility of high-level sensory integration across sleep stages.

Mismatch negativity

In waking subjects, the mismatch negativity (MMN) is elicited by deviant stimuli occurring within a stream of monotonous tones, and it is commonly accepted that it reflects the automatic detection of new sensory input that does not "match" the neuronal representation of the preceding stimuli (Näätänen and Alho, 1995). Since the MMN, which is related to the activation of a temporo-frontal network, is thought to reflect preconscious mechanisms of sensory memory, largely independent from attention, its persistence during sleep may be hypothesised.

Most published studies have failed to demonstrate any significant MMN during SWS, even when recordings have been restricted to stage 2 (for a review, see Atienza *et al.*, 2002). Contrary to results in NREM, Campbell (1992) and then other investigators have reported a genuine "mismatch negativity" during PS (Loewy *et al.*, 1996; Atienza *et al.*, 1997). The PS-MMN appeared to be of similar latency, but smaller amplitude relative to its waking counterpart. Interestingly, this component has recently been reported during quiet sleep (equivalent to adult SWS) in newborns (Cheour *et al.*, 2000).

In summary, while the persistence of a system of deviance detection during NREM sleep is supported by a bulk of convergent studies, the available evidence suggest that such detection does not involve the generation of a cerebral response comparable to the waking-MMN. However, a possible influence of technical factors hampering the recordings (i.e., unfavourable signal-to-noise ratio relative to waking) should not be dismissed, since this very small component may be lost within the much higher sleep negativities.

Event-related potentials to frequency deviance

These event related potentials include a positive component, labelled P300 or P3, which appears in response to rare stimuli randomly delivered in a train of frequent ones. Its presence is known to reflect the detection and discrimination of this deviant stimulus. Many generators are involved in the generation of this component, specially in the frontal, temporal and parietal neocortical, and medial temporal lobes (Baudena *et al.*, 1995; Halgren *et al.*, 1995a,b; Brázdil *et al.*, 1999, 2001).

ERP studies have shown that the discrimination of deviant from repetitive auditory tones by the brain persists during all sleep stages under certain circumstances (Figure 1) (for a review, see Bastuji and García-Larrea, 1999). For instance, both in sleep stage 2 (S2) and slow wave sleep (SWS), deviant stimuli elicit K-complexes of higher amplitude than those evoked by monotonous stimuli (Campbell *et al.*, 1985; Ujszászi and Halász, 1988; Nielsen-Bowman *et al.*, 1991; Bastuji *et al.*, 1995; Bastien *et al.*, 2002). This result indicates that (a) the sleeping brain remains able to detect physical dissimilarities among stimuli, thus reacting to stimulus novelty, and (b) that such detection may somehow implicate the evoked K-complex. Even if deviance detection during NREM may be reflected *in the end* by an enhanced K-complex, a critical question is whether such detection operates through the same mechanisms as in wakefulness. Several teams (Nielsen-Bohlman *et al.*, 1991; Sallinen *et al.*, 1994; Bastuji *et al.*, 1995) observed that the "P450" component to deviant stimuli did not increase with deepening of sleep (from stages 2 to 4) contrary to what was observed for the late "N550–P900" waves. Furthermore, Bastuji *et al.* (1995) noted that the "novelty reaction" of evoked K-complexes did not affect sub-components to the same extent, and increased one of the sub-components (the "P450") to a greater extent than other waves. They suggested that, while amplitude recovery of most K-complex waves may have reflected simple dishabituation related

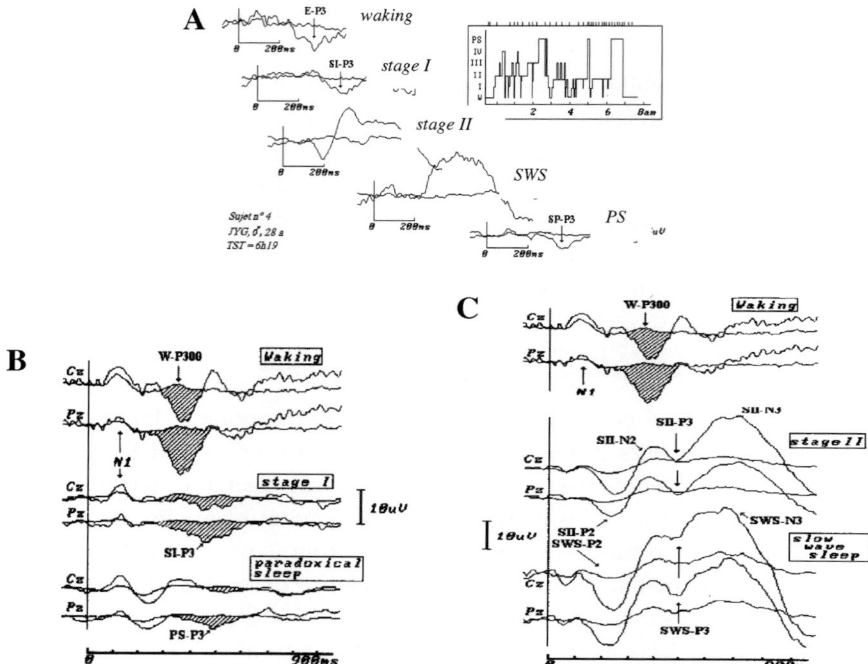

Figure 1. ERPs obtained using pure-tones in a classical odd-ball paradigm. (A) ERPs in one subject during waking and each sleep stage; responses to rare and frequent tones are superimposed. Above the hypnogram (upper right) the small vertical marks indicated the different periods of stimulation. (B) and (C) Grand average ERPs from eight subjects to rare (thick traces) and frequent (thin traces) tones during wakefulness, stage 1, paradoxical sleep, stage 2 and slow wave sleep (negativity up). Note that the morphology of the ERPs are very similar in waking, stage 1 and PS, and differ in stage 2 and SWS with the appearance of new components known to be K complexes. (Adapted from Bastuji *et al.*, 1995.)

to physical deviance, the particular enhancement of P450 might relate to the *relevance* of the stimulus, and therefore to its arousal capacity (Bastuji *et al.*, 1995). It was then suggested that the P450 wave included in the K-complex waveform might be functionally related to the "P3" family of waves sensitive to stimulus discrimination.

During paradoxical (PS or REM) sleep, the morphology of responses to deviant stimuli greatly differs from those obtained in NREM. In particular, deviant stimuli never evoke K-complexes in this sleep stage; they rather give rise to a late positive response at about 450 ms that is reminiscent in latency and scalp topography of the "P3" or "P300" wave recorded during wakefulness in response to task-relevant or meaningful stimuli (Bastuji *et al.*, 1990, 1995; Sallinen *et al.*, 1996; Niiyama *et al.*, 1994; see review, Bastuji and García-Larrea, 1999; Coté, 2002). As illustrated in Figure 1, the P300-like wave recorded during PS is in fact very similar to the one obtained during Stage 1, just following sleep entrance.

Prior familiarisation with the target stimuli during waking facilitates the elicitation of a P300 during paradoxical sleep. Thus, deviant tones of same intensity as background stimuli, appearing with 10% probability, were able to evoke P300-like waves during PS in trained subjects (Bastuji *et al.*, 1990, 1995; Niiyama *et al.*, 1994; Sallinen *et al.*, 1996), but could not evoke PS-P300 in subjects that had not previously learned the task (Coté *et al.*, 2001). In these latter, however, P300-like waves could be triggered during PS by very deviant (delivered at 5% probability) and intrusive stimuli (stimuli much louder than background tones) (Coté and Campbell, 1999; Coté *et al.*, 2001). This leads to the hypothesis that the probability that a given stimulus enters the cognitive level of processing reflected by P300 depends on two phenomena: first, the intrinsic relevance of the stimulus itself, and second its physical intrusiveness. In the case of a previously learned detection task, the significance of the target stimulus is accessible to the subject before going to sleep, and this significance appears to be "transferred" to the ensuing PS. The presence of such a component during PS not only indicates that some stimulus categorisation is possible during this stage, but also that the brain electrophysiological response (and possibly the underlying mechanism of detection) share unique characteristics with those of the waking state.

In summary, a crude detection of physical stimulus salience appears to persist during even the deepest sleep stages, and this contradicts the notion that in NREM each stimulus is treated "as a new one." The mechanisms subserving deviance detection in NREM are reflected by progressive attenuation of K-complexes to repetitive stimuli but recovery of a full-amplitude K-complex to sudden changes in stimulus characteristics. The evoked K-complex appears to be formed by two functionally different "modules," each consisting of a negative–positive complex (N350–P450 and N550–P900), of which the first may be related to the discrimination of relevant information from the external world, while the second appears more related to the stimulus physical salience. Only during PS are the EP reflections of deviance detection (i.e., MMN), and stimulus evaluation (i.e., P300) comparable to those observed during the waking state.

Event-related potentials to subject's own name

In all the studies presented above, the "significant" stimuli delivered differed from the background at least by two features, namely their acoustic properties (i.e., pitch or loudness) *and* their probability of occurrence. In this context, it is difficult to ascertain whether the differential ERPs observed to "rare" stimuli reflect the genuine discrimination of stimulus meaning (access to stimulus intrinsic significance) *or rather* the simple detection of a change in the physical characteristics of the input stream (change in acoustical properties and/or probability of occurrence). To address this dichotomy, more complex stimuli whose intrinsic (i.e., semantic) information is partially independent from their physical attributes — for instance, words — can be used. ERP recording paradigms with verbal material as stimuli are therefore relevant to assess whether and to what extent the detection of a stimulus' intrinsic meaning remains possible during sleep (Bastuji *et al.*, 2002).

The subjects' own names were recently used in ERP sleep studies to answer this question (Pratt *et al.*, 1999; Perrin *et al.*, 1999, 2000). The reasons to choose this type of stimulus were, first, that a person's own name, because of its emotional content and repetition along life, appears as one of the most relevant stimulus for any human subject. Second, there is evidence that hearing our own name during wakefulness produces cognitive brain responses, including a P300, even in the absence of explicit instructions, thus suggesting that a subject's name is automatically and implicitly processed as a target stimulus (Berlad and Pratt, 1995). Indeed, a positive wave peaking between 400 and 500 ms after the beginning of the stimulus has been evoked by the presentation to waking subjects of their own name in "passive" (i.e., "no task") conditions (Berlad and Pratt, 1995; Pratt *et al.*, 1999; Perrin *et al.*, 1999). The characteristics of this wave (latency, amplitude, and scalp topography) are consistent with those of the cognitive "P300" component recorded in target detection tasks (see Figure 2), known to be determined by the task relevance and the unpredictability of the stimulus (for reviews, see Picton, 1992; Hansenne, 2000a).

During sleep, Pratt and co-workers used the subject's own name against a single irrelevant word which acted as "non-target"; probabilities of presentation of both types of words were counterbalanced so as the "target" word could appear with either 30 or 70%. These investigators observed a significant effect of stimulus type (own name versus irrelevant word) during S2 and SWS for different components between 300 and 700 ms, and especially a more prominent P450 during stage 2 in addition to K-complex waveform. They also reported an effect of stimulus probability during PS for the P3 component (rare targets eliciting higher P3s than frequent targets), suggesting a resemblance to the waking P300 wave. Interpretation of their results in terms of detection of stimulus meaning is however uneasy because target and non-target words, although counterbalanced, were not equiprobable (70 versus 30%), thus making the responses sensitive to habituation and "physical novelty" effects, in addition to stimulus significance. To get rid of possible ambiguities linked to these phenomena, Perrin *et al.* (1999) used a paradigm where the subject's own name was presented in strict equiprobable fashion against seven other first names (with 12.5% probability each). Auditory ERPs from ten healthy volunteers were recorded under these conditions, both during wakefulness and all-night

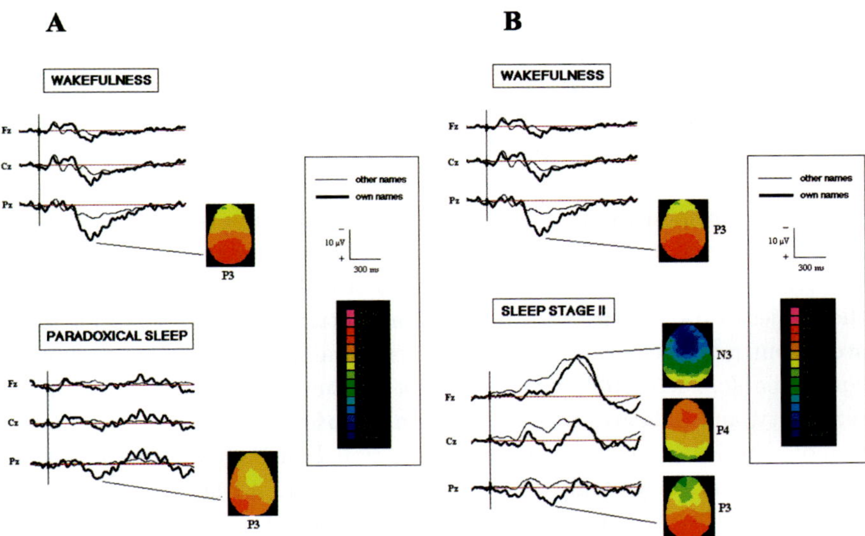

Figure 2. ERPs to own (thick traces) and other (thin traces) names. Averaged traces from 10 subjects. (negativity up). (A) Grand average ERPs during passive pre-sleep waking and paradoxical sleep (PS). Note on the corresponding map the posterior and left maximal amplitude of P3 during PS and the absence of P3 to other names in this stage. (B) Grand average ERPs during passive pre-sleep waking (top) and stage 2 (S2). The topographic maps of P3 are represented for each condition and those of N3 and P4 for S2. (C) Grand average ERPs in S2 of traces without K-complexes. (D) Grand average ERPs in S2 of traces with K-complexes. Note that a P3 to own names was observed in S2 whether K-complexes were or not present, and that a smaller P3 to other names was also recorded during this stage. The amplitude of the N3/P4 was similar in response of both own and other names. (Adapted from Perrin *et al.*, 1999, 2000.)

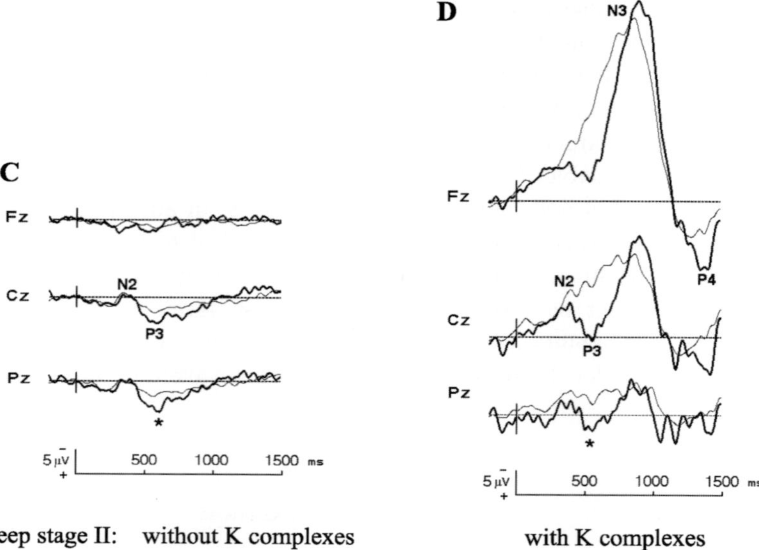

Figure 2. (*Continued*)

sleep (SWS responses not analysed). During wakefulness and paradoxical sleep the general morphology of ERPs was very similar (Figure 2); notably, in both cases a late positive wave at 400–600 ms was selectively evoked by the subject's own name, with maximal amplitude over the posterior scalp areas (but more posterior in PS than during waking). Since all stimuli were equiprobable, such ERP effect could not be due to differences in stimulus regularity, and indicates that the brain mechanisms subserving discrimination of a subject's own name remain operational during paradoxical (REM) sleep, independently of any "physical rarity" effect. We may postulate that the subject's own name constitutes an intrinsically significant stimulus, the knowledge of which needs not be transferred since it is permanently operational; therefore, one's own name can *always* enter a higher level of processing — hence explaining the emergence of a P300 in PS without the need of previous training.

As in all previous studies, the general morphology of ERPs was much more complex during SWS than in waking or PS, most probably because responses in SWS often included K-complexes induced by auditory stimulation (for reviews, see Halász, 1998; Bastuji and García-Larrea, 1999; Bastien *et al.*, 2002). When S2 and SWS ERPs are averaged in the presence of concomitant visible K-complexes on background EEG, the responses include two biphasic consecutive waveforms, commonly labelled "N2/P3" and "N3/P4." When stimuli were proper names, the latencies of these waveforms were delayed as compared to those obtained with tones (Figure 2), probably because of differences in stimulus duration; however, their morphology and scalp distribution were equivalent to those of "N2/P3" and "N3/P4," classically described during S2 and SWS. In the study of Perrin *et al.* (1999) these two biphasic waveforms evolved differentially in response to "subject's own" and "other" names: while the amplitude of the late complex ("N3/P4") was identical for both types of stimuli, the early portion of the K-complex ("N2/P3"), and notably the positive wave P3, were of significantly higher amplitude to the presentation of "own" names. Such differential behaviour strengthens the hypothesis of a "functional duality" of K-complex generating mechanisms, originally put forward by Ujszászi and Halász (1988) who suggested that the early and late K-complex waveforms reflected the activation of two distinct functional systems, of which only the former would be connected to the information processing of external stimuli. Recently, Halász *et al.* (2004) reviewing the data on this topic, have emphasised the "Janus-faced nature of K-complexes" with both activating and sleep preserving properties.

When ERPs are averaged in the absence of concomitant K-complexes in the EEG, only the early portion of the response ("N2–P3"), of low amplitude, is commonly observed (Perrin *et al.*, 2000; see Figure 2). Both latency and scalp distribution strongly suggest that these N2–P3 waves, when evoked alone, do correspond to the early portion of the K-complex described previously. Perrin *et al.* (2000) analysed these two early components with and without the presence of a concomitant K-complex, and showed that they were significantly enhanced in response to the subjects' own name relative to other first names, to a similar degree whether they were part of a K-complex or not. The P3 wave sensitivity to the subject's own name, both in presence and in absence of a K-complex, suggests that the processing of such stimulus significance during S2 is effective even when the high amplitude N3–P4, which corresponds to the typical form of K-complex, is not elicited. This also means that the differential response to the own name is not contingent of the "full" K-complex. Therefore, even if the K-complex might be elicited by an auditory stimulus, its evocation is not necessary to the electrophysiological detection of a relevant stimulus.

Are sleep and waking P3s functionally equivalent?

The persistence of "P3" (or "P300-like") component to the subject's own name during S2 and PS indicates that some cognitive processing of relevant stimuli also persists during sleep. However, the existence of sleep-P3s does not necessarily imply that their underlying processes are equivalent to those of waking, and the question whether waking and sleep P3s can be considered as functionally equivalent remains open.

Paradoxical (REM) sleep

During paradoxical sleep, the general morphology of the P3, its latency, specificity to relevant stimuli and scalp distribution are close to that observed during wakefulness. Waking P300 occurs when the subject is actively engaged in a detection task; it is related to stimulus categorisation and may represent a post-decisional "cognitive closure" mechanism (for reviews, see Picton, 1992; Hansenne, 2000a,b). Considering the PS-P3 as a functional equivalent of the waking P300 assumes therefore that stimulus selection and categorisation remain active during this sleep stage. This also implies that some top-down processes remain operational during paradoxical sleep, since comparison of incoming stimulus against some pre-existing template is necessary for stimulus selection. These assumptions are not incompatible with current thoughts about the cognitive capabilities of paradoxical sleep (Hobson, 1990; Paré and Llinás, 1995). However, although the PS-P3 and the waking-P3 may have some common functional significance, their respective cerebral generators do not appear to be strictly the same. Indeed, the scalp topography of PS-P3 consistently differs from that of waking P3: frontal subcomponents are lacking during PS, resulting in a significant "shift" of PS-P3 towards the posterior regions of the scalp (Niiyama *et al.*, 1994; Bastuji *et al.*, 1995; Cote and Campbell, 1999; Perrin *et al.*, 1999). Such topographical changes might reflect a deficit in the activation of frontal P3 generators thought to subserve attentional control and orienting during waking P3 (Baudena *et al.*, 1995; Brázdil *et al.*, 1999), such attenuation leading to a anterior-posterior disbalance during P3 generation, with predominance of posterior (visual) and parieto-temporal P3-related processes. This suggestion fits with recent neuroimaging results showing a deficit in frontal activation during paradoxical sleep, concomitant with an enhancement of the temporo-posterior metabolism (for a review, see Maquet, 2000).

From a neurochemical point of view, the balance between noradrenergic and cholinergic cerebral systems also changes critically from wakefulness to PS, with decrease in noradrenergic activity and activation of cholinergic processes (Siegel and Rogawski, 1988; Hobson, 1990; Steriade *et al.*, 1990). Taking account that both systems are important for P300 generation during waking (Hammond *et al.*, 1987; Harrison *et al.*, 1988; Pineda *et al.*, 1989; Swick *et al.*, 1994), and that the noradrenergic projections, notably from the locus coeruleus, are largely distributed over the prefrontal cortex (Oken and Salinsky, 1992; Arnsten *et al.*, 1996), it may be hypothesised that topographic changes observed in electrophysiological and metabolic studies during PS may also be related to the decrease of noradrenergic tone during this stage. Thus, while keeping close functional significance, PS and waking P3 activities may be sustained by generating mechanisms with only partial overlap. Such differences might in turn help to explain the disparities in the processing of sensory information, notably stimulus awareness and memory encoding, during the two stages, as animal data suggest that memory storage is regulated by an interaction of noradrenergic and cholinergic influences (e.g., Introinicollison *et al.*, 1996).

Sleep stage 2

The comparisons between sleep stage 2 and waking P3s are more difficult, the significance of "P3" during this stage remaining still subject to controversy. Indeed, even if in stage 2 a "P3" component ("S2-P3") is enhanced in response to subjects' own name, this component may also be observed, with lower amplitude, in response to other names (Perrin *et al.*, 1999, 2000) (see Figure 2), and even in response to repetitive monotonous tones (Ujszászi and Halász, 1988; Nielsen-Bohlman *et al.*, 1991; Bastuji *et al.*, 1995; Hull and Harsh, 2001). The "S2-P3" thus seems to be much less selective to relevant stimuli than the PS-P3, and considering the family of S2-P3s as pure reflects of the discrimination of a relevant stimulus is hardly tenable. Weakening of P300 selectivity to relevant stimuli has been reported in some pathological contexts such as schizophrenia (Wagner *et al.*, 1997; Nieman *et al.*, 1998; Knott *et al.*, 1999), and interpreted as a deficit in non-target inhibition. Similar conclusions were proposed on a patient with blindsight (Shefrin *et al.*, 1988), in whom a P300 was observed in response to both rare and frequent stimuli delivered in the blind hemifield, suggesting that both relevant and irrelevant stimuli were processed as targets. Although these results may be reminiscent of those observed during sleep S2, they can hardly be integrated in a same model, since their unique convergence stands in the unselective behaviour of P300. During SWS, the whole metabolic activity of the cortex is decreased (Maquet, 2000) and there is some experimental evidence to suppose a specific inhibition of thalamo-cortical connectivity (Steriade, 1994). The extent to which a reduced capability for selective stimulus processing in stage 2 would be related to the functional changes in thalamo-cortical network during this stage needs further investigation. A further difference between S2 and waking P3 is the presence, during S2 exclusively, of "N3" and "P4" potentials corresponding to the late portions of the K-complex. The N2/P3 and N3/P4 complexes may reflect the occurrence of two parallel mechanisms in response to stimulus presentation, of which only the first would be sensitive to the stimulus' intrinsic relevance, the second being related to its salience or physical deviance (Perrin *et al.*, 2000; Halász *et al.*, 2004).

P300, consciousness and memory encoding

During wakefulness, P300 has been considered as an electrophysiological event concomitant to the access of information to consciousness and memory (for reviews, see Picton, 1992; Hansenne, 2000). In favour of this hypothesis stands the fact that, in waking, the P300 is a response to events requiring controlled processing, which is both effortful and conscious. Several teams have shown a relationship between P300 characteristics and subsequent memory of the stimulus (Johnson *et al.*, 1985; Howard and Polich, 1985), and drugs with deleterious effects on memory, such as anticholinergics, are also deleterious for P300 (Potter *et al.*, 1992). From results obtained during sleep, it is obvious that *the mere presence of a P3 in average traces does not warrant the access of stimulus to stable memory stores*, since this component can be recorded during PS (and probably S2) even if subjects will not remember the stimulus after awakening. A similar dissociation between P3 and conscious awareness has been described in a few patients with very particular cognitive disorders, such as the prosopagnosic patient recorded by Renault *et al.* (1989) and the patient with blindsight reported by Shefrin *et al.* (1988). These results among others suggest different levels of stimulus encoding, and notably the possibility of dissociation between instantaneous and long-term awareness. Damasio's model of consciousness appears relevant in this context: in this author's view (Damasio, 1998), a "low" level of consciousness, or *core consciousness*, would correspond to the transient process that is incessantly generated relative to any object with which an organism interacts, and during which a transient "core self," or transient sense of knowing, are automatically generated. A second, higher level, *or "extended consciousness"* would depend upon the build-up of an autobiographical self and a set of memories of past and anticipated experiences. Only this extended consciousness would require conventional memory. A dissociation between "core" and "extended" consciousness during sleep may be hypothesised, but not directly evaluated since this would imply to have subjects awakened immediately after the stimulus sessions, which was not done in previous ERP studies. The question whether some form of "core consciousness" is preserved in association to the evocation of P3 cannot, therefore, be answered at this stage. However, studies showing incorporation of external stimulus to the oniric content (Burton *et al.*, 1988; Nielsen, 1993) give indirect arguments to the possibility that core consciousness might be preserved at least during paradoxical sleep. Further evidence in this line could be gathered in the future if the incorporation of external stimuli to dreams could to be related to P3 generation. Recently, we developed a "forced awakening" test (Bastuji *et al.*, 2003) which allows us to explore the relationship between ERPs, stimulus awareness and subsequent recall, subjects being aroused by the stimuli after 3 min of sleep. In subjects whose quality of recall on forced awakening was excellent, P3 was equal to that obtained before sleep. When recall was degraded, P3 was found attenuated and delayed; finally, absence of any recall was associated with absence of P3, which was replaced by sleep negativities or full K-complexes (Garcia-Larrea *et al.*, 2002). These results suggest that the presence of a P3 is crucial to ensure stimulus encoding, and that the quality of encoding is related to the characteristics of the P3 wave. This component might reflect the passage between "instant awareness" of the stimulus and a more permanent mode of encoding giving access to memory retrieval, while sleep negativities may act as "erasers" preventing accurate memory encoding and retrieval of the stimulus.

Semantic discrimination during sleep

The studies reviewed in previous paragraphs demonstrated that the sleeping brain remains able to discriminate between words varying in their intrinsic meaning (Perrin *et al.*, 1999, 2000; Pratt *et al.*, 1999). However, the stimuli used in those studies were *proper names*, which do not have a strict semantic content as compared with common names. From a linguistic point of view, the question whether the processing of proper names is or not strictly semantic remains controversial (Frege, 1949; Searle, 1967; Muller and Kutas, 1996). Work on neuropsychological disorders (Semenza and Zettin, 1988;

Yasuda *et al.*, 2000), neuroimaging investigations (Damasio *et al.*, 1996) and ERP studies (Proverbio *et al.*, 2001), have provided increasing evidence that common names and proper names do not activate identical cerebral networks. Therefore, even if the subject's own names were certainly "discriminated" during sleep, the actual level of discrimination, i.e., phonological versus semantical, performed by the sleeping brain cannot be specified by these studies.

Two different teams have recently addressed this question, investigating the "N400" wave of ERPs in response to common words devoid of emotional context. During wakefulness, the N400 wave is enhanced in response to words that are semantically irrelevant relative to a given context, the amplitude of this effect being correlated to the degree of semantic incongruence (Kutas and Hillyard, 1980; Bentin *et al.*, 1985). Brualla *et al.* (1998) were the first to report that a negative deflection similar to the N400 persisted during S2 and PS in response to semantically unrelated words, suggesting that a simple semantic association of common words remains operative during these sleep stages. Our team further studied how linguistic and pseudo-linguistic stimuli were categorised during sleep as compared to waking (Perrin *et al.*, 2002). Different sequences of auditory stimuli containing pairs of words which included a "prime" followed by either a semantically congruous word or by an incongruous word (50% each) were presented during waking, S2, and PS. Between each pair, we inserted a "pseudo-word," a disyllabic sound without meaning, which allowed to compare the N400 in response to (a) congruous or (b) incongruous words following a prime, (c) pseudo-words following a real word, and (d) primes following a pseudo-word. During wakefulness, the N400 wave developed higher amplitude for pseudo-words than for real but semantically incongruous words, as previously described (Bentin *et al.*, 1985). The N400 response to incongruous words persisted during stage 2 and PS (Figure 3). During S2, all discordant stimuli, regardless of their category (incongruous words, "prime" words following pseudo-words and pseudo-words following words) yielded enhanced N400 responses relative to congruous words. However, no significant difference existed between different levels of discordance, suggesting a loss in this sleep stage of the hierarchic processes observed in wakefulness.

A hierarchic process of discordance reappeared in PS, which however differed from that of the waking state. While incongruous and "prime" words yielded, as in S2, higher N400 amplitudes than congruous words, N400 amplitude to pseudo-words was surprisingly similar to that elicited

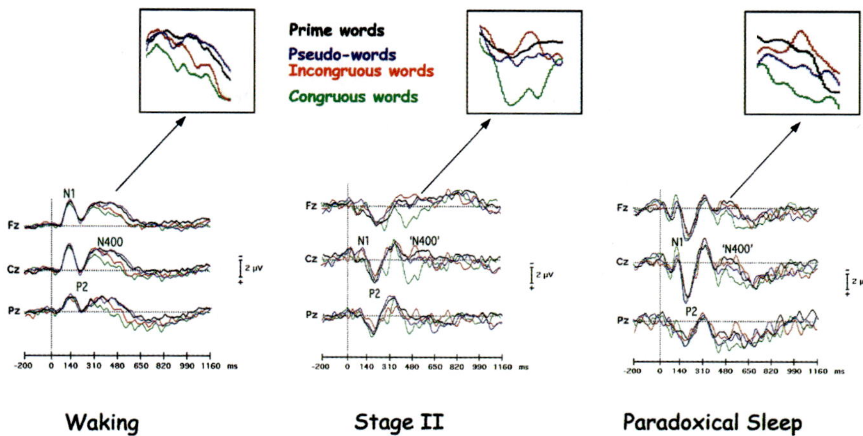

Figure 3. ERPs to words. Grand average ERPs to congruous (green traces), incongruous (red traces), pseudo-words (blue traces) and prime words during wakefulness (left), stage 2 (middle) and paradoxical sleep at Fz, Cz, and Pz (negativity up). Note that the amplitude of N400 was higher in response to pseudo-words during wakefulness, and to incongruous words during PS, while it was similar for incongruous and pseudo-words during S2.

by congruous words, suggesting that pseudo-words were not detected as "incongruous" stimuli during PS. These results are in accordance with the fact that linguistic absurdity (such as onomatopoeia) is accepted in a different manner during paradoxical sleep than during waking, and this might contribute to explain why absurd contents are so naturally incorporated into otherwise plausible dream stories.

In conclusion, studies on evoked potentials during human sleep support the view that relatively sophisticated auditory information processing persists during all sleep stages. Sensory inputs reach primary auditory cortical areas, as it has been reported in animal studies (Velluti and Pedemonte, 2002) and a salient stimulus seems to be detected even in deep SWS. During stage 2 and PS, analysis of semantic information remains possible, and this has also been suggested by metabolic studies (Portas *et al.*, 2000). The similarities and differences between the sleep cognitive responses and the waking P300 have been stressed and the functional significance of this component discussed especially in relation with consciousness and memory of the stimulus. However, even if the sleeping brain remains able to analyse auditory information, further studies are warranted to elucidate the extent and limits of these capabilities.

References

Amadeo, M. and Shagass, C. (1973). Brief latency with evoked potentials during wake and sleep in man. *Psychophysiology*, 10: 244–250.

Amzica, F. and Steriade, M. (1998). Cellular substrates and laminar profile of sleep K-complex. *Neuroscience*, 82: 671–686.

Aristotle (trad. 1955). Parva naturalia. De divinatione per somnum. In Ross, W.D. (Ed.). Oxford: Clarendon Press.

Arnsten, A.F.T., Steere, J.C., and Hunt, R.D. (1996). The contribution of alpha(2) noradrenergic mechanisms to prefrontal cortical cognitive function — potential significance for attention-deficit hyperactivity disorder. *Arch. Gen. Psychiatry*, 53: 448–455.

Atienza, M., Cantero, J.L., and Gomez, C.M. (1997). The mismatch negativity component reveals the sensory memory during REM sleep in humans. *Neurosci. Lett.*, 237: 21–24.

Atienza, M., Cantero, J.L., and Gomez, C.M. (2002). Mismatch negativity (MMN): an objective measure of sensory memory and long-lasting memory during sleep. *Int. J. Psychophysiol.*, 46: 215–225.

Bastien, C. and Campbell, K. (1992). The evoked K-Complex: all-or-none phenomenon? *Sleep*, 15: 236–245.

Bastien, C., Croewley, K.E., and Colrain, I.M. (2002). Evoked potential components unique to non-REM sleep: relationship to evoked K-complexes and vertex sharp waves. *Int. J. Psychophysiol.*, 46: 257–274.

Bastuji, H., García-Larrea, L., Bertrand, O., and Mauguière, F. (1988). BAEP latency changes during nocturnal sleep are not correlated with sleep stages but with body temperature variations. *Electroencephalogr. Clin. Neurophysiol.*, 70: 9–15.

Bastuji, H. and García-Larrea, L. (1999). Evoked potentials as a tool for the investigation of human sleep. *Sleep Med. Rev.*, 3: 23–45.

Bastuji, H., García-Larrea, L., Franc, C., and Mauguière, F. (1990). Influence of sleep on auditory cognitive potentials. *Neurophysiol. Clin.*, 20: 29s.

Bastuji, H., García-Larrea, L., Franc, C., and Mauguière, F. (1995). Brain processing of stimulus deviance during slow-wave and paradoxical sleep: a study of human auditory evoked responses using the oddball paradigm. *J. Clin. Neurophysiol.*, 12: 155–167.

Bastuji, H., Perrin, F., and García-Larrea, L. (2002). Semantic analysis of auditory input during sleep: studies with event related potentials. *Int. J. Psychophysiol.*, 46: 243–255.

Bastuji, H., Perrin, F., and García-Larrea, L. (2003). Event related potentials during forced awakening: a tool for the study of acute sleep inertia. *J. Sleep Res.*, 12: 189–206.

Baudena, P., Halgren, E., Heit, G., and Clarke, J.M. (1995). Intracerebral potentials to rare target and distractor auditory and visual stimuli. III. Frontal cortex. *Electroencephalogr. Clin. Neurophysiol.*, 94: 251–264.

Bentin, S., McCarthy, G., and Wood, C.C. (1985). Event-related potentials, lexical decision and semantic priming. *Electroencephalogr. Clin. Neurophysiol.*, 60: 343–355.

Berlad, I. and Pratt, H. (1995). P300 in response to the subject's own name. *Electroencephalogr. Clin. Neurophysiol.*, 96: 472–474.

Brázdil, M., Rektor, I., Dufek, M., Daniel, P., Jurák, P., and Kuba, R. (1999). The role of frontal and temporal lobes in visual discrimination task — depth ERP studies. *Neurophysiol. Clin.*, 29: 339–350.

Brázdil, M., Rektor, I., Daniel, P., Dufek, M., and Jurak, P. (2001). Intracerebral event-related potentials to subthreshold target stimuli. *Clin. Neurophysiol.*, 112: 650–661.

Brualla, J., Romero, M.F., Serrano, M., and Valdizan, J.R. (1998). Auditory event-related potentials to semantic priming during sleep. *Electroencephalogr. Clin. Neurophysiol.*, 108: 283–290.

Burdach, K.F. (1830). *Die Physiologie als Erfahrungswissenschaft*. Leipzig, vol. 3, p. 460.

Burton, S.A., Harsh, J.R., and Badia, P. (1988). Cognitive activity in sleep and responsiveness to external stimuli. *Sleep*, 11: 61–68.

Campbell, K. (1992). Evoked potential measures of information processing during natural sleep. In: Broughton, R. and Ogilvie, R. (Eds.). *Sleep, Arousal and Performance*. Boston: Birkhäuser, pp. 88–116.

Campbell, K. and Bartoli, E. (1986). Human auditory evoked potentials during natural sleep: the early components. *Electroencephalogr. Clin. Neurophysiol.*, 65: 142–149.

Campbell, K., Bell, I., and Deacon-Elliott, D. (1985). Stimulus related influences in the evoked K-complex. In: Koella, W.P., Ruther, E., and Schulz, H. (Eds.). *Sleep 84*, New York: Raven Press, pp. 235–237.

Cheour, M., Leppanen, P.H., and Kraus, N. (2000). Mismatch negativity (MMN) as a tool for investigating auditory discrimination and sensory memory in infants and children. *Clin. Neurophysiol.*, 111: 4–16.

Cote, K.A. and Campbell, K.B. (1999). P300 to high intensity stimuli during REM sleep. *Clin. Neurophysiol.*, 110: 1345–1350.

Cote, K.A., Etienne, L., and Campbell, K.B. (2001). Neurophysiological evidence for the detection of external stimuli during sleep. *Sleep*, 24: 791–803.

Cote, K.A. (2002). Probing awareness during sleep with auditory odd-ball paradigm. *Int. J. Psychophysiol.*, 46: 227–241.

Damasio, A.R. (1998). Investigating the biology of consciousness. *Philos. Trans. R. Soc. Lond. B. Biol. Sci.*, 353: 1879–1882.

Damasio, H., Grabowski, T.J., Tranel, D., Hichwa, R.D., and Damasio, A.R. (1996). A neural basis for lexical retrieval. *Nature*, 380: 499–505.

Davis, H., Davis, P.A., Loomis, A.L., Harvey, E.N., and Hobart G. (1939). Electrical reactions of the human brain to auditory stimulation during sleep. *J. Neurophysiol.*, 2: 500–514.

Deiber, M.P., Ibanez, V., Bastuji, H., Fischer, C., and Mauguière, F. (1989). Changes of middle latency auditory evoked potentials during natural sleep in humans. *Neurology*, 39: 806–813.

de Lugt, D.R., Loewy, D.H., and Campbell, K.B. (1996). The effect of sleep onset on event related potentials with rapid rates of stimulus presentation. *Electroencephalogr. Clin. Neurophysiol.*, 98: 484–492.

Erwin, R. and Buchwald, J.S. (1986). Midlatency auditory evoked responses: differential effects of sleep in the human. *Electroencephalogr. Clin. Neurophysiol.*, 65: 383–392.

Formby, D. (1967). Maternal recognition of infant's cry. *Devel. Med. Child Neurol.*, 9: 293–298.

Frege, G. (1949). On sense and nominatum. In: Feigl, H. and Sellars, W. (Eds.). *Readings in Philosophical Analysis*. New York: Appleton Century Crofts, pp. 85–102.

García-Larrea, L., Artru, F., Bertrand, O., Pernier, J., and Mauguière, F. (1992). The combined use of brainstem auditory potentials and intracranial pressure monitoring in coma. A study of 57 patients. *J. Neurol. Neurosurg. Psychiatry*, 55: 792–798.

García-Larrea, L., Perrin, F., and Bastuji, H. (2002). Memory encoding, stimulus awareness and event related potentials. Lessons from a forced awakening test. 11th European Congress of Clinical Neurophysiology, Barcelona, 24–28 August 2002. *Clin. Neurophysiol.*, 113: S34.

Halász, P. (1988). Information processing during sleep. In: Koella, W.P., Obàl, F., Schulz, H., and Visser, P. (Eds.). *Sleep'86*. Stuttgart: Gustav Fischer Verlag, pp. 77–78.

Halász, P. (1998). Hierarchy of micro-arousals and the microstructure of sleep. *Neurophysiol. Clin.*, 28: 461–475.

Halász, P. and Ujszászi, J. (1988). A study of K-complexes in humans: are they related to information processing during sleep. In: Koella, W.P., Obàl, F., Schulz, H., and Visser, P. (Eds.). *Sleep'86*. Stuttgart: Gustav Fischer Verlag, pp. 79–83.

Halász, P., Terzano, M., Parrino, L., and Bodizs, R. (2004). The nature of arousal in sleep. *J. Sleep Res.*, 13: 1–23.

Halgren, E., Baudena, P., Clarke, J.M., Heit, G., Liegeois, C., Chauvel, P., and Musolino, A. (1995a). Intracerebral potentials to rare target and distractor auditory and visual stimuli. I. Superior temporal plane and parietal lobe. *Electroencephalogr. Clin. Neurophysiol.*, 94: 191–220.

Halgren, E., Baudena, P., Clarke, J.M., Heit, G., Marinkovic, K., Devaux, B., Vignal, J.P., and Biraben, A. (1995b). Intracerebral potentials to rare target and distractor auditory and visual stimuli. II. Medial, lateral and posterior temporal lobe. *Electroencephalogr. Clin. Neurophysiol.*, 94: 229–250.

Hammond, E.J., Meador, K.J., Aung-Din, R., and Wilder, B.J. (1987). Cholinergic modulation of human P3 event-related potentials. *Neurology*, 37: 346–350.

Hansenne, M. (2000a). The p300 cognitive event-related potential. II. Individual variability and clinical application in psychopathology. *Neurophysiol. Clin.*, 30: 211–231.

Hansenne, M. (2000b). The p300 cognitive event-related potential. I. Theoretical and psychobiologic perspectives. *Neurophysiol. Clin.*, 30: 191–210.

Harrison, J.B., Buchwald, J.S., Kaga, K., Woolf, N.J., and Butcher, L.L. (1988). 'Cat P300' disappears after septal lesions. *Electroencephalogr. Clin. Neurophysiol.*, 69: 55–64.

Hobson, J.A. (1990). Sleep and dreaming. *J. Neurosci.*, 10: 371–382.

Horne, J. (1989). Functional aspects of human slow wave sleep (hSWS). In: Wauquier, A. (Ed.). *Slow Wave Sleep: Physiological, Pathological and Functional Aspects.* New York: Raven Press, pp. 109–118.

Howard, L. and Polich, J. (1985). P300 latency and memory span development. *Dev. Psychol.*, 21: 283–289.

Hull, J. and Harsh, J. (2001). P300 and sleep-related positive waveforms (P220, P450, and P900) have different determinants. *J. Sleep Res.*, 10: 9–17.

Introinicollison, I.B., Dalmaz, C., and Mcgaugh, J.L. (1996). Amygdala beta-noradrenergic influences on memory storage involve cholinergic activation. *Neurobiol. Learning Memory*, 65: 57–64.

Johnson, R., Pfefferbaum, A., and Kopell, B.S. (1985). P300 and long-term memory: latency predicts recognition performance. *Psychophysiology*, 22: 497–507.

Jones, B.E. (1991). Paradoxical sleep and its chemical/structural substrates in the brain. *Neuroscience*, 40: 637–656.

Knott, V., Mahoney, C., Labelle, A., Ripley, C., Cavazzoni, P., and Jones, B.E. (1999). Event-related potentials in schizophrenic patients during a degraded stimulus version of the visual continuous performance task. *Schizophr. Res.*, 35: 263–278.

Kutas, M. and Hillyard, S.A. (1980). Reading senseless sentences: brain potentials reflect semantic incongruity. *Science*, 207: 203–205.

Loewy, D.H., Campbell, K.B., and Bastien, C. (1996). The mismatch negativity to frequency deviant stimuli during natural sleep. *Electroencephalogr. Clin. Neurophysiol.*, 98: 493–501.

Loomis, A.L., Harvey, E.N., and Hobart, G.A. (1939). Distribution of disturbance patterns in the human encephalogram, with special reference to sleep. *J. Neurophysiol.*, 2: 413–430.

Maquet, P. (2000). Functional neuroimaging of normal human sleep by positron emission tomography. *J. Sleep Res.*, 9: 207–231.

Maury, A. (1878). *Le sommeil et les rêves.* 4th ed. Paris: Didier, pp. 161–162.

Mendel, M.I. and Goldstein, R. (1971). Early components of the averaged electroencephalographic response to constant level clicks during all night sleep. *J. Speech Hear. Res.*, 14: 829–840.

Muller, H.M. and Kutas, M. (1996). What's in a name? Electrophysiological differences between spoken nouns, proper names and one's own name. *Neuroreport*, 8: 221–225.

Näätänen, R. and Alho, K. (1995). Mismatch negativity — a unique measure of sensory processing in audition. *Int. J. Neurosci.*, 80: 317–337.

Nielsen, T.A. (1993). Changes in the kinesthetic content of dreams following somatosensory stimulation of leg muscles during REM sleep. *Dreaming*, 3: 99–113.

Nielsen-Bohlman, L., Knight, R.T., Woods, D.L., and Woodward, K. (1991). Differential auditory processing continues during sleep. *Electroencephalogr. Clin. Neurophysiol.*, 79: 281–290.

Nieman, D.H., Devisser, B.W.O., Koelman, J.H.T.M., Hofman, W.F., and Linszen, D.H. (1998). The P3 event-related potential in young recent-onset schizophrenic patients. *Int. Clin. Psychopharmacol.*, 13: S67–S73.

Niiyama, Y., Fujiwara, R., Satoh, N., and Hishikawa, Y. (1994). Endogenous components of event-related potential appearing during NREM stage 1 and REM sleep in man. *Int. J. Psychophysiol.*, 17: 165–174.

Niiyama, Y., Fushimi, M., Sekine, A., and Hishikawa, Y. (1995). K-complex evoked in NREM sleep is accompanied by a slow negative potential related to cognitive process. *Electroencephalogr. Clin. Neurophysiol.*, 95: 27–33.

Niiyama, Y., Satoh, N., Kutsuzawa, O., and Hishikawa, Y. (1996). Electrophysiological evidence suggesting that sensory stimuli of unknown origin induce spontaneous K-complexes. *Electroencephalogr. Clin. Neurophysiol.*, 98: 394–400.

Ogilvie, R.D., Simons, I.A., Kuderian, R.H., MacDonald, T., and Rustenberg, J. (1991). Behavioral, event-related potential, and EEG/FFT changes at sleep onset. *Psychophysiology*, 28: 54–64.

Oken, B.S. and Salinsky, M. (1992). Alertness and attention. *J. Clin. Neurophysiol.*, 9: 480–494.

Osselton, J.W., Binnie, C.D., Cooper, R., Fowler, C.J., Mauguière, F., and Prior, P.F. (Eds.) (1995). *Clinical Neurophysiology.* Vol. 1: *EMG, Nerve Conduction and Evoked Potentials.* Part 1 *Origins and Techniques*; Part 3: *Evoked Potentials.* London: Butherworth-Heinemann.

Osterhammel, P.A., Shallop, J.K., and Terkildsen, K. (1985). The effect of sleep on the auditory brainstem response (ABR) and the middle latency response (MLR). *Scand. Audiol.*, 14: 47–50.

Paré, D. and Llinás, R. (1995). Conscious and pre-conscious processes as seen from the standpoint of sleep-waking cycle neurophysiology. *Neuropsychologia*, 33: 1155–1168.

Perrin, F., García-Larrea, L., Mauguière, F., and Bastuji, H. (1999). A differential brain response to the subject's own name persists during sleep. *Clin. Neurophysiol.*, 110: 2153–2164.

Perrin, F., Bastuji, H., Mauguière, F., and García-Larrea, L. (2000). Functional dissociation of the early and late portions of human K-complexes. *Neuroreport*, 11: 1637–1640.

Perrin, F., Bastuji, H., and García-Larrea, L. (2002). Detection of verbal discordances during sleep. *Neuroreport*, 13: 1345–1349.

Picton, T.W. (1992). The P300 wave of the human event-related potential. *J. Clin. Neurophysiol.*, 9: 456–479.

Pineda, J.A., Foote, S.L., and Neville, H.J. (1989). Effects of locus coeruleus lesions on auditory, long-latency, event-related potentials in monkey. *J. Neurosci.*, 9: 81–93.

Pompeiano, O. (1970). Mechanisms of sensory-motor integration during sleep. *Prog. Physiol. Psychol.*, 3: 1–179.

Portas, C.M., Krakow, K., Allen, P., Josephs, O., Armony, J.L., and Frith, C.D. (2000). Auditory processing across the sleep–wake cycle: simultaneous EEG and fMRI monitoring in humans. *Neuron*, 28: 991–999.

Potter, D.D., Pickles, C.D., Roberts, R.C., and Rugg, M.D. (1992). The effects of scopolamine on event-related potentials in a continuous recognition memory task. *Psychophysiology*, 29: 29–37.

Pratt, H., Berlad, I., and Lavie, P. (1999). 'Oddball' event-related potentials and information processing during REM and non-REM sleep. *Clin. Neurophysiol.*, 110: 53–61.

Proverbio, A.M., Lilli, S., Semenza, C., and Zani, A. (2001). ERP indexes of functional differences in brain activation during proper and common names retrieval. *Neuropsychologia*, 39: 815–827.

Renault, B., Signoret, J.L., Debruille, B., Breton, F., and Bolgert, F. (1989). Brain potentials reveal covert facial recognition in prosopagnosia. *Neuropsychologia*, 27: 905–912.

Sallinen, M., Kaartinen, J., and Lyytinen, H. (1994). Is the appearance of mismatch negativity during stage 2 sleep related to the elicitation of K-complex? *Electroencephalogr. Clin. Neurophysiol.*, 91: 140–148.

Sallinen, M., Kaartinen, J., and Lyytinen, H. (1996). Processing of auditory stimuli during tonic and phasic periods of REM sleep as revealed by event-related brain potentials. *J. Sleep Res.*, 5: 220–228.

Searle, J.R. (1967). Proper names and descriptions. In: Edward, P. (Ed.). *The Encyclopedia of Philosophy*. New York: MacMillan.

Semenza, C. and Zettin, M. (1988). Generating proper name: a case of selective inability. *Cogn. Neuropsychologia*, 5: 711–721.

Shefrin, S.L., Goodin, D.S., and Aminoff, M.J. (1988). Visual evoked potentials in the investigation of "blindsight". *Neurology*, 38: 104–109.

Siegel, J.M. and Rogawski, M.A. (1988). A function for REM sleep: regulation of noradrenergic receptor sensitivity. *Brain Res. Rev.*, 13: 213–233.

Sohmer, H., Gafni, M., and Chisin, R. (1978). Auditory nerve and brain stem responses: comparison in awake and unconscious subjects. *Arch. Neurol.*, 35: 228–230.

Steriade, M. (1994). The thalamus and sleep disturbances. In: Guilleminault, C., Lugaresi, E., Montagna, P., and Gambetti, P., (Eds.). *Fatal Familial Insomnia. Inherited Prion Diseases, Sleep and the Thalamus*. New York: Raven Press, pp. 177–189.

Steriade, M. (1997). Synchronized activities of coupled oscillators in the cerebral cortex and thalamus at different levels of vigilance. *Cerebral Cortex*, 7: 583–604.

Steriade, M., Gloor, P., Llinas, R.R., Lopes de Silva, F.H., and Mesulam, M.M. (1990). Report of IFCN Committee on Basic Mechanisms. Basic mechanisms of cerebral rhythmic activities. *Electroencephalogr. Clin. Neurophysiol.*, 76: 481–508.

Swick, D., Pineda, J.A., Schacher, S., and Foote, S.L. (1994). Locus coeruleus neuronal activity in awake monkeys: relationship to auditory P300-like potentials and spontaneous EEG. *Exp. Brain Res.*, 101: 86–92.

Ujszászi, J. and Halász, P. (1986). Late component variants of single auditory evoked responses during NREM sleep stage 2 in man. *Electroencephalogr. Clin. Neurophysiol.*, 64: 260–268.

Ujszászi, J. and Halász, P. (1988). Long latency evoked potential components in human slow wave sleep. *Electroencephalogr. Clin. Neurophysiol.*, 69: 516–522.

Velluti, R.A. and Pedemonte, M. (2002). In vivo approach to the cellular mechanisms for sensory processing in sleep and wakefulness. *Cell. Mol. Neurobiol.*, 22: 501–516.

Wagner, P., Roschke, J., Fell, J., and Frank, C. (1997). Differential pathophysiological mechanisms of reduced P300 amplitude in schizophrenia and depression: a single trial analysis. *Schizophr. Res.*, 25: 221–229.

Yasuda, K., Nakamura, T., and Beckman, B. (2000). Brain processing of proper names. *Aphasiology*, 14: 1067–1089.

Chapter 24

COGNITIVE ASPECTS OF SLEEP: PERCEPTION, MENTATION, AND DREAMING

Chiara M. Portas[1]

Cognitive activities are closely related to the nebulous concept of consciousness (e.g., Velmans, 1991; Chalmers, 1996). Functions like perception, thinking, and memory merge one in another as conscious mental activity shapes up. Due to their introspective nature the study of these functions is complex, making this task even more impractical during sleep. In fact, fluctuation of brain activation, sensory gating, and changes in neuromodulation dramatically alter the expression of human cognition during sleep. Since sleep takes a third of human life (about 25 years in the average life span) it is fundamental to understand what happens in the sleeping mind during this extended period of time.

Sleep is a very heterogeneous state. Different psycho-physiological phases alternate during each sleep cycle. At present, states are classified as rapid eye movement (REM) sleep appearing at the end of each sleep cycle, and light (S1 and S2) and deep sleep (S3 and S4) constituting non-REM sleep (NREM). These phases are characterized by specific EEG landmarks (see Chapter 5). Moreover, new animal and human studies have shown extremely low frequency oscillations ($<1\,\mathrm{Hz}$) associated to NREM sleep, delta and spindles activity (Steriade, 1997; Acherman and Borbely, 1998)

---

[1] chiara.portas@fys.uib.no

535

and fast gamma frequencies, cortical oscillations associated with REM sleep similar to the ones observed in the waking state (e.g. Steriade and Amzica, 1996). Imaging studies have also shown distinct patterns of activation in REM and NREM sleep: REM sleep is mainly associated with reactivation of fronto-limbic areas and deactivation of prefrontal regions, while NREM sleep is characterized by a global deactivation (Maquet *et al.*, 1996; Braun *et al.*, 1997).

Thus, it is crucial to grant full consideration to the way sleep stage physiology relates to distinctive cognitive activities. This chapter reviews the current knowledge on sensory information processing and mentation/dreaming taking place during sleep.

Perception

There is no direct access to the mental state of a sleeping person. Whatever the sleeper experiences can only be reported upon awakening. The application of techniques like EEG and especially evoked potentials during sleep allowed us to analyze immediate response to stimuli presentation in the form of brain waves.

Studies of evoked potentials

The accessibility of the auditory system during sleep explains why auditory perception is the sensory modality more exploited during sleep. More limited information exists for sensory processing in modalities other than auditory, such as like somatosensory and visual.

It has been known for a long time that sensory stimulation during NREM sleep, especially in stage 2, evokes the appearance in the EEG of a large biphasic waveform named K-complex (Roth *et al.*, 1956). Studies of auditory evoked potentials (AEPs) — (brain waves time-locked to a specific sensory event) — have shown that early latency responses (within 10 ms) are present throughout sleep (Mendel and Kupperman, 1974; Campbell and Bartoli, 1986). These early AEPs are generated in the acoustic nerve and in the brainstem and are very sensitive to the physical properties of the auditory stimulus (Buchwald, 1983). Middle-latency AEPs (10–100 ms), having origin in the thalamocortical neurons (Picton *et al.*, 1974) and primary auditory cortex, are affected in one or more components during NREM sleep, while returning to the profile of wakefulness during REM sleep (Deiber *et al.*, 1989). For example, P1 (a positive wave appearing around 80 ms) disappears during NREM and reappears during REM sleep with an amplitude similar to that observed during wakefulness (Erwin and Buchwald, 1986).

P50, a mid-latency component of the AEPs has been shown to reflect the so-called "auditory gating", a mechanism the brain uses to filter out useless information typically as a function of stimulus repetition (habituation effect). This means that stimulus redundancy produces during waking a decrease in the amplitude of P50. Such decrement is lost in conditions like acute stress and schizophrenia (Adler *et al.*, 1982; Johnson and Adler, 1993). Kisley *et al.* (2001) assessed the effect of vigilance on auditory gating by monitoring the P50. Their results show that sensory gating for unnecessary information (e.g., repeated stimuli) operates during REM sleep similarly to waking.

Finally, late components are sometime present but delayed or altered at some degree. Atienza *et al.* (2001) and Campbell and Colrain (2002) reviewed a large group of studies in relation to late potentials, including N1, mismatch negativity (MMN), P300, and sleep.

N1 is a negative deflection (also defined N1–P2 waveform; e.g., Cote *et al.*, 2001) appearing between 75 and 150 ms mainly generated in the supratemporal auditory cortex with a contribution of frontal regions (Giard *et al.*, 1994). It encodes stimulus features such as frequency, intensity, and location. This pre-conscious sensory analysis is held as a memory trace for at least 150–200 ms (Loveless *et al.*, 1996) and may trigger involuntary attention switch leading to conscious perception (e.g., appearance of P300). During NREM sleep, N1 decreases in amplitude while its latency increases, showing a small recovery in REM sleep (Bastuji *et al.*, 1995). This early stage of processing is altered during sleep and may in turn affect later potentials like MMN and P300. N1 impoverished persistence proves nevertheless that during sleep some information of stimuli features is available for further analysis.

MMN is a negative potential appearing between 100 and 200 ms as a consequence of any variation in a repetitive stream of stimuli. Its generators are in the superior temporal plane of the auditory cortex (review, Alho *et al.*, 1995) with the addition of a frontal component (Giard *et al.*, 1990). As for N1 the frontal component may be related to the involuntary switch of attention leading eventually to conscious perception. It has been suggested that MMN underlies a change-detector system that uses memory traces to detect change and make such information available for further processing (Näätänen *et al.*, 1992). Latency of later AEPs components like

     C. M. Portas

N2 and P300 are directly affected by its latency (Novak *et al.*, 1992). In most studies, MMN is not detectable during NREM sleep, it reappears during REM sleep with characteristics similar to wakefulness but with smaller amplitude (Atienza *et al.*, 1997). The smaller amplitude during REM sleep is perhaps due to decrease of the frontal component (possibly linked to the functional deactivation of prefrontal regions during REM sleep — Maquet *et al.*, 1996). Atienza also proposed that sensory memory trace reflected in MMN has a shorter duration during sleep (Atienza *et al.*, 2000), in the author words "neural representation of repetitive stimuli vanishes faster in REM sleep than in wakefulness, probably as a result of unstable representation". Once again, information processing and sensory memory seem to be present, even if impoverished, at least during REM sleep.

P300, a positive component peaking between 220 and 350 ms, is usually associated with attention and discrimination. P300 is elicited by novel and by deviant stimuli and is usually preceded by N1 and MMN. Dorso-lateral prefrontal cortex, temporal and parietal cortices, the hippocampus, and the cingulate gyrus all contribute to its generation (Escera *et al.*, 2000). Latency of P300 increases and amplitude decreases from wakefulness through sleep (Wesensten and Badia, 1988; Nielsen-Bohlman *et al.*, 1991; Harsh *et al.*, 1994; Atienza *et al.*, 2001). More recent studies used an odd-ball task to probe the presence of P300 during sleep (review, Cote, 2002). It appears that P300 can be recorded during the transition from wakefulness to sleep (stage 1) and then reappears in REM sleep. Such effect is more consistent with rare and intrusive stimuli. However, as for the MMN, the frontal component of the P300 is lost during sleep. This is consistent with the concept of hypofrontality (frontal deactivation, functional deafferentation of the forebrain) described in REM sleep (Maquet *et al.*, 1996; Braun *et al.*, 1997; Hobson *et al.*, 1998a,b). The lack of the frontal component of P300 may support the notion of semi-automatic (pre-conscious) detection of stimuli during sleep. It has been suggested that only privileged (salient) stimuli may produce frontal activation and full awareness (Perrin *et al.*, 1999).

A positive potential peaking at about 200–250 ms (considered by many as an early P300 — also called P3a) has been described in many studies following presentation of deviant stimuli during sleep stages 1 and 2 (review, Atienza *et al.*, 2001). In addition, two groups recorded a positive wave showing high amplitude in REM sleep at 210 and 250 ms latency (Sallinen *et al.*, 1996; Squires *et al.*, 1975, respectively).

P300 response can also vary during sleep as a function of subject personality. Recently, it has been shown that subjects can behave as blunters or monitors. Monitors are more responsive to stimuli during wakefulness and sleep stage 1 showing in addition a larger P300 response (Voss and Harsh, 1998). Blunters and monitors aside, P300 data in sleep speak for preserved information processing during light and REM sleep.

N300 (or N350)/P400 and N550/P900 are AEP components present in sleep only (stages 1 and 2). The first complex reflects the presence of vertex sharp waves in the EEG (Gora *et al.*, 2001) and is affected by intensity, novelty, probability (Nielsen-Bohlman *et al.*, 1991), and relevance of the stimulus (Harsh *et al.*, 1994; Perrin *et al.*, 1999). The second complex, N550/P900, reflects the occurrence of K-complexes in the EEG (Gora *et al.*, 2001) and may be considered similar to the orienting response (facilitating stimulus processing) of wakefulness (Bastien and Campbell, 1992; Bastien *et al.*, 2002).

Therefore, even if auditory information processing is severely affected during sleep, it maintains the capability to monitor the outside environment at some degree (N1, MMN, P300, etc.) extracting meaningful clues (a kind of sub-consciousness?) and eventually producing arousal. From an evolutionary point of view the relevance of this capability is obvious. During sleep, hearing is the sensory modality more accessible and sleep disruption due to intrusive and dangerous stimuli highly increases chances of survival.

Somatosensory processing in sleep has largely been studied by recording somatosensory evoked potentials (SEPs). Early SEPs, e.g., P50 and P20, show minor changes between wakefulness and sleep according to Colon and Weerd (1986). However, Emerson reported that early SEPs' amplitude decreases from wakefulness to stage 2 sleep (Emerson *et al.*, 1988). Late cortical components are maximally attenuated in NREM stage IV and REM sleep (Colon and de Weerd, 1986). Nakano *et al.* (1995) also reported that NREM sleep affects the latency, amplitude, and morphology of N16 and early cortical components while the latencies and morphologies of SEPs during REM sleep are similar to wakefulness. Noguchi *et al.* (1995) reported that frontal and parietal SEP components are affected differentially as sleep progresses. In general, the amplitudes of frontal components, notably P22, were increased in sleep, whereas the amplitudes of parietal components were decreased. Latencies of all components except P14 and frontal N18 showed progressive increase from REM to deep sleep. The SEP waveforms and latencies in REM sleep approximated those in wakefulness. Somatosensory evoked magnetic field (SEFs) studies showed that the early components, 1M, 2M, and 3M, which are generated in the primary sensory cortex controlateral to the stimulated nerve, do not change latency or amplitude in stage 1 or 2 sleep as compared with those in wakefulness. However, the long-latency response, 4M whose latency is about 100 ms, is significantly enhanced in stage 2 but restricted to the primary sensory cortex while the secondary sensory cortex produced no sign of 4M either ipsi or controlateral. These findings can be interpreted as difference in activity between primary and secondary sensory cortex during sleep, that is, an increase of sensitivity to somatosensory stimulation in the primary cortex but a decrease or disappearance in the secondary cortex (Kitamura *et al.*, 1996). In addition to SEPs, somatosensory perception has been explored using painful stimuli. Painful thermal stimulation has been shown to produce arousal from NREM or REM sleep at higher temperatures than during wakefulness (Bentley *et al.*, 2003).

Visual perception has been largely investigated using visual evoked potentials (VEPs). Whyte *et al.* (1987) reported that, in newborns, the vigilance state dramatically affects the amplitude, latency, and waveform of the transient luminance flash VEP. The N300 is the most stable component across sleep states but shows a significant decrease in amplitude in quiet sleep. The P200 disappears in both active and quiet sleep states; the P400 is variable. When a distinction is made between quiet sleep and other vigilance states, significant differences emerge. Similar conclusions were reached by another group (Apkarian *et al.*, 1991). Okusa and Kakigi (2002) measured visual evoked magnetic field (VEF) during sleep in humans. By comparing the magnetic components between the awake and sleep conditions, three components for the sleep condition were found to be enhanced (those at 55, 80–100, and 100–110 ms of the waking VEF). Other components of the waking VEF were reduced or disappeared during sleep. This large change in the VEF during sleep suggests that some qualitative changes occur in the cortical visual processing. In particular, the authors suggest a reduction in the inhibitory activities operating in waking.

Functional imaging studies

The development of functional imaging techniques has provided a different perspective to the field of sensory processing during sleep. Results from these studies are not univocal (Portas *et al.*, 2000; Born *et al.*, 2002; Czisch *et al.*, 2002; Tanaka *et al.*, 2003). Portas and collaborators using functional magnetic resonance (fMRI) showed that presentation of auditory stimuli in NREM sleep produces a significant bilateral activation in the auditory cortices, thalamus, and caudate similar to wakefulness (Figure 1). However, the overall degree and extent of activation (especially in the thalamus) was higher in wakefulness and also included activation of parietal and frontal

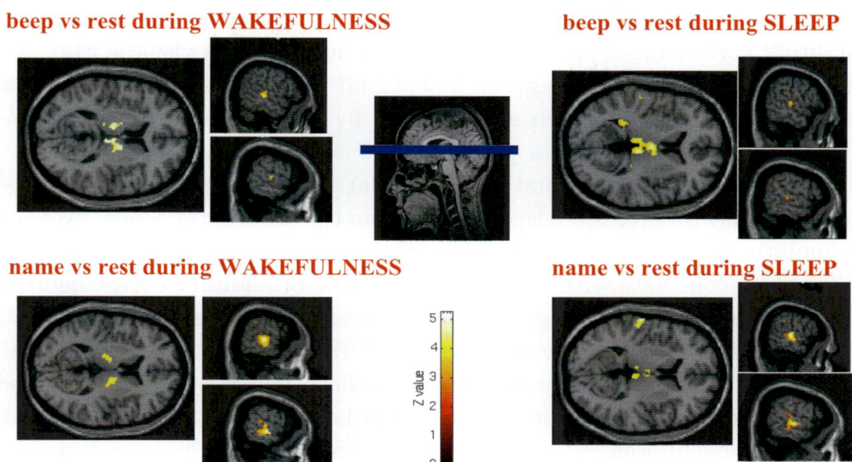

Figure 1. Brain activation during auditory stimulation during wakefulness (left panels) and sleep (right panels).

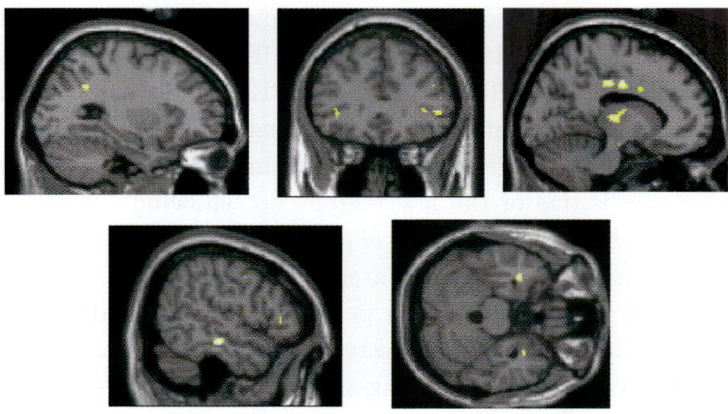

Figure 2. Difference in processing a stimulus in wakefulness compared to sleep: changes in activation are present in the left parietal and prefrontal cortices, thalamus, cingulate gyrus, and temporal regions bilaterally.

regions (Figure 2). Tanaka *et al.* (2003) using fMRI reported a significant decrease of signal intensity percentage after presentation of a pure tone stimulus in the right and left transverse temporal gyri (0.49% and 0.43% during wakefulness vs. 0.05% and 0.07% during stage 1 sleep).

Czisch *et al.* (2002, 2004), using fMRI, found reduced activation in the auditory cortex and a pronounced negative signal in the visual cortex and precuneus during sleep stages 1 and 2 and during deep sleep. Acoustic stimulation during sleep was accompanied by an increase in the number of K-complexes and EEG delta power.

The groups of Tanaka and Czisch similarly conclude that the decreased response may protect the sleeping brain from the arousing effects of external stimulation and facilitate deepening of the sleep stage. These results are difficult to conciliate with the notion that 50% of auditory cortex neurons do not change firing passing from wakefulness to NREM sleep (Peña *et al.*, 1999). In both studies (by the groups of Tanaka and Czisch) the small evoked activity in auditory cortex during sleep is largely underestimated and poorly discussed by the authors. This is in contrast with the view of Portas and collaborators that consider any evoked activity in sleep as a most challenging finding. Thus, the difference between the earlier studies (Portas *et al.*, 2000) and the latter ones may be more speculative than substantial. It should also be considered that the type of stimuli presented in the different studies may have played a role in the degree of evoked activity elicited during sleep. Portas alternated neutral to salient stimuli, perhaps eliciting a greater response due to a more "aroused" (interested?) brain. Notably, activation of the auditory cortex during stimulus presentation has been also shown by a positron emission tomography (PET) study in vegetative state patients (Laureys *et al.*, 2000). An fMRI/PET study has recently shown decreased activation of sensory cortex during visual stimulation in sleep (Born *et al.*, 2002). However, from previous imaging studies we know that the visual cortex is one of the few regions not showing a decrease in flow rate during NREM sleep (Braun *et al.*, 1998; Kajimura *et al.*, 1999). Thus, the latter data may be difficult to interpret.

Despite some incongruities, the peculiarity of the auditory system as a sleep sentinel has also been suggested by data demonstrating privileged access of relevant information during sleep. In 1830, the German physiologist Burdach wrote: "an indifferent word does not arouse the sleeper, but if called by name he awakens ... the mother awakens to the faintest sound from her child ... the miller wakes when the mill stops ... hence the psyche differentiates sensations during sleep". Oswald was the first to demonstrate in a controlled experiment that personal names evoke more K-complexes in the sleeper than any other name or sounds of same intensity (Oswald, 1960). Similarly, Voss and Harsh (1998) have shown that presentation of the subject's own name produces the greatest number of K-complexes and arousals relative to other tones and names.

More recent evoked potentials studies have reported a differential cognitive response to the presentation of the subject's own name during sleep stage 2 and REM sleep (Berlad and Pratt, 1995; Perrin *et al.*, 1999). Complex processing of words has been shown by Brualla *et al.* (1998) and more recently by Wilke *et al.* (2003). In Brualla's study semantic priming was induced and tested during sleep stage 2 and REM sleep by monitoring N400, a negative component of the evoked potentials responsive to this type of tasks. Wilke and colleagues used fMRI to show that during sleep language areas are activated during a story listening task.

Portas *et al.* (2000), using fMRI combined with EEG recording, also showed a specific response to the subject's own name during NREM sleep. In addition, presentation of the subject's own name during sleep was associated with selective activation of the left amygdala and left prefrontal cortex (Figure 3). The authors speculate that following the detection of an emotionally relevant stimulus during sleep, the amygdala may trigger activation of the dorsolateral prefrontal cortex, inducing arousal and sustaining a basic level of sensory awareness. This is in line with the crucial role of the amygdala in processing of emotional stimuli (Le Doux, 1996; Nader *et al.*, 2000). The prefrontal cortex would in turn determine the consequences of

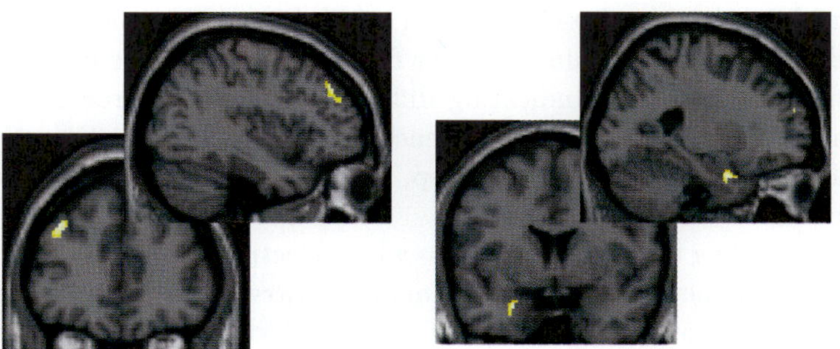

Figure 3. Difference in processing a salient stimulus compared to an irrelevant one during sleep: when the name vs. beep-related brain activity during sleep is compared to name vs. beep-related brain activity during wakefulness, a significant difference in activation is shown in the left prefrontal cortex and in the left amygdala.

the alarm effect either progressing to full awakening or to sensory neglect. The role of the prefrontal cortex in "selection" is well established (Frith *et al.*, 1991; Hyder *et al.*, 1997).

Animal studies

Coenen introduced the concept of transfer ratio to describe the differential access of information to the cortex across the sleep–wake cycle (Coenen and Vendrik, 1972). During wakefulness sensory inputs produce continuous stimulation of thalamocortical neurons inducing a low threshold of depolarization and forcing them to fire in a tonic mode. The flow of transmission from the relay thalamus to the relevant sensory cortex varies accordingly. When thalamo-cortical neurons are excited (tonic firing) the ratio between output and the input varies between 0.7 to 1.0, implying that all or most action potentials of presynaptic neurons produce a post-synaptic action potential (high transfer rate). Decreasing activity of the activating reticular formation during drowsiness and successive sleep allows thalamic interneurons to hyperpolarize (inhibit) thalamo-cortical neurons coupling them in a "burst" or "oscillatory" mode. Hence, during NREM sleep the transfer ratio drops to 0.3–0.4. Thus, the transfer ratio decreases from wakefulness through NREM sleep. It is notable that the ratio never decreases below approximately 0.3, meaning that some information reaches the cortex even in the deepest stages of sleep. This level of processing is probably excluded from integrated awareness. More complex is the transfer ratio during REM sleep. Awakening thresholds and transfer ratio fluctuate according to time of the night and stage. Roschke *et al.* (1995) showed that there is a functional difference in the brain's transfer functions between the first and the following REM episodes, indicating different information processing during consecutive paradoxical sleep. Hence, despite the high activity of the thalamo-cortical neurons in REM sleep, the fate of inputs is also shaped by other factors.

Unit recording studies (in animals) where electrodes were placed at different levels of the auditory system (auditory nerve, cochlear nucleus, olivar nucleus, inferior colliculus, brainstem, auditory cortex) showed shifts in spontaneous firing and in response to pure tones to be closely related to waking, NREM and REM (Velluti *et al.*, 1989; Peña *et al.*, 1992; Pedemonte *et al.*, 1994; Morales-Cobas *et al.*, 1995; Velluti *et al.*, 1990, Velluti, 1997; Peña *et al.*, 1999, respectively). In the Inferior colliculus, 55% of auditory neurons did not show any change in the spontaneous firing rate during

NREM as compared to the previous waking period, while 22% exhibited a discharge increase and 23% decreased their firing. During REM sleep, 14 out of 17 cells increased their spontaneous firing rate. However, 63% of the recorded neurons showed changes, increasing or decreasing in the number of *evoked discharges* during the animal's transitions between wakefulness and NREM (Morales-Cobas *et al.*, 1995). Hence, spontaneous firing and evoked activity can be dissociated, as also reported by other authors (Peña *et al.*, 1999; Edeline *et al.*, 2000).

In the auditory cortex of the cat, Murata and Kameda (1963) have shown a reduced firing in NREM compared to wakefulness. More recent data obtained in guinea pigs showed that approximately 50% of neurons do not change spontaneous firing in relation to the state of vigilance. The other half either increase or decrease activity, e.g., 29% of cells decrease firing passing from wakefulness to NREM, 17% increase firing. Similarly, the evoked response shows that 58% cells are insensitive to state change (from wakefulness to NREM), 24% decrease firing, 18% increase it (Peña *et al.*, 1999). This implies that a large number of neurons do not change firing activity during sleep and are therefore fully operative. Similar effects are shown in the spontaneous and evoked response of auditory cells passing from NREM to REM sleep (Peña *et al.*, 1999). An important methodological issue is that the preferred type of auditory stimulus may not be known for each neuron.

Velluti and Pedemonte observed that firing of sensory units shows phase locking to the hyppocampal theta rhythm, perhaps adding a temporal dimension to incoming information. This correlation is also present during sleep (review, Velluti and Pedemonte, 2002). The existence of an internal clock (called temporal oscillator or multiple oscillators) and its involvement in information processing has been postulated in humans also (Treisman *et al.*, 1990, 1992, 1994; Burle and Bonnet, 1999). These data support the idea that the temporal oscillator allows the transfer of information from one stage to the next one at definite intervals only. A temporal reference is certainly maintained during sleep (Hawkins, 1989).

The *quantity* of information reaching the cortex during sleep is not the only factor determining the amount of on-going information processing. Another aspect to be considered is the *quality* of the information. Edeline *et al.* (2000) demonstrated that different features of information processing are differentially affected by sleep. Neuronal threshold, response latency, frequency selectivity, receptive field size, signal-to-noise ratio, etc., are among the features taken into account by this group. They recorded auditory thalamic cells *in vivo* (guinea pigs) across waking and sleep. Results show that spontaneous activity was decreased in NREM sleep compared to wakefulness whereas it was increased in REM sleep. Mean evoked activity was decreased in NREM sleep and during REM sleep cells showed a dual behavior: 60% decreased their activity and 40% fired at a level similar to wakefulness (independent on stimulus tone intensity). Frequency selectivity increased (narrowed band) in NREM compared to wakefulness and REM sleep. Receptive field size was decreased during NREM sleep compared to wakefulness. During REM sleep the average receptive field size did not differ significantly from wakefulness in the cells in which the evoked response was similar to the wakefulness response. It was reduced, however, in the cells that showed a decrease in the evoked responses. In other words, when evoked activity is reduced there is increased frequency selectivity and decreased receptive field size whatever the vigilance state. Mean response latency increased from wakefulness to NREM to REM sleep (26.7 ms, 28.2 ms, 31.1 ms, respectively). Threshold also changed as a function of vigilance shift: 41 dB in wakefulness, 51 dB in NREM sleep, and 64 dB in REM sleep. The neurons' tendency to "burst" as expected increased in NREM sleep compared to wakefulness or REM sleep. All these effects were similar in different divisions of the auditory thalamus. From these results Edeline and colleagues concluded that the message sent to the cortex is quite impoverished but the preserved intensity coding, neuron selectivity, and organized receptive field (even if smaller) justify the assumption that the cortex has enough information to discriminate stimuli relevance.

The altered quantity and quality of information reaching the perceptual cortices during sleep adds up to the functional deafferentation of the frontal cortex possibly related to reduced noradrenergic output (Hobson *et al.*, 1998a,b). Hobson claims that during sleep (REM sleep in particular) the brain is largely "cholinergic" while during wakefulness is driven by monoaminergic neuromodulation. In fact, the transition from wakefulness to sleep is promoted by a shift of activity of the monoaminergic brainstem nuclei that almost cease firing during sleep (Hobson, 1999). Noradrenaline and serotonin show a clear cortical decrease during sleep and especially REM sleep (e.g., Kalen *et al.*, 1989; Portas *et al.*, 1998). The decrease in noradrenergic activity may also contribute to disinhibition of the cortical dopaminergic system producing the hallucinatory oneiric experience (Hobson, 2004). Monoaminergic activity rapidly reemerges at the transition with wakefulness. The functional deafferentation of frontal regions is highlighted by imaging data showing a marked deactivation of frontal regions and prefrontal cortex during NREM and REM sleep despite the significant activation of other brain regions during REM sleep (Maquet *et al.*, 1996; Braun *et al.*, 1997). The hypo-frontality associated with REM and NREM sleep may be responsible for the characteristic lack of volition, bizarreness, incoherent reasoning of sleep mentation (see section Dreaming and Sleep mentation). Altered cognition during REM sleep (including decreased meta-awareness, incongruous representations in time, space, people, unstable representations, etc.) may also result from lack of intra-hemispheric coherence, e.g., uncoupled gamma activity between frontal and perceptual cortices (Pérez-Garci *et al.*, 2001). In fact, coherent gamma frequency oscillations between neuronal assemblies have been suggested to produce sensory binding in wakefulness (Ribary *et al.*, 1991; Joliot *et al.*, 1994). Inter-hemispheric coherence is maintained in REM sleep but unlike wakefulness, the oscillatory activity is not reset by incoming sensory inputs suggesting that perceptual integration is not taking place (Llinás and Ribary, 1993).

The frontal deafferentation during sleep may also explain the existence of pathological sleep disorders like sleep walking (disorders of arousal). These patients while asleep present complex behavior (they walk, get dressed, eat, act violently, etc.) in the absence of real consciousness. Only a certain degree of awareness of the external environment is retained in order to navigate in space (Espa *et al.*, 2000).

The overall understanding from all the presented data is that a discrete level of processing and some sort of sensory integration is maintained during at least light and REM sleep; however, occurrence of conscious perception is unlikely.

Dreaming and Sleep Mentation

Dreaming is a concept familiar to everybody, only about 1% of the overall population do not experience any oneiric activity (Pagel, 2003). Dreaming and sleep mentation reflect a more or less complex sequence of sensory and emotional events produced by the sleeper's mind. Dreaming is more often associated with REM sleep being present in 90% of REM sleep episodes (Rechtschaffen, 1978). However, dream-like mentation is also observed at sleep onset when EEG shows prevalence of alpha waves (30–40%; e.g., Cicogna *et al.*, 1991), during stages 1 and 2 (70–75%), during stages 3 and 4 (50%), and during relaxed wakefulness (25%) the so-called day dreaming (Foulkes and Fleisher, 1975). Thus, oneiric activity of some sort is almost continuous throughout sleep (Foulkes, 1962; Rechtschaffen *et al.*, 1963; Cicogna *et al.*, 1991).

REM dreaming is usually considered as the classic dream presenting six main features: hallucinoid imagery, narrative structure, bizarreness (e.g., temporal and geographical discontinuity, incongruity), hyperemotionality, delusional acceptance (the dream is mistaken for reality), and deficient memory of its content (about 1 h of dreaming vanishes every night) (Hobson and Stickgold, 1994). On the other hand, NREM sleep mentation reflects a less organized activity and NREM reports are usually shorter and poorer of prior sleep mentation than REM reports (Cicogna *et al.*, 1991; Stickgold *et al.*, 2001). It has been claimed that REM sleep is a paradox from a physiological point of view because it does not generate the type of cognitive responses we would expect from the associated cortical activation. However, it must be considered that the high cortical activity and high frequency oscillations (Steriade and Amzica, 1996) associated with REM sleep coexist with a marked hypofrontality (Maquet *et al.*, 1996; Braun *et al.*, 1997), and temporal uncoupling between sensory cortices and frontal regions (Pérez-Garci *et al.*, 2001). These deficiencies might per se justify the paradox of REM sleep. In addition, REM sleep is characterized by a cholinergic but hypoaminergic brain compared to a highly monoamine-driven brain of waking (Hobson, 1992, 1999; Hobson *et al.*, 1998a,b). The functional and chemical frontal deafferentation may be responsible for some features characteristic of REM sleep mentation like illogical reasoning, disorientation, lack of volition, e.g., inability to plan and act accordingly, lack of reflective evaluation, e.g., unawareness of the dreamer of being hallucinating, also called single-mindeness (Rechtschaffen, 1978), or failure of reality testing (Bosinelli, 1995). These features are also present to some degree in NREM sleep mentation (Cicogna *et al.*, 1991; Nielsen, 1999).

Hobson and colleagues tend to highlight the differences between REM and NREM sleep mentation on the basis of the physiological differences shown by EEG and imaging data (Hobson *et al.*, 1998b). However, the dychotomy REM dreaming vs. NREM sleep mentation is not universally accepted and other scientists consider the difference as quantitative instead of qualitative (Cicogna *et al.*, 1991).

The sequence of complex hallucinations characterizing the oneiric activity develops around a central theme (Rechtschaffen, 1978) that is usually preserved throughout the dream (only changing between dreams of the same night). The visual hallucinations in REM sleep are possibly related to activation of unimodal visual association areas (Braun *et al.*, 1998). The "story" usually includes different sensory modalities. The most common are visual (100%), followed by auditory (65%), vestibular (8%), tactile (1%), olfactory (1%), and gustatory (1%) (McCarley and Hoffman, 1981). Vestibular input fed in by activation of brainstem vestibular nuclei during waking track and direct body position in relation to the environment. Their stimulation during sleep is likely to be related to the sensation of flying, spinning, or falling experienced in dreams.

Motor activity is usually weak during dreaming. This is due to the state of paralysis of the muscles during deep and REM sleep. Evarts (1960) showed that pyramidal tract neurons increase their bursting property during REM sleep. However, a pontine inhibitory mechanism blocks the spinal cord alpha motoneurons producing atonia (Pompeiano *et al.*, 1967; Lai and Siegel, 1991; Lai *et al.*, 2001; Kodama *et al.*, 2003).

Motivational and emotional contents are more frequent in REM than NREM sleep, even after controlling for the greater word count of REM reports (Smith *et al.*, 2004). Typically, dreams have a high emotional component showing anxiety (14% of reports), surprise (9%), anger (9%), joy (7%), sadness (5%), shame (2%) (Hartmann, 1998; Zadra and Donderi, 2000; Nguyen *et al.*, 2002; Schredl, 2003).

Negative emotional dreams (e.g., fearful) are remembered more easily because fear tends to awake the sleeper allowing the dream to be stored in memory (Schredl and Doll, 1998). Pleasant emotional dreams may include sexual interaction and orgasm. Sexual interaction is reported only in 12% of dreams of male subjects (Hall and Van de Castle, 1966) despite the fact that erections are present in 80–90% of REM sleep episodes (Fischer *et al.*, 1965; Karacan *et al.*, 1966). Activation of the amygdala and limbic regions during REM sleep may explain the emotional intensity of dreams (Maquet *et al.*, 1996).

Individual psychological traits emerge at some degree during dreaming (Cernovsky, 1984). Depressed patients report more often than average unpleasant dreams (Blagrove *et al.*, 2004), schizophrenics report dreams with a disorganized structure and incoherent themes similarly to their wakefulness mentation (Hartmann *et al.*, 1987; Claridge *et al.*, 1997). Events that produce anxiety or strong emotions during wakefulness may be revisited during sleep (Blagrove *et al.*, 2004), violence in particular may become a common content of nightmares (Krakow *et al.*, 2002).

However, it is not easy to influence dreams' content by presleep stimulation. Events related to the pre-sleep environment seem to enter the dream imagery in only one-third of cases (Rechschaffen, 1978). Presleep presentation of movies has variable consequenses (Foulkes and Rechtschaffen, 1964). It is likely that different personality traits and life experience play a role in filtering out fictional events.

Sensory stimulation presented during sleep is differently incorporated in dreams: sounds (9% of cases), flashlights (24%), cold water sprays (47%) (Dement and Wolpert, 1958), wrist electrical shocks (20%) (Koulack, 1969).

The most interesting feature of dreaming from this writer's point of view is the role-play developed by the dreamer. As in a virtual theater one or more actors (in addition to the dreamer) act according to a "text" provided on-line by the dreamer. The capacity to read other minds (anticipating their thoughts) is one of the most striking skills of human cognition. In their review "Interacting Minds" the Friths give an account on the far-reaching implications of such skills (Frith and Frith, 1999). The possibility to understand another mind relies on analytical skills, judgment competence, comparison of thoughts, and empathy. Even dream reports from illuminated sleep scientists contain examples of the "Interacting Minds" property. Rechtschaffen (1978) reports a conversation he had during dreaming with his dead father. Rechtschaffen junior asserts that in the dream he is aware of his father's death but is not appalled about his return from the grave (this is in accordance with the common delusional acceptance of dreaming). What comes out unexpected is that the conversation between Rechtschaffen senior and Rechtschaffen junior possess all the characteristics of a sensible and realistic dialog. The dead father "speaks his mind" according to his style and wit, as he would have done in life, although the text of such conversation is improvised by the mind of Rechtschaffen junior. Thus, with this dream report, Rechtschaffen junior clearly proves that an isolated sleeping mind can anticipate other minds' thoughts and opinions. In other words, the dreamer makes up the questions and answers appropriate for the speakers (like playing chess alone). Unfortunately, there are not many studies addressing such aptitude of the oneiric brain. Most dream studies stick to the "deficiency rule" pointing out what does not work in the sleeping brain compared to the wakeful brain. Hopefully, future cognitive studies of sleep will take into account "the interactive minds" issue.

Dreams, as well as thoughts, reflect a private territory of our minds, where complex images, sounds, actions, and actors are not witnessed by anybody but the sleeper. That is why it is very difficult to have objective measurements of such subjective experiences.

Quantitative and qualitative analysis of dream reports have been carried out by sleep researchers. Dream diaries have been largely used in past centuries. Despite the merit of such accurate reports of oneiric activity, they lack any information of sleep stage. On the other hand, data collected in sleep laboratories provide state control (EEG measurements) and systematic investigation of dream features. However, the environment of the sleep laboratory lacks of the naturalness of the home setting (Hobson, 1988). A new way to study dreams has been introduced by the use of Nightcap. This is a simple technique that uses surface sensors to monitor eye and muscle movements allowing one to distinguish REM from NREM sleep. Nightcap is also capable of eliciting awakenings from the two states. Since this tool can be easily used in the home setting it represents a good compromise between the old and modern ways to collect dreams (Stickgold *et al.*, 1994a). Some unanswered issues in dream research might find solution by digging in the large dream database created with the use of Nightcap in sleep laboratories worldwide.

Neuro-psychology dream analysis distinguishes between feature, form, and content. Feature refers to the modality involved (e.g., sensory, motor aspects, orientation, plot, memory, emotion). Form refers to the way the emerging feature develops (e.g., predominance of vision over other senses, character of movement, emotional lability, etc.). Content is made up of story details in the domain of the form analyzed (e.g., what is seen, what is mistaken, what is prompted by the feelings, thematic incoherence, etc.) (Hobson and Hoffman, 1984). More or less any formal analysis of dreams has developed around these cardinal points (Foulkes, 1978; McCarley and Hoffman, 1981; Hobson and Hoffman, 1984; Porte and Hobson, 1996; Stickgold *et al.*, 1994b). Several researchers have investigated dream bizarreness at length (Hobson *et al.*, 1987; Cipolli *et al.*, 1993; Sutton *et al.*, 1994). Despite the impressive amount of work done on the subject, a comprehensive theory of sleep mentation it still missing.

An interesting approach in the study of dreaming has come from "lucid dreaming"

Lucid dreaming means being aware of dreaming and controlling one's dream as it is happening. The term was coined by Frederik van Eeden (1913). Lucid dreaming implies that the dreamer acquires awareness of his dream. The awareness of dreaming occurs seldom in the overall population and in about 3% of subjects monitored in sleep laboratories (Bosinelli, 1995). However, even subjects more prone to lucid dreaming experience this phenomenon in a fraction of their dreams (Rechschaffen, 1978).

Stephen LaBerge (1985) had focused his research on the methods available to develop lucid dreaming. LaBerge is convinced that it is possible to learn how to control the oneiric experience similarly to how it is possible to control thoughts by meditation. Notably, lucid dreaming is an ancient art and the percentage of lucid dreamers may be greater in various cultures and groups who practice spiritual traditions such as shamanism (a form of American Indian medicine), Taoism, Buddhism, Tibetan dream yoga and other disciplines aimed at developing the "witnessing consciousness" of enlightenment. One of the best sources is a 1000-year-old text on Dream Yoga written by Tibetan Monks (see Chuang Tzu, alt. Zhuangzi, 1891). The potential for developing personal goals or achieving "consciousness" while asleep offers great promise for the future. The area of application of dream control is wide, what is difficult to have during wakefulness could be perhaps available through dreaming while such experience mantains a rewarding sense of reality. "Lucid dreaming could provide the handicapped and other disadvantaged people with the nearest thing to fulfilling their impossible dreams: paralytics could walk again in their dreams, to say nothing of dancing and flying" (LaBerge, 1985).

In the western tradition several authors described this phenomenon long before the use of formal dream analysis: Alfred Maury (1861), Jean Marie Leon d'Hervey de Saint Denis (1867), Mary Arnold Forster (1921) all pioneered the field of dream content control and autosuggestion. Thus, lucid dreaming represents a stimulating crossroad in the relationship between consciousness, sleep, and dream (Gackenbach and LaBerge, 1988).

Origin and function of oneiric activity

Dreams have fascinated ancient and modern cultures due to their metaphysical nature. They reflect a virtual reality experience having many features of the real word mixed with unrealistic circumstances (e.g., flying or breathing underwater). In this regard, more than an impoverished cognitive activity dream represents an explorative modality of brain function: a way to analyze possible scenarios of every day life as well as very exciting or scary situations. This perspective of dreaming is discussed in the "rehearsal for behavior" theory, one of the several functional hypothesis of dreaming discussed in the subsequent paragraphs.

Activation-synthesis theory

Hobson and McCarley (1977) proposed this theory after the discovery of the connection between REM-on neurons activation and tonic and phasic events of REM sleep. According to the activation-synthesis hypothesis dreams are the by-product of bursts of activity (e.g., PGO) spreading from subcortical areas (e.g., REM-on neurons of the pons) to the forebrain (e.g., occipital cortex) during REM sleep. Hence, the forebrain would integrate disparate sensory, motor, emotional elements and condense them into a (chaotic) story-like experience. Dream bizarreness in the view of Hobson and McCarley is related to two mechanisms: on the one hand the chaotic synthesis of the oneiric experience and, on the other hand, to a change in neuromodulation producing functional frontal deafferentation and consequent loss of typical frontal lobe cognitive functions like volition and judgment capabilities. The chaotic oneiric synthesis cannot account, however, for the occurrence of repetitive dreams. In a revision of the activation-synthesis theory Hobson and Schmajuk (1988) suggest that the oneiric synthesis is not enterily chaotic but is based on meaningful and affective events (mnemonic units) reflected in activation of hippocampal, amygdala, and limbic areas during REM sleep.

Dreaming as psychopathological state and the dopaminergic hypothesis

Dreaming is a great model of psychopathology, it includes the hallucinatory experiences and delusions of functional psychosis (e.g., schizophrenia) and the disorientation and memory loss of the organic dementias (Hobson, 1988, 2004). Hallucinations and delusions of schizophrenia are likely related to altered functionality of the mesolimbic-cortical dopaminergic system (Csernansky *et al.*, 1991; Glenthoj *et al.*, 1993; Viggiano *et al.*, 2003) perhaps linked to a noradrenergic or trimonoamine imbalance (Nurse *et al.*, 1984; Friedman *et al.*, 1999; Linner *et al.*, 2002; Pralong *et al.*, 2002). In parallel, it has been proposed that reduced noradrenergic modulation of frontal cortex during sleep and REM sleep may produce disinhibition of the dopaminergic system (Hobson *et al.*, 1998a,b; Hobson, 2004). In such contest endogenous or exogenous inputs would induce the hallucinatory and delusional experiences of dreaming (possibly reflected in the activation of unimodal visual association areas; Braun *et al.*, 1998). Notably, dopaminergic drugs (e.g., levo-dopa) produce vivid dreams and nightmares (Sharf *et al.*, 1978).

The second type of symptoms (disorientation and memory loss) has also been related to the neuromodulatory shift from the monoaminergic mode of waking to the cholinergic mode of sleep (Flicker *et al.*, 1981). Hobson has discussed at length the role of neuromodulation in the production of these mental aberrations (Hobson *et al.*, 1998a,b). In Hobson's view, the aminergic demodulation is likely responsible for frontal cortical deactivation observed during REM sleep (PET studies: e.g., Maquet *et al.*, 1996; Braun *et al.*, 1997) and consequently associated with frontal lobe symptoms like disorientation and memory loss whereas the activation of limbic and posterior associative cortices may result from enhanced cholinergic neuromodulation. Some animal data support, in part, this hypothesis (Nuñez, 1996).

Another study supporting the parallel between psychopathology and dreaming comes from Mark Solmes (1997). Solmes analyzed dream report data from 250 patients having focal brain lesions. In his study, bilateral thalamic and limbic-frontal lesions were commonly associated with dream reality confusion or defective reality monitoring. These patients lose the capability to distinguish the waking events from dreams because the oneiric activity acquires vivid characteristics. Solmes also showed that total cessation of dreaming is associated with deep bifrontal lesions or parietal lobe lesions whereas cessation of visual dream imagery is associated with bilateral occipito-temporal lesions. In these patients, REM sleep is present without dreams even when the brainstem is spared. In another group of 25 patients with brainstem lesions the oneiric activity was preserved despite REM sleep being abolished. Hence, Solmes argues that brainstem generated REM sleep is not a sufficient condition to sustain dreaming. Solmes concludes his dream generation analysis suggesting that the common pathway for eliciting dream synthesis in a sleeping brain is represented by frontal dopaminergic circuits (Solmes, 1997).

From Solmes' study it can be derived that brain function/pathology and dream production are closely related. Consistent with this possibility, data from congenitally blind people (having a functional occipital cortex) show a retained capacity for visual imagery in dreaming (Zimler and Keenan, 1983; Aleman *et al.*, 2001; Bertolo *et al.*, 2003; Lopes da Silva, 2003). However, damage of the sensory-motor cortex (e.g., producing hemiplegia) does not affect dream reports (Mach, 1959; Solmes, 1997).

Finally, Schwartz and Maquet (2002) pointed out that several bizarre features of normal dreams have similarities with well-known neuropsychological syndromes after brain damage, such as delusional misidentifications for faces and places. They believe that neuropsychological analysis of dream content might grant new ways of interpreting neuroimaging maps of sleep. Infact, altough brain activation during REM sleep is usually read in relation to underlying physiological and cellular mechanisms, the regional distribution observed in imaging studies might also be linked to specific dream features.

AIM model of Hobson

Hobson's group (Kahn *et al.*, 1997) proposed that the mental activity is a psychophysiological state with no clear boundaries between waking, sleep, meditation, etc. Such mental activity can be defined in a tridimensional (or multidimensional) space where the three dimensions are A, representing the degree of cortical activation (e.g., as shown by single unit recording, EEG, and imaging studies); I, the internal or external stimuli intensity (subject to sensory gating and attentional gain); M, the modulatory influence operated by neurotransmitters. Thus, there would not be a single state of waking or sleep but hundreds or thousands of states that merge one in another. Neuromodulatory influence on brain activity has been discussed above (Hobson, 1988; Hobson *et al.*, 1998a,b). Hence, the system that generates thoughts and images during waking would be the same generating thoughts and images during dreaming given associated difference in local brain activation and neuromodulation. These changes would produce the continuous fluctuation of mind states and the uniqueness of sensorial perception. In fact, no identical perceptions can ever be elicited.

Virtual reality hypothesis

It has been claimed that knowledge of the external world is based on sensory perception and is identified as reality. This suggests that, theoretically, the world might only exist as complex sensory perception encoded in our neural networks. This perceptual "image" reflects the coordinated work of an infinite number of neurons. There are neurons that estimate object color, (Zeki, 1980) others the position, the orientation (Zeki, 1983), others respond to face presentation (Eifuku, *et al.*, 2004) or to the danger associated to them (Phillips, *et al.*, 1997). It has been possible to simulate perceptual experiences by electrically stimulating specific brain regions (Delgado *et al.*, 1968; Delgado, 1969; Moan and Heath, 1972). From this point of view the fictive cognitive experience of dreaming would share the same nature of the waking experience: a fictive reality in a self-contained brain.

This type of reasoning is found in many philosophical essays from Descartes (1637) to Putnam (1982). Many philosophers are fascinated by the idea of subjective versus objective proof of existence, an argument today called *the problem of the brain in the vat*. This theory discusses the possibility that one is just a disembodied brain maintained in life by a feeding fluid and attached through wires to a supercomputer feeding in electrical inputs and simulating the existence of an outside world. Putnam thinks there are no differences in the experience but only in the source of the representation. Hence, if thoughts, perceptions, and reactions are the consequences of neuronal networks' function it is possible that waking mental activity, meditation, lucid dreaming, and oneiric activity are forms more or less complex of virtual reality. This theme has recently become ground for a famous movie called *MATRIX* where humans try to regain control of their lives after discovering that all their experiences are fed in by an evil computer. The provocative argument of "the brain in the vat" intends to challenge old-fashioned ideas on consciousness and cognition.

Computational neurocognitive models

Several efforts have been made to reproduce perceptual integration in computational network (Tononi *et al.*, 1992). Hinton and colleagues have designed a wake–sleep neural network to map waking and sleep imagery (Hinton *et al.*, 1995; Hinton and Dayan, 1996). Their model takes into account the high ratio of top-down to bottom-up connections of the visual cortex. Such prevalence of top-down influences is supposed to shape the way sensory input enters consciousness. In other words, sensory perception is the result of bottom-up processing (analysis of physical characteristics of the stimuli) integrated with top-up mechanisms based on sensory knowledge, saliency, attention, etc. Antrobus (1991), with the DREAMIT-BT model, managed to simulate some characteristics of dreaming. Antrobus considers dreams as sequences of visual images and responses of the dreamer to those images. This would produce the continuity or story-like effect of dreaming. Antrobus claims that visual event sequences are learned during waking perception (e.g., a jam jar is on the shelf — the jar falls from the shelf to the floor — noise of glass breakage — the jam slowly spreads over the floor — and so on and so forth); such knowledge would be applied then in the synthesis of perceptual sequences in sleep in the absence of any external inputs. The sensory sequences would be quite rigid when the learned associations have a high predictability (e.g., they have been experienced hundreds of times in waking: like eating, getting dressed, driving to work, etc.). However, sequences could have sudden "twists" when the learned associations are less predictable (e.g., they have not been experienced often in waking or they have shown different outcomes: running into the woods — seeing the neighbor's dog or a wolf or an oak or something else). These twists are perhaps reflected in the discontinuity and the bizarreness of dreaming. DREAMIT-BT was programmed in a simulated waking state with sequences of events having high or low "predictability" and its performance was then observed in a simulated sleep state (in the absence of any external input). The model reproduced the postulated effect of sequence interruption for low predictability response events (see also Rumelhart *et al.*, 1986). Hence, development of more sophisticated computational models may provide crucial information on the way dreams are synthesized.

Dream as rehearsal for behavior

Contrary to the view of dreaming as a sequence of pre-learned sensory events, other scientists interpret dreams as rehearsal for behavior.

Rosalind Cartwright (1974) considers rehearsal for future behavior as one of the main functions of dreaming. Her view is expressed in the four Rs of dream function: review, revise, rehearse, and repair. Review and revise stand for reediting near-past experiences in order to find solutions for present threats and find emotional balance (repair).

In the same line of reasoning, Bosinelli (1995) suggests that "sleep among its other functions allows the mental apparatus to experiment original productive itineraries that are hardly suitable for to the waking life".

Revonsuo (2000) argues that the biological function of dreaming is to simulate threatening events, and to rehearse threat perception and threat avoidance. From an evolutionary point of view such a mechanism would have been valuable for development and survival. It is likely that in modern times threatening circumstances to be rehearsed include wake stressors and responsabilities.

Bottom-up and top-down mechanisms of oneiric synthesis

An Italian group suggested that whatever the dreaming input source, the result is the activation of mnemonic units, which in turn are material for interpretation and elaboration by top-down cortical mechanisms. The product of this bottom-up first and top-down then processing would constitute the hallucinatory experience of dreaming (Bosinelli, 1995; Cicogna and Cavallero, 1993). However, the source of the bottom-up stimulation cannot be underestimated since it represents the core question in dream research.

Dreaming and reprogramming

In *The Paradox of Sleep: The Story of Dreaming*, Jouvet considers that while sleeping is clearly an essential body function, dreaming might simply be an accidental by-product of brain activity. In fact, paradoxical sleep can be suppressed in humans for very long periods with no discernible detrimental effects. Another interesting option discussed by Jouvet is that during dreaming the brain is genetically "reprogrammed"; in other words any learning unrelated to one's biological individuality would be erased (Jouvet, 1999). This hypothesis is not directly supported by facts and it impossible at the moment to design studies able to investigate such possibility.

Conclusions

It seems evident that a certain degree of mental activity is present throughout sleep. This is shaped as information processing, oneiric synthesis, emerging emotional memories. Notably, during sleep affective inputs find a privileged access to awareness. Thus, while asleep a virtual reality world is shaped by residual brain activation associated to past and present emotions taking advantage of our impoverished will and short-term memory.

References

Achermann, P. and Borbely, A.A. (1998). Temporal evolution of coherence and power in the human sleep electroencephalogram. *J. Sleep Res.*, 7 (Suppl): 36–41.

Adler, L.E., Pachtman, E., Franks, R.D., Pecevich, M., Waldo, M.C., and Freedman, R. (1982). Neurophysiological evidence for a defect in neuronal mechanisms involved in sensory gating in schizophrenia. *Biol. Psychiatry*, 17: 639–654.

Aleman, A., van Lee, L., Mantione, M.H., Verkoijen, I.G., and de Haan, E.H. (2001). Visual imagery without visual experience: evidence from congenitally totally blind people. *Neuroreport*, 12: 2601–2604.

Alho, K., Huotilainen, M., and Näätänen, R. (1995). Are memory traces for simple and complex sounds located in different regions of auditory cortex? Recent MEG studies. *Electroencephalogr. Clin. Neurophysiol.*, 44: 197–203.

Antrobus, J. (1991). Dreaming: cognitive processes during cortical activation and high afferent thresholds. *Psychol. Rev.*, 98: 96–121.

Apkarian, P., Mirmiran, M., and Tijssen, R. (1991). Effects of behavioural state on visual processing in neonates. *Neuropediatrics*, 22: 85–91.

Atienza, M., Cantero, J.L., and Gomez, C.M. (1997). The mismatch negativity component reveals the sensory memory during REM sleep in humans. *Neurosci. Lett.*, 14: 21–24.

Atienza, M., Cantero, J.L., and Gomez, C.M. (2000). Decay time of the auditory sensory memory trace during wakefulness and REM sleep. *Psychophysiology*, 37: 485–493.

Atienza, M., Cantero, J.L., and Escera, C. (2001). Auditory information processing during human sleep as revealed by event-related brain potentials. *Clin. Neurophysiol.*, 112: 2031–2045.

Bastien, C. and Campbell, K. (1992). The evoked K-complex: all-or-none phenomenon? *Sleep*, 15: 236–245.

Bastien, C.H., Crowley, K.E., and Colrain, I.M. (2002). Evoked potential components unique to non-REM sleep: relationship to evoked K-complexes and vertex sharp waves. *Int. J. Psychophysiol.*, 46: 257–274.

Bastuji, H., García-Larrea, L., Franc, C., and Mauguiere, F. (1995). Brain processing of stimulus deviance during slow-wave and paradoxical sleep: a study of human auditory evoked responses using the oddball paradigm. *J. Clin. Neurophysiol.*, 12: 155–167.

Bentley, A.J., Newton, S., and Zio, C.D. (2003). Sensitivity of sleep stages to painful thermal stimuli. *J. Sleep Res.*, 12: 143–147.

Berlad, I. and Pratt, H. (1995). P300 in response to the subject's own name. *Electroencephalogr. Clin. Neurophysiol.*, 96: 472–474.

Bertolo, H., Paiva, T., Pessoa, L., Mestre, T., Marques, R., and Santos, R. (2003). Visual dream content, graphical representation and EEG alpha activity in congenitally blind subjects. *Brain Res. Cogn. Brain Res.*, 15: 277–284.

Blagrove, M., Farmer, L., and Williams, E. (2004). The relationship of nightmare frequency and nightmare distress to well-being. *J. Sleep Res.*, 13: 129–136.

Born, A.P., Law, I., Lund, T.E., Rostrup, E., Hanson, L.G., Wildschiodtz, G., Lou, H.C., and Paulson, O.B. (2002). Cortical deactivation induced by visual stimulation in human slow-wave sleep. *Neuroimage*, 17: 1325–1335.

Bosinelli, M. (1995). Mind and consciousness during sleep. *Behav. Brain Res.*, 69: 195–201.

Braun, A.R., Balkin, T.J., Wesenten, N.J., Carson, R.E., Varga, M., Baldwin, P., Selbie, S., Belenky, G., and Herscovitch, P. (1997). Regional cerebral blood flow throughout the sleep-wake cycle. An H2(15)O PET study. *Brain*, 120: 1173–1197.

Braun, A.R., Balkin, T.J., Wesensten, N.J., Gwadry, F., Carson, R.E., Varga, M., Baldwin, P., Belenky, G., and Herscovitch, P. (1998). Dissociated pattern of activity in visual cortices and their projections during human rapid eye movement sleep. *Science*, 279: 91–95.

Brualla, J., Romero, M.F., Serrano, M., and Valdizan, J.R. (1998). Auditory event-related potentials to semantic priming during sleep. *Electroencephalogr. Clin. Neurophysiol.*, 108: 283–290.

Buchwald, J.S. (1983). Auditory evoked responses in clinical populations and in the cat. *Auris Nasus Larynx*, 10: 87–95.

Burle, B. and Bonnet, M. (1999). What's an internal clock for? From temporal information processing to temporal processing of information. *Behav. Process.*, 45: 59–72.

Campbell, K.B. and Bartoli, E.A. (1986). Human auditory evoked potentials during natural sleep: the early components. *Electroencephalogr. Clin. Neurophysiol.*, 65: 142–149.

Campbell, K.B. and Colrain, I.M. (2002). Event-related potential measures of the inhibition of information processing: II. The sleep onset period. *Int. J. Psychophysiol.*, 46: 197–214.

Cartwright, R.D. (1974). The influence of a conscious wish on dreams: a methodological study of dream meaning and function. *J. Abnorm. Psychol.*, 83: 387–393.

Cernovsky, Z.Z. (1984). Life stress measures and reported frequency of sleep disorders. *Percept. Mot. Skills*, 58: 39–49.

Chalmers, D. (1996). *The Conscious Mind.* Oxford: Oxford University Press.

Chuang, Tzu, alt. Zhuangzi (1891). *The Writings of Chuang Tzu.* Oxford: Oxford University Press (James Legge, translation).

Cicogna, P. and Cavallero, C. (1993). Coscienza e sogno. *Riv. Psicol.*, 78: 27–33.

Cicogna, P., Cavallero, C., and Bosinelli, M. (1991). Cognitive aspects of mental activity during sleep. *Am. J. Psychol.*, 104: 413–425.

Cipolli, C., Bolzani, R., Cornoldi, C., De Beni, R., and Fagioli, I. (1993). Bizarreness effect in dream recall. *Sleep*, 16: 163–170.

Claridge, G., Clark, K., and Davis, C. (1997). Nightmares, dreams, and schizotypy. *Br. J. Clin. Psychol.*, 36: 377–386.

Coenen, A.M. and Vendrik, A.J. (1972). Determination of the transfer ratio of cat's geniculate neurons through quasi-intracellular recordings and the relation with the level of alertness. *Exp. Brain Res.*, 14: 227–242.

Colon, E.J. and de Weerd, A.W. (1986). Long-latency somatosensory evoked potentials. *J. Clin. Neurophysiol.*, 3: 279–296.

Cote, K.A. (2002). Probing awareness during sleep with the auditory odd-ball paradigm. *Psychophysiology*, 46: 227–241.

Cote, K.A., Etienne, L., and Campbell, K.B. (2001). Neurophysiological evidence for the detection of external stimuli during sleep. *Sleep*, 24: 791–803.

Csernansky, J.G., Murphy, G.M., and Faustman, W.O. (1991). Limbic/mesolimbic connections and the pathogenesis of schizophrenia. *Biol. Psychiatry*, 15: 383–400.

Czisch, M., Wetter, T.C., Kaufmann, C., Pollmacher, T., Holsboer, F., and Auer, D.P. (2002). Altered processing of acoustic stimuli during sleep:

reduced auditory activation and visual deactivation detected by a combined fMRI/EEG study. *Neuroimage*, 16: 251–258.

Czisch, M., Wehrle, R., Kaufmann, C., Wetter, T.C., Holsboer, F., Pollmacher, T., and Auer, D.P. (2004). Functional MRI during sleep: BOLD signal decreases and their electrophysiological correlates. *Eur. J. Neurosci.*, 20: 566–574.

Deiber, M.P., Ibanez, V., Bastuji, H., Fischer, C., and Mauguière, F. (1989). Changes of middle latency auditory evoked potentials during natural sleep in humans. *Neurology*, 39: 806–813.

Delgado, J.M.R. (1969). *Physical Control of the Mind, Toward a Psychocivilized Society.* New York: Harper & Row.

Delgado, J.M., Mark, V., Sweet, W., Ervin, F., Weiss, G., Bach-Y-Rita, G., and Hagiwara, R. (1968). Intracerebral radio stimulation and recording in completely free patients. *J. Nerv. Ment. Dis.*, 147: 329–340.

Dement, W. and Wolpert, E.A. (1958). The relation of eye movements, body motility, and external stimuli to dream content. *J. Exp. Psychol.*, 55: 543–553.

Descartes, R. (1991). *Discourse on Method and Meditations on First Philosophy.* Indianapolis, USA: Hackett Publisher (Donald A. Cress, translation).

Descartes (1641). *Meditations on First Philosophy.*

Edeline, J.M., Manunta, Y., and Hennevin, E. (2000). Auditory thalamus neurons during sleep: changes in frequency selectivity, threshold, and receptive field size. *J. Neurophysiol.*, 84: 934–952.

van Eeden, F. (1913). *Proc. Society Psychical Res.*, Vol. 26.

Eifuku, S., De Souza, W.C., Tamura, R., Nishijo, H., and Ono, T. (2004). Neuronal correlates of face identification in the monkey anterior temporal cortical areas. *J. Neurophysiol.*, 91(1): 358–371.

Emerson, R.G., Sgro, J.A., Pedley, T.A., and Hauser, W.A. (1988). State-dependent changes in the N20 component of the median nerve somatosensory evoked potential. *Neurology*, 38: 64–68.

Erwin, R. and Buchwald, J.S. (1986). Midlatency auditory evoked responses: differential effects of sleep in the human. *Electroencephalogr. Clin. Neurophysiol.*, 65: 383–392.

Escera, C., Alho, K., Schroger, E., and Winkler, I. (2000). Involuntary attention and distractibility as evaluated with event-related brain potentials. *Audiol. Neurootol.*, 5: 151–166.

Espa, F., Ondze, B., Deglise, P., Billiard, M., and Besset, A. (2000). Sleep architecture, slow wave activity, and sleep spindles in adult patients with sleepwalking and sleep terrors. *Clin. Neurophysiol.*, 111: 929–939.

Evarts, E.V. (1960). Effects of sleep and waking on spontaneous and evoked discharge of single units in visual cortex. *Fin. Lakaresallsk Handl.*, 19: 828–837.

Fisher, C., Gorss, J., and Zuch, J. (1965). Cycle of penile erection synchronous with dreaming (REM) sleep. *Arch. Gen. Psychiatry*, 12: 29–45.

Flicker, C., McCarley, R.W., and Hobson, J.A. (1981). Aminergic neurons: state control and plasticity in three model systems. *Cell. Mol. Neurobiol.*, 1: 123–166.

Forster, A.M. (1921). *Studies in Dreams*. New York: Macmillan.

Foulkes, W.D. (1962). Dream reports from different stages of sleep. *J. Abnorm. Soc. Psychol.*, 65: 14–25.

Foulkes, D. (1978). *A Grammar of Dreams*. Hassocks: Harvester Press.

Foulkes, D. and Fleisher, S. (1975). Mental activity in relaxed wakefulness. *J. Abnorm. Psychol.*, 84: 66–75.

Foulkes, D. and Rechtschaffen, A. (1964). Presleep determinants of dream content: effect on two films. *Percept. Mot. Skills*, 19: 983–1005.

Friedman, J.I., Adler, D.N., and Davis, K.L. (1999). The role of norepinephrine in the pathophysiology of cognitive disorders: potential applications to the treatment of cognitive dysfunction in schizophrenia and Alzheimer's disease. *Biol. Psychiatry*, 46: 1243–1252.

Frith, C.D., Friston, K., Liddle, P.F., and Frackowiak, R.S. (1991). Willed action and the prefrontal cortex in man: a study with PET. *Proc. R. Soc. Lond. B. Biol. Sci.*, 244: 241–246.

Frith, C.D. and Frith, U. (1999). Interacting minds — a biological basis. *Science*, 286: 1692–1695.

Gackenbach, J. and LaBerge, S. (1988). *Conscious Mind, Sleeping Brain: Perspectives on Lucid Dreaming*. New York: Plenum Press.

Giard, M.H., Perrin, F., Pernier, J., and Bouchet, P. (1990). Brain generators implicated in the processing of auditory stimulus deviance: a topographic event-related potential study. *Psychophysiology*, 27: 627–640.

Giard, M.H., Perrin, F., Echallier, J.F., Thevenet, M., Froment, J.C., and Pernier, J. (1994). Dissociation of temporal and frontal components in the human auditory N1 wave: a scalp current density and dipole model analysis. *Electroencephalogr. Clin. Neurophysiol.*, 92: 238–252.

Glenthoj, B., Mogensen, J., Laursen, H., Holm, S., and Hemmingsen, R. (1993). Electrical sensitization of the meso-limbic dopaminergic system in rats: a pathogenetic model for schizophrenia. *Brain Res.*, 13: 39–54.

Gora, J., Colrain, I.M., and Trinder, J. (2001). The investigation of K-complex and vertex sharp wave activity in response to mid-inspiratory occlusions and complete obstructions to breathing during NREM sleep. *Sleep*, 24: 81–89.

Hall and Van de Castle (1966). *The Content Analysis of Dreams*. New York: Appleton, pp. 320.

Harsh, J., Voss, U., Hull, J., Schrepfer, S., and Badia, P. (1994). ERP and behavioral changes during the wake/sleep transition. *Psychophysiology*, 31: 244–252.

Hartmann, E. (1998). Nightmare after trauma as paradigm for all dreams: a new approach to the nature and functions of dreaming. *Psychiatry*, 61: 223–238.

Hartmann, E., Russ, D., Oldfield, M., Sivan, I., and Cooper, S. (1987). Who has nightmares? The personality of the lifelong nightmare sufferer. *Arch. Gen. Psychiatry*, 44: 49–56.

Hawkins, J. (1989). Sleep disturbance in intentional self-awakenings: behavior-genetic and transient factors. *Percept. Mot. Skills*, 69: 507–510.

d'Hervey de Saint Denis, J.M.L. (1867). *Les rêves et les moyens de les diriger.* Paris: Amyot.

Hinton, G.E. and Dayan, P. (1996). Varieties of Helmholtz machine. *Neural Networks.*, 9: 1385–1403.

Hinton, G.E., Dayan, P., Frey, B.J., and Neal, R.M. (1995). The "wake–sleep" algorithm for unsupervised neural networks. *Science*, 268: 1158–1161.

Hobson, J.A. (1988). *The Dreaming Brain.* USA: Basic Books.

Hobson, J.A. (1992). Sleep and dreaming: induction and mediation of REM sleep by cholinergic mechanisms. *Curr. Opin. Neurobiol.*, 2: 759–763.

Hobson, J.A. (1999). Arrest of firing of aminergic neurones during REM sleep: implications for dream theory. *Brain Res. Bull.*, 50: 333–334.

Hobson, A. (2004). A model for madness? *Nature*, 430: 21.

Hobson, J.A. and Hoffman, S.A. (1984). Picturing dreaming: some features of the drawings in a dream journal. In: Bosinelli, M. and Cicogna, P. (Eds.). *Psychology of Dreaming.* Bologna, Italy: CLUEB.

Hobson, J.A. and McCarley, R.W. (1977). The brain as a dream state generator: an activation-synthesis hypothesis of the dream process. *Am. J. Psychiatry*, 134: 1335–1348.

Hobson, J.A. and Schmajuk, N.A. (1988). Brain state and plasticity: an integration of the reciprocal interaction model of sleep cycle oscillation with attentional models of hippocampal function. *Arch. Ital. Biol.*, 126: 209–224.

Hobson, J.A. and Stickgold, R. (1994). Dreaming: a neurocognitive approach. *Consciousness Cogn.*, 3: 1–15.

Hobson, J.A., Hoffman, S.A., Helfand, R., and Kostner, D. (1987). Dream bizarreness and the activation-synthesis hypothesis. *Hum. Neurobiol.*, 6: 157–164.

Hobson, J.A., Stickgold, R., and Pace-Schott, E.F. (1998a). The neuropsychology of REM sleep dreaming. *Neuroreport*, 9: R1–R14.

Hobson, J.A., Pace-Schott, E.F., Stickgold, R., and Kahn, D. (1998b). To dream or not to dream? Relevant data from new neuroimaging and electrophysiological studies. *Curr. Opin. Neurobiol.*, 8: 239–244.

Hyder, F., Phelps, E.A., Wiggins, C.J., Labar, K.S., Blamire, A.M., and Shulman, R.G. (1997). "Willed action": a functional MRI study of the human prefrontal cortex during a sensorimotor task. *Proc. Natl. Acad. Sci. USA*, 94: 6989–6994.

Johnson, M.R. and Adler, L.E. (1993). Transient impairment in P50 auditory sensory gating induced by a cold-pressor test. *Biol. Psychiatry*, 33: 380–387.

Joliot, M., Ribary, U., and Llinás, R. (1994). Human oscillatory brain activity near 40 Hz coexists with cognitive temporal binding. *Proc. Natl. Acad. Sci. USA*, 91: 11748–11751.

Jouvet, M. (1999). *The Paradox of Sleep: The Story of Dreaming.* Boston, MA: The MIT Press (Laurence Garey, trans.).

Kahn, D., Pace-Schott, E.F., and Hobson, J.A. (1997). Consciousness in waking and dreaming: the roles of neuronal oscillation and neuromodulation in determining similarities and differences. *Neuroscience*, 78: 13–38.

Kalen, P., Rosegren, E., Lindvall, O., and Bjorklund, A. (1989). Hippocampal noradrenaline and serotonin release over 24 hours as measured by the dialysis technique in freely moving rats: correlation to behavioural activity state, effect of handling and tail-pinch. *Eur. J. Neurosci.*, 1: 181–188.

Kajimura, N., Uchiyama, M., Takayama, Y., Uchida, S., Uema, T., Kato, M., Sekimoto, M., Watanabe, T., Nakajima, T., Horikoshi, S., Ogawa, K., Nishikawa, M., Hiroki, M., Kudo, Y., Matsuda, H., Okawa, M., and Takahashi, K. (1999). Activity of midbrain reticular formation and neocortex during the progression of human non-rapid eye movement sleep. *J. Neurosci.*, 19: 10065–10073.

Karacan, I., Goodenough, D.R., Shapiro, A., and Starker, S. (1966). Erection cycle during sleep in relation to dream anxiety. *Arch. Gen. Psychiatry*, 15: 183–189.

Kisley, M.A., Olincy, A., and Freedman, R. (2001). The effect of state on sensory gating: comparison of waking, REM and non-REM sleep. *Clin. Neurophysiol.*, 112: 1154–1165.

Kitamura, Y., Kakigi, R., Hoshiyama, M., Koyama, S., and Nakamura, A. (1996). Effects of sleep on somatosensory evoked responses in human: a magnetoencephalographic study. *Brain Res. Cogn. Brain Res.*, 4: 275–279.

Kodama, T., Lai, Y.Y., and Siegel, J.M. (2003). Changes in inhibitory amino acid release linked to pontine-induced atonia: an in vivo microdialysis study. *J. Neurosci.*, 23: 1548–1554.

Koulack, D. (1969). Effects of somatosensory stimulation on dream content. *Arch. Gen. Psychiatry*, 20: 718–725.

Krakow, B., Schrader, R., Tandberg, D., Hollifield, M., Koss, M.P., Yau, C.L., and Cheng, D.T. (2002). Nightmare frequency in sexual assault survivors with PTSD. *J. Anxiety Disord.*, 16: 175–190.

LaBerge, S. (1985). *Lucid Dreaming.* New York: Ballantine.

Lai, Y.Y. and Siegel, J.M. (1991). Pontomedullary glutamate receptors mediating locomotion and muscle tone suppression. *J. Neurosci.*, 11: 2931–2937.

Lai, Y.Y., Kodama, T., and Siegel, J.M. (2001). Changes in monoamine release in the ventral horn and hypoglossal nucleus linked to pontine inhibition of muscle tone: an in vivo microdialysis study. *J. Neurosci.*, 21: 7384–7391.

Laureys, S., Faymonville, M.E., Degueldre, C., Fiore, G.D., Damas, P., Lambermont, B., Janssen, N., Aerts, J., Franck, G., Luxen, A., Moonen, G., Lamy, M., and Maquet, P. (2000). Auditory processing in the vegetative state. *Brain*, 123: 1589–1601.

Le Doux, J. (1996). *The Emotional Brain.* New York: Simon and Schuster.

Linner, L., Wiker, C., Wadenberg, M.L., Schalling, M., and Svensson, T.H. (2002). Noradrenaline reuptake inhibition enhances the antipsychotic-like effect of raclopride and potentiates D2-blockage-induced dopamine release in the medial prefrontal cortex of the rat. *Neuropsychopharmacology*, 27: 691–698.

Lopes da Silva, F.H. (2003). Visual dreams in the congenitally blind? *Trends Cogn. Sci.*, 7: 328–330.

Loveless, N., Levanen, S., Jousmaki, V., Sams, M., and Hari, R. (1996). Temporal integration in auditory sensory memory: neuromagnetic evidence. *Electroencephalogr. Clin. Neurophysiol.*, 100: 220–228.

Llinás, R. and Ribary, U. (1993). Coherent 40-Hz oscillation characterizes dream state in humans. *Proc. Natl. Acad. Sci. USA*, 90: 2078–2081.

Mach, E. (1959). *The Analysis of Sensation and the Relation of the Physical to the Psychical.* New York: Dover Publications (original work published 1906) (Williams, C. and Waterlow, S. trans.).

Maquet, P., Peters, J., Aerts, J., Delfiore, G., Degueldre, C., Luxen, A., and Franck, G. (1996). Functional neuroanatomy of human rapid-eye-movement sleep and dreaming. *Nature*, 383: 163–166.

Maury, A. (1861). *Le sommeil et les rêves.* Paris.

McCarley, R.W. and Hoffman, E. (1981). REM sleep dreams and the activation-synthesis hypothesis. *Am. J. Psychiatry*, 138: 904–912.

Mendel, M.I. and Kupperman, G.L. (1974). Early components of the averaged electroencephalic response to constant level clicks during rapid eye movement sleep. *Audiology*, 13: 23–32.

Moan, C.E. and Heath, R.G. (1972). Septal stimulation for the initiation of heterosexual activity in a homosexual male. *J. Behav. Ther. Exp. Psychiatry*, 3: 23–30.

Morales-Cobas, G., Ferreira, M.I., and Velluti, R.A. (1995). Firing of inferior colliculus neurons in response to low-frequency sound stimulation during sleep and waking. *J. Sleep Res.*, 4: 242–251.

Murata, K. and Kameda, K. (1963). The activity of single cortical neurons of unrestrained cats during sleep and wakefulness. *Arch. Ital. Biol.*, 101: 306–331.

Nakano, S., Tsuji, S., Matsunaga, K., and Murai, Y. (1995). Effect of sleep stage on somatosensory evoked potentials by median nerve stimulation. *Electroencephalogr. Clin. Neurophysiol.*, 96: 385–389.

Näätänen, R., Teder, W., Alho, K., and Lavikainen, J. (1992). Auditory attention and selective input modulation: a topographical ERP study. *Neuroreport*, 3: 493–496.

Nader, K., Schafe, G.E., and Le Doux, J.E. (2000). Fear memories require protein synthesis in the amygdala for reconsolidation after retrieval. *Nature*, 406: 722–726.

Nguyen, T.T., Madrid, S., Marquez, H., and Hicks, R.A. (2002). Nightmare frequency, nightmare distress, and anxiety. *Percept. Mot. Skills*, 95: 219–225.

Nielsen, T.A. (1999). Mentation during sleep: The REM/NREM distinction. In: Lydic, R. and Baghdoyan, H.A. (Eds.). *Handbook of Behavioral State Control: Cellular and Molecular Mechanisms.* Boca Raton: CRC Press, pp. 101–128.

Nielsen-Bohlman, L., Knight, R.T., Woods, D.L., and Woodward, K. (1991). Differential auditory processing continues during sleep. *Electroencephalogr. Clin. Neurophysiol.*, 79: 281–290.

Noguchi, Y., Yamada, T., Yeh, M., Matsubara, M., Kokubun, Y., Kawada, J., Shiraishi, G., and Kajimoto, S. (1995). Dissociated changes of frontal and parietal somatosensory evoked potentials in sleep. *Neurology*, 45: 154–160.

Novak, G., Ritter, W., and Vaughan, H.G. Jr. (1992). The chronometry of attention-modulated processing and automatic mismatch detection. *Psychophysiology*, 29: 412–430.

Nuñez, A. (1996). Unit activity of rat basal forebrain neurons: relationship to cortical activity. *Neuroscience*, 72: 757–766.

Nurse, B., Russell, V.A., and Taljaard, J.J. (1984). Alpha 2 and beta-adrenoceptor agonists modulate [3H]dopamine release from rat nucleus accumbens slices: implications for research into depression. *Neurochem. Res.*, 9: 1231–1238.

Okusa, T. and Kakigi, R. (2002). Structure of visual evoked magnetic field during sleep in humans. *Neurosci. Lett.*, 328: 113–116.

Oswald, I., Taylor, A.M., and Treisman, M. (1960). Discriminative responses to stimulation during human sleep. *Brain*, 83: 440–453.

Pagel, J.F. (2003). Non-dreamers. *Sleep Med.*, 4: 235–241.

Pedemonte, M., Peña, J.L., Morales-Cobas, G., and Velluti, R.A. (1994). Effects of sleep on the responses of single cells in the lateral superior olive. *Arch. Ital. Biol.*, 132: 165–178.

Peña, J.L., Pedemonte, M., Ribeiro, M.F., and Velluti, R. (1992). Single unit activity in the guinea-pig cochlear nucleus during sleep and wakefulness. *Arch. Ital. Biol.*, 130: 179–189.

Peña, J.L., Pérez-Perera, L., Bouvier, M., and Velluti, R.A. (1999). Sleep and wakefulness modulation of the neuronal firing in the auditory cortex of the guinea pig. *Brain Res.*, 816: 463–470.

Pérez-Garci, E., del Río-Portilla, Y., Guevara, M.A., Arce, C., and Corsi-Cabrera, M. (2001). Paradoxical sleep is characterized by uncoupled gamma activity between frontal and perceptual cortical regions. *Sleep*, 24: 118–126.

Perrin, F., García-Larrea, L., Mauguière, F., and Bastuji, H. (1999). A differential brain response to the subject's own name persists during sleep. *Clin. Neurophysiol.*, 110: 2153–2164.

Phillips, M.L., Young, A.W., Senior, C., Brammer, M., Andrew, C., Calder, A.J., Bullmore, E.T., Perrett, D.I., Rowland, D., Williams, S.C., Gray, J.A., and David, A.S. (1997). A specific neural substrate for perceiving facial expressions of disgust. *Nature*, 389(6650): 495–498.

Picton, T.W., Hillyard, S.A., Krausz, H.I., and Galambos, R. (1974). Human auditory evoked potentials. I. Evaluation of components. *Electroencephalogr. Clin. Neurophysiol.*, 36: 179–190.

Pompeiano, O. (1967). The neurophysiological mechanisms of the postural and motor events during desynchronized sleep. *Res. Publ. Assoc. Res. Nerv. Ment. Dis.*, 1967: 351–423.

Portas, C.M., Bjorvatn, B., Fagerland, S., Gronli, J., Mundal, V., Sorensen, E., and Ursin, R. (1998). On-line detection of extracellular levels of serotonin in dorsal raphe nucleus and frontal cortex over the sleep/wake cycle in the freely moving rat. *Neuroscience*, 83: 807–814.

Portas, C.M., Krakow, K., Allen, P., Josephs, O., Armony, J.L., and Frith, C.D. (2000). Auditory processing across the sleep-wake cycle: simultaneous EEG and fMRI monitoring in humans. *Neuron*, 28: 991–999.

Porte, H.S. and Hobson, J.A. (1996). Physical motion in dreams: one measure of three theories. *J. Abnorm. Psychol.*, 105: 329–335.

Pralong, E., Magistretti, P., and Stoop, R. (2002). Cellular perspectives on the glutamate–monoamine interactions in limbic lobe structures and their relevance for some psychiatric disorders. *Prog. Neurobiol.*, 67: 173–202.

Putnam, H. (1982). Brains in a vat. In: *Reason, Truth, and History*. Cambridge: Cambridge University Press, pp. 1–21.

Rechtschaffen, A., Verdone, P., and Wheaton, J. (1963). Reports of mental activity during sleep. *Can. Psychiatr. Assoc. J.*, 8: 409–414.

Rechtschaffen, A. (1978). The single-mindedness and isolation of dreams. *Sleep*, 1: 97–109.

Revonsuo, A. (2000). The reinterpretation of dreams: an evolutionary hypothesis of the function of dreaming. *Behav. Brain Sci.*, 23: 877–901.

Ribary, U., Ioannides, A.A., Singh, K.D., Hasson, R., Bolton, J.P., Lado, F., Mogilner, A., and Llinás, R. (1991). Magnetic field tomography of coherent thalamocortical 40-Hz oscillations in humans. *Proc. Natl. Acad. Sci. USA*, 88: 11037–11041.

Roth, M., Shaw, J., and Green, J. (1956). The form voltage distribution and physiological significance of the K-complex. *Electroencephalogr. Clin. Neurophysiol.*, 8: 385–402.

Roschke, J., Mann, K., Riemann, D., Frank, C., and Fell, J. (1995). Sequential analysis of the brain's transfer properties during consecutive REM episodes. *Electroencephalogr. Clin. Neurophysiol.*, 96: 390–397.

Rumelhart, D.E., Smolensky, P., McClelland, J.L., and Hinton, G.E. (1986). Schemata and sequential thought processes in PDP models. In: Rumelhart, D.E. and McClelland, J.L. (Eds.). *Parallel Distributed Processing*. Cambridge, MA: MIT Press, pp. 7–57.

Sallinen, M., Kaartinen, J., and Lyytinen, H. (1996). Processing of auditory stimuli during tonic and phasic periods of REM sleep as revealed by event-related brain potentials. *J. Sleep Res.*, 5: 220–228.

Schredl, M. (2003). Effects of state and trait factors on nightmare frequency. *Eur. Arch. Psychiatry Clin. Neurosci.*, 253: 241–247.

Schredl, M. and Doll, E. (1998). Emotions in diary dreams. *Conscious. Cogn.*, 7: 634–646.

Schwartz, S. and Maquet, P. (2002). Sleep imaging and the neuro-psychological assessment of dreams. *Trends Cogn. Sci.*, 6: 23–30.

Sharf, B., Moskovitz, C., Lupton, M.D., and Klawans, H.L. (1978). Dream phenomena induced by chronic levodopa therapy. *J. Neural Transm.*, 43: 143–151.

Smith, M.R., Antrobus, J.S., Gordon, E., Tucker, M.A., Hirota, Y., Wamsley, E.J., Ross, L., Doan, T., Chaklader, A., and Emery, R.N. (2004). Motivation and affect in REM sleep and the mentation reporting process. *Conscious. Cogn.*, 13: 501–511.

Solmes, M. (1997). *The Neuropsychology of Dreams*. Mahwah, NJ: Lawrence Erlbaum Associates.

Squires, N.K., Squires, K.C., and Hillyard, S.A. (1975). Two variants of long-latency positive waves evoked by unpredictable auditory stimuli in man. *Electroencephalogr. Clin. Neurophysiol.*, 38: 387–401.

Steriade, M. (1997). Synchronized activities of coupled oscillators in the cerebral cortex and thalamus at different levels of vigilance. *Cereb. Cortex*, 7: 583–604.

Steriade, M. and Amzica, F. (1996). Intracortical and corticothalamic coherency of fast spontaneous oscillations. *Proc. Natl. Acad. Sci. USA*, 93: 2533–2538.

Stickgold, R., Pace-Schott, E., and Hobson, J.A. (1994a). A new paradigm for dream research: mentation reports following spontaneous arousal from REM and NREM sleep recorded in a home setting. *Conscious. Cogn.*, 3: 16–29.

Stickgold, R., Rittenhouse, C.D., and Hobson, J.A. (1994b). Dream slicing: a new technique for assessing thematic coherence in subjective reports of mental activity. *Conscious. Cogn.*, 3: 114–128.

Stickgold, R., Malia, A., Fosse, R., Propper, R., and Hobson, J.A. (2001). Brain-mind states: I. Longitudinal field study of sleep/wake factors influencing mentation report length. *Sleep*, 24: 171–179.

Sutton, J.P., Rittenhouse C.D., Pace-Schott, E., Stickgold, R., and Hobson, J.A. (1994). A new approach to dream bizarreness: graphing continuity and discontinuity of visual attention in narrative reports. *Conscious. Cogn.*, 3: 61–88.

Tanaka, H., Fujita, N., Takanashi, M., Hirabuki, N., Yoshimura, H., Abe, K., and Nakamura, H. (2003). Effect of stage 1 sleep on auditory cortex during pure tone stimulation: evaluation by functional magnetic resonance imaging with simultaneous EEG monitoring. AJNR. *Am. J. Neuroradiol.*, 24: 1982–1988.

Tononi, G., Sporns, O., and Edelman, G.M. (1992). Reentry and the problem of integrating multiple cortical areas: simulation of dynamic integration in the visual system. *Cereb. Cortex*, 2: 310–335.

Treisman, M., Faulkner, A., Naish, P.L., and Brogan, D. (1990). The internal clock: evidence for a temporal oscillator underlying time perception with some estimates of its characteristic frequency. *Perception*, 19: 705–743.

Treisman, M., Faulkner, A., and Naish, P.L. (1992). On the relation between time perception and the timing of motor action: evidence for a temporal oscillator controlling the timing of movement. *Q. J. Exp. Psychol. A*, 45: 235–263.

Treisman, M., Cook, N., Naish, P.L., and MacCrone, J.K. (1994). The internal clock: electroencephalographic evidence for oscillatory processes underlying time perception. *Q. J. Exp. Psychol. A*, 47: 241–289.

Velluti, R.A. (1997). Interactions between sleep and sensory physiology. *J. Sleep Res.*, 6: 61–77.

Velluti, R.A. and Pedemonte, M. (2002). In vivo approach to the cellular mechanisms for sensory processing in sleep and wakefulness. *Cell. Mol. Neurobiol.*, 22: 501–516.

Velluti, R., Pedemonte, M., and García-Austt, E. (1989). Correlative changes of auditory nerve and microphonic potentials throughout sleep. *Hearing Res.*, 39: 203–208.

Velluti, R.A., Pedemonte, M., and Peña, J.L. (1990). Auditory brain stem unit activity during sleep. In: Horne, J. (Ed.). *Sleep '90*. Bochum: Ponteanagel Press, pp. 94–96.

Velmans, M. (1991). Is human information processing conscious? *Behav. Brain Sci.*, 14: 651–726.

Viggiano, D., Vallone, D., Ruocco, L.A., and Sadile, A.G. (2003). Behavioral, pharmacological, morpho-functional molecular studies reveal a hyperfunctioning mesocortical dopamine system in an animal model of attention deficit and hyperactivity disorder. *Neurosci. Biobehav. Rev.*, 27: 683–689.

Voss, U. and Harsh, J. (1998). Information processing and coping style during the wake/sleep transition. *J. Sleep Res.*, 7: 225–232.

Wesensten, N.J. and Badia, P. (1988). The P300 component in sleep. *Physiol. Behav.*, 44: 215–220.

Whyte, H.E., Pearce, J.M., and Taylor, M.J. (1987). Changes in the VEP in preterm neonates with arousal states, as assessed by EEG monitoring. *Electroencephalogr. Clin. Neurophysiol.*, 68: 223–225.

Wilke, M., Holland, S.K., and Ball, W.S. Jr. (2003). Language processing during natural sleep in a 6-year-old boy, as assessed with functional MR imaging. *AJNR Am. J. Neuroradiol.*, 24: 42–44.

Zadra, A. and Donderi, D.C. (2000). Nightmares and bad dreams: their prevalence and relationship to well-being. *J. Abnorm. Psychol.*, 109: 273–281.

Zeki, S. (1980). The response properties of cells in the middle temporal area (area MT) of owl monkey visual cortex. *Proc. R. Soc. Lond. B Biol. Sci.*, 207(1167): 239–248.

Zeki, S. (1983). Colour coding in the cerebral cortex: the responses of wavelength-selective and colour-coded cells in monkey visual cortex to changes in wavelength composition. *Neuroscience*, 9(4): 767–781.

Zimler, J. and Keenan, J.M. (1983). Imagery in the congenitally blind: how visual are visual images? *J. Exp. Psychol. Learn. Mem. Cogn.*, 9: 269–282.

Chapter 25

INTERACTIONS BETWEEN SLEEP, WAKEFULNESS AND THE OLFACTORY SYSTEM

Jorge M. Affanni[1] and Claudio O. Cervino

This chapter addresses three main issues aimed at contributing to answer three kinds of questions: (1) What happens in the olfactory system during sleep and wakefulness? (2) How does the stimulation of the olfactory system influence some phenomena of sleep and wakefulness? (3) What happens with some phenomena of sleep and wakefulness when the olfactory system is damaged?

The treatment of those questions will be restricted mainly to the electrical activity of the main olfactory system (OS) of mammals with exclusion of the vomeronasal system. The recording of the electrical activity of the olfactory bulb (OB) and the primary olfactory cortex is relatively easy. It is a precious method that superbly facilitates the chronic study of free unanesthetized animals. Of course, there are other approaches but this is a mandatory previous step for investigating the modulation exerted by the waking/sleep cycle and its transitional states.

The Biological Significance of Olfaction. Specific and Nonspecific Aspects

Olfaction is a primal sense for humans as well as for animals. From an evolutionary standpoint, it is one of the most ancient of senses. It allows

---

[1]jorgeaffanni@uolsinectis.com.ar

vertebrate and invertebrate organisms possessing olfactory receptors to detect and identify food, mates, and predators. In humans, it also has an important role that provides sensual pleasures from the odors of flowers and perfume. This sense gives warnings of danger providing information about food condition or the presence of hazardous chemicals. Mammals can recognize thousands of odors, some of which prompt powerful responses (Axel, 1995). The endothermic abilities of mammals allow them to occupy nocturnal niches for which the sense of smell is particularly useful. There are two facts reflecting the primal importance of olfaction in mammalian life: (1) The enormous amount of genetic information devoted to this sensory system (Zhang and Firestein, 2002). (2) The large number of different centrifugal fibers which provide control of the OB activity from a striking number of brain structures (see references in Kratskin, 1995).

Intensive research on the gen family of human olfactory receptors has been done (Malnic *et al.*, 2004). The olfactory neurons have unique features: (1) They are in direct contact with the ambient and are regenerated during the whole adult life. (2) They have the ability to transport varied materials from the nasal cavity into the brain. Some of these materials arrive at the dorsal raphe nucleus, locus coeruleus and the horizontal limb of the diagonal band by retrograde neuronal transport (Baker, 1995). It must be noted that the latter structures are involved in the mechanisms of sleep and wakefulness.

The OS was usually regarded as concerned exclusively with information about odors. This specific role determined in past years a tendency to exclude other possible functions, which were suggested by the anatomical arrangements of the OS: the so-called nonspecific functions. The concept of nonspecific functions is due to J. Herrick. In his comparative study of the central connections of the olfactory nerve he observed that they were "characteristically diffuse, widely dispersed and interconnected" (Herrick, 1933). He then made the brilliant deduction that such anatomical arrangement was suggesting some function beyond simply transmitting specific sensory information. Since the time of Herrick several papers were published giving support to that concept. When the effects of peripheral olfactory damage are compared to those of bulbectomy certain general modulatory functions of the OB are strongly suggested. Donald Cain in an inspiring article (Cain, 1974) reviewed the existing data and proposed that the OB is involved in a forebrain arousal mechanism comprised mainly of hypothalamus and limbic system. Later, another inspiring article was published showing that the OS is not one system but many systems each with a different combination of connections and physiological properties to collaborate in the control of different types of behavior (Shepherd *et al.*, 1981). Of course the importance of these concepts for improving our knowledge on the interactions between sleep (S), wakefulness (W) and the OB appears quite obvious. However, little attention was given to this problem.

Overview of the organization of the olfactory system

The outputs from the olfactory receptors pass to the OB and after leaving it through axons from mitral and tufted cells, they reach the olfactory cortex without previously passing through the thalamus. However, this unique feature does not mean that olfactory influences do not reach neocortical structures because the olfactory cortex projects both directly and via the medial dorsal thalamic nucleus to areas of the orbitofrontal neocortex. The structures receiving direct input from the OB are named as primary olfactory cortex. This cortex may be divided into three groups (Shipley *et al.*, 1995): (1) The anterior olfactory nucleus. (2) The rostral olfactory cortex including the induseum griseum, the anterior hippocampal continuation, taenia tecta, infralimbic cortex and olfactory tubercle (OT). (3) The lateral olfactory cortex including the piriform cortex, periamygdaloid cortex, transitional cortices, and entorhinal cortex.

The piriform cortex projects to the mediodorsal thalamus, which in turn, projects to the frontal lobe. The amygdala by contrast projects preferentially to the hypothalamus. The entorhinal cortex projects to the hippocampus. There is a direct projection of the OB to the supraoptic region. Some specific nuclei of the amygdala also receive direct projection from the OB. The above mentioned areas constitute the major sites of processing olfactory information. In monkeys the lateroposterior and central centroposterior orbitofrontal cortices also receive olfactory information through connections with different regions of the ipsilateral primary olfactory cortex (Tanabe *et al.*, 1975). There are connections of the OB with the hypothalamus, septal area, diagonal band, amygdala, hippocampus, thalamus, raphe nuclei, and locus coeruleus. The sole mention of connections with these structures suggests that the olfactory system might play a role in sleep mechanisms or be influenced by them.

In addition to studies on anatomical connectivity there are electrophysiological studies showing that the 15–60 Hz induced waves appearing during inspiration of odororized air are recorded in various limbic and hypothalamic structures: prepiriform and piriform cortices, OT, amygdala, hypothalamus and hippocampus. Other tertiary areas also receive olfactory information: lateral preoptic area, diagonal band of Brocca, lateral habenular nuclei, mediodorsal and medioventral nuclei of the thalamus, and medial forebrain bundle (Powell *et al.*, 1965).

The Potentials of the Olfactory System are Instrumental in the Study of the Variations Introduced by Sleep and Wakefulness

The field potentials

Before describing the changes produced by sleep (S) and wakefulness (W) on these potentials, we wish to summarize the properties of the different types of electrical activities together with the conditions of their occurrence. Five types of field potentials of the OB were described:

1. Induced waves (Adrian, 1950).
2. Intrinsic activity (Adrian, 1950).
3. Slow potentials (Ottoson, 1959).
4. "Arousal discharges" (Hernandez Peón *et al.*, 1960).
5. The rhino-central rhythm (Affanni and García Samartino, 1984).

The first three were seen in all the mammals thus far studied. The fourth was described in cats. The fifth is seen in the armadillo and the opossum.

Induced waves (gamma activity) and intrinsic activity

Adrian (1950) in a classical paper studied the electrical activity of the OB in anesthetized cats, rabbits, and hedgehogs. This paper paved the way for all that is presently known about the electrical activity of the OS. The potential waves were classified by him into two main types: (a) Large sinusoidal oscillations usually at a fixed frequency appearing at each inspiration of quiet breathing or set up by strong stimuli. If no air flowed through the nose, the waves were absent. (b) Smaller and less regular waves occurring in the absence of stimulation and related to the intrinsic activity of the OB. The first type of response was termed by Adrian as "induced activity," to distinguish it from the second one or background activity ("intrinsic activity") of higher frequency seen during the absence of stimulation. The integrity of the olfactory epithelium was essential for the induced activity to appear. In contrast, the intrinsic activity required neither the integrity of the olfactory epithelium nor the nervous connections between the OB and the forebrain. This oscillatory activity represents one of the most striking phenomena of the olfactory system.

The induced waves are also termed "olfactory bursts," Adrian's induced waves, or "sinusoidal activity." They belong to a group of electrical oscillations widely observed in the cerebral cortex occurring in association with behavioral, sensory and cognitive activities. The frequency of such oscillations varies in different species and cortical areas, but in most mammals oscillates between 30–90 Hz. They were also termed gamma waves or gamma activity (GA). The latter is the term adopted in the present chapter. The presence or absence, the duration or the amplitude of the gamma activity represents one of the most important signals to be considered when assessing the functional state of the olfactory system during sleep and wakefulness.

Slow waves of Ottoson

These waves were described in the OB of frogs and rabbits (Ottoson, 1959). They are elicited by blowing odor laden air over the olfactory mucosa (OM). They last for the duration of the stimulus. Gault and Leaton (1963) because of the correspondence between the record of airflow and Ottoson's slow waves demonstrated the value of the latter as a measure of nasal respiration.

"Arousal discharges"

Lavin *et al.* (1959) and Hernandez Peón *et al.* (1960) observed GA in cats during alertness or when the mesencephalic reticular formation was stimulated. That activity was termed "arousal discharges." According to those investigators, the discharges were radically different from Adrian's induced waves in spite of their similar form. They were also different from the intrinsic activity. The authors based their opinion on two facts: (1) The induced activity persisted after the OB was disconnected from the brain. (2) The intrinsic activity was still observed after the elimination of the OM and the separation of the OB from the brain. In contrast, the "arousal discharges" required the integrity of both the OM and of the connections with some brain regions.

The rhino-central rhythm

A peculiar and conspicuous rhythm was observed in the OB of the armadillo and the opossum (Affanni and García Samartino, 1984). It is clearly seen in the band of 8–12 Hz only during W and especially during relaxed W (Figure 1). The elimination of the OM or respiration through a tracheal tube provokes its disappearance. The same effect is obtained by the transverse section of the olfactory peduncles (OP). Therefore, for appearing, the rhythm

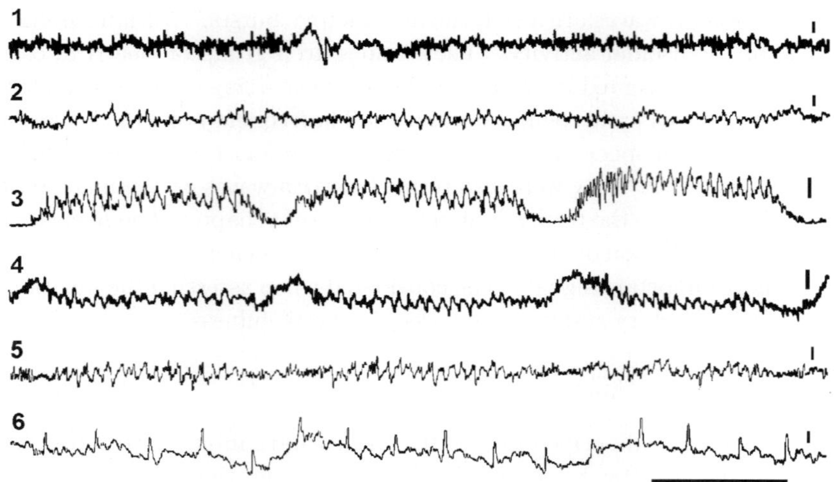

Figure 1. Electrical activity during wakefulness. 1. Neocortex; 2, 3. Right olfactory bulb; 4, 5. Left olfactory bulb. 6 EKG. Vertical bar, 50 μV; horizontal bar, 1 s. Note the Ottoson slow waves in 3–4 and the rhino-central rhythm in 3-4-5. (From Affanni and García Samartino, Comparative study of electrophysiological phenomena in the olfactory bulb of some South American marsupials and edentates, In: Bolis, L., Keynes, R.D., and Maddrell, S.H.P. (Eds.). *Comparative Physiology of Sensory Systems*. Cambridge: Cambridge University Press, 1984. Reproduced with permission.)

needs both the stimulation of the OM by the nasal airflow and the integrity of the connections between the OB and brain. From the fact that the rhythm needs peripheral influences coming from the nose and central influences coming from the brain we suggested that it could be termed rhino-central rhythm. It was also found in the OT (García Samartino *et al.*, 1987).

An overview of the participation of peripheral and central connections of the OB in the generation of the different electrical activities reveals the following facts: (1) The appearance of Adrian's GA only needs peripheral afferences. The elimination of the OM provokes its disappearance. (2) The intrinsic activity needs neither the peripheral nor the central connections. (3) Ottoson's waves need only the peripheral connections. (4) The rhino-central rhythm needs both peripheral and central connections. (5) The "arousal discharges" also need both peripheral and central connections.

Unitary activity

Simultaneous records from the surface and the deeper layers of the OB show that the oscillatory waves do not develop until some time after the mitral cell discharge has started. Once developed the discharges are grouped with a frequency corresponding to that of the waves (Adrian, 1950). There is continuous discharge of axon spikes in the deeper layers of the OB when the intrinsic activity is going on undisturbed by olfactory stimuli. The latter fact is important for interpreting the effects of eliminating the OM or the OB (see below). During W and S, the nutritional state and respiration (see below) modify the activity of mitral units.

Influences Acting on the Electrical Activity of the Olfactory System during Wakefulness and Sleep

The electrical activity of the OS is modulated by the S/W cycle. However, when considering the changes introduced by that cycle, the first thing that must be considered is that the changes are highly variable in their details or even in their gross features. There are variations in the same animal, between different animals and between animals of different species. Behind that variability, there is a multiplicity of ambient parameters and behavioral or physiological conditions. During S and W there are different sources of variation. Some of them operate exclusively during W. Others are active during both phases of the cycle. The following can be cited: (1) the degree of alertness and attention; (2) respiratory cycles; (3) sniffing; (4) breath holding (irritant substances, alarm, increased attention); (5) changes in the vasomotor activity of the nasal mucosa by emotional factors; (6) the presence or absence of odorants in the room air; (7) the influences exerted by the multiple centrifugal inputs to the OB; (8) the probable and almost unknown role of the "nasal cycle" as a source of variation for the electrical activity of the olfactory system; (9) mouth breathing; (10) stimuli to different sensory modalities (visual, acoustic, somatic, tactile); (11) the nutritional state (hunger or satiety); and (12) the position of the snout (when it is lying on the animal's coat).

The influence of some of those sources of variation can be easily understood even if they have not been studied systematically. Before summarizing the changes of the olfactory potentials, we shall refer specifically to a pair of the sources of variation. One is the "nasal cycle" about which precise information regarding its influence on the OS electrical activity is lacking. Research is needed on this subject. The other is the complex set of centrifugal inputs to the OB. Their influence during S and W is of primary importance particularly when the peripheral olfactory input is lacking (see below). This is why we dedicate the following lines to them.

The possible influence of the nasal cycle

The nasal cycle is a periodic, simultaneous, and opposing change in the volume of each nasal cavity. It is due to the nasal turbinate swelling controlled by the autonomic vasculature of the nasal mucosa. It is an ultradian rhythm having a periodicity ranging from 40 min to 4 h and has been reported in humans and laboratory animals. This cycle rhythm is thought to be originated in the hypothalamus. References can be found in Frye (1995). The influence of this cycle on the electrical activity of the OS has not been studied. In any case, we think that the existence of a reciprocal change in airway resistance might have important consequences for the electrical activity of the olfactory system during W and S. Additionally, it might determine asymmetry between the olfactory regions of the right and left brain hemispheres. Apart from the cycle there is evidence suggesting that changes in the volume of the nasal mucosa may suppress the Ottoson's waves during paradoxical sleep (PS) (Homeyer *et al.*, 1995).

The influence of centrifugal inputs to the olfactory bulb

Regarding the influence of centrifugal inputs to the OB, many unsolved questions are still waiting for systematic research especially in their relation to W and S. One of the most outstanding characteristics of those inputs is the diversity of their sites of origin (see references in Kratskin, 1995).

Two systems project to the OB: one is originated in higher olfactory structures whereas the other projects to the OB from nonolfactory regions. In the first one, bulbopetal fibers arise from the anterior olfactory nucleus, the nucleus of the lateral olfactory tract, the anterior and posteromedial cortical nuclei, the piriform cortex, the periamigdaloid area and the entorhinal cortex. This indicates the existence of reciprocal connections between those structures and the OB. In the second system, the fibers arise mainly from the basal forebrain regions and the brainstem: the horizontal and vertical limbs of the diagonal band of Brocca, sustantia innominata, ventral pallidum, lateral and dorsomedial hypotalamic areas, zona incerta, raphe nuclei, and locus coeruleus. It is worth noting that projections from the raphe nuclei are part of the reticular ascending system and provide a basis for the reticular control of the olfactory input. Through those connections, the bulbar neurons receive excitatory and inhibitory inputs. These inputs are probably tonic in their nature. There is evidence that the GA can be modulated by centrifugal influences since the section of one or both OP increases its amplitude and duration (Scaravilli *et al.*, 1971; Affanni *et al.*,

1973, 1974; Panizza *et al.*, 1973). Centrifugal influences on the OB were revealed by DC potentials in that structure (Carreras *et al.*, 1967).

Some of the regions from which centrifugal fibers are projected to the olfactory bulb appear directly involved in the S/W mechanisms. Therefore, functional changes in the olfactory system are to be expected during S and W. In the same way, the elimination of peripheral olfactory input or the destruction of components of the olfactory system is expected to produce changes in S/W phenomena. It is surprising, in view of these considerations, the scanty information regarding this subject.

Modulation of the Field Potentials of the Olfactory System during Wakefulness and Sleep

We shall now refer to the changes occurring in some OS structures. The OB and the piriform cortex were the most intensively studied due to the relatively large OB volume and the relatively large palleocortical areas of the macrosmatic animals mostly used in the laboratories. The OB is easily accessible in most of the experimental animals and its connections with the brain can be easily severed.

As a generalization, it can be affirmed that during wakefulness, there are abundant high amplitude bursts of gamma activity. The same happens with Ottoson's slow waves and with the rhino-central rhythm. Contrarily, during slow wave sleep (SWS) and PS, the GA greatly decreases or disappears and so do Ottoson's slow waves. During SWS, abundant slow waves (not those of Ottoson) similar to those seen in the neocortex are observed. Neither during SWS nor during PS the conspicuous rhino-central rhythm characteristic of wakefulness is observed.

Changes in gamma activity

Changes in the "arousal discharges"

The study of GA during W and S requires the use of chronically implanted animals. Hernández-Peón and his collaborators (Hernández-Peón *et al.*, 1960) initiated an accurate study of the electrical activity of the OB during those physiological states, especially during W. The OB of awake and relaxed cats showed GA around 40 Hz similar to that observed by Adrian. Intermittent bursts of even faster frequency and amplitude appeared during alertness and specially during sniffing (Lavin *et al.*, 1959). Stimuli of different sensory modalities (visual, acoustic, olfactory, somatic, gustatory) provoked the appearance of GA around 34–48 Hz in the OB of cats

(Hernández-Peón *et al.*, 1960). An association between that activity and the degree of arousal was observed. Attention increased the bursts. The electrical stimulation of the mesencephalic reticular formation also elicited them. When sensory stimulation (auditory, visual, and tactile) was applied to tracheotomized cats, a conspicuous GA was observed (Peñaloza Rojas and Alcocer-Cuarón, 1967). Since tracheotomy prevents the flow of air through the nose, it is evident that the effect of sensory stimulation could not be due to modifications of the airflow. Consequently, a central influence active during W must be admitted.

Changes in the induced activity of Adrian

Olfactory bulb. Adrian's GA can be observed during W, SWS, and PS. However, during both phases of S they appear greatly diminished in amplitude being often undetectable.

The GA of the OS was also observed in cats, rabbits and rats (Bressler and Freeman, 1980); rabbits (Bressler, 1984); rabbits, cats, and hedgehogs (Adrian, 1950); viscaches (*Lagostomus maximus*) (Scaravilli *et al.*, 1971); dogs and monkeys (Domino and Ueki, 1960); opossums (Vaccarezza and Affanni, 1964; Affanni *et al.*, 1968); armadillos (Affanni and García Samartino, 1984; Cervino, 1997); and humans (Hughes *et al.*, 1969).

Piriform cortex. Olfactory-like responses to non olfactory stimulation were observed in the prepiriform cortex (MacLean *et al.*, 1952). The spontaneous electrical activity of the prepiriform cortex deserves special attention for it represents an important part of the primary olfactory cortex where processing of the olfactory signals takes place. There is evidence that a large proportion of the spontaneous electrical activity of the basal forebrain of cats is bilaterally generated by the prepiriform cortex. This activity is not generated by the subcortical structures in which the electrodes are placed (Freeman, 1957). This suggests that such propagation might have functional significance.

During active W, the dominant waveform of the prepiriform cortex of cats is a sinusoidal wave with a dominant frequency of 34–38 Hz appearing in bursts. Additionally, there are waves of the same amplitude but of half the dominant frequency. There is also a repetitive wave in the low-frequency range, the frequency of which is related to that of respiration. The bursts of the dominant frequency are closely related to the slow wave (Freeman, 1959). The amplitude of the GA is related to a wide range of behavior. Three classes of behavior were distinguished: rest, anticipation, and action. Rest provides the baseline amplitude of the oscillations. During anticipation, there is augmentation of the amplitude. During action, the amplitude varies according to the kind of response. It is higher than during rest in oral activities (chewing, lapping, licking, etc). The amplitude is still of greater magnitude during locomotor activities (Freeman, 1960).

During S intense changes are observed. There is suppression of the electrical activity at the dominant frequency and appearance of irregular slow waves, which are aperiodic and not related to respiration (Freeman, 1959). The prepiriform cortex needs the input from the OB for the normal generation of GA. Bulbar ablation disrupts the 40-Hz oscillations and produces a marked diminution of the EEG amplitude in that cortex (Becker and Freeman, 1968). In the rat piriform cortex, low levels of GA are associated with spontaneous apnea and higher levels with sniffing. Closing one nostril results in the ipsilateral disappearance of GA but persists in the contralateral side (Vanderwolf, 2000). According to the author who made his study during W, the GA is entirely dependent on olfactory input and the previously reported relations to conditioning, arousal, etc., are a consequence of changes in the airflow through the upper airway.

Amygdala–prepiriform. Lesse (1960) and Freeman (1960) presented evidence suggesting that the GA of 40 Hz in the amygdala–prepiriform region is associated with the extreme states of arousal.

Simultaneous records of GA from the OB and the basolateral amygdala in were made in cats (Gault and Leaton, 1963). Whenever a burst of GA was seen in the amygdala, it coincided quite closely with GA in the OB. This was clearly seen during exploratory activity and sniffing. However, it was possible for GA to occur in the OB without activation of the amygdala thus suggesting that some other influence was acting to regulate GA in the amygdala.

There are significant changes in the amygdala oscillations in association with different levels of S including PS (Adey *et al.*, 1963) although in this study the oscillations were of very low frequency.

Pagano and Gault (1964) presented data concerned with developing a measure of the amygdala activity. They investigated the 40-Hz GA oscillations at various levels of arousal (light S, relaxed, alert, arousal) in an attempt to derive a quantified central measure of arousal. The recordings correlated with behavioral and cortical measures of arousal. The amygdala GA appeared quite sensitive throughout the arousal continuum (PS excluded) and was stable over time. These data led the authors to consider the GA as a central measure of arousal. Lesse (1960) and Freeman (1960) presented evidence suggesting that the 40-Hz GA in the amygdala–prepiriform region is associated with the extreme states of arousal.

Gault and Coustan (1965) by the application of nasal insuflation in acute preparations or by blowing air into the nose of awake chronic cats could obtain GA of the OB at a frequency of 40 Hz. In the amygdala–prepiriform GA could also be observed. Nevertheless, it seems clear that some central factor controls the 40-Hz activity, if the activity is simultaneously present in the olfactory bulbs. The response of single units of the rat amygdala to different odors was studied by Cain and Bindra (1972). Neurons that increase their overall rates of discharge during S were found in the amygdala (Jacobs and McGinty, 1971). The human amygdala responds with bursts of GA with each inspiration of odorants (Hughes and Andy, 1979).

Entorhinal cortex. The entorhinal cortex also shows GA in waking cats. It was shown that the propagation of activity through the cortical circuits and the oscillations depend upon the background of neuronal activity. The disconnection of the OB stops the background excitatory input incident to the entorhinal cortex. After the disconnection, this cortex retains the ability for developing evoked responses but without its characteristic oscillations. Consequently, a nonzero background appears as necessary and sufficient to maintain the normal oscillatory responses of the entorhinal cortex (Ahrens and Freeman, 2001). If we consider that the entorhinal cortex is a site of convergence for the other sensory inputs, the relevance of inputs from the OB appears evident, especially when GA seems crucial for brain function.

The abrupt changes of the electrical activity of the olfactory system and chaos. The importance of general arousal

The GA appears and disappears abruptly. This abruptness is one of the most distinctive features of the olfactory responses. The oscillations appear under varied circumstances during W, SWS, or PS: synchronously with nasal respiration or after the application of olfactory, visual, tactile, somatic or auditory stimuli. They also appear abruptly in arousal from both SWS and PS, being usually observed after each sniff. Because of this property, the system became an excellent model for studying one of the most fascinating aspects of neurobiology: the recognition of chaos operating in the nervous system. Chaos is undeniable in the propensity of neuronal populations to shift simultaneously and abruptly from one activity pattern to another in response to the smallest stimuli (Freeman, 1991). This author proposed that chaos is the very property that makes perception possible. The ability of bulbar neuronal populations to jump globally from a non oscillatory state to an oscillatory one and then back again is an important clue to the presence of chaos. According to Freeman (1991) for a fast oscillation to occur in response to some odorant the neuronal assemblies of the OB and the olfactory cortex must be "primed" to respond strongly to input. In his opinion, the factors enabling that priming are represented by the general arousal and the olfactory input itself. In this way, when the animals are sexually aroused, hungry and thirsty or threatened, the OB is prepared to respond strongly.

Changes in Ottoson's slow waves

Gault and Leaton (1963) simultaneously recorded the nasal airflow and Ottoson's slow waves in cats. Under these conditions, there was a clear correspondence between the record of airflow and the Ottoson's slow potentials. Consequently, the waves are a measure of respiration. Records during resting and active periods of W were taken. During W, the amplitude of the slow waves was maximal in consonance with what is known of the tidal volume during arousal and W. With tracheal breathing or when the nose was experimentally blocked, the waves disappeared. When the cats were drowsy, the slow potentials of the OB were of very low amplitude compared with the potentials seen after arousal stimuli.

Changes in the rhino-central rhythm

During wakefulness and only during this state, the olfactory bulb of the armadillo shows a very conspicuous 8–12 Hz rhythm. When the animals are in relaxed W it clearly dominates the tracings and very often, it is the sole type of activity seen. This is the state in which it appears maximally conspicuous. When the animals sniff or get excited Adrian's GA and Ottoson's waves dominate the tracings. However, the rhythm sometimes coexists with those activities.

During SWS, the rhythm is never observed and is replaced by the Adrian's GA of small amplitude or by the large slow waves, characteristic of SWS in this and other mammals. During PS it is never observed. The unique presence during wakefulness is in sharp contrast with Adrian's and Ottoson's waves. The latter, permanently or occasionally, may be seen during W, SWS, and PS, with variable amplitude.

The finding of this rhythm indicates the importance of exploring the electrical activities of the olfactory structures in different species. In this case, the finding of a different rhythm, occurring clearly during a specific phase of the S/W cycle, may reveal new operating mechanisms and physiological conditions.

Modulation of the Unitary Activity of the Olfactory System during Wakefulness and Sleep

The influence of the nutritional state

There are combined modulating effects of the general level of arousal and specific hunger arousal on the rat OB responses (Gervais and Pager, 1979). These effects can be demonstrated recording the vigilance state parameters and the multi-unit mitral cell activity. Nutritionally modulated OB responses for food odor are seen only during W. During SWS, there is either high responsiveness with cortical arousal or general inexcitability. There are no responses during PS. During SWS, each odorous stimulus elicits higher cortical arousal in the hungry than in the satiated state. The feeding schedule appears significant since rats fed 2 h a day display a reversed circadian sleep-waking cycle and a lower SWS proportion compared with that of rats fed *ad libitum*.

Food deprived control rats with recordings of cortical EEG and multiunit mitral cell activity were submitted to the three following parameters (Gervais and Pager, 1982) with these results: (1) In a two-choice test they explore significantly more the side of the cage odorized by food odor than the nonodorized one. (2) The presentation of food odor during SWS arouses them significantly more often than in the food satiated condition. (3) During W, the multiunit mitral cell responsiveness towards food presentation is enhanced. The same three parameters were tested in rats with one olfactory peduncle completely sectioned or intact either in the medial or in the lateral part of the other olfactory peduncle. Under these conditions, waking rats need both medial and lateral pathways in order to perform normally the detection task. During SWS, only the medial pathway is needed to mediate cortical arousal response to food odor presentation.

The influence of the respiratory cycle

The multiunit activity from mitral cells in the OB of anesthetized rats is modulated in accordance with the respiratory cycle. This cycle and neuronal activity still coincide in tracheotomized animals provided the OP is left intact (Pager, 1980). These experiments suggest that centrifugal influences are responsible for the coincidence.

Influence of sensory stimulation on the amygdala

Most units of the amygdala show spontaneous firing in the absence of experimental stimulation. The firing is modified by sensory stimulation (smoke and other stimuli). Spontaneous sleep reduces the rate of spontaneous firing, decreases the facilitatory and increases the inhibitory effects of sensory stimulation (Sawa and Delgado, 1963).

Influence of the reticular formation

There is reticular control of single neurons in the OB (Mancia *et al.*, 1962).

The Effect of the Stimulation of the Olfactory System on Sleep and Wakefulness

Peripheral olfactory stimulation

The arousal mechanisms are readily accessible for the action of olfactory stimuli. Arduini and Moruzzi (1953) used acute *cerveau isolé* cats to study the olfactory arousal reactions. These preparations have only two sensory modalities available: the main and accessory OS and the visual system. Bright flickering light failed to desynchronize the EEG in spite of the integrity of the visual system. In sharp contrast, when room air was blown into the nose or simply if an odorant was added to the naturally respired air, there was an arousal reaction. After the stimulation, the normally synchronized cerveau isolé showed cortical arousal and desynchronization of the intrathalamic reticular formation. The experiments of Villablanca (1965) with chronic cerveau isolé cats confirmed the original findings of Arduini and Moruzzi. While visual stimuli were not capable of eliciting arousal, olfactory stimulation produced a clear one. These experiments were interpreted as suggesting the existence of an autonomous arousal system independent of the midbrain reticular formation. The existence of two arousal systems has been postulated (Routtenberg, 1971). One is represented by the ascending reticular activating system of Moruzzi and Magoun (1949). The other is the limbic-midbrain system of Nauta (1958) concerned with incentive and reward. The central olfactory areas are thought a part of this second system. It is worth noting that the olfactory system appears as the only sensory system that has direct access to this forebrain arousal system. However, we suggest that the vomeronasal system might probably have the same property.

There is evidence in sleeping cats that olfactory stimuli will desynchronize the high-voltage cortical slow waves (Hernandez Peón *et al.*, 1960). Surprisingly, according to these authors, olfactory stimulation applied to cats during W provokes the suppression of the "arousal discharges." In freely moving rats, mitral cells multiunit activity and vigilance states were recorded during stimulation by odorants known to provoke emotional behavior. The greatest awakening influence was for odor of fox (predator of the rat) and for odor of grouped rats. The response of mitral cells is not only modulated by the biological significance of the stimulus but by the arousal level. It decreases from W to SWS (Catarelli and Chanel, 1979). Badia *et al.* (1990) reported that humans react behaviorally, autonomically, and centrally to olfactory stimuli applied while sleeping in stage 2. Although the percentage of overall responsivity was low, significant differences in response to odor periods *vs* non odor periods were found for microswitch closures, EEG, EMG, and heart rate. A time-of-night effect was additionally observed in that responsivity tended to be greatest early in the night. An interesting phenomenon is represented by the existence of "blind smell" which we think it would be better to term it "anosmic smell." EEG and behavioral evidence suggests that airborne chemicals can affect the nervous system without being consciously detected (Sobel *et al.*, 1999). Magnetic resonance imaging (MRI) was used to localize brain activation induced by an airborne chemical. The inferior frontal gyrus and anterior medial thalamus were activated by the undetectable airborne chemical. The prandial state (from hunger to satiety) and the stimulus familiarity modulate facial and autonomic responses to milk odors applied during S episodes in human neonates (Soussignan *et al.*, 1999).

Recently, it has been shown that exposure to relevant odor reveals differential characteristics of the GA in the rat central olfactory pathways (Chabaud *et al.*, 2000). Local field recordings of the OB, anterior and posterior piriform cortex, and lateral entorhinal cortex of freely moving rats show that odor presentation is associated with changes in a wide 15–90 Hz frequency band in each olfactory structure. However, two interesting phenomena occur: (1) The nutritional state modulates the initial responses (before habituation) to odor presentation because the OB and the entorhinal cortex respond selectively in the frequency of 15–30 Hz. (2) When the olfactory stimuli are repeated the habituation that follows is also modulated by the nutritional state. It is differentially expressed with a dissociation of the oscillatory activities of the anterior and posterior parts of the piriform cortex.

Electrical stimulation of the olfactory tubercle

The random stimulation of the OT in chronically prepared cats produces decrease of the time spent in W (Obál *et al.*, 1980). Bilateral lesions of the olfactory tubercles primarily suppressed SWS with a gradual increase in W. On the second week after the lesions the latter increase reached 80–90%. These results were interpreted as suggesting that the OT has a tonic hypnogenic effect.

Deprivation of the Olfactory System

What happens to the OS when it is deprived of odor stimulation? This deprivation occurs in several experimental conditions: (1) Suppression of nasal airflow (closure of the nostrils, tracheal breathing). (2) Decrease in number of olfactory receptors, elimination of the OM. (3) Total ablation or lesions of olfactory structures. (4) Exposure to odor-free environments.

Several papers were published describing changes in morphology, neurochemistry and metabolism after those procedures (see references, Maruniak, 1995). However, studies of the effects on W and S are extremely scanty.

The effect of olfactory deafferentation on the electrical activity of the olfactory system during wakefulness and sleep

We must clearly define what is understood by olfactory deafferentation. This point is of the outmost importance since in past years a considerable confusion was generated on this matter. Olfaction is very important in many aspects of mammalian life. It is therefore not surprising that numerous investigators tried to assess the physiological and behavioral effects of smell suppression. However, this was done by bilateral bulbectomy. They obtained a variety of interesting results, which in many cases were simply attributed to the absence of olfaction. However, bulbectomy implies the suppression of millions of neurons, including those of the accessory olfactory bulb. The neurons of the latter bulb exhibit central connections and centrifugal inputs different from those of the OB (Shipley *et al.*, 1995). The

OB is continuously displaying its intrinsic activity and sending impulses to the higher olfactory centers even after the elimination of the olfactory receptors. Consequently, bulbectomy implies suppression of olfaction plus "something else" which corresponds to a still rather unknown function of the OB (Cain, 1974). We consider that in the interpretation of the results of bulbectomy, special attention must be dedicated to the concomitant elimination of the accessory olfactory bulb. To avoid confusion we use the expression "peripheral olfactory deafferentation" when only the olfactory receptors are eliminated, to distinguish this operation from bulbectomy.

Peripheral olfactory deafferentation

Regarding the effects of the elimination of the OM, a distinction must be made between short- and long-term effects. The elimination of the OM leads to degeneration of the OB with intense loss of neurons. Therefore, when examining long-term effects the deficit in bulbar function and perhaps of primary olfactory cortex must be taken into account. Contrarily, if a change in electrical activity is observed shortly after the mucosal ablation, the effect might probably be attributed to the loss of olfactory receptors. As we shall see in this chapter the elimination of the OM in the armadillo produces a striking change in the electrical activity of the OB, which is clearly observable as soon as the animal recovers from anesthesia.

The long-term effects of the destruction of the OM were studied by Beteleva and Novikova (1961) in waking rabbits, not during S. During 3–4 months they observed generalized changes in the electrical activity of the brain. The authors reported the following changes: (1) disappearance of the OB GA and development of slow waves of frequency 3–4 Hz together with depression and slowing of its basic activity. (2) Depression and slowing of the hippocampal activity and of the sensory, motor and visual cortical regions. (3) Increase in the amplitude of the electrical activity of the reticular formation. Obviously, in the results of Beteleva and Novikova the participation of degenerative phenomena in the OB cannot be excluded. In any way, those findings suggest a powerful influence of the OS on brain activity during W.

Peripheral olfactory deafferentation in the armadillo

We studied this deafferentation in a macrosmatic animal, the armadillo, *Chaetophractus villosus*, with some unexpected results. The armadillo is an excellent model for studies on the OS because of the great size of the olfactory bulbs, olfactory tubercles, and piriform cortex. The high position of the rhinal fissure on the lateral brain surface determines the great extension of the palleocortical areas (Benítez *et al.*, 1994; Ferrari *et al.*, 1998). It is also an excellent model for S studies. It is a heavy sleeper, which under laboratory conditions sleeps during approximately 85.4% of the day (García Samartino *et al.*, 1974). It shows perfectly distinguishable periods of SWS and PS. It also shows absence of penile erection during PS and peculiar penile movements during SWS (Affanni *et al.*, 2001). When these animals are experimentally covered with soil they do not stop their breathing due to a remarkable adaptation of the nostrils which permits the use of the air trapped between the particles of soil (Affanni *et al.*, 1987). While being covered with soil, the GA of the OB disappears. The disappearance is due to the modification of the nasal air flow and to centrifugal influences on the OB (Affanni *et al.*, 1986).

After the elimination of the OM or when submitted to tracheal breathing, the armadillo shows dramatic changes in the electrical activity of the OB during W and S. However, there is a remarkable difference between the recordings of both states. That difference is one of the most striking facts revealed by the use of this animal (Affanni and García Samartino, 1984). During W, Adrian's GA, Ottoson's waves, and the rhino-central rhythm disappear. This is not surprising in view of what is known about the crucial role of peripheral afferences on those electrical activities (see above). What appears surprising is a striking phenomenon occurring during SWS and PS: the olfactory bulb is invaded by high amplitude gamma activity in spite of the absence of olfactory mucosa which suppresses the peripheral olfactory input (Figure 2). This stands in stark contrast with the decrease or disappearance of GA observed during S when the OM is intact and the animal is breathing through its nose. The section of the OP eliminates the oscillations indicating that their generation is due to the centrifugal input to the OB. Our recent results (unpublished) indicate that the invasion is not restricted to the OB. In fact, the dorsal part of the frontal cortex, the OT and several regions of the piriform cortex are also invaded by GA. An example of this fact is shown in (Figure 3). Taking into account that those areas represent approximately two thirds of the brain surface of armadillos (Benitez *et al.*, 1994; Ferrari *et al.*, 1998) the relevance of this sleep phenomenon is quite evident. In direct relation with our results, studies in waking rats (Vanderwolf, 2000) showed that the generation of GA in the piriform cortex is entirely dependent on olfactory input. Our results

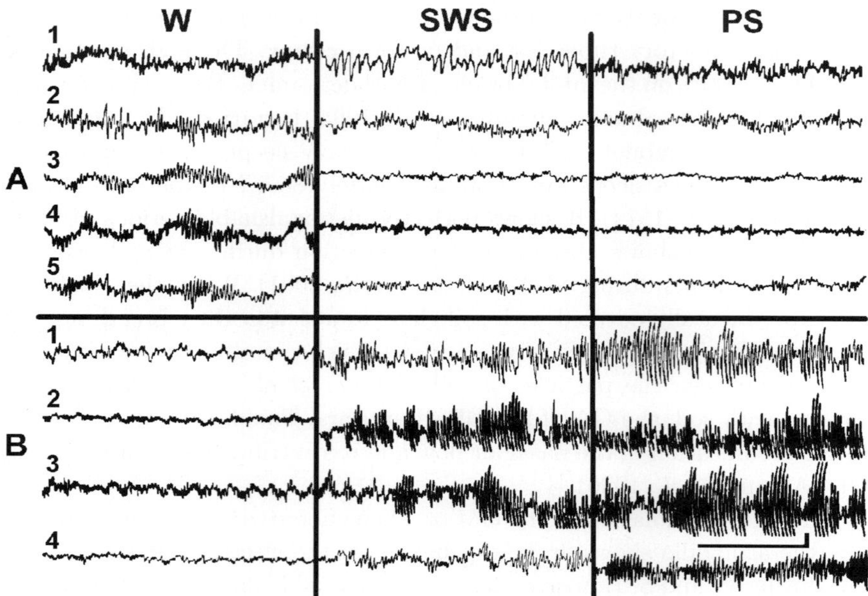

Figure 2. Electrical activity of the olfactory bulb. (A) Before destruction of olfactory mucosa: 1. Neocortex; 2, 3. Right olfactory bulb; 4, 5. Left olfactory bulb. (B) After destruction of olfactory mucosa. 1, 2. Right olfactory bulb; 3, 4. Left olfactory bulb. W. Wakefulness. SWS. Slow wave sleep. PS. Paradoxical sleep. Vertical bar, 50 μV; horizontal bar, 1 s. (Modified from Affanni and García Samartino, Comparative study of electrophysiological phenomena in the olfactory bulb of some South American marsupials and edentates. In: Bolis, L., Keynes, R.D., and Maddrell, S.H.P. (Eds.). *Comparative Physiology of Sensory Systems*. Cambridge: Cambridge University Press, 1984. Reproduced with permission.)

apparently are in opposition to those findings. However, Vanderwolf made his study during W whereas our phenomenon was found during S. Of course, species differences cannot be discarded.

Another interesting phenomenon is the immediate disappearance of the gamma activity after the application of arousing stimuli (visual, auditory, tactile, etc.) (Figure 4). This suggests that the brain systems responsible for the arousal reaction directly or indirectly block the influence of the centrifugal system. These findings indicate that during S, the nasal airflow impinges upon the intact OM initiating events, which impede the generation of GA in the OB. This indicates the importance of nasal breathing for the maintenance of the normal electrophysiological patterns of S. It is evident that during S the OS remains "open" to the subtle influence of

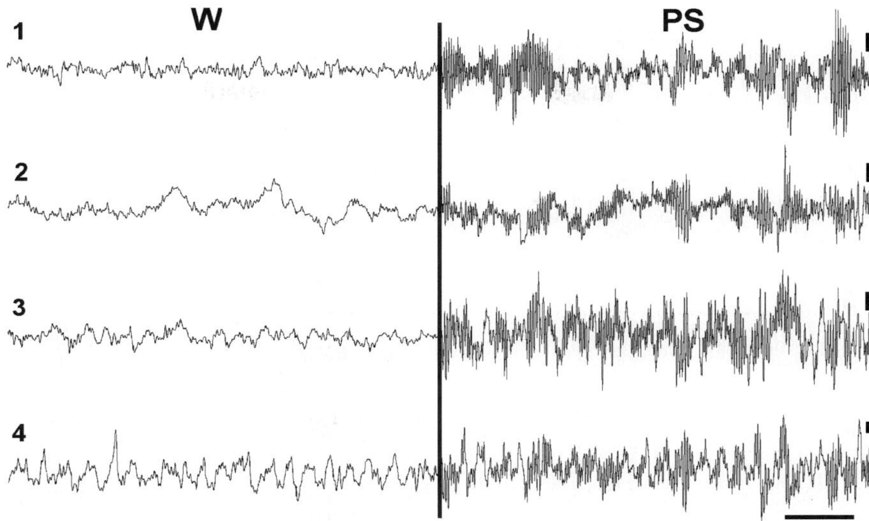

Figure 3. Electrical activity after the elimination of olfactory mucosa. W. Wakefulness. PS. Paradoxical sleep. 1. Left olfactory bulb. 2. Dorsal aspect of frontal cortex. 3. Olfactory tubercle. 4. Piriform cortex. Vertical bar, 50 µV; horizontal bar, 1 s. (Unpublished results.)

nasal airflow. In the absence of nasal airflow or when the OM is eliminated such an impediment is removed and consequently the GA reappears. We do not know how this is accomplished. It might be possible that the nasal airflow initiates a direct action on the OB, which blocks its response to the centrifugal input. Another possibility is that the influence initiated by the nasal airflow blocks the centrifugal impulses at their site of origin. We wish to emphasize that the presence of GA during S when the OM is lacking or during tracheal breathing suggests that sleep can serve as a valuable research "tool." Indeed, it might continue to reveal new feedback relations between centrifugal fibers and the olfactory structures.

Last but not least another finding is worth mentioning. We found a small number of normal armadillos (10 out of 130) which exhibited the invasion of GA in the OB and piriform cortex during SWS and PS. This occurred in spite of not having been submitted to the elimination of the OM (García Samartino *et al.*, 1981). In all of them the section of one OP suppressed the GA on the side of the section. During W, the OB showed Adrian's GA indicating that the OM was in good functional condition. Therefore, it cannot be ascertained that the oscillatory waves are purely of central origin.

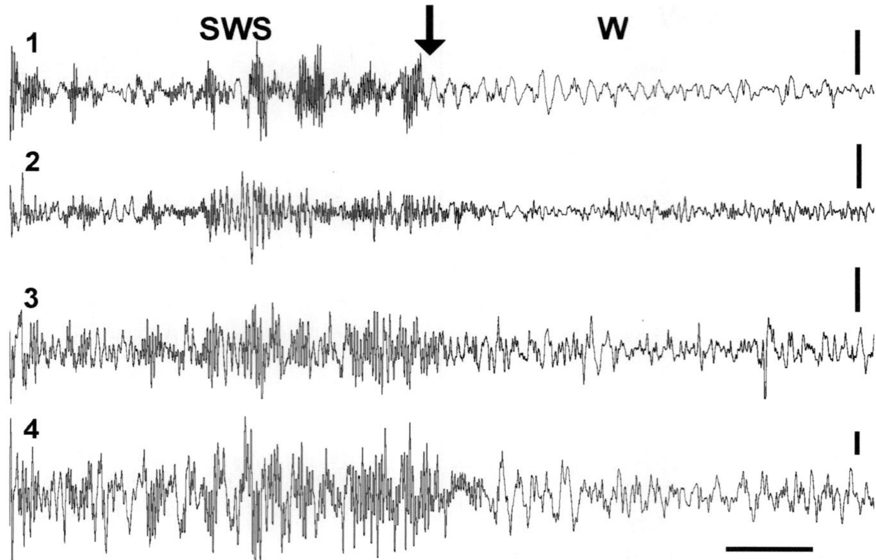

Figure 4. Arousal from SWS in the peripherally deafferented armadillo. SWS. Slow wave sleep. W. Wakefulness. 1. Left olfactory bulb. 2. Dorsal aspect of frontal cortex. 3. Olfactory tubercle. 4. Piriform cortex. Arrow indicates application of an auditory stimulus. Note the theta rhythm characteristic of peripheral olfactory deafferentation in 1 and 4. Vertical bar, 50 μV; horizontal bar, 1 s. (Unpublished results.)

However, at least the participation of central influences is undeniable. These findings suggest that under some still unknown conditions SWS and PS can trigger the appearance of GA.

These results with armadillos indicate the convenience of extending the observations to other animals not frequently adopted for experimental research. Nobody knows how many new phenomena are still waiting to be discovered in some species. However, we think that it would be convenient to investigate the more commonly used laboratory animals in association with what happens during SWS and PS when the peripheral olfactory input is suppressed. Regarding the latter point it must be remembered that rodents are obligatory nasal breathers. This might cause different ways of responding to the lack of olfactory input.

As far as we know there are in the literature at least two examples of GA suggesting that they were produced by the sole influence of centrifugal inputs to the OB: (1) The OB oscillations observed in tracheotomized awake cats during sensory stimulation (Peñaloza-Rojas and

Alcocer-Cuaron, 1967). (2) The oscillations of the OB, piriform lobe, and amygdaloid nuclei of intact dogs during PS; that GA persisted while the dogs were submitted to tracheal breathing (Ganzha and Bogach, 1975). However, these experiments only showed that the GA was not due to changes in the nasal airflow. The exclusive influence of centrifugal fibers would only be demonstrated by the persistence of the GA after the elimination of the OM.

The effects of bulbectomy or of the section of the olfactory peduncles

Our team provided the first evidence that the olfactory bulbs are involved in the regulation of S (Vaccarezza and Affanni, 1966). In opossums, the bilateral section of the olfactory peduncles separating the bulbs from the rest of the brain produces striking changes in the S patterns, particularly in PS. The following facts were observed; (1) increase of the percentage of SWS in total sleep time; (2) decrease in the percentage of PS in total sleep time; and (3) decrease in the mean duration of PS episodes. The reduction in PS does not last long and after some days the normal values are restored. Sham operated animals and those with longitudinal or incomplete section of the olfactory peduncles show no changes in the sleep patterns. In that paper, we wrote that our results suggested that "the olfactory bulb plays an important role in the regulation of the functional organization of the structures involved in the production and maintenance of sleep. This participation seems to be independent of impulses coming from the olfactory receptors since their destruction was unable to elicit the changes observed after the section of the olfactory peduncles." Cain (1974) commenting on our results suggested that "olfactory bulb activity, apart from any specific olfactory stimulation, may modulate sleep patterns in marsupials and possibly other mammals."

The changes in the 24-h S/W pattern and emotionality after bilateral bulbectomy in rats were studied by Araki *et al.* (1980). On the third and seventh day after the ablation of the OB, no significant difference was found in SWS throughout the whole experimental period. Instead, PS was significantly decreased during the 24-h and light period. However, those changes returned to normal values on the 15th day after the bulbectomy. The rats displayed hiperemotionality and an increase in locomotor activity. These behavioral changes were gradually produced following bulbectomies and were maintained during over 15 days. One interesting observation is represented by the fact that the time course of the PS decrease was not consistent with the time course of hiperemotionality. The same happened with locomotor activity. This was interpreted by the authors as suggesting that the reduction in PS may play a role in the initiation of hiperemotionality but not in its maintenance. Our results (Vaccarezza and Affanni, 1966) and those of Araki *et al.* (1980) coincide in showing that PS is particularly sensible to the separation or the ablation of the OB. Moreover, both groups report the transient quality of the changes observed.

It is worth noting that the olfactory bulbs influence chronobiological processes: bulbectomy unmasks the photoperiodic response (i.e., light controlled seasonal reproduction) in animals that normally do not exhibit photoperiodism (Nelson and Zucker, 1981). Additionally, bulbectomy lengthens the circadian period of locomotor activity (Pieper and Lobocki, 1991).

Where Goes Future Research?

We have seen some differences between the effects of eliminating the OM and those of eliminating or separating the OB from the brain. The elimination of the OM changes mainly the electrophysiological patterns of SWS and PS whereas the elimination or separation of the OB changes not only the electrophysiological patterns but the percentages and duration of the sleep phases. Probably, deeper studies will reveal some degree of overlapping of those effects. We do not know if some of these effects can be translated to microsmatic animals like humans. Furthermore, we think that research concerning the latter point is badly needed in view of the fact that in humans there are pathological conditions — Alzheimer's disease, Parkinson's disease, etc. (Ferreyra-Moyano and Barragán, 1994; Bylsma *et al.*, 1997; Mesholam *et al.*, 1998) in which there are serious olfactory deficits and lesions in olfactory structures. Does this affect the quality of sleep? Of course, this might have far-reaching consequences for brain development and brain health. The lesson from animal research on OS deprivation is that it is advantageous to have enough patience to wait for the initiation of sleep.

References

Adey, W.R., Kado, R.T., and Rhodes, J.M. (1963). Sleep: cortical and subcortical recordings in the chimpanzee. *Science*, 6: 932–933.
Adrian, E. (1950). The electrical activity of the mammalian olfactory bulb. *Electroencephalogr. Clin. Neurophysiol.*, 2: 377–388.

Affanni, J.M. and García Samartino, L. (1984). Comparative study of electro-physiological phenomena in the olfactory bulb of some South American marsupials and edentates. In: Bolis, L., Keynes, R.D., and Maddrell, S.H.P. (Eds.). *Comparative Physiology of Sensory Systems*. Cambridge: Cambridge University Press, pp. 315–333.

Affanni, J.M., Morita, E., and García Samartino, L. (1968). Efecto de la sección de los pedúnculos olfatorios de la comisura anterior sobre la actividad eléctrica del bulbo olfatorio del marsupial *Didelphys azarae*. *Rev. Soc. Argent. Biol.*, 44: 183–188.

Affanni, J.M., García Samartino, L., Scaravilli, A.M., and Panizza, J.S. (1973). Cambios en la actividad sinusoidal inducida después de la sección de los pedúnculos olfatorios en *Chaetophractus villosus* (Mammalia, Dasypodidae). *Physis*, 32: 101–105.

Affanni, J., Gori, A., Scaravilli, A., and García Samartino, L. (1974). Aumento bilateral de la duración de respuestas olfatorias por sección de un pedúnculo olfatorio en *Chaetophractus villosus* (Mammalia, Dasypodidae). *Physis*, 33: 151–155.

Affanni, J., Casanave, E., García Samartino, L., and Ferrari, R. (1986). Neocortical and olfactory bulb activity, in armadillos submitted to covering with soil. *Arch. Int. Physiol. Biochim.*, 94: 271–279.

Affanni, J.L., García Samartino, E., Casanave, E., and Dezi, R. (1987). Absence of apnea in armadillos covered by soil. *Respir. Physiol.*, 67: 239–243.

Affanni, J.M., Cervino, C.O., and Aldana Marcos, H. (2001). Absence of penile erections during paradoxical sleep. Peculiar penile events during wakefulness and slow sleep in the armadillo. *J. Sleep Res.*, 10: 219–228.

Ahrens, K.F. and Freeman, W.J. (2001). Response dynamics of entorhinal cortex in awake, anesthetized, and bulbectomized rats. *Brain Res.*, 911: 193–202.

Araki, H., Yamamoto, T., Watanabe, S., and Ueki, S. (1980). Changes in sleep-wakefulness pattern following bilateral olfactory bulbectomy in rats. *Physiol. Behav.*, 24(1): 73–78.

Arduini, A. and Moruzzi, G. (1953). Sensory and thalamic synchronization in the olfactory bulb. *Neurophysiology*, 5: 235–242.

Axel, R. (1995). Molecular logic of smell. *Sci. Am.*, 273: 154–159.

Badia, P., Wesensten, N., Lammers, W., Culpepper, J., and Harsh, J. (1990). Responsiveness to olfactory stimuli presented in sleep. *Physiol. Behav.*, 48: 87–90.

Baker, H. (1995). Transport phenomena within the olfactory system. In: Doty, R. (Ed.). *Handbook of Olfaction and Gustation*. New York: Marcel Dekker Inc., pp. 173–190.

Becker, C.J. and Freeman, W.J. (1968). Prepyriform electrical activity after loss of peripheral or central input or both. *Physiol. Behav.*, 3: 597–599.

Benítez, I., Aldana Marcos, H., and Affanni, J. (1994). The encephalon of *Chaetophractus villosus*. A general view of its most salient features. *Comun. Biol.*, 12: 57–73.

Beteleva, T. and Novikova, L. (1961). Electrical activity in various cortical regions and in the reticular formation after elimination of the olfactory analyser. *Zh. Vyssh. Nerv. Deiat. Im. I. P. Pavlova*, 3: 527–535.

Bressler, S.L. (1984). Spatial organization of EEGs from olfactory bulb and cortex. *Electroencephalogr. Clin. Neurophysiol.*, 57: 270–276.

Bressler, S.L. and Freeman, W.J. (1980). Frequency analysis of olfactory system EEG in cat, rabbit, and rat. *Electroencephalogr. Clin. Neurophysiol.*, 50: 19–24.

Bylsma, F.W., Moberg, P.J., Doty, R.L., and Brandt, J. (1997). Odor identification in Huntington's disease patients and asymptomatic gene carriers. *J. Neuropsychiatry Clin. Neurosci.*, 9: 598–600.

Cain, D.P. (1974). The role of the olfactory bulb in limbic mechanisms. *Psychol. Bull.*, 81: 654–671.

Cain, D.P. and Bindra, D. (1972). Responses of amygdala single units to odors in the rat. *Exp. Neurol.*, 35: 98–110.

Carreras, M., Mancia, D., and Mancia, M. (1967). Centrifugal control of the olfactory bulb as revealed by induced DC potential changes. *Brain Res.*, 6: 548–560.

Cattarelli, M. and Chanel, J. (1979). Influence of some biologically meaningful odorants on the vigilance states of the rat. *Physiol. Behav.*, 23: 831–838.

Cervino, C.O. (1997). Estudio cuantitativo de dos nuevos ritmos bioeléctricos de los bulbos olfatorios registrados en el armadillo sudamericano *Chaetophractus villosus* (Mammalia, Dasypodidae). Doctoral Thesis (MS), University of Buenos Aires, Argentina.

Chabaud, P., Ravel, N., Wilson, D.A., Mouly, A.M., Vigouroux, M., Farget, V., and Gervais, R. (2000). Exposure to behaviourally relevant odour reveals differential characteristics in rat central olfactory pathways as studied through oscillatory activities. *Chem. Senses*, 25: 561–573.

Domino, E.F. and Ueki, S. (1960). An analysis of the electrical burst phenomenon in some rhinencephalic structures of the dog and monkey. *Electroencephalogr. Clin. Neurophysiol.*, 12: 635–648.

Ferrari, C.C., Aldana Marcos, H.J., Carmanchahi, P.D., Benitez, I., and Affanni, J.M. (1998). The brain of the armadillo *Dasypus hybridus*. A general view of its most salient features. *Biocell*, 22: 123–140.

Ferreyra-Moyano, H. and Barragan, E. (1994). Environmental factors in the etiology of Alzheimer's dementia and other neurodegenerative diseases. In: Isaacson, R. and Jensen, K. (Eds.). *The Vulnerable Brain and Environmental Risks, Volume 3: Toxins in Air and Water*. New York: Plenum Press, pp. 43–63.

Freeman, W.J. (1957). Oscillating corticonuclear dipole in the basal forebrain of the cat. *Science*, 126: 1343–1344.

Freeman, W.J. (1959). Distribution in time and space of prepyriform electrical activity. *J. Neurophysiol.*, 22: 644–665.

Freeman, W.J. (1960). Correlation of electrical activity of prepyriform cortex and behavior in cat. *J. Neurophysiol.*, 23: 111–131.

Freeman, W.J. (1991). The physiology of perception. *Sci. Am.*, 264: 78–85.

Frye, R. (1995). Nasal airwall dynamics and olfactory function. In: Doty, R. (Ed.). *Handbook of Olfaction and Gustation*. New York: Marcel Dekker Inc., pp. 471–490.

Ganzha, B.L. and Bogach, P.G. (1975). Electrical reaction of olfactory structure and the amygdaloid complex of the brain of dogs in a paradoxical stage of sleep. *Neirofiziologiia*, 7: 227–233.

García Samartino, L., Scaravilli, A., Affanni, J., and Cinto, R. (1974). Estudio cuantitativo de la vigilia y el sueño en *Chaetophractus villosus* (Mammalia, Dasypodidae). *Physis*, 33: 145–150.

García Samartino, L., Gori, A., Scaravilli, A., and Affanni, J. (1981). Participación central en el aumento espontáneo de las ondas sinusoidales inducidas del bulbo olfatorio y area piriforme durante el sueño de *Chaetophractus villosus*. *Physis*, 39: 25–30.

García Samartino, L., Affanni, J.M., Casanave, E.B., Ferrari, R., and Iodice, O. (1987). On the presence of a peculiar alpha rhythm in the olfactory tubercle of waking armadillos. *Electroencephalogr. Clin. Neurophysiol.*, 66: 185–190.

Gault, F. and Leaton, R. (1963). Electrical activity of the olfactory system. *Electroencephalogr. Clin. Neurophysiol.*, 15: 299–304.

Gault, F. and Coustan, D. (1965). Nasal air flow and rhinencephalic activity. *Electroencephalogr. Clin. Neurophysiol.*, 18: 617–624.

Gervais, R. and Pager, J. (1979). Combined modulating effects of the general arousal and the specific hunger arousal on the olfactory bulb responses in the rat. *Electroencephalogr. Clin. Neurophysiol.*, 46: 87–94.

Gervais, R. and Pager, J. (1982). Functional changes in waking and sleeping rats after lesions in the olfactory pathways. *Physiol. Behav.*, 29: 7–15.

Hernandez-Peón, R., Lavin, A., Alcocer-Cuarón, C., and Marcelin, J.P. (1960) Electrical activity of the olfactory bulb during wakefulness and sleep. *Electroencephalogr. Clin. Neurophysiol.*, 12: 41–58.

Herrick, J. (1933). The functions of the olfactory parts of the cerebral cortex. *Proc. Natl. Acad. Sci. USA*, 19: 7–14.

Homeyer, P., Sastre, J.P., Buda, C., and Jouvet, M. (1995). Suppression of Ottoson waves in the isolated olfactory bulb during sleep in the pontine cat. *Neuroreport*, 27: 773–776.

Hughes, J.R. and Andy, O.J. (1979). The human amygdala. I. Electrophysiological responses to odorants. *Electroencephalogr. Clin. Neurophysiol.*, 46: 428–443.

Hughes, J.R., Hendrix, D.E., Wetzel, N., and Johnston, J.W. (1969). Correlations between electrophysiological activity from the human olfactory bulb and the subjective response to odoriferous stimuli. In: Pfaffmann, C. (Ed.). *Olfaction and Taste III*. New York: Pergamon Press, pp. 172–191.

Jacobs, B.L. and McGinty, D.J. (1971). Amygdala unit activity during sleep and wakefulness. *Exp. Neurol.* 33: 1.

Kratskin, I. (1995). Functional anatomy, central connections, and neurochemistry of the mammalian olfactory bulb. In: Doty, R. (Ed.). *Handbook of Olfaction and Gustation*. New York: Marcel Dekker, Inc., pp. 103–126.

Lavin, A., Alcocer-Cuarón, C., and Hernández-Peón, R. (1959). Centrifugal arousal in the olfactory bulb. *Science*, 129: 332–333.

Lesse, H. (1960). Rhinencephalic electrophysiological activity during "emotional behavior" in cats. *Rass Giuliana Med.*, 12: 224–237.

Malnic, B., Godfrey, P.A., and Buck, L.B. (2004). The human olfactory receptor gen family. *Proc. Natl. Acad. Sci. USA*, 101: 2584–2589.

Mancia, M., Green, J.D., and von Baumgarten, R. (1962). Reticular control of single neurons in the olfactory bulb. *Arch. Ital. Biol.*, 100: 463–475.

Maruniak, J. (1995). Deprivation and the olfactory system. In: Doty, R. (Ed.). *Handbook of Olfaction and Gustation.* New York: Marcel Dekker Inc., pp. 455–469.

Mesholam, R.I., Moberg, P.J., Mahr, R.N., and Doty, R.L. (1998). Olfaction in neurodegenerative disease: a meta-analysis of olfactory functioning in Alzheimer's and Parkinson's diseases. *Arch. Neurol.*, 55: 84–90.

McLean, P., Horwitz, N., and Robinson, F. (1952). Olfactory-like responses in pyriform area to non-olfactory stimulation. *Yale J. Biol. Med.*, 25: 159–172.

Moruzzi, G. and Magoun, H. (1949). Brain stem reticular formation and activation of the EEG. *Electroencephalogr. Clin. Neurophysiol.*, 1: 455–473.

Nauta, W.J. (1958). Hippocampal projections and related neural pathways to the midbrain in the cat. *Brain*, 81: 319–340.

Nelson, R.J. and Zucker, I. (1981). Photoperiodic control of reproduction in olfactory-bulbectomized rats. *Neuroendocrinology*, 32: 266–271.

Obál, F. Jr, Benedek, G., Reti, G., and Obál, F. (1980). Tonic hypnogenic effect of the olfactory tubercle. *Exp. Neurol.*, 69: 202–208.

Ottoson, D. (1959). Studies on the potentials in the rabbit's olfactory bulb and nasal mucosa. *Acta Physiol. Scand.*, 47: 136–148.

Pagano, R.R. and Gault, F.P. (1964). Amygdala activity: a central measure of arousal. *Electroencephalogr. Clin. Neurophysiol.*, 17: 255–260.

Pager, J. (1980). An efferent respiratory modulation demonstrated in the olfactory bulb of the rat. *C.R. Seances Acad. Sci. D*, 290: 251–254.

Panizza, J., Affanni, J., García Samartino, L., and Scaravilli, A. (1973). Características electrofisiológicas del bulbo olfatorio de la vizcacha *Lagostomus maximus*. *Physis*, 32: 423–436.

Penaloza-Rojas, J.H. and Alcocer-Cuarón, C. (1967). The electrical activity of the olfactory bulb in cats with nasal and tracheal breathing. *Electroencephalogr. Clin. Neurophysiol.*, 22: 468–472.

Pieper, D.R. and Lobocki, C.A. (1991). Olfactory bulbectomy lengthens circadian period of locomotor activity in golden hamsters. *Am. J. Physiol.*, 261: 973–978.

Powell, T., Cowan, W., and Raisman, G. (1965). The central olfactory connexions. *J. Anat.*, 99: 791–813.

Routtenberg, A. (1971). Stimulus processing and response execution: a neurobehavioral theory. *Physiol. Behav.*, 6: 589–596.

Sawa, M. and Delgado, J. (1963). Amygdala unitary activity in the unrestrained cat. *Electroencephalogr. Clin. Neurophysiol.*, 15: 637–650.

Scaravilli, A., Affanni, J., Panizza, J., and García Samartino, L. (1971). Efecto de la interrupción de las conexiones de un sistema cortical simple (bulbo olfatorio) con el resto del cerebro. Estudio comparado en *Chaetophractus villosus* y *Lagostomus maximus*. *Rev. Soc. Argent. Biol.*, 47: 249–258.

Shepherd, G.M., Nowycky, M.C., Greer, C.A., and Mori, K. (1981). Multiple overlapping circuits within olfactory and basal forebrain systems. In: Székey, G., Lábos, E., and Damjanovich, S. (Eds.). *Neural Communication and Control. Adv. Physiol. Sci.*, 30: 263–278.

Shipley, M.T., McLean, J.H., and Ennis, M. (1995). Olfactory system. In: Paxinos, G. (Ed.). *The Rat Nervous System*. 2nd edn. Sydney: Academic Press, pp. 899–926.

Sobel, N., Prabhakaran, V., Hartley, C.A., Desmond, J.E., Glover, G.H., Sullivan, E.V., and Gabrieli J.D. (1999). Blind smell: brain activation induced by an undetected air-borne chemical. *Brain*, 122: 209–217.

Soussignan, R., Schaal, B., and Marlier, L. (1999). Olfactory alliesthesia in human neonates: prandial state and stimulus familiarity modulate facial and autonomic responses to milk odors. *Dev. Psychobiol.*, 35: 3–14.

Tanabe, T., Yarita, H., Iino, M., Ooshima, Y., and Takagi, S.F. (1975). An olfactory projection area in orbitofrontal cortex of the monkey. *J. Neurophysiol.*, 38: 1269–1283.

Vaccarezza, O. and Affanni, J. (1964). Actividad bioeléctrica del bulbo olfatorio del marsupial (*Didelphis azarae*), comadreja o zarigüeya. *Rev. Soc. Argent. Biol.*, 40: 9–13.

Vaccarezza, O. and Affanni, J. (1966). Influencia de los bulbos olfatorios sobre el sueño del marsupial (*Didelphis azarae*). *Rev. Soc. Argent. Biol.* 42: 106–111.

Vanderwolf, C.H. (2000). What is the significance of gamma wave activity in the pyriform cortex? *Brain Res.*, 877: 125–133.

Villablanca, J. (1965). The electrocorticogram in the chronic cerveau isole cat. *Electroencephalogr. Clin. Neurophysiol.*, 19: 576–586.

Zhang, X. and Firestein, S. (2002). The olfactory receptor gene superfamily of the mouse. *Nat. Neurosci.*, 5: 124–133.

Chapter 26

SLEEP AND MEMORY

Carlo Cipolli[1]

The view that sleep plays an important role in the processing of information to be retained for further recall dates back to the beginning of the theory of memory consolidation (Muller and Pilzecker, 1900; for a review, see McGaugh, 2000). The actual nature of the relationship between sleep and memory, however, has been debated since the first experimental demonstration of a positive influence of sleep on the retention of new information (Jenkins and Dallenbach, 1924).

Three distinct phases can be identified in the experimental investigation into this relationship with respect to the aspect focussed. They are (a) a "naturalistic" phase (from 1924 to discovery of cyclic organization of sleep), where the influence of sleep on memory was considered as an effect of sleep as a whole; (b) a stage-related phase (from late 1950s to the early 1990s), where the influence of sleep was hypothesized to differ with respect to stages and/or cycles; (c) a task-related phase (from late 1990s up to the present, where the two main systems of knowledge (declarative and non-declarative, that is knowledge of "what" and of "how") were hypothesized to be influenced in a different manner by sleep.

The studies carried out in the third phase are characterized by a much deeper awareness of the methodological constraints involved in sleep investigations, regardless of the fact that sleep has been taken into account as a whole or a sequence of stages and cycles. This awareness has two

---

[1] carlo.cipolli@unibo.it

implications. First, the specific limits of the adopted paradigm of research are considered in a more accurate way than before. Second, in any attempt to provide a comprehensive account for the relationships between sleep and memory it is widely agreed that several indications from recent findings cannot be generalized because some important methodological problems raised by the studies carried out in the first and second phases remain unresolved.

In presenting the main lines of the evidence as yet collected, the most important indications provided by early studies will be also examined, in order to put into focus more clearly the theoretical frameworks of the main findings obtained. Therefore, the indications in favor of a positive role of sleep as a whole and as a sum of distinct components (stages and cycles) will be examined together with the methodological constraints involved in investigation into the relationship between sleep and memory.

The Naturalistic Studies on the Sleep Effect

The first experimental evidence that sleep has a positive effect on delayed retention of new information (the so-called "sleep effect") was provided by Jenkins and Dallenbach (1924). They observed that the subjects who slept for 8 h following a learning session remembered a list of paired words better than subjects who remained awake. This effect was explained within the framework of the interference theory of memory and thus considered as the outcome of the minor interference experienced during sleep compared to that encountered in waking.

This explanation, however, was the object of serious criticism from several researchers who studied the retention over intervals longer than 8 h, covering one or more 24-h periods (Graves, 1937; Newman, 1939). These studies showed that sleep has a positive effect only when it follows the learning session, against the prediction of the interference theory that the retention rate depends on the amount of sleep over the interval between the learning session and the recall test. Were this hypothesis correct, the retention rate should not depend on whether sleep or waking follows the learning session.

To overcome the discrepancy between the predictions of the interference theory and the available data, the possibility was considered that the superior retention following sleep is a consequence of the functioning of memory processes at work during sleep. Such processes could either decrease the decay of the information acquired during learning session in previous waking or actively enhance retention. The latter possibility corresponds to a key prediction of the consolidation theory of memory. This theory, which has been put forward at the beginning of 20th century, has been reformulated several times (for a review, see McGaugh, 2000), in order to make it as comprehensive enough to account for several types of data collected not only in waking, but also in sleep condition.

Naturalistic studies (considering sleep as a whole, regardless of the different neurophysiological characteristics of its stages and cycles, which however became known to researchers only after the discovery of REM sleep and cyclic organization of sleep: Aserinky and Kleitman, 1953; Dement and Kleitman, 1957) did not bring conclusive evidence in favor of the consolidation rather than of the interference theory and, thus, of the consolidation power of sleep, notwithstanding the elegance of the experimental design of some studies. For example, Benson and Feinberg (1977) tested retention after 8, 16, and 24 h from learning session using five measures of recall. They found that retention is enhanced only when sleep immediately follows the learning session and, complementarily, that recall is less dependent on whether sleep or waking follows the learning session when the material has been learnt by rote. However, these findings do not entail the degree of consolidation being enhanced properly during sleep, and the possibility is not excluded that over-learnt materials are less affected by decay and interference than weakly learnt materials.

More direct evidence in favor of the consolidation function of sleep was searched for by analyzing the effects of specific types of sleep on retention of materials (i.e., stimuli) delivered mostly during previous waking and, in some studies, during sleep.

The Stage-Related Phase

From the time of the discovery of REM sleep and cyclic organization of sleep, physiological and psychological distinctive features of REM sleep (such as higher brain activation, postural muscle atonia, bursts of rapid eye movements, large rebound after deprivation, more frequent occurrences of dream-like experiences than in other stages) prompted researchers to speculate about its functional properties. Among other possible functions, the processing of recently acquired information for organization and retention was considered a plausible function of REM sleep, both in animals (for a review, see Hennevin *et al.*, 1995) and humans (for a review, see Smith, 1995).

In humans, the hypothesis of (re-)processing function of rapid eye movement (REM) sleep was investigated overall by comparing the retention rate of well-controlled materials (such as verbal stimuli differing in length and complexity) at the end of the learning session and after equivalent periods of sleep and waking. The influence of sleep on retention of stimuli was measured by adopting two main strategies based on the comparison of retention rates after equivalent intervals characterized (a) by different proportion of sleep stages, or (b) by uninterrupted sleep or sleep deprivation. These strategies are clearly complementary, so in some experiments they were combined (Ekstrand *et al.*, 1977; Tilley, 1979).

The results of the experiments adopting the first strategy suggested a more positive effect of stages 3 and 4 of non-rapid eye movement (NREM) sleep (which are more represented in the first half of the night) than of REM sleep (which is more represented in the second half) on the retention of simple materials such as word pairs and short sentences, while REM sleep seemed more important for the retention of complex (such as prose paragraphs) and emotionally loaded materials (Empson and Clarke, 1970). Instead, experiments in which subjects were deprived of sleep showed greater negative effects after REM than NREM sleep deprivation, thus suggesting that it is REM sleep that facilitates retention more strongly (for a review, see Lewin and Glaubman, 1975)

Also these investigations did not provide definitive evidence for the superiority of one main type of sleep (NREM and REM) in enhancing retention, as pointed out recently by some researchers (Vertes and Eastman, 2000; Siegel, 2001). The enhancement in retention has been shown to be influenced by several factors, such as the types of materials to be retained for delayed recall test, the time of night when sleep occurs (Hockey *et al.*, 1972; Lammers *et al.*, 1991), the length of the interval between learning and sleep onset (Portnoff *et al.*, 1966).

In attempting to estimate more directly the influence of specific sleep stages on retention of new information, some researchers adopted the strategy of measuring the capacity of specific stages of sleep for the online processing of new information. This strategy was applied by delivering simple stimuli (such as words, personal names, short sentences, short sequences of digits, or visual flashes) and assessing their retention rate after next awakening or examining their insertion rate as contents into the ongoing dream experience. This strategy led to ascertain that retention is better when stimuli are delivered during REM rather than NREM sleep, and that such superiority persists at least for 15 min following stimulus presentation (Shimizu *et al.*, 1977). There is also a strong correlation between the retention rate and the level and duration of EEG activation (possibly resulting in short waking periods, as indicated by the alpha pattern) after stimulus presentation (Lehmann and Koukkou, 1974; Oltmann *et al.*, 1977).

Complementary evidence was gathered by investigations where the delivery of poorly organized stimuli (such as olfactory stimuli: Badia *et al.*, 1990) aimed to trigger specific behavioral responses that had been learned in previous waking. The analysis of behavioral responsiveness to external stimuli provided important support for the possibility that complex operations of information processing take place during sleep (such as the recording of the stimulus, the selection of the appropriate motor response, and the realization of that response) (Bonnet, 1982; Lammers *et al.*, 1991). Such indications have been confirmed by subsequent studies in which the activation level of specific brain areas when a meaningful stimulus (personal names) or simple tone was delivered during REM sleep was examined using neuroimaging techniques (Portas *et al.*, 2000). Moreover, short-term retention of external stimuli has shown to be possible in both sleep types (albeit superior in REM sleep), as is the access to old information in long-term memory (e.g., appropriate motor responses), even though long-term retention seems to presuppose a period of high EEG activation (Shimizu *et al.*, 1977; Burton *et al.*, 1988).

The possibility that an external stimulus can be retained in short-term memory and, thus, be available for operations potentially enhancing the degree of consolidation seemed crucial in order to understand not only whether, but also how consolidation is improved during sleep. Some pieces of pertinent, albeit preliminary, evidence have been gathered by examining the main outcome of the processing of stimuli delivered before and during sleep, namely the contents of dream experiences in which they appear incorporated. Burton *et al.* (1988) showed that the presentation of a tone alternately leads to elicit the appropriate motor response (a deep breath) or to insert it as content into the ongoing dream experience. This possibility will be examined in detail later.

In general terms, the study of long-term retention of such well-controlled materials as stimuli delivered before or during sleep has shown that the occurrence and magnitude of the sleep effect are influenced by several factors, the actual power of which, however, is difficult to estimate. Such factors are the characteristics of sleep *per se* (namely, the occurrence and proportion of NREM and REM sleep, the total amount of sleep, the sleep efficiency) and in the interaction with circadian rhythms (namely, the varying proportions of sleep stages in the cycles occurring at different moments through the 24-h interval), and the length of waking period preceding the sleep onset (during which such operations as rehearsal and recoding of stimuli may facilitate the following recall test). Although some pieces of evidence have been gathered in favor of specific factors related to sleep length and organization, it appears however difficult to plan experiments capable of disentangling the proportions of sleep effect that are due, respectively, to the protection from interference and the enhancement in retention because of further consolidation (Ekstrand *et al.*, 1977; for a methodological discussion, see also Born and Gais, 2000). The main difficulty depends on the impossibility of manipulating the architecture of sleep (NREM sleep precedes REM sleep in each cycle) and on the unpredictability of the length of the interval between storage of new information and sleep onset (as well as of the intrusions of waking periods during sleep), where operations relevant for retention, such as rehearsal and encoding of stimuli, may occur (Cipolli and Salzarulo, 1979).

The Task-Related Phase

Until the early 1990s, the materials used to assess the influence of sleep on memory were mainly verbal in nature, albeit with some difference in complexity (word lists, sentences, prose paragraphs, logical dilemma) and task to perform (free recall, cued recall, recognition: for a review, see Cipolli, 1995). Only in a small part of experiments the elaboration of pre-sleep materials (or instructions) for the acquisition of motor abilities, artificial languages, or visuo-perceptual skills was required (for a review, see Smith, 1995). The latter studies, however, were of potentially equal (or even greater) interest, as regarding distinct types of implicit knowledge, the acquisition of which appears as important as that of explicit knowledge, which is conveyed usually by verbal materials.

The importance of studying the influence of sleep on the implicit knowledge relies on several pieces of experimental and clinical neuropsychological evidence in favor of the existence of two memory systems, respectively, declarative and non-declarative in nature. The acquisition of knowledge concerning events (recent or remote) and semantic (i.e., general and abstract) information is more conscious, more voluntary, and faster than the acquisition of knowledge concerning procedural (i.e., perceptual, motor, and phonological) skills, priming, and conditioning. Moreover, the two memory systems can also be functionally dissociated, as indicated by the possibility of improving procedural skills in amnesic patients (for a review, see Squire, 1993). This makes it apparent that the pieces of evidence gathered on the

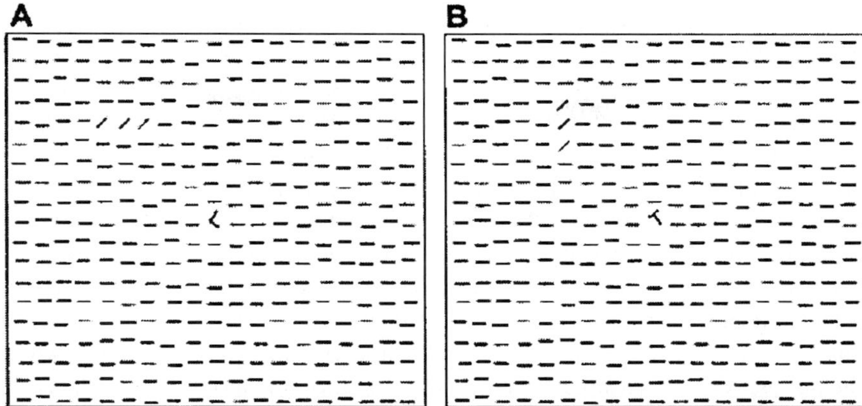

Figure 1. Example of a texture discrimination task (TDT), originally described by Karni and Sagi (1991). Screens consist of a background of horizontal bars with a rotated letter ("T" or "L") at the central fixation point and an array of three diagonal bars (in either a horizontal row or a vertical column) in the upper left visual field. (Adapted from Stickgold *et al.*, 2002.)

retention of declarative information (such as words, sentences, and prose paragraphs) cannot be automatically considered valid for non-declarative memory during sleep. Finally, Karni *et al.* (1994) showed that after a training session a substantial delayed learning of a texture discrimination task occurs during a night of uninterrupted sleep, while selective disruption of REM sleep (but not of NREM sleep) prevents the improvement in performance (Figure 1). This demonstration of the usefulness in distinguishing the two types of memory systems also in studying the relationship between sleep and memory suggested to reconsider the role of sleep as a whole and as a sequence of stages and cycles in the consolidation of new items of declarative and non-declarative knowledge.

Consolidation of procedural knowledge

The findings obtained by Karni *et al.* (1994) generated a large number of studies in the late 1990s and early 2000s, with the primary aim to corroborate the hypothesis that the acquisition of non-declarative knowledge (such as visual skills) is at some extent sleep-dependent. To investigate the improvement of visual skills, all studies used the Karni and Sagi's (1991) task of texture discrimination, while for motor learning various tasks were used (also by the same group of researchers). For example, Born's group used a task of reversed reproduction (or mirror tracing: Plihal and Born, 1997, 1999), then one of finger-to-thumb opposition (Fischer *et al.*, 2002).

The most important indications provided by these studies were the following: (a) improvement in motor as well as visual skills is actually (albeit not exclusively) sleep-dependent (Plihal and Born, 1997, 1999); (b) the benefit in delayed performance relies on the fact that during the first night after the training session subjects sleep rather than remain awake, while the length of waking interval between training and sleep does not entail any additional benefit for delayed performance (Stickgold *et al.*, 2000c); (c) the level of performance is further improved over the subsequent nights if the first one following acquisition is spent in sleep, while no improvement occurs when the subject remains awake during the first night (Stickgold *et al.*, 2000a).

The sleep-dependence rather than time-dependence of the gain in performance has been made further plausible by the demonstrations that the diurnal decrement in the performance level obtained at the end of the training session can be contrasted in an effective way by a period of diurnal sleep (i.e, a nap, Mednick *et al.*, 2002), and that the contrastive effect is more conspicuous if the period of diurnal sleep is long enough to include not only NREM but also REM sleep (i.e., a long nap, Mednick *et al.*, 2003).

Some studies have provided support for an exclusive relationship between the improvement of delayed performance in tasks of non-declarative memory and REM sleep (Plihal and Born, 1997, 1999). However, other studies have shown that besides REM sleep other stages, in particular slow-wave sleep (SWS, stages 3 and 4 of NREM-sleep of the first half of the night: Stickgold *et al.*, 2000c), concur to improve performance. As a consequence, the attribution of a specific role to REM sleep in the consolidation of procedural (motor and perceptual) skills is slightly different according to whether it is considered *per se* or in combination with other stages. In the former case, it is suggested that REM sleep enhances consolidation overall in the late part of the night, where it is present to a greater extent, while in the latter case it is suggested that REM sleep enhances the consolidation level, which has been triggered by SWS-related processes (Gais *et al.*, 2000).

A more complex picture has been provided by studies on the relationship between delayed learning of motor skills and sleep. Plihal and Born (1997, 1999) observed a more accurate level of performance in a mirror tracing task after a period of sleep rather than after waking and, overall, after a greater proportion of REM sleep. Similar data were obtained by Fischer *et al.* (2002) in another motor task (sequences of finger-to-thumb opposition), with the additional indication that sleep on the first night following training is critical to improve the performance level. Moreover, Walker *et al.* (2002) found that subjects trained in a task of finger tapping further improve performance after a period of sleep (about 20%), but not after a period of waking; however, this improvement of performance is correlated with the percentage of stage 2 NREM sleep, which is particularly frequent in the second half of the night. This indication seems important, albeit partially in contrast with those of other studies, as it was obtained in a well-designed experiment, in which subjects were tested at the end of training session either in the morning or in the evening and retested after a 12-h interval following wake or sleep. Improvement of performance was observed for the subjects who spent a period of sleep in this interval.

In a further study where the finger-tapping task was used and subjects were retested across 3 days after the training session, Walker *et al.* (2003a) showed that following the initial training, a small practice (i.e., exercise)-dependent improvement is possible before, but not after, the large sleep-dependent gain consequent to a night of sleep (see Figure 2). Moreover,

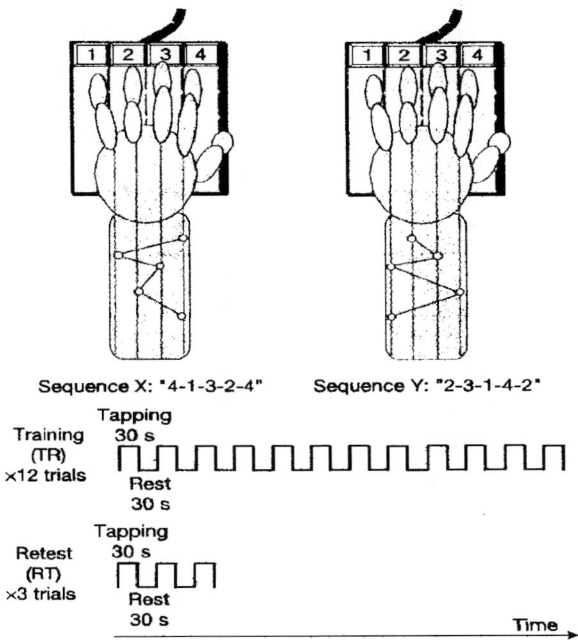

Figure 2. Example of a finger-tapping task, with distinct sequences to be learned. (Adapted from Walker *et al.*, 2003.)

the amount of this sleep-dependent learning is not modified by variation in the amount of initial training, with which it is not significantly correlated. Finally, the sleep-dependent motor-skill learning is not exclusively developed during the night following training: additional nights of sleep may further improve motor skills, consistently with what has been observed for visual skills (Stickgold *et al.*, 2000a).

In recent studies, the notion that sleep is a necessary condition for the consolidation of procedural memory and gain in performance at later retrieval has been complemented by examining the subject's awareness of the task to perform. This aspect corresponds to a fairly crucial dimension of learning, given that procedural skill learning can occur in an implicit (or incidental) way, or in an explicit (intentional) manner; that is, with awareness of and attention to task rules and structures. Explicit and implicit processes are usually entwined, above all in the initial phases of learning, before the skills become highly automated. However, the two types of learning can be experimentally disentangled, as shown by Robertson *et al.* (2004), who assessed skill improvement in implicit and explicit sequence-learning tasks before and after a 12-h interval. The task consisted in reacting as fast and as accurately as possible to cues appearing in one of four positions, which changed according to an underlying fixed 12-item sequence (repeatedly presented). In the explicit condition awareness of this sequence was prompted by signaling to the subjects whenever the repeating sequence was reintroduced, while in the implicit condition subjects were told only that a four-choice reaction task was to be performed. A dependence of procedural learning (i.e., decrease in reaction time) on sleep was observed only for the explicit condition. This finding, which is consistent with the indications of previous studies, where subjects were fully aware of the type of skill being trained, raises the question of the role of awareness in activating a sleep-dependent memory process (Born and Wagner, 2004). Awareness is not an independent system, but interacts with declarative and non-declarative memory systems in a complex way, as shown by Wagner *et al.* (2004). Prior to sleep subjects had to process strings of digits without awareness of an underlying structure. More than twice as many subjects gained explicit knowledge of the hidden structure of the digit strings in this sleep-dependent learning, as compared with waking control conditions. However, the subjects gaining explicit knowledge did not improve response time, while those who did not gain such knowledge showed an improvement in response time, thus suggesting that sleep enhances declarative memory at the expense of procedural memory formation.

Consolidation of declarative knowledge

In the studies carried out over the last 10 years the evidence gathered in favor of a consolidation improvement of declarative knowledge during sleep has been undoubtedly less consistent. This may depend on several reasons, the most important of which appears to be the much shorter time needed to store items of declarative knowledge in long-term memory (and, thus, to execute the most crucial operations for consolidation) compared with the time needed for non-declarative knowledge. Therefore, the role of sleep could be more difficult to disentangle from that of other factors, above all for the easier tasks regarding items of declarative information.

After Karni *et al.*'s (1994) demonstration of the consolidation function of REM sleep for procedural knowledge, attempts have been renewed to establish, using thorough techniques, whether sleep influences consolidation of declarative knowledge and what specific stages are involved. In this line of research, Plihal and Born (1997, 1999) showed matched retention rates after the first or second half of the night spent in sleep or in waking. Recall of lists of paired words proved to be enhanced when subjects slept in the first half of the night, while no significant difference was observed in retention rates after sleep or waking in the second half of the night (the contrary being true for non-declarative memory for a task such as mirror tracing). From these studies it has been argued that overall SWS, which occurs above all in the first half of the night, improves consolidation of declarative knowledge.

More recently, Born and colleagues have shown that a low cholinergic tone during SWS is essential for declarative memory consolidation of semantically related words (paired-associate words list), but not for procedural memory (mirror tracing task, Gais and Born, 2004a). Moreover, an intensive learning of word pairs can modify sleep characteristics, with a substantial increase of spindles (Gais *et al.*, 2002). It should be established, however, if the effect observed depends on the nature of the task, as in these studies related words were used, instead of unrelated word pairs, as in previous studies. Were this hypothesis corroborated, the positive influence of sleep should be attributed to the strengthening of previously formed associations rather than to the formation and retention of novel associations. This would indicate, as suggested by Walker and Stickgold (2004), that the role of sleep in consolidation of declarative knowledge depends on fairly subtle aspects of declarative tasks, such as task difficulty (as first shown by Empson and Clarke, 1970) and emotional salience (more emotional items being better retained after periods of REM than NREM sleep,

Wagner *et al.*, 2001). It is apparent that a more detailed examination of different categories of declarative memory may further clarify the apparently contradictory indications gathered up to now, namely the role of both SWS (and stage 2 NREM sleep) and REM sleep in memory consolidation (for reviews, see Smith, 2001; Gais and Born, 2004b).

Finally, the consolidation of strictly episodic memories (characterized by so-called autonoetic consciousness, which allows an individual to recollect vivid spatiotemporal and phenomenological details of a previous event) seems to require REM rather than SWS sleep, above all for the spatial component of episodic memory (Rauchs *et al.*, 2004). This finding is potentially of great interest, as it raises the question of how consolidation of recent events is improved by reprocessing during sleep, in particular for the development of dream experiences, a large proportion of contents of which appear to derive from some elaboration of recent or remote events.

General Hypotheses of How Sleep Influences Memory Consolidation

The amount of data collected over the last 10 years has repeatedly raised a typical issue of the second phase of the investigations as to the relationship between sleep and memory, namely whether consolidation depends on specific stages of sleep rather than on sleep as a whole. In the task-related phase the question has been posited in terms of stage-dependence of the consolidation for information related to the two-memory systems. It is apparent that the responses to this question have several implications for the explanation of how consolidation is improved during sleep.

The two most comprehensive accounts regarding the recently gathered evidence correspond to the "dual-process hypothesis" and "two-step (or sequential) hypothesis." The former, which was originally put forward by Plihal and Born (1997), is apparently supported by the greater amount of data collected in the 1990s and posits that procedural memory benefits mainly from REM sleep and that declarative memory is advantaged by NREM (in particular, SWS) sleep. It is apparent that this hypothesis relies above all on the earlier observations that procedural tasks are better improved in the second half of the night (richer in REM sleep) (Plihal and Born, 1997, 1999). It seems worth stressing that the same group then observed that the consolidation of emotional–verbal (declarative) stimuli also occurs during REM sleep (Wagner *et al.*, 2001), and that the consolidation of procedural knowledge is also influenced by NREM sleep (Fischer *et al.*, 2002). Taken together with those of other groups, these findings suggest the possibility of a complex interaction between the characteristics of the tasks to perform (and materials) and the stages and cycles of sleep: the greater improvement in performance in a visual learning task having been observed as related to the product of the amount of SWS in the first cycle and of REM sleep in the fourth cycle (Stickgold *et al.*, 2000c). This possibility is made further plausible by the indication that other stages of NREM sleep can improve consolidation of procedural skills (for example, stage 2 of NREM sleep for visual skills or the amount of spindles for motor skills, Fischer *et al.*, 2002; Gais and Born, 2004a).

Several data among those made available by investigations carried out both before and after the distinction of the two-memory systems (for two reviews carried out from different theoretical perspectives, see Smith, 2001; Vertes, 2004) can be interpreted as supporting or contrasting the possibility of the interaction between sleep stages and task characteristics. This fact does not provide support to the recurrent criticism as to the role of sleep in consolidation of new information (Siegel, 2001; Vertes, 2004), but rather indicates the need to reformulate the original question of stage-dependence of the consolidation function of distinct memory tasks.

An alternative (so-called two-step or sequential) hypothesis was put forward by Giuditta *et al.*, 1995 on the basis of evidence mostly following experiments on animals. This two-step hypothesis assumes that the occurrence of both SWS and REM sleep is required to improve consolidation of adaptive memories and, in humans, especially of procedural knowledge (Stickgold *et al.*, 2000b). A large body of data collected in the last 10 years is compatible with this frame, the explanatory power of which, however, stems from neurophysiological rather than from behavioral correlates of improved performance in procedural tasks (Maquet, 2001; Peigneux *et al.*, 2003).

A possibility that appears widely complementary has been suggested by Ficca and Salzarulo (2004) in terms of cooperation between NREM and REM sleep within the cycle of sleep. Postulating that this cooperation is maintained throughout the cycles developed over the night, the consolidation improvement may be accounted for not as a sum of the distinct contributions of the stages of sleep, but as the outcome of their interaction within one or more cycles of sleep. This possibility implies that improvement in retention is related (a) to the amount of cycles of sleep over the night and (b) to the preservation of the interaction of the two main types of sleep within each cycle. Both these conditions received some support from

Salzarulo and colleagues as regards declarative knowledge. They observed that delayed retention of word lists (the next morning) is impaired when the number of cycles completed during the previous night is small (as often happens in older people; Mazzoni *et al.*, 1999) and when the NREM–REM organization has been experimentally disrupted over the night (Ficca *et al.*, 2000).

So far, however, no piece of evidence has been collected in favor of the consolidation power of cycle organization for non-declarative (in particular, procedural) knowledge during night sleep. At best, Mednick *et al.*'s (2003) findings that longer naps (with both NREM and REM sleep) prevent deterioration of the learning advantage in a visual texture discrimination task more than short naps (with only NREM sleep) can be considered as indirect evidence in favor of the role of sleep cycle in consolidation improvement.

Notwithstanding their theoretical interest, the two hypotheses above have not been as yet stated in such a firm way as to generate studies aiming to test their specific predictions. Rather, several researchers tend toward one of the two hypothesis on the basis of the most recent data made available by their studies. It is apparent, however, that the question of the stage- or cycle-dependent nature of the consolidation improvement is strictly entwined with that of the mechanism(s) responsible for this improvement, so that the question cannot be adequately resolved before we have understood how consolidation is improved.

A fairly comprehensive explanatory hypothesis has been put forward by Stickgold (1998), namely that the improvement in consolidation of memories acquired in previous waking is due to the off-line reprocessing that they undergo during sleep. This hypothesis is compatible with the more general view of an "interplay" during sleep between different brain structures (the so-called "neocortex–hippocampus dialogue" postulated by Buzsaki, 1996) and has already received support at some of the different (from cellular to behavioral) levels of the processing leading to memory formation and consolidation. At a neurobiological level, neuroimaging studies (using positron emission tomography techniques) have shown that brain regions (left premotor area and bilateral cuneus) specifically involved in the execution of a serial reaction time task (regarding procedural memory) during the training phase are reactivated during (exclusively) REM sleep in previously trained subjects and that the performance level on the same task after a period of sleep is higher in trained rather than in untrained subjects (Maquet *et al.*, 2000). This experience-dependent change may be attributed to an increased functional connectivity during REM sleep, which would optimize the networks subtending the subject's visual and motor responses. Peigneux *et al.* (2003) have argued that recent memory traces, embodied in the networks challenged by new environmental conditions, are processed during subsequent periods of (REM) sleep, while leaving the question open of how this processing serves to consolidate these traces.

Some pieces of at least indirect evidence in favor of the hypothesis that processing of recent information during sleep has some consolidation effect are available also at a behavioral level. These pieces come from studies on reactivation during sleep of stimuli which have been stored in memory during previous waking. Using the paradigm of cued recall it has been shown that next-day retention of new information is enhanced by repeated delivery during REM (but not NREM) sleep of external cues (such as auditory clicks) with which that information has been associated in previous waking (Guerrien *et al.*, 1989; Smith and Weeden, 1990). These findings indicate that rehearsal, which is one of the basic mechanisms to enhance the consolidation level of items of new information in waking (Benjamin and Biork, 2000), remains effective even also during sleep. This possibility was earlier supported by Tilley (1979), who observed some consolidation improvement during REM as well as stage 2 of NREM sleep by re-delivering during such sleep stages the paired words presented in previous waking.

The question of the residual effectiveness of rehearsal during sleep seems crucial for the explanatory power of the hypothesis of an off-line reprocessing of memories during sleep. At a behavioral level, some plausible implications of this hypothesis can be tested in a pertinent manner at least for memories that are declarative in nature. Indeed, a lot of studies on the so-called dream sources have shown that contents of dream experiences (or, in more general terms, mental sleep experiences, MSEs) widely derive from transformation of several types of declarative knowledge, such as recent and remote events and items of semantic information (for a meta-analysis, see Baylor and Cavallero, 2001). Moreover, the amount of MSEs developed over each night of sleep is impressive. Psychophysiological studies carried out after Foulkes' (1962) demonstration of the presence of MSE, albeit with some difference in content and complexity, in all stages of NREM sleep have consistently indicated that MSE reports can be obtained in more than 80% of awakenings provoked during REM sleep and in about 50% of awakenings from NREM sleep (for a review, see Nielsen, 1999). Such frequencies of MSEs warrant the interest of examining the fate of the items of information that are transformed into their contents.

Dream Experience as the Output of a System of Information Processing

Some insights into the possible consolidation improvement of reprocessing of recently acquired items of declarative knowledge are offered by some studies on dream production and recall. This hypothesis was first suggested by Pivik and Foulkes (1968) and then put forward again from time to time. MSEs are not only usually perceptually vivid and sometimes bizarre in content, but also organized into relatively lengthy and coherent narratives of quite plausible and complex events. Such a prominent characteristic suggests that MSE is the result of a much more complex production system than supposed in early studies (Dement and Kleitman, 1957). Moreover, MSEs vary in length and content features (such as bizarreness and vividness) with respect to stage and cycle of sleep, being longer and more bizarre ("dreamlike") in REM than in NREM sleep and in the second rather than first half of the night (Foulkes and Schmidt, 1983; Cipolli *et al.*, 1998).

Given these characteristics, MSEs have been considered as the output of a complex multilevel system of information processing (Foulkes, 1982, 1985), the functioning of which involves several memory processes, taking place at three basic levels:

1. *recruitment of information* relevant to the ongoing MSE;
2. *insertion of contents* on a moment-by-moment basis, providing the sequential character of the ongoing MSE;
3. *hierarchical organization of contents*, providing the coherence and connection of episodes of MSE.

A number of indications as to the functioning of memory processes supposedly operative at these levels have been provided by delayed recall of MSE contents, in particular those resulting from transformation of well-controlled memory sources such as pre-sleep stimuli (so-called incorporation contents) and from repeated access and transformation of the same sources in distinct MSEs of the same night (so-called interrelated contents, see below). The main processes are the following: at the first level, there is the *access* (possibly repeated at different moments of the same period of sleep) to various types of memory sources (semantic, episodic, habits), with slight variations in their proportions with respect to sleep stage and cycle (Baylor and Cavallero, 2001).

At the second level comes the *insertion* of the accessed items of information into MSE contents through the complex operations of matching their features with those of the frame of the ongoing MSE. These operations have been identified above all by analyzing the incorporation of various kinds of pre-sleep stimuli into dream contents (Antrobus and Arkin, 1991; Cipolli *et al.*, 1983a,b) and do not seem to vary with respect to sleep stage or cycle or to perceptual features of the stimuli, but rather with respect to their semantic characteristics.

At the third, higher level, there is the *planning of the narrative frame* (in which single contents are inserted) of the MSE. Story-like organization appears a reliable characteristic of MSEs, although it is more marked in those developed during REM sleep rather than those elaborated in stage 2 of NREM sleep (Foulkes and Schmidt, 1983). This organization shows an increasing complexity over the night (Cipolli *et al.*, 1998). Such stage- and cycle-related variations in length and complexity (Cipolli and Poli, 1992) of MSEs point to a varying effectiveness of the production system, plausibly due to different amounts of cognitive resources available for the structural (both sequential and hierarchical) organization of MSEs.

Studies on the relationships between the narrative frame and content units of MSEs and their memory sources have consistently indicated that both frame and contents hardly ever come from direct reproduction (i.e., "replay"), but rather from transformation of memory sources (Stickgold *et al.*, 2000c; Baylor and Cavallero, 2001; Fosse *et al.*, 2003). These indications lead to the argument that the processing underlying MSE production is active in nature and, thus, may improve consolidation in a way similar to that involved in the so-called "generation effect." This effect, observed in information elaborated in waking, consists of better long-term retention for items that are actively elaborated in tasks such as solving anagrams, completing word fragments, translating from one language to another (Mulligan, 2001), compared with items that are only acquired passively. Moreover, where strong associative relationships are formed between the sources and outcomes of performed tasks (Marsh *et al.*, 2001; Mulligan, 2002), active processing appears to improve the consolidation level for the items in the input as well as those in the processing output. This consolidation advantage has been attributed to the deeper rehearsal undergone when items are actively elaborated rather than passively acquired (through elaborative and mechanic rehearsal respectively, Benjamin and Bjork, 2000).

Some evidence that rehearsal remains effective even during sleep is provided by cued-recall studies, which have shown that next-day retention of new items of information is enhanced by repeated delivery during REM sleep of external cues (such as auditory clicks) with which that information has been associated in previous waking (Guerrien *et al.*, 1989; Smith and Weeden, 1990).

To substantiate the above hypothesis more fully, the effectiveness of internally triggered rehearsal — that is, by cues deriving from MSE production — has to be demonstrated. Postulating that the processing of recent information during sleep improves consolidation both of the input (the pre-sleep stimulus) and output (the dream content) during sleep as well as in waking, it follows that delayed recall ought to be better (a) for processed stimuli rather than for unprocessed ones and, thus, for contents of dreams that incorporate stimuli rather than for those that do not, and (b) for those contents of distinct MSEs resulting from the presumable repeated access to the same or similar sources (so-called interrelated contents, see below).

In testing these predictions, however, also the repetitive nature of MSE processing has to be taken into account. The repeated incorporation into successive dream experiences of pre-sleep stimuli (Cipolli *et al.*, 1983a,b) and day residues (such as performed tasks, Stickgold *et al.*, 2000b) suggests that the consolidation level of the stimuli may be enhanced progressively. The coexistence of these two characteristics of the processing makes it unlikely that both the effects (i.e., on the input and the output) will be observable in the same experimental context. Demonstrating consolidation of the output requires that the likelihood of processing a pre-sleep stimulus be higher than for other items of information where an MSE to be reported at scheduled awakening is produced; demonstrating consolidation of the input requires that the likelihood of processing the stimulus remain higher than for other items of information during an uninterrupted lengthy period of sleep.

However, by experimentally manipulating the likelihood of pre-sleep stimuli being processed during sleep, the consolidation effect of the act of processing causing rehearsal (and insertion as content) can be dissociated from the consolidation effect of repeated processing of the same items over the night. Indeed, when a cognitive concern (such as the requirement that a recall task be performed after awakening) is associated to a sentence-stimulus delivered prior to sleep, this enhances the likelihood that the stimulus will be incorporated into MSE contents (without modifying the ordinary modalities of access and elaboration of the items involved). Thus, if the stimulus with which a cognitive concern is associated is repeatedly changed, its likelihood of incorporation is high until the associated task is completed, and then reduced to a chance level when concern is associated with a different stimulus (Cipolli *et al.*, 2001); while the task is uncompleted, the likelihood of incorporation remains uniformly high (Cipolli *et al.*, 2003).

Such a procedure can weaken the probability that contents involving previously incorporated stimuli be further consolidated through reprocessing of the stimulus and incorporation into subsequent MSEs.

In a recent study (Cipolli *et al.*, 2004) the immediate (i.e., in night report collected after provoked awakening during REM sleep) and delayed recall (i.e., in morning report) of contents incorporating a pre-sleep stimulus associated to a cognitive concern (induced by a recall task to be completed after the next awakening) was compared with recall of other contents. Prior to each of the three sleep onsets planned over the experimental night, subjects were asked to retain a semantically incoherent sentence for recall after the subsequent provoked awakening. This type of stimulus was chosen to exclude the possibility of previous by-chance acquisition and to trigger deep elaboration of the various parts of the stimulus for insertion into MSE contents. The cognitive concern so induced was expected not only to persist during the subsequent period of sleep and to guide (re)processing, but also to facilitate incorporation of the current stimulus into the MSE, and thus improve consolidation of the content(s) that were therein incorporated. To enhance the likelihood of retention, subjects were also required to recall the stimulus immediately after its delivery, and thereby indirectly invited to rehearse it before falling asleep.

The findings obtained have provided partial, but coherent support for the general hypothesis that the active nature of (re-)processing of recently acquired items of declarative knowledge during sleep improves consolidation. The consolidation advantage provided by (re-)processing of pre-sleep stimuli at their output seems widespread (more than 80% of REM-MSEs), and extendable to other types of recent declarative knowledge. The proportion of reports with incorporations was close to that observed using similar types of verbal stimuli (Cipolli *et al.*, 2001), among others, such as single words (Hoelscher *et al.*, 1981), sentences (Cipolli *et al.*, 1983a,b), and prose paragraphs (Cipolli *et al.*, 1988a). Report length and proportions of common (i.e., present in both night and morning reports and, thus, better consolidated) non-incorporation units were fully comparable with those obtained in other studies using the same techniques of report analysis (Cipolli *et al.*, 1984, 1992).

This study provides three main indications: (i) The consolidation advantage for contents with valid incorporations (that is, of the stimulus currently to be retained) is conspicuous, their retention rate in morning reports being about three times that of other contents (see Figure 3c) and about twice that of by-chance similar contents (forward and backward

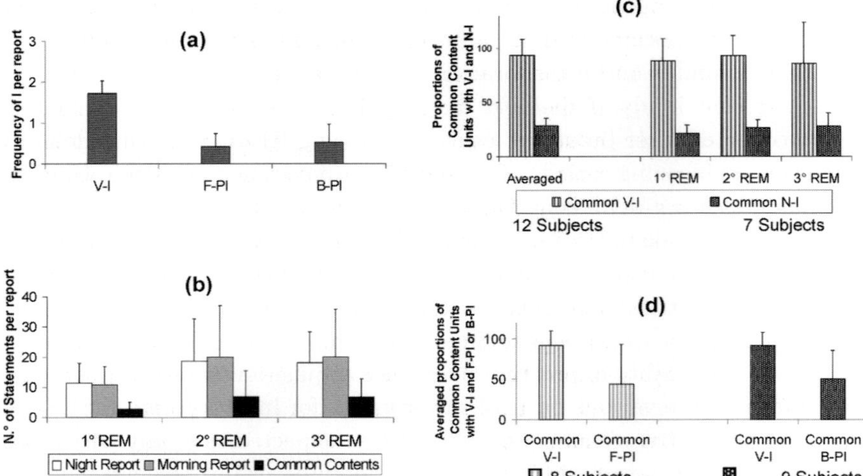

Figure 3. Rates of incorporation of pre-sleep stimuli in REM-MSEs and long-term retention. Legends: I = incorporations; V-I = valid incorporations; F-PI = forward pseudo-incorporations; B-PI = backward pseudo-incorporations; N-I = non-incorporations; Common = content units common to night and morning reports. Error bars = standard deviations.

pseudo-incorporations, regarding contents similar to stimuli not yet delivered or no longer to be retained (Figure 3d).

(ii) The effect found appears reliable, since the observed decrease in chance levels of the frequency of incorporation of pre-sleep stimuli dissociated from cognitive concern (backward pseudo-incorporations: Figure 3a), goes against the possibility that this effect was an artifact. Complementarily, the better long-term retention of valid incorporation units, compared with by-chance similar content units (Figure 3d), strengthens the possibility that the effect depends on the properties of the processing rather than on the characteristics of the stimulus.

(iii) The comparable frequencies of valid incorporations per report in the three periods of REM sleep (Figure 3b) indicate that during all periods of REM sleep the arousal level remains adequate for deep processing of the stimulus currently to be retained.

These indications complement those from cued-recall studies as evidence of the effectiveness of rehearsal during sleep. However, given that recent items of knowledge are usually re-activated internally rather than externally during sleep, they provide a potentially much more general indication as to how sleep improves consolidation. Indeed, recently acquired items of declarative knowledge are often associated, at least implicitly, with cognitive concerns induced by tasks (such as further recall and reorganization) to be completed during the next waking (Fowler *et al.*, 1973). Moreover, the cognitive concern induced by these tasks remains operative across sleep stages and cycles (potentially until morning awakening, when not manipulated as in the present study; Cipolli *et al.*, 1983b, 1988b).

The two supposedly concomitant effects of reprocessing on the input and the output cannot be simultaneously observed, as the elaboration to which recent information is subjected is also iterative. This means that any consolidation advantage given to a stimulus by the processing leading to its incorporation into the MSE reported after scheduled awakening may be counterbalanced by the advantage provided to other stimuli (or other parts of the stimulus) by the processing leading to incorporation into other, non-reported, MSEs. Therefore, the complementary prediction that delayed recall ought to be better for processed stimuli rather than for unprocessed ones should be tested in further studies. Retention of pre-sleep stimuli for which the likelihood of (re)processing has been manipulated should be assessed after long enough periods of uninterrupted sleep to suppose that some stimuli have been repeatedly processed (and incorporated) while others have not. If placed in competition for access and elaboration during sleep, the stimuli associated to the most compelling task should be more frequently accessed and elaborated for incorporation into MSEs and, thus, better retained at delayed recall than those associated with the least compelling task. It is apparent that, were the generation effect also confirmed for the input of the processing, a further distinction between REM and stages of NREM sleep would be necessary, insofar as they may exert separate effects on the consolidation of declarative knowledge (for a review, see Gais and Born, 2004b).

The hypothesis of a generation effect on the output of MSE processing has been further supported by findings of another recent experiment (Cipolli *et al.*, in press), carried out on delayed recall of so-called "interrelated contents." These contents, which correspond to the identical or similar contents occurring in two of more MSEs developed over the same night (Rechtschaffen *et al.*, 1963; Kramer *et al.*, 1964), are present in about two-thirds of pairs of reports collected after sequences of awakenings provoked during REM–REM, NREM–NREM, and NREM–REM sleep (for a review, see Cipolli *et al.*, 2003). Since interrelated contents share all or several semantic features, they are likely to derive from repeated access to, and elaboration of, the same items of declarative knowledge. Therefore, if the improvement of consolidation is somehow related to the amount of processing that given items undergo, interrelated contents should be better retained at delayed recall than non-interrelated ones, as a consequence of the repeated rehearsal involved.

This hypothesis was tested by comparing the proportion of interrelated and non-interrelated contents that were common to night and morning reports (and thus better consolidated; Cipolli *et al.*, 1984, 1992) of the MSEs of the same and different subjects. MSEs were collected in two experimental nights where subjects were asked to recall MSE after awakening during the first four periods of REM sleep (night reports) and to re-recall MSEs the next morning (morning reports).

The findings obtained further strengthen the hypothesis that rehearsal (the amount of which is plausibly greater for interrelated than non-interrelated contents) involved in MSE processing maintains some effectiveness for consolidation. Indeed, the proportion of report pairs with interrelated contents, and above all their frequency per report pair (see Figure 4), proved to be much higher in the MSEs of the same subjects than in those of different subjects (and, thus, of the chance level). As the occurrence of interrelated contents appears an ordinary outcome of the MSEs

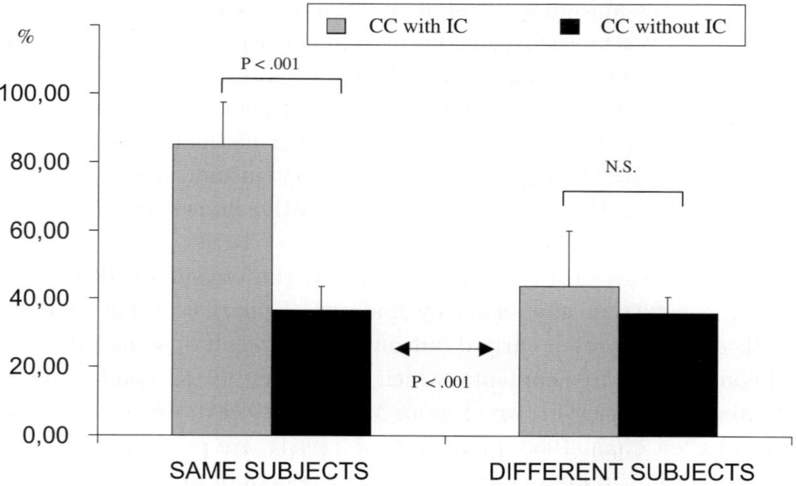

Figure 4. Retention rates of interrelated and non-interrelated contents in morning report pairs. Legends: CC = contents common to night and morning report pairs of mental sleep experiences; IC = interrelated contents.

elaborated over the night, it can be argued that the mechanisms supposed to be operative for their production are usually operative during sleep.

A demonstration that retention is also improved for the input of inter-related contents is needed to definitively argue in favor of the consolidation power of rehearsal involved in the repeated processing of items of declarative knowledge during sleep. Such a demonstration may be obtained by comparing the retention rates of target items (for example, pre-sleep verbal stimuli) before and after a period of sleep during which their likelihood of being processed, and thus rehearsed, has been manipulated experimentally (using the procedure applied by Cipolli *et al.*, 2004). The expected indication that long-term retention is improved also for the input of the processing would be of general interest, as it would be obtained without modifying the ordinary modality of processing during sleep, where items of declarative knowledge are usually re-activated internally rather than externally.

Conclusion

The pieces of evidence available for declarative knowledge (in particular, those presented in the previous paragraph) are far to be conclusive, although they have provided a partial support for the possibility to enlighten also at a behavioral level how reprocessing of recent information improves consolidation level. However, it seems now more plausible to posit that insertion into MSE contents and improvement of consolidation level are non-independent, albeit distinct, outcomes of a system of information processing that is more general and effective than usually assumed.

In particular, it seems urgent that, together with the effectiveness of rehearsal involved in MSE processing, also the time course of consolidation improvement is examined. This issue has been approached so far only for non-declarative knowledge (for both perceptual and motor skills: Stickgold *et al.*, 2000a; Walker *et al.*, 2003b). Recent memories are reprocessed for insertion into MSE contents not only during the following night, but also after several nights, as shown by dream reports collected at home and compared with daytime experiences with a different temporal delay (1–7 days, Nielsen *et al.*, 2004). This finding makes it further plausible that also for declarative knowledge the improvement of consolidation involves several steps and perhaps interacts with retrieval and organization processes occurring in subsequent waking periods. Clarifying this issue seems a crucial step in the understanding of how MSE processing can influence consolidation and organization of episodic and semantic information.

                    C. Cipolli

Acknowledgment

This study was supported in part by a grant from the National Project Funds (MM06244347/2001). The author is indebted to M. Mazzetti for her useful comments on a previous version of the manuscript.

References

Antrobus, J.S. and Arkin, A.M. (1991). The effects of external stimuli applied prior to and during sleep on sleep experience. In: Ellman, S.J. and Antrobus, J.S. (Eds.). *The Mind in Sleep: Psychology and Psychophysiology.* Oxford: J. Wiley & Sons, pp. 265–307.

Aserinsky, E. and Kleitman, N. (1953). Regularly occurring periods of eye motility and concomitant phenomena during sleep. *Science*, 118: 273–274.

Badia, P., Wesensten, N., Lammers, W., Culpepper, J., and Harsh, J. (1990). Responsiveness to olfactory stimuli presented in sleep. *Physiol. Behav.*, 48: 87–90.

Baylor, G.W. and Cavallero, C. (2001). Memory sources associated with REM and NREM dream reports throughout the night: a new look at the data. *Sleep*, 24: 165–170.

Benson, K. and Feinberg, I. (1977). The beneficial effect of sleep in an extended Jenkins and Dallenbach paradigm. *Psychophysiology*, 14: 375–384.

Benjamin, A.S. and Bjork, R.A. (2000). On the relationship between recognition speed and accuracy for words rehearsed via rote versus elaborative rehearsal. *J. Exp. Psychol. LMC*, 26: 638–648.

Bonnet, M.H. (1982). Performance during sleep. In: Webb, W. (Ed.). *Biological Rhythms, Sleep and Performance.* Chichester: J. Wiley & Sons, pp. 205–237.

Born, J. and Gais, S. (2000). REM sleep deprivation: the wrong paradigm leading to wrong conclusions. *Behav. Brain Sci.*, 23: 912–913.

Born, J. and Wagner, U. (2004). Awareness in memory: being explicit about the role of sleep. *Trends Cogn. Sci.*, 8: 242–244.

Burton, S.A., Harsch, J.R., and Badia, P. (1988). Cognitive activity in sleep and responsiveness to external stimuli. *Sleep*, 11: 61–68.

Buzsaki, G. (1996). The hippocampo-neocortical dialogue. *Cereb. Cortex*, 6: 81–92.

Cipolli, C. (1995). Sleep, dreams and memory: an overview. *J. Sleep Res.*, 4: 2–9.

Cipolli, C. and Poli, D. (1992). Story structure in verbal reports of mental experience after awakening in REM sleep. *Sleep*, 15: 133–142.

Cipolli, C. and Salzarulo, P. (1979). Sentence memory and sleep: a pilot study. *Sleep*, 2: 193–198.

Cipolli, C., Fagioli, I., Maccolini, S., and Salzarulo, P. (1983a). Associative relationships between pre-sleep sentence stimuli and reports of mental sleep experience. *Percept. Mot. Skills*, 56: 223–234.

Cipolli, C., Salzarulo, P., Baroncini, P., Fagioli, I., Fumai, A., Maccolini, S., and Tuozzi, G. (1983b). Incorporation of pre-sleep sentence stimuli in different halves of the night. In: Koella, W.P. (Ed.). *Sleep 1982*. Basel: Karger, pp. 375–377.

Cipolli, C., Calasso, E., Maccolini, S., Pani, R., and Salzarulo, P. (1984). Memory processes in morning recall after multiple night awakenings. *Percept. Mot. Skills*, 59: 435–446.

Cipolli, C., Baroncini, P., Cavallero, C., Cicogna, P., and Fagioli, I. (1988a). Incorporation of cognitive stimuli into mental sleep experience and contextual emotive stress. In: Koella, W.P., Obàl, F., Schulz, H. and Visser, P. (Eds.). *Sleep 1986*. Stuttgart: Fischer, pp. 388–390.

Cipolli, C., Fagioli, I., Baroncini, P., Fumai, A., Marchiò, B., and Sancini, M. (1988b). The thematic continuity in mental experiences in REM and NREM sleep. *Int. J. Psychophysiol.*, 6: 307–313.

Cipolli, C., Fagioli, I., Baroncini, P., Fumai, A., Marchiò, B., Sancini, M., Tuozzi, G., and Salzarulo, P. (1992). Recall of mental experience with or without prior verbalization. *Am. J. Psychol.*, 10: 385–407.

Cipolli, C. Bolzani, R., and Tuozzi, G. (1998). Story-like organization of dream experience in different periods of REM sleep. *J. Sleep Res.*, 7: 13–19.

Cipolli, C., Bolzani, R., Fagioli, I., and Tuozzi, G. (2001). Active processing of declarative knowledge during REM-sleep dreaming. *J. Sleep Res.*, 10: 277–284.

Cipolli, C., Cicogna, P., Mattarozzi, K., Mazzetti, M., Natale, V., and Occhionero, M. (2003). Continuity of the processing of declarative knowledge during human sleep: evidence from interrelated contents of mental sleep experiences. *Neurosci. Lett.*, 342: 147–150.

Cipolli, C., Fagioli, I., Mazzetti, M., and Tuozzi, G. (2004). Incorporation of presleep stimuli into dream contents: evidence for a consolidation effect on declarative knowledge during REM sleep? *J. Sleep Res.*, 13: 317–326.

Cipolli, C., Fagioli, I., Mazzetti, M., and Tuozzi, G. (2005). Consolidation effect of the processing of declarative knowledge during human sleep: evidence from long-term retention of interrelated contents of mental sleep experiences. *Brain Res. Bull.* 65: 97–104.

Dement, W. and Kleitman, N. (1957). Cyclic variations in EEG during sleep and their relation to eye movements, body motility, and dreaming. *Electroencephalogr. Clin. Neurophysiol.*, 9 (Suppl.): 673–690.

Ekstrand, B.R., Barrett, T.R., West, J.N., and Maier, W.G. (1977). The effect of sleep on human long-term memory. In: Drucker-Colin, R.R. and Mc Gaugh, J.L. (Eds.). *Neurobiology of Sleep and Memory*. New York: Academic Press, pp. 419–438.

Empson, J.A. and Clarke, P. (1970). Rapid eye movements and remembering. *Nature*, 227: 287–288.

Ficca, G. and Salzarulo, P. (2004). What in sleep is for memory. *Sleep Med.*, 5: 225–230.

Ficca, G., Lombardo, P., Rossi, L., and Salzarulo, P. (2000). Morning recall of verbal material depends on prior sleep organization. *Behav. Brain Res.*, 112: 159–163.

Fischer, S., Hallschmid, M., Elsner, A.L., and Born, J. (2002). Sleep forms memory for finger skills. *Proc. Natl. Acad. Sci. USA*, 99: 11987–11991.

Fosse, M.J., Fosse, R, Hobson, J.A., and Stickgold, R. (2003). Dreaming and episodic memory: a functional dissociation? *J. Cogn. Neurosci.*, 15: 1–9.

Foulkes, D. (1962). Dream report from different stages of sleep. *J. Abnorm. Soc. Psychol.*, 65: 14–25.

Foulkes, D. (1982). A cognitive-psychological model of REM dream production. *Sleep*, 5: 169–187.

Foulkes, D. (1985). *Dreaming: A Cognitive-Psychological Analysis*. Hillsdale, NJ: Erlbaum.

Foulkes, D. and Schmidt, M. (1983). Temporal sequence and unit composition in dream reports from different stages of sleep. *Sleep*, 6: 265–280.

Fowler, M.J., Sullivan, M.G., and Ekstrand, B.R. (1973). Sleep and memory. *Science*, 179: 302–304.

Gais, S. and Born, J. (2004a). Low acetylcholine during slow-wave sleep is critical for declarative memory consolidation. *Proc. Natl. Acad. Sci. USA*, 101: 2140–2144.

Gais, S. and Born, J. (2004b). Declarative memory consolidation: mechanisms acting during human sleep. *Learn. Mem.*, 11: 679–685.

Gais, S., Molle, M., Helms, K., and Born, J. (2002). Learning-dependent increases in sleep spindle density. *J. Neurosci.*, 22: 6830–6834.

Gais, S., Plihal, W., Wagner, U., and Born, J. (2000). Early sleep triggers memory for early visual discrimination skills. *Nat. Neurosci.*, 3: 1335–1339.

Giuditta, A., Ambrosini, M.V., Montagnese, P., Mandile, P., Cotrugno, M., Grassi, Z.G., and Vescia S. (1995). The sequential hypothesis of the function of sleep. *Behav. Brain Res.*, 69: 157–166.

Graves, E.A. (1937). The effect of sleep on retention. *J. Exp. Psychol.*, 19: 316–322.

Guerrien, A., Dujardin K., Mandai, O., Sockeel, P., and Leconte, P. (1989). Enhancement of memory by auditory stimulation during postlearning REM sleep in humans. *Physiol. Behav.*, 45: 947–950.

Hennevin, E., Hars, B., Maho. C., and Bloch, V. (1995). Processing of learned information in paradoxical sleep: relevance for memory. *Behav. Brain Res.*, 69: 125–135.

Hockhey, G.R., Davies, S., and Gray, M.M. (1972). Forgetting as a function of sleep at different times of day. *Q. J. Exp. Psychol.*, 24: 386–393.

Hoelscher, T.J., Klinger, E., and Barta, S. (1981). Incorporation of concern- and nonconcern-related verbal stimuli into dream content. *J. Abnorm. Psychol.*, 90: 88–91.

Karni, A. and Sagi, D. (1991). The time course of learning a visual skill. *Nature*, 365: 250–252.

Karni, A., Tanne, D., Rubenstein, B.S., Askenasy, J.J.M., and Sagi, D. (1994). Dependence on REM-sleep of overnight improvement of a perceptual skill. *Science*, 265: 679–682.

Kramer, M., Whitman, R.M., Baldrigde, B.J., and Lansky, L.M. (1964). Patterns of dreaming: the interrelationship of the dreams of a night. *J. Nerv. Ment. Dis.*, 139: 426–439.

Jenkins, J.K. and Dallenbach, K.M. (1924). Obliviscence during sleep and waking. *Am. J. Psychol.*, 35: 605–612.

Lammers, W.J., Badia, P. Hughes, R., and Harsh, J. (1991). Temperature, time-of-night of testing, and responsiveness to stimuli presented while sleeping. *Psychophysiology*, 28: 463–467.

Lehmann, D. and Koukkou, M. (1974). Computer analysis of EEG wakefulness-sleep patterns during learning of novel and familiar sentences. *Electroencephalogr. Clin. Neurophysiol.*, 37: 73–84.

Lewin, I. and Glaubman, H. (1975). The effect of REM deprivation: is it detrimental, beneficial or neutral? *Psychophysiology*, 12: 349–353.

Maquet, P. (2001). The role of sleep in learning and memory. *Science*, 294: 1048–1052.

Maquet, P., Laureys, S., Peigneux, P., Fuchs, S., Petiau, C., Phillips, C., Aerts, J., Del Fiore, G., Degueldre, C., Meulemans, T., Luxen, A., Franck, G., Van Der Linden, M., Smith, C., and Cleeremans, A. (2000). Experience-dependent changes in cerebral activation during human REM sleep. *Nat. Neurosci.*, 3: 831–836.

Marsh, E.J., Edelman, G., and Bower, G.H. (2001). Demonstrations of a generation effect in context memory. *Mem. Cognit.*, 29: 798–805.

Mazzoni, G., Gori, S., Formicola, G., Gneri, C., Massetani, R., Murri, L., and Salzarulo, P. (1999). Word recall correlates with sleep cycles in elderly subjects. *J. Sleep Res.*, 8: 185–188.

McGaugh, J.L. (2000). Memory — a century of consolidation. *Science*, 287: 248–251.

Mednick, S., Nakayama, K., Cantero J.L., Atienza, M., Levin, A., Pathak, N., and Stickgold, R. (2002). The restorative effect of naps on perceptual deterioration. *Nat. Neurosci.*, 5: 677–681.

Mednick, S., Nakayama, K., and Stickgold, R.J. (2003). Sleep-dependent learning: a nap is as good as a night. *Nat. Neurosci.*, 6: 697–698.

Muller, G.E. and Pilzecker, A. (1900). Experimentelle Beitrage zur lehre vom Gedachtnis. *Z. Psychol. Physiol. Sinnes.*, 1: 1–300.

Mulligan, N.W. (2001). Generation and hypermnesia. *J. Exp. Psychol. LMC*, 27: 436–450.

Mulligan, N.W. (2002). The generation effect: dissociating enhanced item memory and disrupted order memory. *Mem. Cognit.*, 30: 850–861.

Newman, E.B. (1939). Forgetting of meaningful material during sleep and waking. *Am. J. Psychol.*, 52: 65–71.

Nielsen, T.A. (1999). Mentation during sleep: the NREM/REM distinction. In: Lydic, R. and Baghdoyan, H.A. (Eds.). *Handbook of Behavioral State Control*. Boca Raton, FL: CRC Press, pp. 101–128.

Nielsen, T.A., Kuiken, D., Alain, G., Stenstrom, P., and Powell, R.A. (2004). Immediate and delayed incorporations of events into dreams: further replication and implications for dream function. *J. Sleep Res.*, 13: 327–336.

Oltman, P.K., Goodenough, D.R., Koulack, D., Maclin, F., Schroeder, H.R., and Flannagan, M.J. (1977). Short-term memory during Stage 2 sleep. *Psychophysiology*, 14: 439–444.

Peigneux, P., Laureys, S., Fuchs, S., Destrebecqz, A., Collette, F., Delbeuck, X., Phillips, C., Aerts, J., Del Fiore, G., Degueldre, C., Luxen, A., Cleeremans, A., and Maquet, P. (2003). Learned material content and acquisition level modulate cerebral reactivation during posttraining rapid-eye-movements sleep. *Neuroimage*, 20: 125–134.

Pivik, T. and Foulkes, D. (1968). NREM mentation: relation to personality, orientation time and time of night. *J. Cons. Clin. Psychol.*, 32: 144–151.

Plihal, W. and Born, J. (1997). Effects of early and late nocturnal sleep on declarative and procedural memory. *J. Cogn. Neurosci.*, 9: 534–547.

Plihal, W. and Born, J. (1999). Effects of early and late nocturnal sleep on priming and spatial memory. *Psychophysiology*, 36: 571–582.

Portas, C., Krakow, K., Allen, P., Josephs, O., Armony, J.L., and Frith, C.D. (2000). Auditory processing across the sleep-wake cycle: simultaneous EEG and fMRI monitoring in humans. *Neuron*, 28: 991–999.

Portnoff, G., Baekeland, F., Goodenough, D., Karacan, I., and Shapiro, A. (1966). Retention of verbal materials perceived immediately prior to onset of non-REM sleep. *Percept. Mot. Skills*, 22: 751–758.

Rauchs, G., Bertran, F., Guillery-Girard, B., Desgranges, B., Kerrouche, N., Denise, P., Foret, J., and Eustache, F. (2004). Consolidation of strictly episodic memories mainly requires rapid eye movement sleep. *Sleep*, 27: 395–401.

Rechtschaffen, A., Vogel, G., and Shaikun, G. (1963). Interrelatedness of mental activity during sleep. *Arch. Gen. Psychiatry*, 9: 536–547.

Robertson, E.M., Pascual-Leone, A., and Press, D.Z. (2004). Awareness modifies the skill-learning benefits of sleep. *Curr. Biol.*, 14: 208–212.

Shimizu, A., Takehashi, H., Sumitsuji, N., Tanaka, M., Yoshida, I., Kaneko, Z. (1977). Memory retention of stimulations during REM and NREM stages of sleep. *Electroencephalogr. Clin. Neurophysiol.*, 43: 658–665.

Siegel, J.M. (2001). The REM sleep-memory consolidation hypothesis. *Science*, 294: 1058–1063.

Smith, C. (1995). Sleep states and memory processes. *Behav. Brain Res.*, 69: 137–145.

Smith, C. (2001). Sleep states and memory processes in humans: procedural versus declarative memory systems. *Sleep Med. Rev.*, 5: 491–506.

Smith, C. and Weeden, K. (1990). Post training REMs coincident auditory stimulation enhances memory in humans. *Psychiatr. J. Univ. Ottawa*, 15: 85–90.

Squire, L.R. (1993). The organization of declarative and nondeclarative memory. In: Ono, T., Squire, L.R., Raichle, M.E., Perrett, D.I., and Fukuda, M. (Eds.). *Brain Mechanisms of Perception and Memory: From Neuron to Behavior*. New York: Oxford University Press, pp. 219–227.

Stickgold, R. (1998). Sleep: off-line memory reprocessing. *Trends Cogn. Sci.*, 2: 484–492.

Stickgold, R., Fosse, R., and Walker, M.P. (2002). Linking brain and behavior in sleep-dependent learning and memory consolidation. *Proc. Natl. Acad. Sci. USA*, 99: 17137–17142.

Stickgold, R., LaTanya, J., and Hobson, J.A. (2000a). Visual discrimination learning requires sleep after training. *Nat. Neurosci.*, 3: 1237–1238.

Stickgold, R., Malia, A., Maguire, D., Roddenberry, D., and O'Connor, M. (2000b). Replaying the game: hypnagogic images in normals and amnesics. *Science*, 290: 350–353.

Stickgold, R., Whidbee, D., Schirmer, B., Patel, V., and Hobson, J.A. (2000c). Visual discrimination task improvement: a multi-step process occurring during sleep. *J. Cogn. Neurosci.*, 12: 246–254.

Tilley, A.J. (1979). Sleep learning during Stage 2 and REM sleep. *Biol. Psychol.*, 9: 155–161.

Vertes, R.P. (2004). Memory consolidation in sleep: dream or reality. *Neuron*, 44: 135–148.

Vertes, R.P. and Eastman, K.E. (2000). The case against memory consolidation in REM sleep. *Behav. Brain Sci.*, 23: 867–876.

Wagner, U., Gais, S., and Born, J. (2001). Emotional memory formation is enhanced across sleep intervals with high amounts of rapid eye movement sleep. *Learn. Mem.*, 8: 112–119.

Wagner, U., Gais, S., Haider, H., Verleger, R., and Born, J. (2004). Sleep inspires insight. *Nature*, 427: 352–355.

Walker, M.P. and Stickgold, R. (2004). Sleep-dependent learning and memory consolidation. *Neuron*, 44: 121–133.

Walker, M.P., Brakefield, T., Morgan, A., Hobson, J.A., and Stickgold, R. (2002). Practice with sleep makes perfect: sleep dependent motor skill learning. *Neuron*, 35: 205–211.

Walker, M.P., Brakefield, T., Hobson, J.A., and Stickgold, R. (2003a). Dissociable stages of human memory consolidation and reconsolidation. *Nature*, 425: 616–620.

Walker, M.P., Brakefield, T., Seidman, J., Morgan, A., Hobson, J.A., and Stickgold, R. (2003b). Sleep and the time course of motor skill learning. *Learn. Mem.*, 10: 275–284.

INDEX